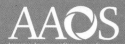

Sixth Edition

Emergency Medical Responder

Your First Response in Emergency Care

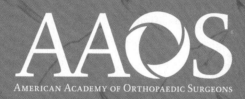

AMERICAN ACADEMY OF ORTHOPAEDIC SURGEONS

Series Editor:
Andrew N. Pollak, MD, FAAOS

Author:
David Schottke, RN, NRP, MPH

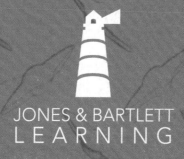

JONES & BARTLETT
LEARNING

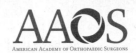
AMERICAN ACADEMY OF ORTHOPAEDIC SURGEONS

World Headquarters
Jones & Bartlett Learning
5 Wall Street
Burlington, MA 01803
978-443-5000
info@jblearning.com
www.jblearning.com

Substantial discounts on bulk quantities of Jones & Bartlett Learning publications are available to corporations, professional associations, and other qualified organizations. For details and specific discount information, contact the special sales department at Jones & Bartlett Learning via the above contact information or send an email to specialsales@jblearning.com.

Jones & Bartlett Learning books and products are available through most bookstores and online booksellers. To contact Jones & Bartlett Learning directly, call 800-832-0034, fax 978-443-8000, or visit our website, www.jblearning.com.

34843-9

Production Credits
General Manager, Safety and Trades: Doug Kaplan
General Manager, Executive Publisher: Kimberly Brophy
VP, Product Development and Executive Editor: Christine Emerton
Director, PSG Editorial Development: Carol B. Guerrero
Acquisitions Editor—EMS and Emergency Care: Tiffany Sliter
Senior Development Editor: Alison Lozeau
Editorial Assistant: Jessica Sturtevant
VP, Sales, Public Safety Group: Matthew Maniscalco
Director of Sales, Public Safety Group: Patricia Einstein
Director of Production: Jenny L. Corriveau

Production Editor: Lori Mortimer
Director of Marketing Operations: Brian Rooney
VP, Manufacturing and Inventory Control: Therese Connell
Composition: diacriTech
Cover Design: Kristin E. Parker
Director of Rights & Media: Joanna Gallant
Rights & Media Specialist: Robert Boder
Media Development Editor: Shannon Sheehan
Cover Image: © Mike Legeros. Used with permission; (skid plate) © Photos.com
Printing and Binding: LSC Communications
Cover Printing: LSC Communications

Library of Congress Cataloging-in-Publication Data
Names: Schottke, David, author. | American Academy of Orthopaedic Surgeons, issuing body.
Title: Emergency medical responder : your first response in emergency care / American Academy of Orthopaedic Surgeons; author, David Schottke.
Description: Sixth edition. | Burlington, MA : Jones & Bartlett Learning, [2018] | Includes index.
Identifiers: LCCN 2016035884 | ISBN 9781284107272
Subjects: | MESH: Emergencies | Emergency Treatment | Emergency Medical Technicians—education | Emergency Medical Technicians—standards | Examination Questions
Classification: LCC RC86.7 | NLM WB 18.2 | DDC 616.02/5—dc23
LC record available at https://lccn.loc.gov/2016035884

ISBN: 9781284107272
6048

Printed in the United States of America
21 20 19 18 17   10 9 8 7 6 5 4 3

Brief Contents

Contents

Skill Drills

Prepare for Class with Navigate 2 Digital Curriculum Solution Packages

Navigate 2 resources offer unbeatable value with mobile-ready course materials to help you prepare for your EMR class.

Purchase access to the Advantage, Preferred, or Premier option at 25% off!*

ADVANTAGE PACKAGE

Navigate 2 Advantage Access Includes:

- eBook
- Study Center
- Assessments
- Analytics

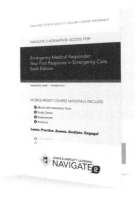

ISBN: 978-1-284-11662-5

PREFERRED PACKAGE

Navigate 2 Preferred Access Includes:

- eBook
- Study Center
- Assessments
- Analytics
- TestPrep

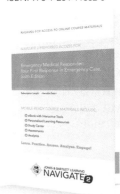

ISBN: 978-1-284-11671-7

PREMIER PACKAGE

Navigate 2 Premier Access Includes:

- eBook
- Study Center
- Assessments
- Analytics
- TestPrep
- Lectures

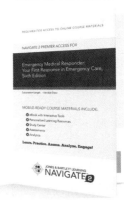

ISBN: 978-1-284-13417-9

Order today at www.jblearning.com

*Prices subject to change. Access codes to Navigate 2 course materials are available at 25% off the cost of the textbook.

Acknowledgments

Jones & Bartlett Learning and the American Academy of Orthopaedic Surgeons would like to acknowledge the contributors and reviewers of *Emergency Medical Responder: Your First Response in Emergency Care, Sixth Edition*.

◼ Contributors and Reviewers

Mike Alt, NREMT-P, AHA
Instructor & RESA Instructor (Fire & EMS)
RESA 8
Upper Tract, West Virginia

Christine Alvarez, BS, EMT-P
Director Prehospital Care Programs
LaGuardia Community College, CUNY
LIC, New York

Rebecca C. Anhold, VATL, ATC, AEMT, EMS Educator
Education Coordinator
Fort Defiance High School
Fort Defiance, Virginia

Jorge Anzardo, EMT-P
Program Director
American Medical Academy
Miami, Florida

Hector D. Arroyo, Jr., EMT-P, CIC
FDNY Bureau of Training
Bayside, New York

Kenneth Ashley, MS, ATC, AEMT
Educator & Athletic Trainer
Prince Edward County High School
Farmville, Virginia
Appomattox, Virginia

Stephen Barney, NRP
EMS Coordinator
Vance Granville Community College
Henderson, North Carolina

Ken Bartz, AEMT I/C
Southwest Wisconsin Technical College
Fennimore, Wisconsin

Dana Baumgartner, NRP, WI EMS I/C
Nicolet College
Rhinelander, Wisconsin

Jason Baumgartner, CCEMTP, IC-II
Nicolet College
Rhinelander, Wisconsin

Edward L. Bays, BS, NRP
EMS Education Director
Mountwest Community & Technical College
Huntington, West Virginia

Shelly Beck, MS, AEMT
University of Utah Center for Emergency
    Programs
Salt Lake City, Utah

David S. Becker, LNHA, MA, LP, EFO
Columbia Southern University
Orange Beach, Alabama

Daniel Benard, MBA EMT-P IC
Kalamazoo Valley Community College
Kalamazoo, Michigan

Rob Bernini, EMT-P, CCEMT-P
Harrisburg Area Community College
Harrisburg, Pennsylvania

Darren Scott Blackburn, MA, PMP
New Westminster, British Columbia, Canada

Nick Bourdeau, RN, Paramedic I/C
Huron Valley Ambulance
Ann Arbor, Michigan

Karen Bowlin, NREMT
EMT/CPR Director
Mid-Plains Community College – North Platte
North Platte, Nebraska

Christopher T. Boyer, MPA, MA, NR-P FP-C
Delaware Technical Community College
Dover, Delaware

Jason W. Burrow, Lieutenant
Hanover Fire EMS
Hanover, Virginia

Aaron R. Byington, MA, NRP
EMS Faculty and Course Coordinator
Davis Applied Technology College
Kaysville, Utah

Patrick Carr, BS, EMS, NRP
University of New Mexico Pararescue
    Paramedic Program
Albuquerque, New Mexico

Julia Chamberlain, BSN, RN, Paramedic, I/C
EMS Educator
Onondaga Fire Department
Leslie, Michigan

Joshua Chan, BA, NRP, FP-C
Life Link III, Flight Paramedic
Minneapolis, Minnesota
Glacial Ridge Emergency Services and
    Training, EMS Educator
Glenwood, Minnesota

Russ Christiansen, BS, NREMT-P, CCEMTP
Casper College
Casper, Wyoming

Michael A. DeMello, NRP
Fire Chief
Bristol Fire Department
Bristol, Rhode Island

Brent Ellen
Program Specialist
Office of the Fire Marshal and Emergency
    Management Emergency Preparedness
    Response Unit Provincial CBRNE/HUSAR
    Program
Ontario, Canada

Jeffrey L. Foster, EMD, NRP, CCEMTP, IC
CarolinaEast Health Systems
New Bern, North Carolina

Aaron A. Hadley, EMT
EMS Instructor
Davis County Health Department
North Salt Lake, Utah

Keith B. Hermiz, NREMT-A, I/C
Grafton Rescue Squad, Inc.
Grafton, Vermont

Rebecca C. Hill, AS, PN, Paramedic
Georgia Piedmont Technical College
Covington, Georgia

Joseph Hurlburt, BS, NREMT-P, EMT-P I/C
Instructor Coordinator/Training Officer
Rapid Response EMS
Romulus, Michigan

Sue A. Kartman, BS, EMT-P
Adjunct Facility
Wisconsin Indianhead Technical
    College (WITC)
Northcentral Technical College (NTC)
Phillips, Wisconsin

Blake E. Klingle, MS, RN, CCEMT-P
Waukesha County Technical College
Pewaukee, Wisconsin

Joshua Lopez, BS-EMS, NRP, I/C
University of New Mexico School of
    Medicine, Emergency Medical Services
    Academy
Kirtland Air Force Base Pararescue
    Paramedic Program
Albuquerque, New Mexico

Joe Martinez, MN CP, NRP
Hennepin Technical College
Brooklyn Park, Minnesota

Ellen A. Mathein, EMT, CPA
Nicolet Area Technical College
Rhinelander, Wisconsin

Michael McDonald, RN, BSN, NRP, NCEE
Loudoun County Department of Fire
    and Rescue
Leesburg, Virginia

Kristen McKenna, BS, NRP
University of South Alabama EMS Department
Mobile, Alabama

**Beth Ann McNeill, EMT, MS, CIC, Regional
Faculty**
Monroe Community College PSTF
Rochester, New York

**Nicholas J. Montelauro, AAS NRP FP-C
NCEE**
MHP Education and Training
Terre Haute, Indiana

Travis A. Myklebust, Paramedic
Fire Chief
Lewiston Fire Department
Lewiston, Idaho

Brian C. Nees, BS, NRP
University of New Mexico
Albuquerque, New Mexico

Stacey Oho, NREMTP
Assistant Professor Paramedic Instructor
Kapiolani Community College
Honolulu, Hawaii

Michael Osterman, FF/EMT-P
Lead Instructor
American Medical Academy
Miami, Florida

Stephen P. Rice, MS, EMT-B
EMS Instructor
Shrewsbury, Massachusetts

Jo Richmond, NRP
Richmond EMS Training Solutions, LLC
Hayes, Virginia

Steve Rollin, AAS, Paramedic
Yavapai College
Prescott Valley, Arizona

Stuart Rosenhaus, BS, EMT CIC
Brooklyn College
City University of New York
Brooklyn, New York

Ian T.T. Santee, MPA
City and County of Honolulu – Emergency
    Services Department
Honolulu, Hawaii

Kenneth Schaaf, NRP, I/C
Sr. Program Manager
University of New Mexico EMSA
Albuquerque, New Mexico

Bernard J. Schweter, PhD, EMTP, EMSI
Cuyahoga Community College
Cleveland, Ohio

**Holly Scribner, AAS, AS, BAS, MSEd,
FF/Paramedic**
Cushing Rescue Squad
Cushing, Maine

Richard Tippelt, Captain, AEMT
Town of Beloit, WI, Fire Department
Fire/EMS/Law Enforcement Instructor
Blackhawk Technical College
Janesville, Wisconsin

Stephen Trala, MPH, RN, NRP, CHS-IV
University of Vermont Health Net Critical
    Care Transport
Burlington, Vermont

Brian Turner, CCEMT-P, RN
Trinity Medical Center
Rock Island, Illinois

Michael Ung, BS-FES, EMT-P
Core Instructor
University of Miami Gordon Center for
    Research in Medical Education
EMS Faculty
Miami-Dade College – Medical Campus
Miami, Florida

Matthew G. Watson, AAS, NREMT-B
Law Enforcement Professional
Winchester, Virginia

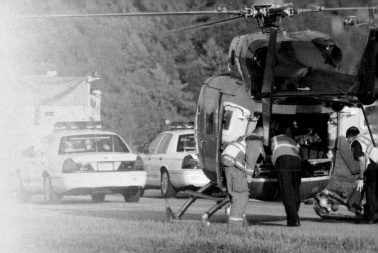

SECTION 1

Preparatory

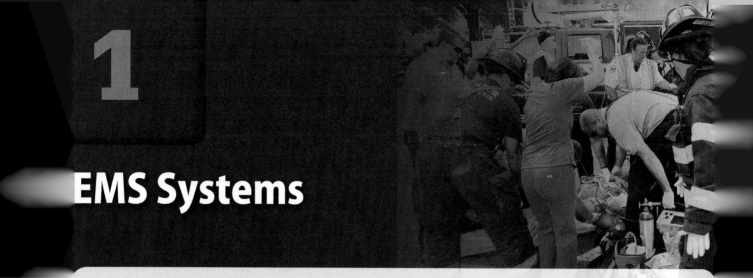

1

EMS Systems

■ Introduction

An **emergency medical responder (EMR)** is often the first medically trained person to arrive on the scene of an emergency. As an EMR, the care you give could mean the difference between life and death. Your care is usually followed by care given by **emergency medical technicians (EMTs)**, **paramedics**, nurses, physicians, and other allied health professionals.

■ The EMS System

The EMS system was developed to improve patient outcomes. Evidence showed that patients who received appropriate emergency medical care before they reached the hospital had a better chance of surviving a major injury or sudden illness than patients who did not receive such care.

It is important that you understand the operation and complexity of your EMS system Figure 1-1 . Personnel from different agencies may provide emergency medical services. For some agencies, providing emergency medical services is a major function. Other agencies have a minimal yet vital role in providing emergency medical care.

Problems during an EMS operation often result from a lack of coordination between resources and personnel. Agencies and personnel need to share an understanding of their roles for an EMS system to operate smoothly. This understanding develops through close cooperation, careful planning, communication, and continual effort. You can best understand the EMS system by examining the sequence of events as an injured or ill patient is cared for in the system.

▶ Reporting

The first step in reporting an emergency is recognizing that an emergency exists. The patient, a relative, or bystander sees a serious illness or injury and decides to call for help. Most emergency calls are made using cellular phones. Other calls are made using landline telephones, two-way radios, or personal emergency call systems. An **emergency response communications center** or **public safety answering point (PSAP)** usually receives the telephone call reporting an incident Figure 1-2 . The communications center may be a fire, police, or EMS agency, a 9-1-1 center,

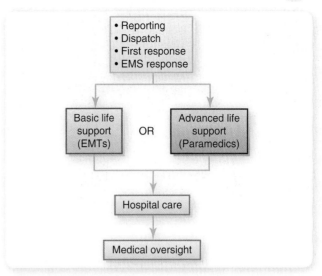

Figure 1-1 The EMS system.
© Jones & Bartlett Learning.

• Reporting
• Dispatch
• First response
• EMS response

Basic life support (EMTs) OR Advanced life support (Paramedics)

Hospital care

Medical oversight

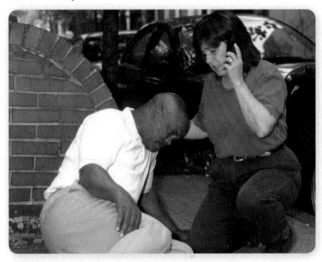

Figure 1-2 Reporting an emergency.
© Jones & Bartlett Learning. Courtesy of MIEMSS.

or a seven-digit emergency telephone number used by one or all of the emergency agencies. Enhanced 9-1-1 centers use computers to determine the location of landline telephones as soon as the telephone in the 9-1-1 center is answered.

▶ Dispatch

Once the emergency response communications center is notified of an incident, appropriate equipment and personnel are dispatched to the scene Figure 1-3 .

YOU are the Provider   CASE 1

A few weeks after completing your EMR course, you are traveling along a freeway in your town. Suddenly the traffic slows down. At the right side of the road you see a station wagon that has just crashed into the wall of a concrete overpass. As you pull over to stop, you see two people dragging a woman by her arms and legs away from the wrecked car.

1. Why is your role as an EMR so important during the first minutes after a crash?
2. Why is it important to know how the components of your EMS system work?
3. How does good interaction between different levels of the EMS team improve the quality of care?

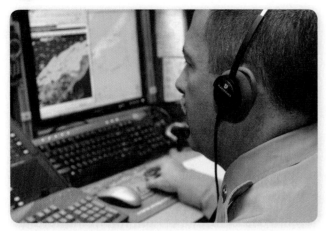

Figure 1-3 An emergency response communications center receives the call.
© Jones & Bartlett Learning. Courtesy of MIEMSS.

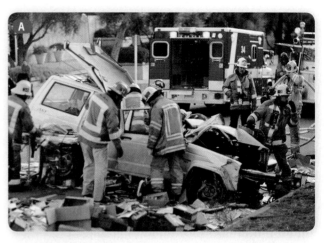

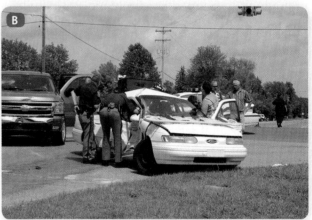

Figure 1-4 Firefighters **(A)** and law enforcement personnel **(B)** are EMRs in many emergencies.
A: © Corbis/Getty; B: Courtesy of Captain David Jackson, Saginaw Township Fire Department.

Dispatch may occur by landline telephone, cellular phone, pager, public safety radio system, computer, or other means. Agencies, personnel, and equipment that are involved in the emergency medical first response vary by community.

▶ First Response

Firefighters (paid or volunteer) or law enforcement personnel, because of their location or speed in responding, are in many cases the first EMRs on scene Figure 1-4 . Most communities have many EMRs but few EMTs and even fewer paramedics. Emergency medical responders may be employed as lifeguards, security officers, teachers, or workers in an industrial setting. A community with four or five fire stations may have only two or three ambulances. The patient's first and perhaps most crucial contact with the EMS system occurs when the trained EMR arrives. For example, a key survival factor for people in cardiac arrest is the length of time between when the heartbeat stops and when manual cardiopulmonary resuscitation (CPR) starts.

▶ EMS Response

The arrival of an emergency medical vehicle (usually an ambulance) staffed by EMTs or paramedics is the patient's second contact with the EMS system Figure 1-5 . A properly equipped vehicle and the EMT staff make up a **basic life support (BLS)** unit. Each EMT has completed at least 150 hours of training. Many complete even longer training courses.

EMTs continue the care begun by EMRs. EMTs stabilize the patient's condition further and prepare the patient for transport to the emergency department of the hospital. Well-trained emergency personnel who can carefully move the patient and provide proper treatment increase the chance that the patient will arrive at the emergency department in the best possible condition.

Advanced emergency medical technicians (AEMTs) are able to perform limited **advanced life support (ALS)**

skills. They have completed at least 300 hours of training. Advanced EMTs may work alone or with a paramedic on an ALS unit.

Paramedics provide advanced life support services. They have received at least 1,000 hours of additional training. They can administer intravenous fluids and certain medications. They can also monitor and treat heart conditions with medications and defibrillation. **Defibrillation** is the administration of an electric shock to the heart of a patient who is experiencing a highly irregular heartbeat, known as ventricular fibrillation. Defibrillation may also be done by specially trained EMTs and EMRs. Paramedics are also trained to place special airway tubes (endotracheal tubes) to keep the patient's airway open.

Each level of skill builds on the one that precedes it: the paramedic's skills originate from those of the EMT, and the techniques used by the EMT depend on those of the EMR. All skill levels are based on what is learned in the EMR course: airway maintenance; bleeding control; and prevention, recognition, and treatment of shock.

The EMS system involves more than emergency medical care. For example, law enforcement personnel may provide protection and control at the scene of an

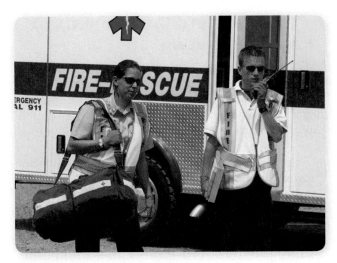

Figure 1-5 EMS responds.
© Jones & Bartlett Learning. Courtesy of MIEMSS.

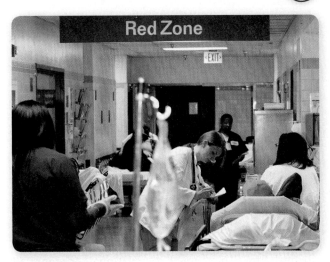

Figure 1-6 Hospital emergency care.
© Ric Feld, Files/AP Photo.

incident. Fire units provide fire protection, specialized rescue, and patient extrication.

▶ Hospital Care

The patient's third contact with the EMS system occurs in the hospital, primarily in the emergency department. After being treated at the scene, the patient is transported to an appropriate hospital, where definitive treatment can be provided **Figure 1-6**. It may be necessary to transport some patients to the closest **appropriate medical facility** first. An appropriate medical facility may be a hospital, trauma center, or medical clinic. They will be stabilized there and then transported to a hospital that provides specialized treatment. Specialized treatment facilities include trauma centers, spinal cord injury centers, hand centers, cardiac centers, stroke centers, burn centers, pediatric centers, poison control centers, and perinatal centers. You must learn and follow your local patient transportation protocols.

▶ Public Health and EMS

The EMS system holds a unique place in our society. In most communities, it is considered part of the public safety function of government. EMS can also be considered a part of public health because these services are available to all people in a community. It is important for you to understand the basic functions of public health agencies because EMS personnel need to interact with public health practitioners.

Public health departments monitor restaurant cleanliness, conduct immunization programs, and determine the incidence of contagious diseases such as influenza, tuberculosis, and hepatitis. Public health departments also work to prevent the incidence or progression of diseases. They monitor the spread of contagious diseases and inform other members of the medical community about the scope of a disease. When people's actions can affect the spread of a disease, public health personnel work hard to educate the community about how to limit the spread of that disease.

Because prevention is better than treatment, public health and public safety departments provide education and screening programs to help prevent injuries and illness. They conduct car seat installation programs, programs to encourage seat belt use, alcohol awareness programs, programs to encourage bicycle and motorcycle helmet use, blood pressure screenings, and diabetes screenings. Public health departments provide support to EMS in certain situations. For example, EMS personnel may receive vaccinations at a public health clinic. In some cases, EMS may be called upon to support certain functions of a public health department. In the event of an epidemic such as influenza, EMS systems may need to work with public health departments to determine the number of people who are sick. The Centers for Disease Control and Prevention (CDC) is one public health agency that monitors the incidence of diseases. They also provide the standard precaution guidelines we use to prevent the spread of contagious diseases.

▶ The History of EMS

As an EMS provider, you should have some understanding of the history of EMS. Many advances in civilian EMS have followed progress initially established in the military medical system. Horse-drawn ambulances were first used to remove wounded patients from the battlefield during the Civil War. Traction splints were first used in World War I, which greatly reduced the death rate from fractured femurs (thigh bones). During World War II, well-trained medical corpsmen and field hospitals helped reduce battlefield mortality (deaths). In the 1950s, during the Korean Conflict, timely helicopter evacuations to mobile army surgical hospitals (MASH units) further reduced battlefield mortality. Additional medical advances were made in the 1960s and 1970s during the Vietnam War. Improved tourniquets, chemical blood clotting agents, and fluid resuscitation protocols helped improve survival during the conflicts in Iraq and Afghanistan.

In the United States during the 1950s and 1960s, funeral homes, hospitals, and volunteer rescue squads provided most ambulance service. The only training available for ambulance attendants was basic first aid.

Even interns who staffed hospital-based ambulances had no special training for their prehospital duties. Hearses were commonly used to transport ill and injured patients. The mortality rate from trauma to civilians was much higher than the mortality experienced by military personnel.

Some physicians recognized that civilian prehospital medical care lagged behind military emergency medical care. They urged the National Academy of Sciences to investigate this situation. In 1966, the National Academy of Sciences/National Research Council produced a landmark paper, *Accidental Death and Disability: The Neglected Disease of Modern Society*. This paper described the deficiencies in emergency medical care. It recommended the development of a national course of instruction for prehospital emergency care personnel. It also called for nationally accepted textbooks, ambulance vehicle design guidelines, ambulance equipment guidelines, state regulations for ambulance services, and improvements in hospital emergency departments. As a result of this effort, in the early 1970s the US Department of Transportation developed a national standard curriculum for training EMS providers. This curriculum was the grandfather of the education guidelines in use today, the *National EMS Education Standards*.

During the 1980s, the use of ALS within EMS became common. Today paramedics are able to perform many procedures that were limited to physicians in the early days of EMS. Currently, cities, counties, fire departments, third-party EMS departments, rescue squads, and hospitals provide most EMS. EMS providers are now trained through standardized courses conducted at accredited training centers. Certified personnel use standardized vehicles to transport patients to hospital emergency departments. Hospital emergency departments provide a high level of care for emergency patients.

▶ Ten Standard Components of an EMS System

EMS systems can be organized in many different ways. Different agencies may provide different parts of the system. For example, first responders in one community may be law enforcement officers. In another community, the first responders may be firefighters. Both function similarly from a medical care perspective.

The National Highway Traffic Safety Administration (NHTSA) of the US Department of Transportation evaluates EMS systems based on the following 10 criteria, which are used primarily in the administration of an EMS system:

1. Regulation and policy
2. Resource management
3. Human resources and training
4. Transportation equipment and systems
5. Medical and support facilities
6. Communications system
7. Public information and education
8. Medical direction
9. Trauma system and development
10. Evaluation

■ A Word About Transportation

As an EMR, your primary goal is to provide immediate care for a sick or injured patient. As more highly trained EMTs or paramedics arrive on the scene, you will assist them in treating the patient and preparing the patient for transportation. Although other EMS personnel usually transport patients, you need to understand when a patient must be transported quickly to a hospital or other medical facility **Figure 1-7**.

This book uses three terms to describe proper patient transportation to an appropriate medical facility:

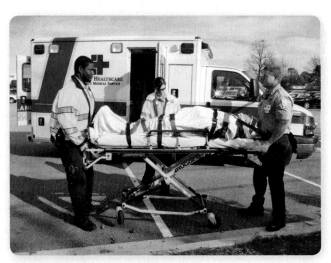

Figure 1-7 Ambulance transport to a hospital or medical facility.
Courtesy of Rhonda Hunt.

Words of Wisdom

In order to prevent confusion, in this text the term *provider* is used to refer to an EMS provider at any level: an EMR, EMT, or paramedic. The term *public safety provider* includes firefighters, law enforcement personnel, and EMS providers. The term *rescuer* refers to public safety providers engaged in the rescue and care of patients at an incident.

- **Transport.** This means that a patient's condition requires care by medical professionals, but speed in getting the patient to a medical facility is not the most important factor. For example, this might describe the transportation needed by a patient who has sustained an isolated injury to an extremity but whose condition is otherwise stable.
- **Prompt transport.** This phrase is used when a patient's condition is serious enough that the patient needs to be taken to an appropriate medical facility in a fairly short period of time. If the patient is not transported fairly quickly, the condition may get worse and the patient may die.
- **Rapid transport.** This phrase is used when EMS personnel are unable to give the patient adequate lifesaving care in the field. The patient may die unless he or she is transported immediately to an appropriate medical facility. This phrase is rarely used in this book.

Each of these three phrases refers to transportation to an appropriate medical facility. An appropriate medical facility may be a hospital, trauma center, or medical clinic. It is essential that you be familiar with the services provided by the medical facilities in your community and that you follow the protocols for your department.

EMS personnel must work closely with their medical director to establish transportation protocols that ensure that patients are transported to the closest medical facility capable of providing adequate care. To provide the best possible care for the patient, all members of the EMS team must remember that they are key components in the total system. Smooth operation of the team ensures the best care for the patient.

EMR Training

This book is written for an emergency medical responder training course. Although the book alone can teach you many things, it is best to use it as part of an approved EMR course. In this EMR course, you will learn how to examine patients and how to use basic emergency medical skills. These skills are divided into two main groups: (1) those needed to treat injured trauma patients and (2) those needed to care for patients experiencing illness or serious

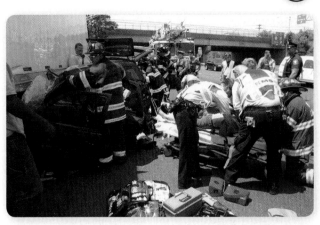

Figure 1-8 A typical emergency scene with injured patients.
© Mark C. Ide.

medical problems. The skills and knowledge you will gain from this course provide the foundation for the entire EMS system Figure 1-8 . Your actions can prevent a minor situation from becoming serious and will sometimes determine whether a patient lives or dies.

You will learn the following skills to stabilize conditions and treat persons who have been injured:

- Controlling airway, breathing, and circulation (Chapters 7 and 8)
- Controlling external bleeding (hemorrhage) (Chapter 14)
- Treating shock (Chapter 14)
- Treating wounds (Chapter 14)
- Splinting injuries to stabilize extremities (Chapter 15)

In addition to these trauma skills, you will learn to recognize, stabilize, and provide initial treatment for the following medical conditions:

- Heart attacks (Chapter 10)
- Seizures (Chapter 10)
- Problems associated with excessive heat or cold (Chapter 13)
- Alcohol and drug abuse (Chapter 11)
- Poisonings (Chapter 11)
- Bites and stings (Chapter 11)
- Altered mental status (Chapter 10)
- Behavioral or psychological crises (Chapter 12)
- Emergency childbirth (Chapter 16)

YOU are the Provider   CASE 2

You are dispatched to 11 North Fourth Street for a report of an injured woman. Your dispatcher reports that the woman was excited and that he was not able to get additional information from her. He indicates that the patient will meet you in front of her house. You arrive at the address and find a 38-year-old woman sitting on the front porch steps crying. After you introduce yourself, you ask her why she called EMS. She tells you that she had a skillet of grease, and as she tried to move it, it caught on fire. She has some blisters and reddening on both hands and redness on her face. You ask her if the fire is out. She says she does not know. She says there is no one else in the house.

1. Why is it so important to get correct information from the emergency dispatcher?
2. What are the first actions you need to take at this emergency scene?

Goals of EMR Training

It is important for you to understand the basic goals of EMR training. This training aims to teach you how to evaluate, stabilize, and treat patients using a minimum of specialized equipment. As an EMR, you will find yourself in situations in which little or no emergency medical equipment is readily available. You must know how to improvise using materials and objects already present at an emergency scene to serve in place of otherwise unavailable medical equipment. Finally, EMR training teaches you what you can do to help EMTs and paramedics when they arrive on the scene.

▶ Know What You Should Not Do

The first lesson you must learn as an EMR is what not to do. For example, it may be better for you to leave a patient in the position found rather than attempt to move him or her without the proper equipment or an adequate number of trained personnel. Sometimes the first priority at an emergency scene is to stabilize the scene or call for more help before beginning patient care. It is also critical that you not judge a patient based on his or her cultural background, religion, color, gender, sexual orientation, age, or socioeconomic status. Doing so may undermine the quality of care you provide. Treat all your patients as you would treat a member of your own family.

▶ Know How to Use Your EMR Life Support Kit

The second goal of EMR training is to teach you to treat patients using limited emergency medical supplies. An EMR life support kit should be small enough to fit in the trunk of an automobile or on almost any police, fire, or rescue vehicle. Although the contents of the kit are limited, such supplies are all you need to provide immediate care for most patients you will encounter. The suggested contents of an EMR life support kit are shown in **Figure 1-9** and described in **Table 1-1**.

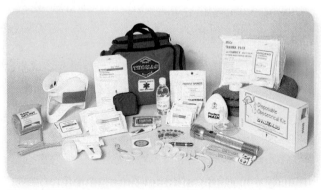

Figure 1-9 Suggested contents of an EMR life support kit.
© Jones & Bartlett Learning. Courtesy of MIEMSS.

Table 1-1	Suggested Contents of an EMR Life Support Kit
Patient examination equipment	1 flashlight
Personal safety equipment	5 pairs nitrile or latex gloves 5 face masks 1 bottle hand sanitizer
Resuscitation equipment	1 mouth-to-mask resuscitation device 1 portable hand-powered suction device 1 set oral airways 1 set nasal airways
Bandaging and dressing equipment	10 gauze adhesive strips, 1-inch (2.5-cm) 10 gauze pads, 4-inch × 4-inch (10-cm × 10-cm) 5 gauze pads, 5-inch × 9-inch (13-cm × 23-cm) 2 universal trauma dressings, 10-inch × 30-inch (25-cm × 76-cm) 1 occlusive dressing for sealing chest wounds 4 conforming gauze rolls, 3-inch × 15-inch (8-cm × 38-cm) 4 conforming gauze rolls, 4.5-inch × 15-inch (11-cm × 38-cm) 6 triangular bandages 1 roll of adhesive tape, 2-inch (5-cm) 1 burn sheet
Patient immobilization equipment	2 (each) cervical collars: small, medium, large *or* 2 adjustable cervical collars 3 rigid conforming splints (structural aluminum malleable [SAM] splints) *or* 1 set air splints for arm and leg *or* 2 (each) cardboard splints 18-inch and 24-inch
Extrication equipment	1 spring-loaded center punch 1 pair heavy leather gloves
Miscellaneous equipment	2 blankets (disposable) 2 cold packs 1 bandage scissors
Other provider equipment	1 set personal protective clothing (helmet, eye protection, EMS jacket) 1 American National Standards Institute (ANSI)-approved reflective vest 1 fire extinguisher (5-lb ABC dry chemical) 1 *Emergency Response Guidebook* 6 flares 1 set of binoculars

© Jones & Bartlett Learning.

▶ Know How to Improvise

The third goal of EMR training is to teach you how to improvise. As a trained EMR, you will often be in situations with little or no emergency medical equipment. Therefore, it is important that you know how to improvise.

This book gives examples of improvisation that can be applied to real-life situations. You will learn, for example, how to use articles of clothing and handkerchiefs to stop bleeding and how to use wooden boards, magazines, or newspapers to immobilize injured extremities.

▶ Know How to Assist Other EMS Providers

Finally, EMR training teaches you how to assist EMTs and paramedics once they arrive on the scene. Many procedures that EMTs and paramedics use require at least three people to be performed correctly. Thus you may have to assist with these procedures and you must know what to do.

■ Additional Skills

EMRs operate in a variety of settings. Many problems encountered in urban areas differ sharply from those found in rural settings. Regional variations in climate not only affect the situations you encounter but also require you to use different skills and equipment in treating patients. Certain skills and equipment mentioned in this book are beyond the essential, minimum knowledge you need to successfully complete an EMR course. However, these supplemental skills and equipment may be required in your local EMS system.

■ Roles and Responsibilities of the EMR

As an EMR, you have several roles and responsibilities. Depending on the emergency situation, you may need to:

- Maintain your body in a healthy physical and mental condition.
- Maintain equipment in a ready state.
- Respond promptly and safely to the scene of an accident or sudden illness.
- Ensure that the scene is safe from hazards.
- Protect yourself.
- Protect the incident scene and patients from further harm.
- Summon appropriate assistance (EMTs, fire department, rescue squad).

- Gain access to the patient.
- Perform patient assessment.
- Administer emergency medical care.
- Provide reassurance to patients and family members.
- Move patients only when necessary.
- Seek and then direct help from bystanders, if necessary.
- Control activities of bystanders.
- Assist EMTs and paramedics, as necessary.
- Maintain continuity of patient care.
- Document your care.
- Keep your knowledge and skills up to date.

Concern for the patient is primary; you should perform all activities with the patient's well-being in mind. Prompt response to the scene is essential if you are to provide quality care to the patient. It is important that you know your response area well so you can quickly determine the most efficient route to the emergency scene.

When you reach the emergency scene, park your vehicle so that it does not create an additional hazard. The emergency scene should be protected, with the least possible disruption of traffic. Do not block the roadway unnecessarily. Assess the scene for hazards such as downed electrical wires, gasoline spills, or unstable vehicles. When operating on highways, take steps to control traffic to prevent additional crashes and injuries. These steps are necessary to ensure that patients experience no further injuries and that rescuers (other than EMS personnel) and bystanders are not hurt.

If the equipment and personnel already dispatched to the scene cannot cope with the incident, you must immediately summon additional help. It may take some time for additional equipment and personnel to reach the scene, especially in rural areas or in communities with systems staffed by volunteers.

Once you have taken the preceding steps, you must gain access to the patient. This may be as simple as opening the door to a car or house or as difficult as squeezing through the back window of a wrecked automobile. Next, examine the patient to determine the extent of the injury or illness. This assessment of a patient is called the patient assessment sequence. Once the patient assessment is completed, you must stabilize the patient's condition to prevent it from getting worse. To do this, you will use techniques you learned in

YOU are the Provider   CASE 3

It is shortly after 1000 hours on a sunny Sunday morning when dispatch interrupts your breakfast with a report of a 37-year-old man who has slipped on a dock and fallen at the local marina. You arrive on scene to find the man lying on the dock clutching his foot, breathing normally. You notice the ankle is deformed.

1. Reaching into your medical kit, you are unable to find a splint. What else could you use to splint the man's ankle?
2. How might you be asked to assist advanced EMS personnel?
3. Why is it important that EMRs know how to improvise?

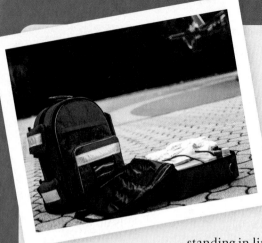

Voices *of* Experience

One day, while running errands, I stopped by the local coffee shop for my usual double latte with extra cream and sugar. While standing in line waiting to place my order, I saw my neighbor, Mrs. Jones. We were talking about her family (who did not live nearby) when she started to experience some type of medical emergency. I was very concerned by this and asked Mrs. Jones if she was okay. She responded, "My, what a gorgeous day it is outside," and began to fall down. I quickly caught her, lowered her to a chair, and told someone to call 9-1-1. After the EMS crew arrived and I told them what I saw, I left.

" Because of you, I am here today. "

As I was walking back home, I thought, "I have lived here for 25 years and think it's time I gave something back to the community." That afternoon I called the EMS system that transported Mrs. Jones. They helped me sign up for an EMR course at the local community center. Upon completion of the course, I volunteered for a couple shifts a month for the EMS system. During the course, I learned how to protect myself while responding to a medical emergency or a traumatic event. I also learned how the EMS system works, how they are notified, how to prepare myself to respond to a call safely and effectively, which skills and procedures I can and cannot do, and what happens when the patient is transported to the hospital. These are all parts of an effective EMS system, starting with personnel training and moving to vehicle staffing and transport of patients. It is important to remember that the system is like a circle that is complete only when the patient is discharged from the facility.

That day at the coffee shop, the EMS crew showed up about 2 or 3 minutes after they were called. They assessed the situation, called for a higher level of care, loaded the patient on the stretcher, and, due to the long transport time, met ALS providers on the way. What I didn't see was what happened when Mrs. Jones arrived at the hospital. A couple of days later, I saw Mrs. Jones back at the coffee shop. She came over to me, gave me a big hug, and said, "Thank you for saving my life. I had an ischemic stroke, but because of you, I am here today."

Greg LaMay, BS, NREMT-P
Education Coordinator
East Texas Medical Center-EMS (ETMC-EMS)
Tyler, Texas

training and the equipment available. Correctly applying these techniques can have a positive effect on the patient's condition.

When EMTs or paramedics arrive to assist, it is important to tell them what you know about the patient's condition and what you have done to stabilize or treat it. Your next task is to assist the EMTs or paramedics.

In some communities or situations, you may be asked to accompany the patient in the ambulance. If CPR is being performed, you may need to assist or relieve the EMT or paramedic, especially if the hospital is far from the scene. In some EMS systems, you may be qualified to drive the ambulance to the hospital so EMS personnel with more advanced training can devote all their efforts to patient care.

▶ The Importance of Documentation

Once your role in treating the patient is finished, it is important that you record your observations about the scene, the patient's condition, and the treatment you provided. Documentation should be clear, concise, accurate, and according to the accepted policies of your organization. Documentation is important because you will not be able to remember the treatment you give to all patients. It also serves as a legal record of your treatment and may be required in the event of a lawsuit. Documentation also provides a basis to evaluate the quality of care given.

Documentation should include:

- The condition of the patient when found
- The patient's description of the injury or illness
- The initial and later vital signs
- The treatment you gave the patient
- The agency and personnel who took over treatment of the patient
- Any other helpful facts

Further information about documentation is included in Chapter 5, *Communications and Documentation.*

▶ Attitude and Conduct

As an EMR, you will be judged on your attitude and conduct, as well as on the medical care you administer. It is important to understand that professional behavior has a positive impact on your patients. To be a good EMR, you need to reflect certain characteristics. You need to be honest and conduct yourself with integrity. You need to be aware of the patient's feelings and have empathy for your patients. You need to be motivated to get the job done and to understand the limits of your training and skills. You must advocate for patients. Unresponsive patients are totally dependent on your skills, knowledge, and the concern you bring to the emergency scene.

Because you will often be the first medically trained person to arrive on the scene of an emergency, it is important to be calm and caring. You will gain the confidence of patients and bystanders more easily by using a courteous and caring tone of voice. Introduce yourself by name and title or position. Show an interest in your patients. Avoid embarrassing your patients and help protect their privacy. Talk with your patients and let them know what you are doing. A good rule of thumb to follow is to treat all your patients the way you would treat a close family member. This attitude will go a long way in helping patients through the emergency and will make your job easier, too.

Remember, medical information about patients is confidential and should not be discussed with your family or friends. This information should be shared only with other medical personnel who are involved in the care of that patient.

Your appearance should be neat and professional at all times. You should be well groomed and clean. A uniform helps identify you as an EMR. If you are a volunteer who responds from home, always identify yourself as an EMR. Your professional attitude and neat appearance help provide much needed reassurance to patients Figure 1-10 . Good EMS personnel learn to keep a cool head and maintain a warm heart while caring for a patient.

YOU are the Provider CASE 4

You are dispatched to a local big box store for the report of a sick man. You are close to this location and arrive on the scene within 2 minutes. A store employee meets you at the front door and directs you to a 73-year-old man who is sitting on a chair close to the checkout area. As you approach, you notice that the patient is pale and sweaty and seems to be short of breath. His wife tells you that he started to have severe chest pains just before she called 9-1-1. She says that his pain is just like the pain he had 3 years ago when he had a heart attack.

1. What should you say as you approach this patient?
2. What level of emergency medical care do you think is best for this patient?
3. With whom can you share information about this patient's history, symptoms, and treatment?

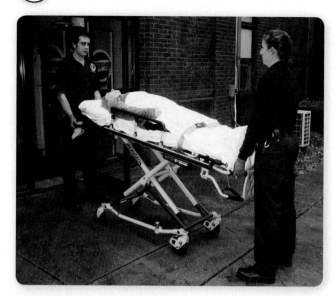

Figure 1-10 A professional attitude and neat appearance reassure patients.
© Jones & Bartlett Learning.

Medical Oversight

The overall leader of the medical care team is the physician or medical director. To ensure that the patient receives appropriate medical treatment, it is important that EMRs receive direction from a physician. Each EMS agency should have a physician who directs training courses, helps set medical policies and procedures, and ensures quality management of the EMS system. This type of medical direction is known as indirect (or offline) medical control.

A second type of medical control is known as direct (or online) medical control. A physician who is in contact with prehospital EMS providers, usually paramedics or EMTs, by two-way radio or wireless telephone provides online medical control. In cases where large numbers of people are injured, physicians may respond to the scene of the incident to provide on-scene medical control.

Quality Improvement

Quality improvement is a process used by medical care systems to evaluate the effectiveness and safety of current treatments and procedures. It is also used to determine the effectiveness and safety of new treatments and procedures. This process is used to evaluate all parts of the health care system, including EMS. The Institute of

Medicine has identified six components of the quality improvement process. These are:

1. **Safety.** The actions of EMRs must not cause harm to patients, bystanders, or EMS providers.
2. **Effectiveness.** EMS care should be based on scientific knowledge and provide the desired benefit to the patient. Refrain from any treatment that does not benefit the patient.
3. **Patient-centeredness.** Emergency medical care must be responsive to the patient's needs. Be responsive to the patient's physical needs as well as to his or her values, religion, and heritage.
4. **Timeliness.** Provide care in a timely manner. Timely patient care is an especially important component of EMS.
5. **Efficiency.** Always strive to deliver care without wasting supplies, equipment, or time.
6. **Equitability.** Strive to deliver your best care to all people. This means patient care should not vary between people of different genders, different sexual orientations, different ethnic backgrounds, different geographic locations, or different socioeconomic levels.

EMS systems should have quality improvement programs to evaluate the care they provide. Evaluations should include the six components listed above. They should consider if errors have occurred because of a gap in skills or knowledge. Your organization uses protocols, continuing medical education, and call debriefing to help improve the quality of care being given to your patients. As part of the quality improvement process, you may be asked to participate in a research study or in data collection in your service. EMS research is an important part of the quality improvement process to ensure good patient care.

Your Certification

Most states require certification, registration, or licensure of emergency medical care providers. **Certification** is the process by which a person, institution, or program is evaluated and recognized as meeting certain standards to ensure safe and ethical patient care. Your state has a lead agency that administers regulations relating to EMS operations. Once certified as an EMR, you must follow the national or state standards for your level of practice. Your employer may set additional requirements for your conduct and practice. You must keep your certification current by meeting continuing education requirements and keeping your skills up to date. Failure to keep your certification current can result in penalties.

You are the Provider: CASE 1

1. Why is your role as an EMR so important during the first minutes after a crash?

In the first few minutes after a crash or other emergency, you may be the only person on the scene who has been trained to deal with a medical emergency. Your initial actions can keep the scene safe until other responders arrive and make a difference in the patient's outcome. Also, you can determine whether additional resources need to be dispatched.

2. Why is it important to know how the components of your EMS system work?

It is important to understand the components of the EMS system because you are a part of the system. You provide a vital function in the system and are supported by and interact with people who fulfill other functions within the system.

3. How does good interaction between different levels of the EMS team improve the quality of care?

Good interactions between different levels of the EMS team improve patient care by relaying vital patient information and improving the efficiency of patient care.

You are the Provider: CASE 2

1. Why is it so important to get correct information from the emergency dispatcher?

You need the correct address to get to the emergency scene. Responding to an incorrect address will result in a delay in stabilizing the scene and providing care for the patient.

2. What are the first actions you need to take at this emergency scene?

The first actions you need to take at this scene include: Ensure that the scene is safe. Do not enter the building to see if the fire is out unless you are properly trained and equipped. Protect yourself. Do not let the patient reenter the house. Call for additional assistance. In this case, that would include fire suppression personnel and to verify that EMS transportation has been dispatched.

You are the Provider: CASE 3

1. Reaching into your medical kit, you are unable to find a splint. What else could you use to splint the man's ankle?

Look around the dock or the man's boat for anything that can be made into a splint—a magazine, a newspaper, a pillow, a towel, or seat cushions.

2. How might you be asked to assist advanced EMS personnel?

Given the man's location, responding EMTs may need assistance with lifting and moving the patient onto a stretcher and into an ambulance.

3. Why is it important that EMRs know how to improvise?

EMRs occasionally face situations where they have little or no medical gear available and must find solutions, such as using a pillow to stabilize a broken ankle when a conventional splint is not available.

You are the Provider: CASE 4

1. What should you say as you approach this patient?

Introduce yourself by name and title. Sometimes it is helpful to say, "I'm here to help you." Include the patient's wife in your introduction to put her at ease. Asking the patient his name can also be helpful. Patients respond better to your questions when you use their name.

2. What level of emergency medical care do you think is best for this patient?

Experienced emergency medical care providers learn to listen to what the patient and patient's family tell them. When the man's wife tells you that the pain is just like the pain he had with a heart attack, there is a good chance that he might be having a heart attack now. When you combine that information with his pain, sweating, and shortness of breath, you can conclude that this is a serious condition that would benefit from advanced life support care, if it is available. It is reasonable for you to relay your findings to the emergency dispatcher and request advanced life support personnel to stabilize this patient and promptly transport him to an appropriate medical facility.

3. With whom can you share information about this patient's history, symptoms, and treatment?

You can share information about this patient such as signs and symptoms of his illness, his medical history, and treatment with other members of the prehospital EMS system who are involved with his care. It is also necessary to share this information with health care workers who are caring for him at the hospital. In addition, it is important to have someone talk with the patient's wife.

Prep Kit

▶ Ready for Review

- The EMR is often the first medically trained person to arrive on the scene. The initial care provided is essential because it is available sooner than more advanced emergency medical care and could mean the difference between life and death.
- EMRs should understand the EMS system. The typical sequence of events of the EMS system is reporting, dispatch, emergency medical response, EMS vehicle response, and hospital care.
- The four basic goals of EMR training are to know what not to do, how to provide care using your EMR life support kit, how to improvise, and how to assist other EMS providers.
- As an EMR, your primary goal is to provide immediate care for a sick or injured patient. As more highly trained personnel (EMTs or paramedics) arrive on the scene, you will assist them in treating and preparing the patient for transportation.
- Once your role in treating the patient is finished, it is important that you record your observations about the scene, the patient's condition, and the treatment you provided. Documentation should be clear, concise, accurate, and according to the accepted policies of your organization.
- Remember that medical information about a patient is confidential and should be shared only with other medical personnel who are involved in the care of that particular patient.
- The overall leader of the medical care team is the physician or medical director. To ensure that the patient receives appropriate medical treatment, it is important that EMRs receive direction from a physician.
- Quality improvement helps to determine the level of care rendered by an EMS service. It measures care in six component areas: safety, effectiveness, patient-centeredness, timeliness, efficiency, and equitability. EMS systems should have an ongoing quality improvement program.

▶ Vital Vocabulary

advanced emergency medical technician (AEMT) A person who is able to perform basic life support skills and limited advanced life support skills.

advanced life support (ALS) The use of specialized equipment (such as cardiac monitors and defibrillators) and specialized techniques (such as intravenous fluid administration, drug infusion, and endotracheal intubation) to stabilize a patient's condition.

appropriate medical facility A hospital or medical clinic with adequate medical resources to provide continuing care to sick or injured patients who are transported after field treatment by emergency medical responders.

basic life support (BLS) Emergency lifesaving procedures performed without advanced emergency procedures to stabilize the condition of patients who have experienced sudden illness or injury.

certification The process by which a person, institution, or program is evaluated and recognized as meeting certain standards to ensure safe and ethical patient care.

defibrillation Process of delivering an electric shock through a person's chest wall and heart for the purpose of ending lethal heart rhythms such as ventricular fibrillation and to help establish normal heart contraction rhythms.

emergency medical responder (EMR) The first medically trained person to arrive on the scene.

emergency medical technician (EMT) A person who is trained and certified to provide basic life support and certain other noninvasive prehospital medical procedures.

emergency response communications center A fire, police, or emergency medical services agency; a 9-1-1 center; or a seven-digit telephone number used by one or all of the emergency agencies to receive and dispatch requests for emergency care; also called a public safety answering point.

paramedic A person trained and certified to provide advanced life support.

public safety answering point (PSAP) A fire, police, or emergency medical services agency; a 9-1-1 center; or a seven-digit telephone number used by one or all of the emergency agencies to receive and dispatch requests for emergency care; also called an emergency response communications center.

Assessment
in Action

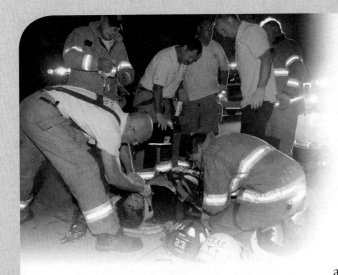

A call comes in on a Friday evening at 1943 hours. You and your partner are dispatched to a local high school for a report of an injured soccer player. As you arrive on the scene you are directed to a 17-year-old female soccer player who is trying not to cry. She states she is in a lot of pain. Upon questioning her, you learn that she was hit from the right side as she was running and now her knee is very painful. She states that she tried to walk, but she cannot put any weight on her right knee. Her right knee shows some deformity and swelling. She tells you nothing else seems to be hurt.

1. What is your initial responsibility when arriving on scene?

   A. Document your patient care.
   B. Summon appropriate assistance.
   C. Protect the incident scene and the patient from further harm.
   D. Move the patient inside a building.

2. If a patient's first contact with the EMS system is interaction with an EMR, and the second occurs when EMTs arrive, the third would be when the patient:

   A. arrives in the emergency department at the hospital.
   B. sees his or her personal physician.
   C. is discharged.
   D. is moved to the ambulance.

3. How can you assist emergency medical providers with more advanced training?

   A. Maintain command of the incident scene.
   B. Interpret cardiac rhythms.
   C. Help prepare the patient for transport.
   D. Give epinephrine.

4. All of the following are standard components of an EMS system EXCEPT:

   A. medical and support facilities.
   B. communications system.
   C. testing.
   D. transportation systems.

5. In the EMS system, a medical director does all of the following EXCEPT:

   A. help set medical policies and procedures.
   B. ensure that the EMRs are properly trained.
   C. direct the staffing for the ambulance fleet.
   D. ensure the quality management of the EMS system.

6. The roles and responsibilities of the EMR include all of the following EXCEPT:

   A. ensuring that the scene is safe from hazards.
   B. sharing the patient's medical condition with the public media.
   C. gaining access to the patient.
   D. protecting the incident scene and patients from further harm.

7. Why is it important for you to know how to improvise certain medical equipment?

8. With whom can you share information about the patient's injuries, illness, and treatment?

9. What should you tell EMTs arriving on the scene about the condition of this soccer player?

10. Why is it important to tell responding EMS personnel about your assessment and treatment of this patient?

Workforce Safety and Wellness

National EMS Education Standard Competencies

Preparatory

Uses simple knowledge of the emergency medical services (EMS) system, safety/well-being of the emergency medical responder (EMR), and medical/legal issues at the scene of an emergency while awaiting a higher level of care.

Workforce Safety and Wellness

> Standard safety precautions (pp 23–29)
> Personal protective equipment (pp 24–25)
> Stress management (pp 19–21)
  • Dealing with death and dying (p 18)
> Prevention of response-related injuries (pp 25–29)

Medicine

Recognizes and manages life threats based on assessment findings of a patient with a medical emergency while awaiting additional emergency response.

Infectious Diseases

Awareness of

> A patient who may have an infectious disease (pp 23–25)
> How to decontaminate equipment after treating a patient (p 29)

Knowledge Objectives

1. Describe the emotional aspects of emergency care encountered by patients, patients' families, and emergency medical responders (EMRs). (p 17)
2. Describe five stages a person may experience when dealing with grief or death. (p 18)
3. Explain how to confront death and dying with integrity, empathy, respect, and careful delivery of service. (p 18)
4. Describe reactions to stress and grief that EMRs must face concerning care of the dying patient, death, and the grieving process of family members. (p 18)
5. List six signs and symptoms of stress. (p 19)
6. Describe the steps that contribute to wellness and their importance in managing stress. (pp 19–21)
7. Explain the types of actions EMRs can take to reduce or alleviate stress. (p 21)
8. List hazards commonly encountered by EMRs. (p 23)
9. Describe three routes of disease transmission. (pp 23–24)
10. Describe the standard precautions for preventing infectious diseases from airborne and blood-borne pathogens. (pp 24–25)
11. Discuss the importance of standard precautions. (p 23)
12. Explain proper handwashing techniques. (p 24)
13. Explain how to remove gloves properly. (pp 25–26)
14. List the steps to take if clothing comes in contact with body fluid from a patient. (p 25)
15. Describe the safety equipment that EMRs should have available for their protection. (p 27)
16. Describe three phases of safety when responding to the scene. (p 25; p 27)
17. Describe 11 types of hazards to look for when assessing the scene for unsafe conditions. (pp 27–29)

Skills Objectives

1. Demonstrate integrity, empathy, respect, and careful delivery of service when confronted with the death of a patient. (p 18)
2. Demonstrate proper handwashing techniques. (p 24)
3. Demonstrate the safe removal of medical gloves. (p 26)
4. Demonstrate proper treatment of clothing that has come into contact with a patient's body fluid. (p 25)
5. Demonstrate the proper use of safety equipment needed for EMRs. (p 27)
6. Demonstrate scene assessment of a real or simulated rescue event for safety hazards. (pp 27–29)

■ Introduction

This chapter provides information that will help you understand the factors that may affect your physical or emotional well-being as an emergency medical responder (EMR).

You and your patients and their families can experience various degrees of stress and grief during and following a medical emergency. This chapter addresses methods for recognizing, preventing, and reducing stress from emergency incidents. It also discusses hazards you may encounter from infectious diseases and outlines procedures you must follow to reduce your risk of infection. Finally, this chapter covers scene safety and how to prevent injury to yourself and further injury to your patients.

To fulfill your duties as an EMR, you must be in good physical condition. As a new EMR, you should have a complete physical examination to ensure that you are healthy enough to do your job. Most public safety departments require this examination as part of their hiring process. If your department does not have this requirement, you should still have periodic physical examinations to ensure continuing good health.

■ Emotional Aspects of Emergency Medical Care

Providing emergency medical care as an EMR is stressful. You will experience stress while handling emergency incidents. You may also experience signs of stress following these incidents. In addition, your patients, their families and friends, and bystanders will often show signs and symptoms of stress. Because stress cannot be completely eliminated, you must learn how to avoid unnecessary stress and how to prevent your stress level from getting too high. Some of the stress-reduction techniques discussed in this chapter will also be helpful when dealing with your patients and their families and friends.

Although all emergency medical calls produce a certain level of stress, some types of calls are more stressful than others. Your past experiences may make it difficult for you to deal with certain types of calls. For example, if a patient with severe injuries reminds you of a close family member, you may have difficulty treating the patient without experiencing a high level of stress. This is especially true if an emergency call involves a very young or a very old patient Figure 2-1 . Calls involving critical patients; death; unusual danger; violence; unusual sights, smells, or sounds; or mass casualties are also likely to produce high levels of stress. Likewise, past experiences may also play a part in reducing (or increasing) your stress during the care of a patient.

Because you work in a stressful environment, you must make a conscious effort to prevent and reduce unnecessary stress. You can do this in several different ways: learn to recognize the signs and symptoms of stress, adjust your lifestyle to include stress-reducing activities, and learn what services and resources are available to help you.

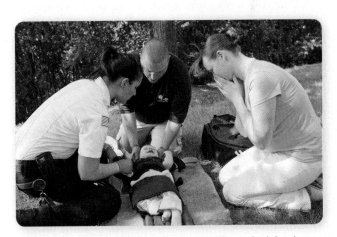

Figure 2-1 Certain kinds of patients may produce a high level of stress.
© Jones & Bartlett Learning. Photographed by Glen E. Ellman.

YOU are the Provider   CASE 1

The past week has been especially busy for you and the other members of your shift. You have been dispatched to an unusually large number of serious medical emergencies. You and your crew have cared for a seriously burned infant, an older woman who was found dead by her caregiver, and a motorcyclist about your age who had severe head injuries. As your crew reviews these calls, you realize that crew members were affected differently by these calls.

1. Why do you think crew members had different reactions to the events of the past week?
2. Which types of calls would be most stressful for you?
3. What changes should you consider to reduce your stress level?

> ### Safety
>
> Do not underestimate the effect that stress can have on you. As a firefighter, EMS provider, or law enforcement officer, you may see more suffering in a year than many people will see in their entire lifetime.

Normal Reactions to Stress

You need to understand how stress can affect you and the people for whom you provide emergency medical care. It is important to realize that a wide variety of stressful events may trigger a grief reaction. These events include a major incident, a serious illness, drug or alcohol addiction, incarceration, the end of a relationship or divorce, loss of a job or income, or a major rejection. Dying is one of the most stressful events people experience. Anyone involved with a person suffering a significant loss will go through some sort of grieving process. This includes a patient, his or her family, and caregivers, including emergency first responders.

One well-recognized model for understanding people's reactions to grief and stress was proposed by Dr. Elisabeth Kübler-Ross. This model defines five stages of grief—denial, anger, bargaining, depression, and acceptance. In studying this model, it is important to understand that people will experience grief in a variety of ways. Some people will exhibit no outward signs of grief. Other people will experience only some of these stages. People do not experience these stages of grief in any order. They can occur at any time during the grieving process.

- **Denial ("Not me!").** The first stage in the grieving process is denial. A person experiencing denial cannot believe what is happening. This stage may serve as a protection for the person experiencing the situation, and it may also serve as a protection for you as the caregiver. Realize that this reaction is normal.
- **Anger ("Why me?").** The second stage of the grieving process is anger. Understanding that anger is a normal reaction to stress can help you deal with anger that is directed toward you by a patient or the patient's family. Do not become defensive; this anger is likely a result of the situation and not a result of your patient care. This realization can enable you to tolerate the situation without letting the patient's anger distract you from performing your duties of providing care.
- **Bargaining ("Okay, but . . .").** The third stage of the grieving process is bargaining. Bargaining is the act of trying to make a deal to postpone death and dying. If you encounter a patient or family member who is in this stage, try to respond with a truthful and helpful comment such as, "We are doing everything we can

and the paramedics will be here in just a few minutes." Remember that bargaining may be a normal part of the grieving process.

- **Depression ("Heavy-hearted").** The fourth stage of the grieving process is depression. Depression is often characterized by sadness or despair. A person who is unusually silent or who seems to retreat into his or her own world may have reached this stage. This may also be the point at which a person begins to accept the situation. It is not surprising that patients and their families get depressed about a situation that involves death and dying—nor is it surprising that you as a rescuer also get depressed. Our society tends to consider death a failure of medical care rather than a natural event that happens to everyone. A certain amount of depression is a natural reaction to a major threat or loss. The depression can be mild or severe, and it can be of short duration or long-lasting. If you have depression that continues, it is important for you to contact qualified professionals who can help you.
- **Acceptance.** The final stage of the grieving process is acceptance. Acceptance does not mean that you are satisfied with the situation. It means that you understand that death and dying cannot be changed. It may require a lot of time to work through the grieving process and arrive at this stage. As an EMS provider, you may see acceptance in family members who have had time to realize that their loved one's illness is terminal. However, not all people who experience grief are able to work through it and accept the loss.

By understanding these five stages, you can better understand the grief reaction experienced by patients, their families, and their friends. You can also better understand your own reaction to stressful situations. Some helpful techniques for dealing with patients in stressful situations are presented in Chapter 12, *Behavioral Emergencies*. These techniques will help you to develop more comfort and skill when dealing with stressful situations.

> ### Words of Wisdom
>
> As you go through the anger phase of the grieving process, you may want to direct your anger at the patient, the patient's family, your coworkers, or your own family. Anger is a normal reaction to unpleasant events. Sometimes it helps to talk out your anger with coworkers, family members, or a counselor. By talking through your anger, you avoid keeping it bottled up inside where it can cause unhealthy physical symptoms or emotional reactions. Directing the energy from your anger in positive ways may help you move forward. For example, at the scene of a motor vehicle crash, you may be angry that a child has been injured. Focusing your energy on providing the best medical care for the injured child may help you work through your feelings.

► Stress Management

Stress management has three components: recognizing stress, preventing stress, and reducing stress.

Recognizing Stress

An important step in managing stress in yourself and others is the ability to recognize its signs and symptoms. Only then can you take steps to prevent or reduce stress.

Signs and Symptoms

The following warning signs should help you recognize stress in your coworkers, friends, or yourself:

- Irritability (often directed at coworkers, family, and friends)
- Inability to concentrate
- Change in normal disposition
- Difficulty in sleeping or nightmares (may be hard to recognize because many emergency care personnel work a pattern of rotating hours that makes normal sleep patterns hard to maintain)
- Anxiety
- Indecisiveness
- Guilt
- Loss of appetite or overeating
- Loss of interest in sexual relations
- Loss of interest in work
- Isolation
- Feelings of hopelessness
- Alcohol or drug misuse or abuse
- Physical symptoms

► Preventing Stress

Three simple-to-remember techniques that can prevent stress are: eat, drink, and be merry (in a healthy, stress-reducing manner).

1. **Eat.** A healthy, well-balanced diet helps prevent and reduce stress. According to the American Heart Association, a healthy daily diet should include 6 to 8 eight servings of grains and whole grains, 4 to 5 servings of vegetables, 4 to 5 servings of fruits, 2 to 3 servings of fat-free or low-fat dairy products, less than 6 ounces (28 g) of lean meats, poultry, and seafood, and 2 to 3 servings of fats and oils. In addition, they recommend 4 to 5 servings of nuts, seeds, and legumes and 5 or fewer servings of sweets per week. An illustration of a healthy diet compiled by the United States Department of Agriculture (USDA) is shown in ▶ Figure 2-2 .

   The amount of food you need is related to your size, your weight, and your level of physical activity. The steps you can take to plan a healthy diet are illustrated in ▶ Figure 2-3 .

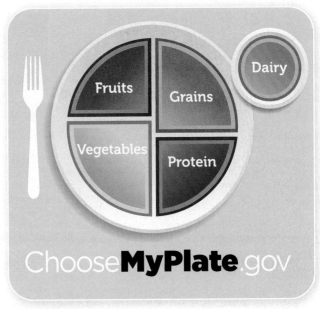

Figure 2-2 A healthy diet is illustrated by the USDA MyPlate food guidance system.
Courtesy of the USDA.

Many people need to cut down on the amount of sweets in their diet. Eating large quantities of sweets puts your energy level on a roller coaster. Your blood glucose level quickly rises, but in a few hours the level drops and you crave more sweets. To maintain more consistent glucose levels, it is much better to eat an adequate amount of whole grain breads, cereals, rice, and pasta. These food products provide energy over a longer period of time and help to reduce the highs and lows brought on by consumption of excess sugars. Reducing your intake of sugars now may help you reduce your chance of developing type 2 diabetes later in life.

EMS providers often find it hard to maintain regular meal schedules. By planning your food intake and having healthy foods available, you can improve your eating habits. Healthy eating not only helps to cut down on your stress level, it also helps reduce your risk of heart and blood vessel diseases, which are the most common causes of death in public safety workers. Keeping your weight at recommended levels helps your body better cope with stress.

2. **Drink.** Active EMS providers need to drink adequate amounts of fluids every day ▶ Figure 2-4 . Law enforcement officers, firefighters, and EMS providers who work in hot environments or wear hot bunker gear or ballistic vests are at special risk for dehydration. The average adult loses about eight glasses of water a day through sweat, exhaling, and elimination. Water in adequate

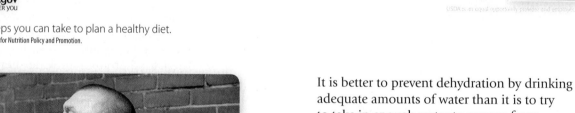

GRAINS	VEGETABLES	FRUITS	MILK	MEAT & BEANS
Make half your grains whole	Vary your veggies	Focus on fruits	Get your calcium-rich foods	Go lean with protein
Eat at least 3 oz. of whole-grain cereals, breads, crackers, rice, or pasta every day 1 oz. is about 1 slice of bread, about 1 cup of breakfast cereal, or ½ cup of cooked rice, cereal, or pasta	Eat more dark-green veggies like broccoli, spinach, and other dark leafy greens Eat more orange vegetables like carrots and sweet potatoes Eat more dry beans and peas like pinto beans, kidney beans, and lentils	Eat a variety of fruit Choose fresh, frozen, canned, or dried fruit Go easy on fruit juices	Go low-fat or fat-free when you choose milk, yogurt, and other milk products If you don't or can't consume milk, choose lactose-free products or other calcium sources such as fortified foods and beverages	Choose low-fat or lean meats and poultry Bake it, broil it, or grill it Vary your protein routine — choose more fish, beans, peas, nuts, and seeds

For a 2,000-calorie diet, you need the amounts below from each food group. To find the amounts that are right for you, go to MyPyramid.gov.

| Eat 6 oz. every day | Eat 2½ cups every day | Eat 2 cups every day | Get 3 cups every day; for kids aged 2 to 8, it's 2 | Eat 5½ oz. every day |

Find your balance between food and physical activity

- Be sure to stay within your daily calorie needs.
- Be physically active for at least 30 minutes most days of the week.
- About 60 minutes a day of physical activity may be needed to prevent weight gain.
- For sustaining weight loss, at least 60 to 90 minutes a day of physical activity may be required.
- Children and teenagers should be physically active for 60 minutes every day, or most days.

Know the limits on fats, sugars, and salt (sodium)

- Make most of your fat sources from fish, nuts, and vegetable oils.
- Limit solid fats like butter, margarine, shortening, and lard, as well as foods that contain these.
- Check the Nutrition Facts label to keep saturated fats, *trans* fats, and sodium low.
- Choose food and beverages low in added sugars. Added sugars contribute calories with few, if any, nutrients.

MyPyramid.gov
STEPS TO A HEALTHIER YOU

U.S. Department of Agriculture
Center for Nutrition Policy and Promotion
April 2005
CNPP-15

USDA

Figure 2-3 Steps you can take to plan a healthy diet.
Courtesy of the USDA Center for Nutrition Policy and Promotion.

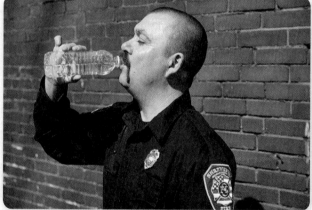

Figure 2-4 Drinking adequate quantities of water is important.
© Jones & Bartlett Learning.

quantities is essential for maintaining proper body function. Natural fruit juices are another good source of fluids. It is important to keep your body hydrated while you are on duty. When you are working in a hot environment or are involved in a strenuous incident, rehydrate yourself by regularly consuming adequate amounts of water or a sports drink.

It is better to prevent dehydration by drinking adequate amounts of water than it is to try to take in enough water to recover from dehydration.

Avoid consuming excessive amounts of caffeine and alcohol. Caffeine is a drug that causes adrenaline to be released in your body. Adrenaline raises your blood pressure and increases your stress level. By limiting your intake of caffeine-containing beverages such as coffee, tea, cola drinks, and energy drinks, you can reduce your tendency toward stress. Caffeine and alcohol also cause dehydration. Using tobacco products and drinking alcoholic beverages are discouraged. Although alcoholic drinks seem to relax you, they can cause depression and reduce your ability to deal with stress. Some people who drink alcohol become addicted to it. Drinking too much alcohol can end your career.

3. **Be merry.** When a person is happy, he or she generally is not experiencing an elevated level of stress. It is important to learn to balance your lifestyle. Assess both your work

environment and your home environment. At work, address problems promptly before they produce major stress. When you are off duty, remember to get an adequate amount of sleep and make time for personal activities. If you are working in a volunteer agency, it is best that personnel not be on call all the time.

Other ways to prevent stress include spending time with your friends and family. In your recreational activities, include friends who are not coworkers. Develop hobbies or activities that are not related to your job. Exercise regularly. Exercise is a great stress reliever. Swimming, running, and bicycling are three types of excellent aerobic exercise. Meditation and religious activities also reduce stress for many people. People who can balance the pressures of work with relaxing activities at home usually enjoy life much more than people who can never leave the stories and stress of work behind. If you are feeling stress away from your job, consider seeking assistance from a mental health professional.

Safety

Because public safety services must be provided 24 hours a day, many law enforcement, fire, EMS, and security personnel work rotating shifts. Firefighters and emergency medical providers may work shifts that are 24 hours or longer with a variety of days off. Emergency responders may be required to alternate between day and night shifts.

These work schedules disrupt normal sleep patterns. In addition, many people in public safety work overtime shifts, have a second job, or commute long distances to work. This combination of factors often means that many public safety personnel do not get enough sleep.

Scientific studies have shown that most people need about 8 hours of uninterrupted sleep per night. If you are not meeting this need, your mental and physical health may suffer and you will be less able to deal with stress. In addition, the care you give to patients may be compromised. It is important to make getting enough sleep a priority in your life.

Reducing Stress

If pressures at work or home are causing you continual stress, you may benefit from the help of a mental health professional. Mental health professionals include psychologists, psychiatrists, social workers, and specially trained clergy. They are trained to listen in a nonjudgmental way and to help you find ways to diminish your stress. You may be able to connect with a mental health professional through your department's employee assistance program. Your medical insurance usually covers this type of care. Contact your employee assistance representative if you are experiencing continuing signs or symptoms of stress.

Critical incident stress management (CISM) is a program available through some public safety departments.

It consists of **preincident stress education**, **on-scene peer support**, and **critical incident stress debriefings (CISDs)**:

1. Preincident stress education provides information about the stresses you will encounter and the reactions you may experience. It is designed to help you understand the normal stress responses you may experience when encountering an abnormal emergency situation.
2. On-scene peer support and disaster support services provide aid for you on the scene of especially stressful incidents. Examples are major disasters or situations that involve the death of a coworker or a child.
3. A debriefing after a stressful emergency situation may help to alleviate the stress reactions caused by the situation. A debriefing is a meeting between emergency responders and specially trained leaders. The purpose of a debriefing is to allow an open discussion of feelings, fears, and reactions to the high-stress situation. A debriefing is not an investigation or an interrogation. Debriefings are usually held within 24 to 72 hours after a major incident. The specially trained leaders can offer suggestions and information on overcoming stress **Figure 2-5**.

Find out if your department has an employee assistance program. Contact this program's representative if you are involved in a high-stress incident such as a call that involves a very young or very old patient, a mass-casualty incident, or a situation that involves unusual violence. If you think you might be experiencing signs or symptoms of stress from such an incident, contact your supervisor or a stress counselor. More information about stress debriefing is presented in Chapter 12, *Behavioral Emergencies*.

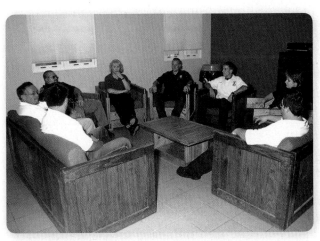

Figure 2-5 A debriefing after a stressful emergency situation may be helpful in relieving stress.
© Jones & Bartlett Learning. Courtesy of MIEMSS.

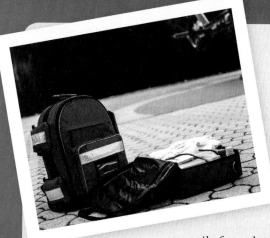

Voices *of* Experience

It was the middle of the night, and we were dispatched to a domestic violence event. The scene was not secure, so we staged a mile from the scene and waited until police arrived and declared the scene secure.

The wife was complaining of head and neck injuries and had been beaten pretty badly. She stated her husband had come home from a bar and started beating her. The husband was not around and could not be found, although his vehicle was still in the driveway. The wife stated that her husband ran out the door when he heard sirens coming. The neighbors had called 9-1-1 as a result of all of the yelling and noise coming from this home.

> **It was a very scary moment—the husband had a shotgun.**

We treated the wife for her injuries. As we proceeded outside to load her into the ambulance, the husband jumped out from the backseat of his car and came toward us. It was a very scary moment—the husband had a shotgun and was waiting to shoot his wife and anyone treating her. Luckily the police were walking with us, and they were able to subdue the husband and secure his firearm.

We then proceeded to load the wife into the ambulance and left the scene heading toward hospital. We drove down the road, stopped, and finished treating our patient with an IV and pain medication. The call could have been so much worse, but fortunately we had police on scene, and they quickly took care of the shooter and kept us safe.

Any domestic violence scene, even one that is considered secure, can change quickly and without warning. Situations occurring in the middle of the night may also contribute to questionable security. Always watch your back in any situation, as the scene could change for the worse quickly and at any time.

Julia Chamberlain BSN, RN, Paramedic, I/C
Onondaga Fire Department
Onondaga, Michigan

■ Workforce Safety

As an EMR, you will encounter a wide variety of hazards at emergency scenes. It is important for you to recognize these hazards and to know what steps to take to minimize the risk they pose to your patients, your partners, and yourself. This section covers common hazards you will encounter, including infectious diseases, traffic, crime and violence, crowds, electrical hazards, fire, hazardous materials, unstable objects, sharp objects, animals, environmental conditions, and special rescue situations.

▶ Infectious Diseases and Standard Precautions

In recent years, Ebola virus disease (Ebola), the acquired immunodeficiency syndrome (AIDS) epidemic, and the growing concern about hepatitis, influenza, tuberculosis (TB), and methicillin-resistant *Staphylococcus aureus* (MRSA) have increased awareness of infectious (communicable) diseases. It is important for you to have some understanding of the most common infectious diseases to allow you to protect yourself from unnecessary exposure to these diseases. It will also prevent you from becoming unduly alarmed when you encounter these diseases. Infectious diseases can be contracted in several different ways, such as eating infected food and through contact with infected blood or infected body fluid. Exposure can take place through a small cut, direct contact with a mucous membrane, or from unprotected sex.

The three most common routes for transmission of infectious diseases are contact with infected blood, contact with airborne droplets, and direct contact with infectious agents. The disease-causing agents that are spread through contact with infected blood are called blood-borne **pathogens**. Human immunodeficiency virus (HIV), the virus that causes AIDS, and the viruses that cause hepatitis B and hepatitis C are blood-borne pathogens. Other infectious diseases are spread through contact with droplets of airborne pathogens. Influenza, TB, and severe acute respiratory syndrome (SARS) fall within this group. A third group of infectious diseases is spread by direct contact. One example is MRSA, an infection that is spread by direct contact with the patient's skin or with contaminated clothing or towels.

Blood-borne Pathogens

HIV is transmitted by contact with infected blood, semen, or vaginal secretions. There is no scientific documentation that the virus is transmitted by contact with sweat, saliva, tears, sputum, urine, feces, vomitus, or nasal secretions, unless these fluids contain visible signs of blood. Exposure can take place in the following ways:

- The patient's blood is splashed or sprayed into your eyes, nose, or mouth or into an open sore or cut.
- You have blood from the infected patient on your hands and then touch your own eyes, nose, mouth, or an open sore or cut.
- A needle that was used to inject the patient breaks your skin.
- Broken glass at a motor vehicle collision or other incident that is covered with blood from an infected patient penetrates your glove and skin.

Remember that some patients who are infected with HIV do not know they are infected. Others who are infected do not show any symptoms. This is why the Centers for Disease Control and Prevention (CDC) recommends that health care workers wear certain types of gloves any time they are likely to come into contact with secretions or blood from any patient. Whenever you are on the job, you should also cover any open wounds you have.

Hepatitis B is also spread by direct contact with infected blood, although it is far more contagious than HIV. EMRs should follow the standard precautions described in the following section to reduce their chance of contracting hepatitis B. Check with your medical director about receiving injections of hepatitis vaccine to protect you against this infection. This vaccine should be made available to you. Meningitis and syphilis are two other diseases that can be spread by contact with contaminated blood.

Airborne Pathogens

TB is a contagious disease that is spread by droplets from the respiratory system. When an infected person coughs or sneezes, the TB virus is spread through the air. Although TB is often hard to distinguish from other diseases, patients who pose the highest risk usually have a cough. This disease is dangerous to EMRs because

YOU ▶ **are the Provider**   **CASE 2**

Three days after being dispatched to the home of a teenage mother whose 4-month-old had died, you notice your partner is not as upbeat as normal. You have also noticed that in the last 2 days your partner has stopped eating during the usual station house meals and has become irritable.

1. What may be causing the changes in your partner's behavior?
2. What can your partner do to alleviate the signs and symptoms?
3. During the initial incident, the mother repeatedly asked rescuers, "Why me?" Which stage of grief was she experiencing?

drug-resistant strains of TB have evolved. To minimize your exposure when you encounter a patient with a cough, wear a face mask or a high-efficiency particulate air (HEPA) respirator **Figure 2-6** and put an oxygen mask on the patient. If no oxygen mask is available, place a face mask on the patient. You should have a skin test for TB every year.

Influenza, whooping cough, and SARS are other diseases that are spread through airborne droplets. Influenza is caused by viruses that change over time. When certain conditions are right, a new strain of the influenza virus may cause many people in a community to become sick. The H1N1 strain of influenza (swine flu) has caused concern because few people have immunity to this strain of virus. When a new strain of an influenza virus develops, your department will need to follow the latest recommendations from the CDC for your protection.

▶ Direct Contact

MRSA infection is caused by the bacterium *Staphylococcus aureus*—often called staph. MRSA is a strain of staph that is resistant to the broad-spectrum antibiotics commonly used for treatment. Most MRSA infections occur in health care settings such as hospitals, dialysis centers, and nursing homes. It most commonly occurs in people with weakened immune systems, where it can be fatal. However, MRSA can also occur in otherwise healthy people. In healthy people, MRSA may show up as a skin sore. As an EMR, you need to be sure you follow standard precautions to avoid contracting MRSA from your patients. In addition, you need to avoid sharing your towels, razors, and other personal care items. Wash your towels in hot water and dry them thoroughly.

Ebola is an example of a disease that is spread by direct contact. The Ebola virus can be spread from an infected person to others by direct contact through broken skin or through mucous membranes such as the eyes, nose, or mouth. The body fluids that can spread this infection include blood, urine, breast milk, and semen. Ebola can also be spread through unprotected contact with a dead person. Although this disease is not normally present in North America, there have been cases of an infected person bringing the disease into the United States from a country where there was an Ebola epidemic. Any emergency provider who will be caring for patients known to have a highly contagious disease such as Ebola must have special training in handling infected patients.

Safety

The most important step you can take to remain healthy and reduce the transmission of disease is to wash your hands. Bacteria and viruses are picked up when you touch any contaminated surface. Examples include keyboards, doorknobs, steering wheels, telephones, head sets, and EMS equipment. Once bacteria and/or viruses are on your hands, touching your eyes, mouth, or nose with your fingers can introduce these microorganisms into your body.

Wash your hands before and after eating, before and after using the toilet, after blowing your nose or sneezing into your hands, before and after preparing food, and before and after touching a patient. After you touch something that might be contaminated, wash your hands as soon as possible. Wearing gloves does not excuse you from the need to wash your hands regularly.

Wash your hands with clean, warm, running water. Apply soap and rub your hands together to make a substantial lather. The soap does not have to be antibacterial; regular soap is sufficient. Be sure to scrub all the surfaces; wash between your fingers, and under your nails, as well as the backs of your hands. Keep rubbing your hands together for at least 20 seconds, about the time it takes to sing "Happy Birthday!" Thoroughly rinse your hands and dry them with a paper towel.

Standard Precautions

Federal regulations require all health care workers, including EMRs, to assume that all patients are potentially infected with blood-borne pathogens. These regulations require that all health care workers use protective equipment to prevent possible exposure to blood and certain body fluids.

You will not always be able to tell whether a patient's body fluids contain blood. Therefore, the CDC recommends that all health care workers use the following **standard precautions**:

1. Always wear approved latex or nitrile gloves when handling patients, and change gloves after contact with each patient. Wash your hands with soap and water immediately after removing gloves. If soap and water are not available, a hand sanitizer can be used as a temporary cleansing agent until soap and warm water are available. Note that leather gloves are not considered safe—leather is porous and traps fluids.

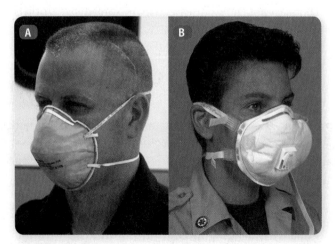

Figure 2-6 Two types of respirators (**A, B**) that reduce the transmission of airborne pathogens.
© Jones & Bartlett Learning. Courtesy of MIEMSS.

2. Always wear a protective mask, eyewear, or a face shield when you anticipate that blood or other body fluids may splatter. Wear a gown/apron, head covering, and shoe covers if you anticipate splashes of blood or other body fluids such as those that occur with childbirth and major trauma.

3. Wash your hands and other skin surfaces immediately and thoroughly with soap and water if they become contaminated with blood and other body fluids **Figure 2-7**. Change contaminated clothes and wash exposed skin thoroughly.

4. Do not recap, cut, or bend used needles. Place them directly in a puncture-resistant container designed for sharps.

5. Even though saliva has not been proven to transmit HIV, you should use a face shield, pocket mask, or other airway adjunct if the patient needs resuscitation.

Proper removal of gloves is important to minimize the spread of pathogens **Skill Drill 2-1**:

1. Begin by partially removing one glove. With the other gloved hand, pinch the first glove at the wrist, being careful to touch only the outside of the glove, and start to roll it back off the hand, inside out **Step 1**.

2. Remove the second glove by pinching the exterior with the partially gloved hand **Step 2**.

3. Pull the second glove inside out toward the fingertips **Step 3**. Grasp both gloves with your free hand, touching only the clean interior surfaces and gently remove the gloves **Step 4**.

Federal agencies such as the Occupational Safety and Health Administration (OSHA) and state agencies such as state public health departments have regulations about standard precautions. Because these regulations are constantly changing, it is important for your department to stay updated on these regulations and provide continuing education to keep you current with the latest changes related to infectious disease precautions.

Immunizations

Certain immunizations are recommended for EMS providers. These include influenza, tetanus prophylaxis, and hepatitis B vaccines. You also should check the status of your varicella (chickenpox) vaccine and your measles, mumps, and rubella (German measles) vaccines. Tuberculin testing may also be recommended. Your medical director can determine which immunizations and tests are needed for members of your department. Being properly immunized protects you from contracting these diseases from patients. In certain cases such as influenza, it also helps to protect patients from getting influenza from you.

▶ Responding to the Scene

Scene safety is a most important consideration to you as an EMR. You must consider your safety and the safety of all the other people at the scene of an emergency. An injured or dead EMR cannot help those in need. He or she becomes someone who needs help, increasing the difficulty of a rescue. Drive safely and always fasten your seat belt when you are in your vehicle. Paying close attention to safety factors can help prevent unnecessary illness, injuries, and death.

> **Safety**
>
> If your clothing comes in contact with body fluid from a patient, remove the clothing as soon as possible. If body fluids have contacted you through your clothing, take a shower, washing thoroughly with hot, soapy water. Your clothing should be placed in a marked plastic bag or handled so that the body fluids are contained. Clothing should be washed as soon as possible in hot, soapy water. Always follow the protocols of your department and the CDC's most recent recommendations for these situations.

Dispatch

Safety begins when you are dispatched to an emergency. Be sure you have correct dispatch information, including the address, before you begin your response. Use your dispatch information to anticipate hazards that may be present and to determine the best way to approach the scene of the emergency.

Response

Vehicle crashes are a major cause of death and disability in law enforcement officials, firefighters, and EMS providers. As you respond to the scene of an emergency, remember the safety information that you learned in your driving courses. Drive safely and always fasten your

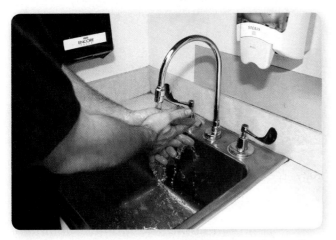

Figure 2-7 Wash your hands thoroughly with soap and water if you are contaminated with blood or other body fluids.
© Jones & Bartlett Learning. Courtesy of MIEMSS.

Skill Drill 2-1

Proper Removal of Medical Gloves

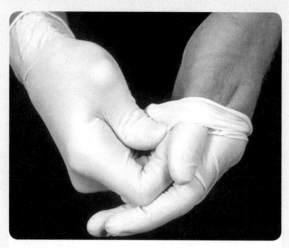

Step 1 Partially remove the first glove by pinching at the wrist. Be careful to touch only the outside of the glove.

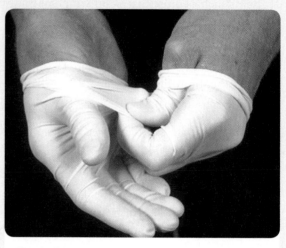

Step 2 Remove the second glove by pinching the exterior with the partially gloved hand.

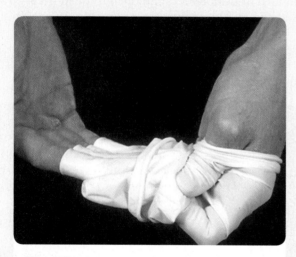

Step 3 Pull the second glove inside out toward the fingertips.

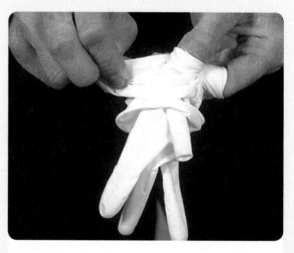

Step 4 Grasp both gloves with your free hand, touching only the clean interior surfaces, and gently remove the gloves.

© Jones & Bartlett Learning. Courtesy of MIEMSS.

YOU are the Provider   CASE 3

You are sent to the home of a 76-year-old man with an unknown medical illness. You walk in and identify yourself as an EMR. You notice that the man is sweating, even though the room temperature is cool. You start your assessment. Each time he starts to answer a question, you notice that he is stopped by a productive cough. He tells you that he has had a temperature of 104°F (40°C) for a few days.

1. Which route of disease transmission are you most concerned about with this patient?
2. What precautions should you take to protect yourself when caring for this patient?
3. What steps do you need to take to protect yourself and others after caring for this patient?

seat belt when you are in your vehicle. Your seat belt can save your life only when it is fastened. Plan the best route and drive quickly but safely to the scene. Be especially careful during periods of rain, snow, or high wind. Slow down your response to make sure you arrive safely. All emergency responders who will be driving should complete an emergency vehicle operator's course.

Parking Your Vehicle

When you arrive at the emergency scene, park your vehicle so that it protects the area from traffic hazards. Check to be sure that the emergency warning lights are operating correctly. Be careful when getting out of your vehicle, especially if you must step into a traffic area.

Federal safety standards require approved safety vests any time you are working on an active highway. These vests enhance your visibility in the daytime, and the reflective material on your safety vest helps make you more visible in the dark Figure 2-8 . If your vehicle is not needed to protect the incident scene, park it out of the way of traffic. Leave room for other arriving vehicles such as ambulances to be positioned near the patient. Above all else, make sure that you have protected the emergency scene from further incidents.

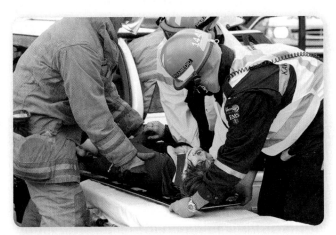

Figure 2-8 Reflective clothing helps make you more visible.
© Murray Wilson/Fotolia.com.

▶ Assessing the Scene

As you approach the emergency scene, scan the entire area carefully to determine what hazards are present. Consider the following hazards based on the type of emergency; address them in the most appropriate order. For example, assess the scene of a motor vehicle crash for downed electrical wires before you check for broken glass.

Traffic

Consider whether traffic is a problem. Sometimes the most important first step you need to take at a motor vehicle crash scene is to control traffic to prevent further collisions. If you need more help to handle traffic, call for assistance before you get out of your vehicle.

Crime or Violence

If your dispatch information leads you to believe that the incident involves violence or a crime, follow your department's protocols for approaching the scene. If you are trained in law enforcement procedures, follow your local protocols. If you are not a law enforcement official, proceed very carefully. If you have any doubts about the safety of the scene, it is better to wait at a safe distance and request help from law enforcement officials. If the scene involves a crime, remember to take a mental picture of the scene and avoid disturbing anything at the scene unless it is absolutely necessary to move objects to provide patient care.

Crowds

Crowds may range in size from a few neighbors or bystanders to a huge mass gathering at a large parade or sporting event. The mood of a crowd may range from friendly and helpful to hostile. Friendly neighborhood crowds may interfere very little with your duties. Unfriendly, unruly, or hostile crowds may require a police presence before you are able to begin assessing and treating patients. Assess the crowd's mood before you get in a position from which there is no exit. Request help from law enforcement officials before the crowd is out of control. Safety considerations may require you to wait for the arrival of police before you approach the patient.

Electrical Hazards

Electrical hazards can be present at many types of emergency scenes. Patients located inside buildings may be in contact with a wide variety of electrical hazards. These can range from a faulty extension cord in a house to high-voltage machinery in an industrial setting. Patients located outside may be in contact with high-voltage electrical power lines that have fallen because of a motor vehicle crash or a storm. Assess the emergency scene for any indications of electrical problems. Inside a building, look for cords, electrical wires, or electrical appliances near or in contact with the patient. When you are outside, look for damaged electrical poles and downed electrical wires. Do not approach an emergency scene if there are indications of electrical problems. Keep all other people away from the source of the hazard. Because electricity is invisible, make sure that the electrical current has been turned off by a qualified person before you get close to the source of the current. Always wear a helmet with a chin strap and face shield in situations that may involve electrical hazards.

Fire

Fire is a hazard to both you and the patient. Contact with a power source can result in severe injury or death. Anytime there appears to be a fire, immediately call for fire department assistance. If you are a trained firefighter, follow rescue and firefighting procedures for your department. If you are not a trained firefighter, do not exceed the limits of your training because any attempt to rescue a person from a burning building is a high-risk undertaking. Do not enter a burning building without proper turnout gear and self-contained breathing apparatus. Recent fire research has shown that during a fire, keeping doors and windows closed until hose streams are in place will slow the growth and spread of fire. Do not open doors and windows before the firefighters arrive. Vehicles that have been involved in collisions also may present a fire hazard from fuel or other spilled fluids. Keep all ignition sources such as cigarettes and road flares away. Carefully assess the fire hazard before you determine your course of action.

Hazardous Materials

Hazardous materials (sometimes referred to as HazMats) may be found almost anywhere. Motor vehicle crashes with large trucks may involve hazardous materials. Hazardous materials may also be found in homes, businesses, and industries. Federal regulations require vehicles that are transporting a certain quantity of hazardous materials to be marked with specific placards **Figure 2-9**.

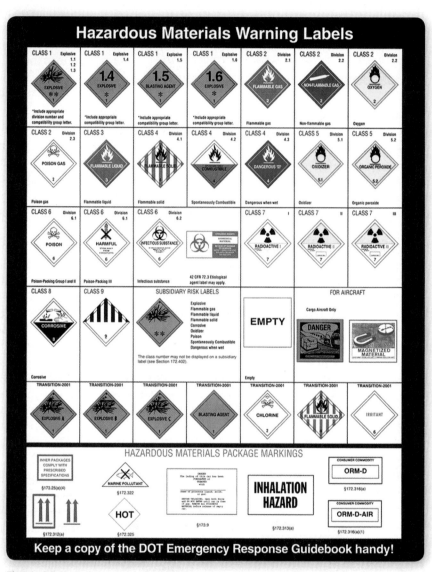

Figure 2-9 Hazardous materials placards.
Courtesy of the US Department of Transportation.

YOU are the Provider   CASE 4

You and your partner are returning to headquarters after lunch when dispatch sends you to the scene of a rented box truck that has rolled over. Injuries are reported, but dispatch is unable to tell you the extent of the injuries or the number of people involved. As you pull up to the scene, you spot a hazardous materials placard.

1. Where should you park your vehicle?
2. What other issues should you consider before leaving your vehicle?
3. Why is your safety a concern?

Be aware that small quantities of certain hazardous materials may be transported without displaying placards. If you believe that a crash may involve hazardous materials, stop uphill and upwind at some distance from the crash. Then determine whether the vehicle is marked with a placard. A pair of binoculars in the life support kit is helpful for this. The placard indicates the class of material being transported. You should carry an *Emergency Response Guidebook* to assist you in determining the hazard involved and follow your department protocols. Also note the presence of leaking fluids. The presence of odors or fumes may be the first indication of hazardous materials located in buildings. If you believe that a hazardous material is present, call for assistance from the agency that handles hazardous materials in your community. Remain far away from any suspected HazMat incident so you do not become an additional casualty. (See Chapter 20, *Vehicle Extrication and Special Rescue*, for more information on handling HazMat incidents.)

Unstable Objects

Unstable objects may include vehicles, trees, poles, buildings, cliffs, and piles of materials. Motor vehicle collisions, wind storms, ice storms, explosions, fires, building collapses, and earthquakes may result in unstable objects. After a collision, a motor vehicle may be located in an unstable position. You may need to stabilize the vehicle before you assess the patient or begin patient extrication. Do not attempt to enter or get under an unstable vehicle. Undeployed air bags are another hazard after a motor vehicle collision. Motor vehicle collisions may result in other unstable objects, including trees or poles that were hit in the collision. Fires and explosions can result in unstable buildings. Assess a building for stability before attempting to enter it. If you are in doubt about the safety of the building, follow your local protocols and call for trained personnel rather than attempting to enter an unsafe building alone.

▶ Sharp Objects

Sharp objects are frequently present at an emergency scene. These objects range from broken glass at the scene of a motor vehicle crash to hypodermic needles in the pocket of a drug addict. Being aware of sharp objects can reduce the chance of injury to you and to your patients. Latex and nitrile medical gloves can help prevent the spread of disease from blood contamination, but they provide no protection against sharp objects. When glass or other sharp objects are present, wear heavy leather or firefighting gloves over your medical gloves to prevent injuries.

Safety

After working at a scene that involves potential infectious exposure, you should clean and disinfect your equipment. Cleaning refers to the removal of dirt, dust, blood, or other visible contaminants. Disinfection requires special chemicals that kill pathogenic agents when applied directly to a surface. Disposable equipment and supplies should be disposed of in a manner that prevents contamination of other objects. Follow your local protocols and the latest recommendations of the CDC and OSHA. It is also important to complete the appropriate documentation of the exposure.

▶ Animals

Animals, whether they are house pets, farm stock, or wild, are found indoors and outdoors. Pets can become very upset in the confusion of a medical emergency. When you need to enter a house to take care of a patient, be sure excited pets have been secured in another part of the house away from the patient. People often travel with their pets, so pets can be part of the scene of a motor vehicle crash. Service dogs may be possessive of their owners. Farm animals, too, can be a safety hazard; be careful when entering a field that may contain livestock. Animals may present hazards such as bites, kicking, or even trampling. Careful assessment of the incident scene can prevent unnecessary injuries.

▶ Environmental Conditions

Weather cannot be changed or controlled; therefore, you should consider the effect weather will have on rescue operations. Dress appropriately for the expected weather and be prepared for precipitation and temperature extremes for you and your patients. Be alert for possible damage from high winds. Keep your patients dry and comfortable. Darkness makes it hard to see all the hazards that may be present, so use any emergency lighting that is available. A bright flashlight is a valuable tool in many rescue situations.

▶ Special Rescue Situations

Special safety considerations are required in situations involving water rescue, ice rescue, confined space or below-grade rescue, terrorism, and mass-casualty incidents. These situations are covered in Chapter 20, *Vehicle Extrication and Special Rescue*. Do not enter an emergency situation that is unsafe unless you have the proper training and equipment.

YOU are the Provider   SUMMARY

You are the Provider: CASE 1

1. **Why do you think crew members had different reactions to the events of the past week?**

Calls that involve young children, older adults, or people your own age may be more difficult for many people. Because young children are not able to take care of themselves, these calls may be more stressful. Older patients may remind you of your parents, neighbors, or grandparents. Calls that involve someone your age may remind you of your own vulnerability. Certain calls will be more difficult for some team members than for others because each of us has different life experiences.

2. **Which types of calls would be most stressful for you?**

It is sometimes helpful to consider which types of calls may be most stressful for you. By engaging in this type of self-reflection, you may be able to reduce your stress on these calls. Talking about your concern with a close friend or supervisor may also be helpful.

3. **What changes should you consider to reduce your stress level?**

Consider your current lifestyle and the stressors in your life. Evaluate your diet, your type and amount of fluid intake, the amount and type of exercise you get, the quality and quantity of sleep you get, and how you deal with the stressors at work and away from work. Then consider how to make changes to reduce your stress level and improve your health.

You are the Provider: CASE 2

1. **What may be causing the changes in your partner's behavior?**

Your partner may be showing signs of job-related stress in connection with the dispatch call that involved the death of an infant. Calls involving children are among the most stressful. Among the signs of post-event stress problems are irritability directed at coworkers, family, and friends; a change in the person's normal disposition; and possibly a loss of appetite.

2. **What can your partner do to alleviate the signs and symptoms?**

There are many methods of handling stress, but it is important to first recognize the signs of job-related stress. EMS personnel experiencing stress also need to maintain proper nutrition when the body's resources are strained. Finally, EMS providers experiencing post-event stress should consider contacting their employee assistance program representative for help.

3. **During the initial incident, the mother repeatedly asked rescuers, "Why me?" Which stage of grief was she experiencing?**

The mother may have been in the second stage of the five stages of grief, which is anger. The other stages are denial, bargaining, depression, and acceptance.

You are the Provider: CASE 3

1. **Which route of disease transmission are you most concerned about with this patient?**

The primary means by which this patient could infect others is through airborne droplets of infected secretions. If this patient is coughing up secretions, you need to avoid contact with these also.

2. **What precautions should you take to protect yourself when caring for this patient?**

By placing a mask on this patient, you may prevent the spread of infectious airborne droplets. However, if the patient is coughing up secretions, this may not be a good option. A second option is for you and the other caregivers to put on masks. You should don gloves and consider donning gowns if available. Also it might be helpful to supply the patient with tissues to cover his mouth when coughing.

3. **What steps do you need to take to protect yourself and others after caring for this patient?**

After caring for this patient, it is important to dispose of your masks, gloves, gowns, and any other objects that may have come in contact with the patient's airborne droplets or secretions. You need to learn your agency's policy for disposing of potentially infected materials. Do not forget to thoroughly wash your hands. Consider changing your uniform if it has come in contact with any infected secretions.

You are the Provider: CASE 4

1. **Where should you park your vehicle?**

The vehicle should be parked to protect the area from traffic hazards. However, because the truck is displaying a hazardous materials placard, you need to consider additional risks. The placard indicates the types of materials that may be carried on the truck. Before approaching the vehicle, check your *Emergency Response Guidebook* to determine the type of hazardous materials that may be involved. Then follow local protocols.

2. What other issues should you consider before leaving your vehicle?

Motor vehicle incidents present many potential hazards for EMRs. Broken glass presents an injury risk to rescuers.

Likewise, leaking fluids and fumes from hazardous materials can also be considered potential hazards.

3. Why is your safety a concern?

An injured or dead EMR will not be able to help people in need. Furthermore, an injured EMR adds to the number of victims, increasing the difficulty of the situation for the other EMRs.

Prep Kit

▶ Ready for Review

- EMRs should understand the role that stress plays in the lives of emergency care providers and patients who have experienced a sudden illness or injury. Stress is a normal part of an EMR's life.
- Five stages of the grieving process following different kinds of loss including death and dying are denial, anger, bargaining, depression, and acceptance. Patients and rescue personnel may experience some or all of these stages. People experience these stages in different orders and at different rates.
- Stress management consists of recognizing, preventing, and reducing critical incident stress.
- Scene safety is an important part of your job. You should understand how airborne and blood-borne diseases are spread and how standard precautions prevent the spread of infection. You should also know the steps you can take to protect yourself from infectious diseases.
- As you arrive on the scene of a collision or illness, you must assess the scene for a wide variety of hazards. Potential hazards include traffic, crime, crowds, unstable objects, sharp objects, electrical problems, fire, hazardous materials, animals, environmental conditions, special rescue situations, and infectious disease exposure. You should understand the safety equipment and precautions needed for the various types of rescue situations.

▶ Vital Vocabulary

acceptance The stage of the grieving process when the person experiencing grief recognizes the finality of the grief-causing event.

anger The stage of the grieving process when the person experiencing grief becomes upset or angry at the grief-causing event or other situation.

bargaining The stage of the grief reaction when the person experiencing grief barters to change the grief-causing event.

critical incident stress debriefing (CISD) A system of psychological support designed to reduce stress on emergency personnel after a major stress-producing incident.

critical incident stress management (CISM) A process that confronts the responses to critical incidents and defuses them, directing the emergency services personnel toward physical and emotional equilibrium.

denial A stage of a grief reaction when the person experiencing grief rejects the grief-causing event.

depression A stage of the grief reaction when the person expresses despair—an absence of cheerfulness and hope—as a result of a grief-causing event.

on-scene peer support Stress counselors at the scene of stressful incidents who help emergency personnel deal with stress.

pathogens Microorganisms that are capable of causing disease.

preincident stress education Training about stress and stress reactions conducted for public safety personnel before they are exposed to stressful situations.

standard precautions An infection control concept that treats all body fluids as potentially infectious.

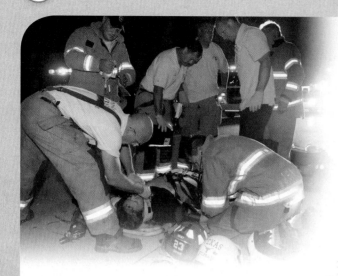

Assessment
in Action

You and your partner are dispatched to a motor vehicle crash on a secondary country road. When you arrive at the scene, you see a car sitting in the roadway with the driver's door open. A man is kneeling beside a 17-year-old boy who is lying in the road. A crumpled bicycle is positioned about 50 feet (15 m) from them. You note that the teenager is wearing a helmet. He is bleeding from a scrape on his forearm, and he complains of pain from his left leg, which is bent at an abnormal angle.

1. Which of the following hazards should you be most concerned about when attempting to help the patients?

   A. Vehicle instability
   B. Downed electrical lines
   C. Broken glass
   D. Uncontrolled traffic

2. What is another hazard you will need to consider when caring for these patients when arriving at the scene of a motor vehicle collision?

   A. Airborne pathogens
   B. Environmental conditions
   C. Blood-borne pathogens
   D. Traffic

3. Because the patient is bleeding, what are the minimum standard precautions you should take?

   A. Handwashing and a mask
   B. Gloves
   C. Shoe covers and a gown
   D. Leather gloves

4. All of the following are signs and symptoms of job-related stress EXCEPT:

   A. irritability.
   B. difficulty sleeping.

   C. alcohol or drug misuse or abuse.
   D. working too hard.

5. A stress-reducing diet includes all of the following EXCEPT:

   A. fruits.
   B. vegetables.
   C. low-fat milk, yogurt, and cheese.
   D. fried fast foods.

6. What personal protective equipment would you incorporate into your care of these patients?

7. How stressful do you think this call would be for you?

8. What should you do if your clothing comes into contact with body fluid from a patient?

9. What are some of the emotional aspects that could impact an EMR's reaction to this call?

10. If, on arrival, you find the patient is trapped by the car, what additional resources would you need to call?

Lifting and Moving Patients

National EMS Education Standard Competencies

Preparatory

Uses simple knowledge of the EMS system, safety/well-being of the EMR, medical/legal issues at the scene of an emergency while awaiting a higher level of care.

Workforce Safety and Wellness

> Standard safety precautions (p 34)
> Personal protective equipment (Chapter 2, *Workforce Safety and Wellness*)
> Stress management (Chapter 2, *Workforce Safety and Wellness*)
  • Dealing with death and dying (Chapter 2, *Workforce Safety and Wellness*)
> Prevention of response-related injuries (pp 34–35)
> Lifting and moving patients (pp 35–42; pp 44–56)

EMS Operations

Knowledge of operational roles and responsibilities to ensure safe patient, public, and personnel safety

Knowledge Objectives

1. Describe the general guidelines for moving patients. (p 34)
2. Explain the purpose and indications for use of the recovery position. (pp 34–35)
3. Discuss the components of good body mechanics. (p 35)
4. Explain how emergency medical responders should decide when emergency movement of a patient is necessary. (p 35)
5. Describe the purpose of each of the following pieces of equipment:
   • Wheeled ambulance stretcher (p 44)
   • Portable stretcher (p 44)
   • Stair chair (p 44)
   • Long backboard (p 45)
   • Short backboard (p 45)
   • Scoop stretcher (p 46)

Skills Objectives

1. Demonstrate the components of good body mechanics. (p 35)
2. Demonstrate the steps needed to perform the following emergency patient drags:
   • Clothes drag (p 35)
   • Blanket drag (p 36)
   • Arm-to-arm drag (p 36)
   • Firefighter drag (p 36)
   • Emergency drag from a vehicle (p 37)
3. Demonstrate the steps needed to perform the following carries for nonambulatory patients:
   • Two-person extremity carry (p 38)
   • Two-person seat carry (p 38)
   • Cradle-in-arms carry (p 39)
   • Two-person chair carry (p 39)
   • Pack-strap carry (p 39)
   • Direct ground lift (pp 40–41)
   • Transfer from a bed to a stretcher (pp 40–41)
4. Demonstrate the steps needed to perform the following walking assists for ambulatory patients:
   • One-person walking assist (pp 41–42)
   • Two-person walking assist (pp 41–42)
5. Demonstrate the steps in each of the following procedures for patients with suspected spinal injuries:
   • Applying a cervical collar (pp 47–48)
   • Moving the patient using a long backboard (p 45)
   • Assisting with a short backboard device (pp 45–46; pp 49–50)
   • Log rolling (pp 49–52)
   • Straddle lifting (p 52)
   • Straddle sliding (p 52)
   • Strapping (pp 52–53)
   • Immobilizing the patient's head (pp 53–54)

Introduction

As an emergency medical responder (EMR), you must analyze a situation, quickly evaluate a patient's condition (under stressful circumstances and often by yourself), and carry out effective, lifesaving emergency medical procedures. These procedures sometimes include lifting, moving, or positioning patients as well as assisting other emergency medical services (EMS) providers in moving patients and preparing them for transport.

Usually you will not have to move patients. In most situations, you can treat the patient in the position found and later assist other EMS personnel in moving the patient. In some cases, however, the patient's survival may depend on your knowledge of emergency movement techniques. You may have to move patients for their own protection (for example, to remove a patient from a burning building), or you may have to move patients before you can provide needed emergency care (for example, to administer cardiopulmonary resuscitation [CPR] to a patient in cardiac arrest who was found in a bathroom). You can perform some of the techniques presented in this chapter with no equipment, whereas other techniques require simple objects that are often available at emergency scenes. With other techniques, you can assist other EMS providers in using the specialized equipment they bring to the emergency scene.

General Principles

Every time you move a patient, keep the following general guidelines in mind:

1. Do no further harm to the patient.
2. Move the patient only when necessary.
3. Move the patient as few times as possible.
4. Move the patient's body as a unit.
5. Use proper lifting and moving techniques to ensure your own safety.
6. Have one rescuer give commands when moving a patient (usually the rescuer at the patient's head).

Also consider the following recommendations:

- Delay moving the patient, if possible, until additional EMS personnel arrive.
- Treat the patient before moving him or her unless the patient is in an unsafe environment.
- Try not to step over the patient (your shoes may drop sand, dirt, or mud onto the patient or you might fall onto the patient).
- Explain to the patient what you are going to do and how. If the patient's condition permits, he or she may be able to assist you.

Unless you must move patients for treatment or protection, leave them in the position in which you found them. There is usually no reason to hurry the moving process. If you suspect the patient has sustained trauma to the head or spine, keep the patient's head and spine immobilized so he or she does not move (discussed later in the chapter).

Safety

Whatever technique you use for moving patients, keep these rules of good body mechanics in mind:

1. Know your own physical limitations and capabilities. Do not try to lift too heavy a load.
2. Keep yourself balanced when lifting or moving a patient.
3. Maintain a firm footing.
4. Lift and lower the patient by bending your legs, not your back. Keep your back as straight as possible at all times and use your large leg muscles to do the work.
5. Try to keep your arms close to your body for strength and balance.
6. Move the patient as few times as possible.

Recovery Position

Place unconscious patients who have not sustained suspected trauma in the sidelying **recovery position** to

YOU are the Provider   CASE 1

At 1023 hours you and your partner are dispatched to a large discount supermarket for the report of a 74-year-old woman who has slipped and fallen after stepping on some grapes in the produce department. As you assess the patient, she tells you she has some tenderness in her right leg. Her right wrist is noticeably deformed and painful. You also note she has a large abrasion and some swelling on her forehead. The nearest ambulance is 8 to 10 minutes away.

1. Under what circumstances would it be necessary to move this patient before the EMS transport unit arrives?
2. Why is it often better for EMRs to delay moving a patient until the arrival of an EMS transport unit?

help keep the airway open 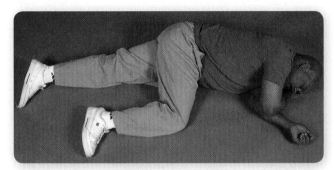 Figure 3-1 . The recovery position also allows secretions to drain from their mouth.

Body Mechanics

Your top priority is to ensure your own safety. Improperly lifting or moving a patient can result in injury to you or to the patient. By exercising good body mechanics, you reduce the possibility of injuring yourself Figure 3-2 .

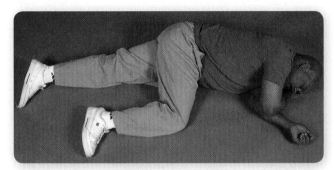

Figure 3-1 A patient in the recovery position.
© Jones & Bartlett Learning. Courtesy of MIEMSS.

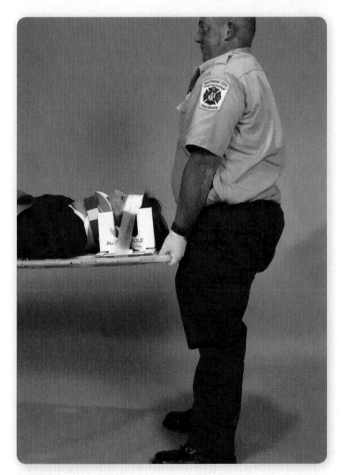

Figure 3-2 An EMR demonstrates good body mechanics. His back is straight and he is lifting using his leg muscles.
© Jones & Bartlett Learning. Courtesy of MIEMSS.

Good body mechanics means using the strength of the large muscles in your legs to lift patients instead of using your back muscles. This practice prevents strains and injuries to weaker muscles, especially in your back. Get as close to the patient as possible so that your back is in a straight and upright position, and keep your back straight as you lift. Do not lift when your back is bent over a patient. Lift without twisting your body. Keep your feet in a secure position and be sure you have a firm footing before you start to lift or move a patient.

To lift safely, keep certain guidelines in mind. Before attempting to move a patient, assess the weight of the patient. Know your physical limitations and do not attempt to lift or move a patient who is too heavy for you to handle safely. Call for additional personnel if needed for your safety and the safety of the patient. Discuss the route of travel prior to lifting. Because you will sometimes need to assist other EMS providers, practice with them so that lifts are handled in a coordinated and helpful manner.

As you lift, make sure you communicate with the other members of the lifting team. Failure to give clear commands or failure to lift at the same time can result in serious injuries to both rescuers and patients. You can never practice too much; perfect your lifts and moves until they become smooth for you and your partner and for the patient.

Emergency Movement of Patients

How do you decide when emergency movement of a patient is necessary? Immediately move a patient in the following situations:

- Danger of fire, explosion, or structural collapse exists.
- Hazardous materials are present.
- The emergency scene cannot be protected.
- It is otherwise impossible to gain access to other patients who need lifesaving care.
- The patient has experienced cardiac arrest and must be moved so you can begin CPR.

▶ Emergency Drags

If the patient is lying on the floor or ground during an emergency situation, you may have to drag the person away from the scene instead of trying to lift and carry the patient. Make every effort to pull the patient in the direction of the long axis of the body to protect the spine as much as possible.

Clothes Drag

The **clothes drag** is the simplest way to move the patient in an emergency Figure 3-3 . If the patient is too heavy for you to lift and carry, grasp the patient's clothing in the neck and shoulder area, rest the patient's head on your arms for protection, and drag the patient out of danger.

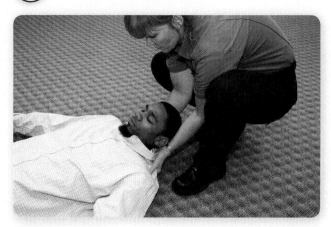

Figure 3-3 Clothes drag.
© Jones & Bartlett Learning. Courtesy of MIEMSS.

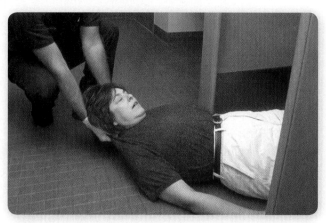

Figure 3-4 Remove the patient from a tight space to administer CPR.
© American Academy of Orthopaedic Surgeons.

Cardiac Patients and the Clothes Drag. In most situations, you can easily determine whether emergency movement is necessary. Cases involving patients in cardiac arrest are the exception. Patients in cardiac arrest are often found in a bathroom or small bedroom. You will have to judge whether basic life support (BLS) or advanced life support (ALS) can be adequately provided in that space. If the room is not large enough, move the patient as soon as you have determined he or she has experienced cardiac arrest.

Drag the patient from the tight space to a larger room (such as a living or dining room) that has space to perform CPR and ALS procedures Figure 3-4. Quickly move furniture out of the way so you and other EMS personnel have room to work. You will be able to provide care with increased efficiency, which will more than make up for the time it took to move the patient. Take time to make adequate room before you begin CPR!

Words of Wisdom

To eliminate distractions at the scene, take a second to turn off any televisions, radios, or music players. Emergency scenes are calmer and less stressful when you are not competing against a loud television program or music to be heard.

Blanket Drag

If the patient is not dressed or is dressed in clothing that could tear easily during the clothes drag (for example, a nightgown), move the patient by using a large sheet, blanket, or rug (**blanket drag**). Place the sheet, blanket, rug, or similar item on the floor and roll the patient onto it. Pull the patient to safety by dragging the sheet or blanket. You can also use the blanket drag to move a patient who weighs more than you do Figure 3-5.

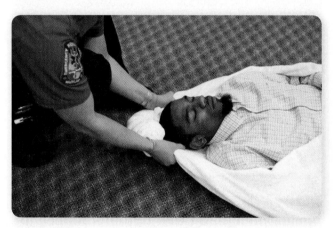

Figure 3-5 Blanket drag.
© Jones & Bartlett Learning. Courtesy of MIEMSS.

Arm-to-Arm Drag

If the patient is on the floor, you can place your hands under the patient's armpits from the back of the patient and grasp the patient's forearms. The **arm-to-arm drag** allows you to move the patient by carrying the weight of the upper part of the patient's body as the lower trunk and legs drag on the floor Figure 3-6. This drag enables you to move a heavy patient and it offers some protection for the patient's head and neck.

Firefighter Drag

The **firefighter drag** enables you to move a patient who is heavier than you are because you do not have to lift or carry the patient. Tie the patient's wrists together with any material that is handy—such as a cravat (a folded triangular bandage), strip of gauze, belt, or necktie—being careful not to impair circulation. Then get down on your hands and knees and straddle the patient. Pass the patient's tied hands around your neck, straighten your arms, and drag the patient across the floor by crawling on your hands and knees Figure 3-7.

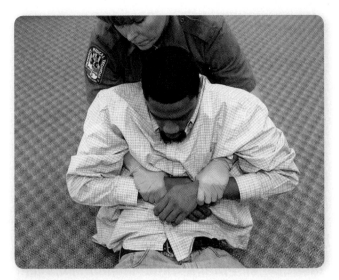

Figure 3-6 Arm-to-arm drag.
© Jones & Bartlett Learning. Courtesy of MIEMSS.

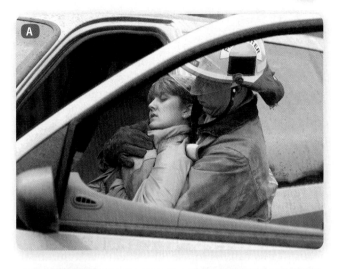

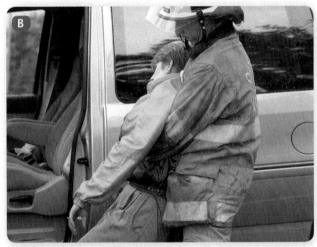

Figure 3-8 Emergency removal from a vehicle. **A.** Grasp the patient under the arms. **B.** Pull the patient down into a horizontal position.
A&B: © Jones & Bartlett Learning. Courtesy of MIEMSS.

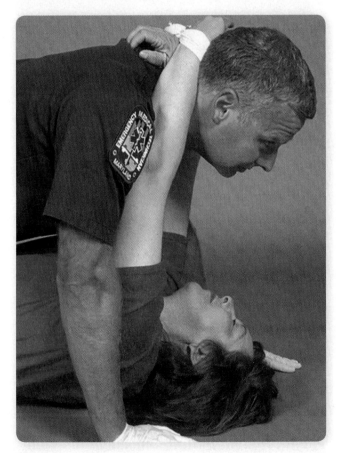

Figure 3-7 Firefighter drag. Tie the patient's wrists together, then drag the patient across the floor by crawling on your hands and knees with the patient's arms around your neck.
© Jones & Bartlett Learning. Courtesy of MIEMSS.

Emergency Drag From a Vehicle

Sometimes you have to use emergency movement techniques in life-threatening situations when no equipment is immediately available (for example, to remove a patient from a motor vehicle that is on fire or to administer CPR). All the basic movement principles apply, but the techniques need to be slightly modified because the patient is sitting instead of lying down. Emergency drags from a vehicle can be performed with one or more rescuers.

One Rescuer. Grasp the patient under the arms and cradle the patient's head between your arms **Figure 3-8** . Pull the patient down into a horizontal position as you ease him or her from the vehicle. Although there is no effective way to remove a patient from a vehicle by yourself without causing some movement, it is important to prevent excessive movement of the patient's neck.

Two or More Rescuers. If you must immediately remove a patient from a vehicle and two or more rescuers are present, have one rescuer support the patient's head and neck, while the second rescuer moves the patient by lifting under the arms. The patient can then be removed in line with the long axis of the body, with the head and neck manually stabilized in a neutral position. If time permits and if you have one available, use a long backboard for patient removal. Procedures for using a long backboard are covered later in this chapter.

► **Carries for Nonambulatory Patients**

Many patients are unable or should not be allowed to move without your assistance. Patients who are unable to move because of injury or illness must be carried to safety. This section describes several useful carrying techniques for nonambulatory patients. Whatever technique you use, remember to follow the rules of good body mechanics.

Two-Person Extremity Carry

The **two-person extremity carry** enables two rescuers with no equipment to move a patient in tight or narrow spaces, such as mobile home corridors, small hallways, and narrow spaces between buildings **Figure 3-9** . The focus of this carry is to use the patient's **extremities** to move the patient. First, the rescuers help the patient sit up. Rescuer One kneels behind the patient, reaches under the patient's arms, and grasps the patient's wrists. Rescuer Two then backs in between the patient's legs, reaches around, and grasps the patient behind the knees. At a command from Rescuer One, the two rescuers stand up and carry the patient away, walking straight ahead.

Two-Person Seat Carry

With the **two-person seat carry**, two rescuers use their arms and bodies to form a seat for the patient.

The rescuers kneel on opposite sides of the patient near the patient's hips. The rescuers then raise the patient to a sitting position and link arms behind the patient's back. The rescuers then place the other arm under the patient's knees and link with each other. If possible, the patient puts his or her arms around the necks and shoulders of the rescuers for additional support. Although the two-person seat carry requires two rescuers, it does not require any equipment **Figure 3-10** .

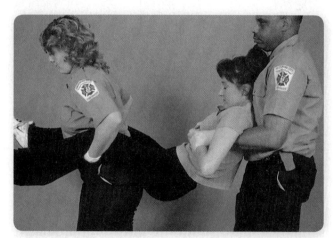

Figure 3-9 Two-person extremity carry.
© Jones & Bartlett Learning. Courtesy of MIEMSS.

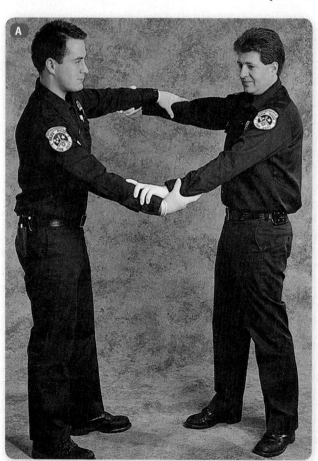 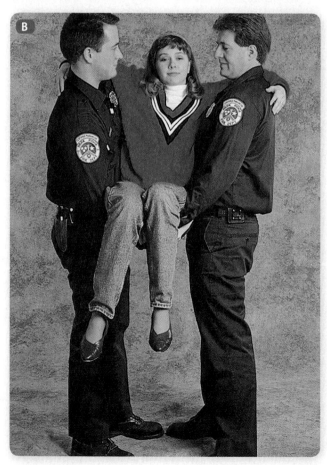

Figure 3-10 Two-person seat carry. **A.** Link arms. **B.** Raise the patient to a sitting position.
A&B: © Jones & Bartlett Learning. Courtesy of MIEMSS.

Cradle-in-Arms Carry

The **cradle-in-arms carry** can be used by one rescuer to carry a child. Kneel beside the patient and place one arm around the child's back and the other arm under the thighs. Lift slightly and roll the child into the hollow formed by your arms and chest. Be sure to use your leg muscles to stand Figure 3-11 .

> **Safety**
>
> Keep your back as straight as possible and use the large muscles in your legs to do the lifting!

Two-Person Chair Carry

In the **two-person chair carry**, two rescuers use a chair to support the weight of the patient. Do not use a folding chair. Test the strength of the chair using a healthy person before moving an ill or injured patient using the chair. The chair carry is especially useful for taking patients up or down stairways or through a narrow hallway. An additional benefit is that because the patient is able to hold on to the chair (and should be encouraged to do so), he or she feels much more secure than with the two-person seat carry.

Rescuer One stands behind the seated patient, reaches down, and grasps the back of the chair close to the seat. Rescuer One then tilts the chair slightly backward on its rear legs so Rescuer Two can step back in between the legs of the chair and grasp the chair's front legs. The patient's legs should be between the legs of the chair. When both rescuers are correctly positioned, Rescuer One gives the command to lift and walk away Figure 3-12 .

Pack-Strap Carry

The **pack-strap carry** is a one-person carry that allows you to carry a patient while keeping one hand free. Have the patient stand (or have other rescue personnel support the patient) and back into the patient so your shoulders fit into the patient's armpits. Grasp the patient's wrists and cross the arms over your chest Figure 3-13 . Now you can hold both wrists in one hand and your other hand remains free.

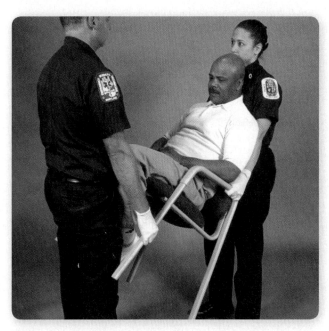

Figure 3-12 Two-person chair carry.
© Jones & Bartlett Learning. Courtesy of MIEMSS.

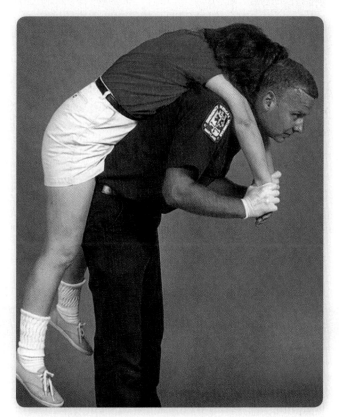

Figure 3-13 Pack-strap carry. After the patient's arms are crossed in front of your chest, you can hold the patient's wrists in one hand, leaving the other hand free if needed.
© Jones & Bartlett Learning. Courtesy of MIEMSS.

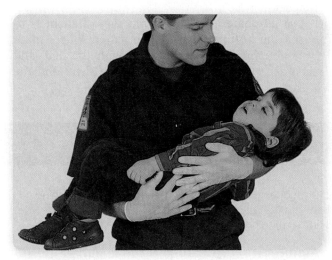

Figure 3-11 Cradle-in-arms carry.
© Jones & Bartlett Learning. Courtesy of MIEMSS.

Optimal weight distribution occurs when the patient's armpits are over your shoulders. Squat deeply to avoid potential injury to your back and pull the patient onto your back. After you position the patient correctly, bend forward to lift the patient off the ground, stand up, and walk away.

> **Safety**
>
> Because the two-person chair carry may force the patient's head forward, have Rescuer Two watch the patient for airway problems.

Direct Ground Lift

Use the direct ground lift to move a patient who is on the ground or the floor to an ambulance stretcher. Use this lift only for those patients who have not sustained a traumatic injury. The direct ground lift requires you to bend over the patient and lift with your back in a bent position. This positioning of your body results in poor body mechanics; therefore, avoid this lift whenever possible. Using a long backboard or portable stretcher is much better for your back and may be more comfortable for the patient. The steps for performing the direct ground lift are described in **Skill Drill 3-2** .

1. Assess the patient. Do not use this lift if the patient has any possible head, spine, or leg injuries.
2. Rescuer One kneels at the patient's chest on the right or left side. Rescuer Two kneels at the patient's hips on the same side as Rescuer One **Step 1** .
3. Place the patient's arms on the chest.
4. Rescuer One places one arm under the patient's neck and shoulder to cradle the patient's head and then places the other arm under the patient's lower back. Rescuer Two places one arm under the patient's knees and the other arm above the buttocks **Step 2** .

5. Rescuer One gives the command: "Ready? Roll!" and both rescuers roll their forearms up so the patient is as close to them as possible.
6. Rescuer One gives the command: "Ready? Lift!" and both rescuers lift the patient to their knees and roll the patient as close to their bodies as possible.
7. Rescuer One gives the command: "Ready? Stand!" and both rescuers stand and move the patient to the stretcher **Step 3** .
8. To lower the patient to the stretcher, the rescuers reverse the steps listed above **Step 4** .

> **Safety**
>
> The direct ground lift requires you to use poor body mechanics, so avoid using it whenever possible. Never use the direct ground lift with a patient who may have sustained any injury to the head, spine, or legs.

Transferring a Patient From Bed to Stretcher

Patients who are ill are often found in their beds. If EMS personnel need to transport these patients to the hospital, they may request your assistance with transferring a patient from the bed to the ambulance stretcher using the draw sheet method **Figure 3-14** .

Place the stretcher next to the bed, making sure it is at the same height as the bed and that the rails are lowered and straps unbuckled. Hold the stretcher to keep it from moving. Loosen the bottom sheet underneath the patient or log roll the patient onto a blanket. Reach across the stretcher and grasp the sheet and blanket firmly at the patient's head, chest, hips, and knees. Gently slide the patient onto the stretcher.

An alternate method for moving a patient is to loosen the bottom sheet of the patient's bed, place the ambulance stretcher parallel with the bed, and reach across the stretcher to pull the sheet and the

---

YOU are the Provider

CASE 2

As you are driving to work, you are shocked to see a driver ahead of you suddenly swerve to the left, cross over the oncoming lane of traffic, and collide with a tree. You park your vehicle and rush toward the wreck. As you approach the crashed vehicle, you find a male driver slumped against the deflated airbag, and he does not seem to be moving. You see smoke starting to come from the engine compartment and can smell burning plastic and oil.

1. How can you quickly remove this patient from the burning vehicle?
2. How do you determine where to place this patient after removal?

Skill Drill 3-1

Direct Ground Lift

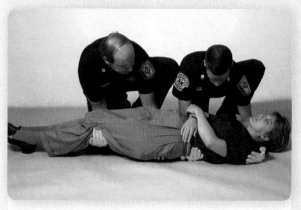

Step 1 Kneel at the patient's side.

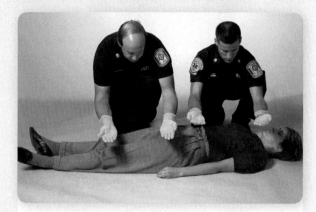

Step 2 Place arms under the patient.

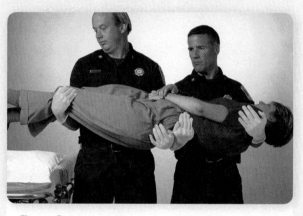

Step 3 Lift the patient.

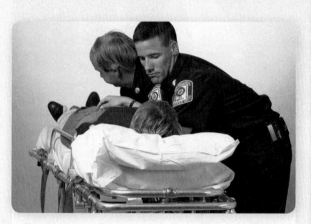

Step 4 Move the patient to the stretcher.

© Jones & Bartlett Learning. Courtesy of MIEMSS.

patient onto the stretcher. However, use this method with caution because it requires you to reach across the stretcher to get to the patient. This action results in poor body mechanics; therefore, avoid using it whenever possible.

▶ Walking Assists for Ambulatory Patients

Frequently, patients simply need assistance to walk to safety. Either one or two rescuers can perform this task. Choose a technique after you have assessed the patient's condition and the scene of the incident. The technique you might use to help a patient walk to a chair is probably not appropriate to help a patient walk up a highway embankment.

One-Person Walking Assist

Use the **one-person walking assist** if the patient is able to bear his or her own weight. Help the patient stand. Have the patient place one arm around your neck and hold the patient's wrist (which he or she should drape over your shoulder). Put your free arm around the patient's waist and help the patient to walk Figure 3-15.

Two-Person Walking Assist

The **two-person walking assist** is the same as the one-person walking assist, except that two rescuers are needed. This technique is useful if the patient cannot bear weight. The two rescuers completely support the patient Figure 3-16.

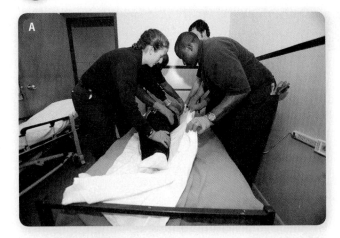

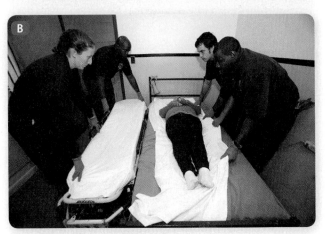

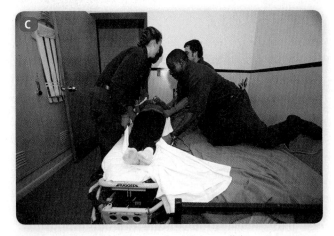

Figure 3-14 The draw sheet method. **A.** Log roll the patient onto a sheet or blanket. **B.** Bring the stretcher in parallel with the bed. Gently slide the patient to the edge of the bed. **C.** Transfer the patient to the stretcher.
A, B, & C: © Jones & Bartlett Learning. Courtesy of MIEMSS.

Safety

Do not use any of the lifts or carries explained in this chapter if you suspect the patient has a spinal injury—unless, of course, it is necessary to remove the patient from an immediately life-threatening situation.

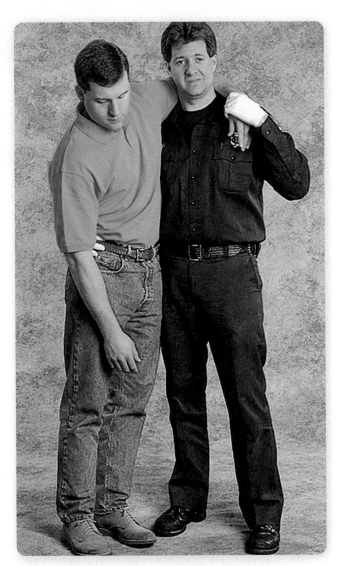

Figure 3-15 One-person walking assist.
© Jones & Bartlett Learning. Courtesy of MIEMSS.

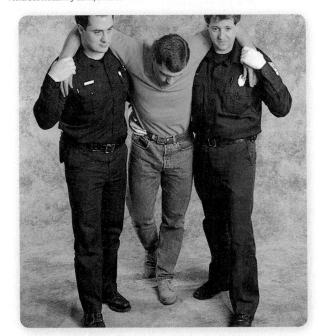

Figure 3-16 Two-person walking assist.
© Jones & Bartlett Learning. Courtesy of MIEMSS.

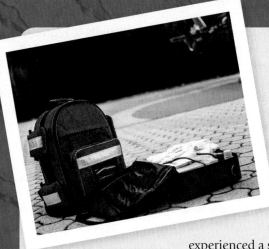

Voices *of* Experience

"How are you going to get me to the ambulance? I'm a big guy!" *Good question*, I thought. He was 350 pounds (159 kg) and had experienced a stroke while in the shower in a dark, upstairs motel room. The stroke had rendered him nonambulatory. He had no clothes to grab onto and was positioned on the floor between the bed and the wall in a right lateral recumbent position. He also needed manual stabilization because of a fall. There was a four-person fire crew, my partner, and myself on scene. The small space was limiting in that not all of us would fit around the patient to appropriately care for or move him.

> **Throughout the move, we stayed in constant communication with each other and with the patient.**

With everyone working together, we used two sheets from the bed: one to cover him and one to position under him. The sheet under the patient would be used for the draw sheet method. The patient was moved with the long axis of his body onto the backboard while manual stabilization was maintained. A firefighter put his tarp/carry-all under the backboard prior to moving the patient, giving us more handles to safely carry him after he was secured to the backboard. The limited space around the patient allowed for only one crew member at the patient's head and one at the feet. The two of them worked together to push and pull, respectively, with the tarp/carry-all to move the patient across the balcony to the landing of the stairs. On the landing, we were able to add two crew members: one on the patient's right side and one on the left. One of the two remaining crew members went to the bottom of the stairs to position and stabilize the gurney while the other stood behind the person who was going backwards down the stairs while moving the patient to ensure the safety of his fellow crew member.

For any successful patient move, the cornerstone is communication. Prior to walking down the stairs, we discussed how the move would be executed and shared our plan with the patient. Throughout the move, we stayed in constant communication with each other and with the patient. This communication reduced the chance of injuring him or ourselves. We successfully made it to the gurney, where we continued to work as a team using a four-person lift to elevate the gurney and load the patient into the ambulance.

"I didn't think you were going to be able to do it, but that wasn't bad at all!" That was the nicest thing I had heard all night.

Lori Gallian, Paramedic
American Medical Response
Sacramento, California

Equipment

Most of the lifts and moves described in the previous section are performed without the use of any specialized equipment. However, EMS departments commonly use various types of patient-moving equipment. To be able to assist other EMS providers, familiarize yourself with the following equipment.

▶ Wheeled Ambulance Stretchers

Wheeled ambulance stretchers are carried by ambulances and are one of the most commonly used EMS devices **Figure 3-17**. These stretchers are also called cots. Each type of stretcher has its own set of levers and controls for raising and lowering the stretcher to different heights. The head end of the stretcher can be raised to elevate the patient's head. These stretchers have belts to secure the patient. Some EMS departments use electronic stretchers, commonly called ambulance stretchers, which can be raised and lowered using a battery-powered system. These stretchers reduce the strain on EMS providers and operate smoothly for patient comfort. If you regularly work with the same EMS unit, it will be helpful for you to learn how their particular type of stretcher operates.

Stretchers can be rolled or they can be carried by two or four people. If the surface is smooth, a wheeled stretcher can be rolled with one person guiding the head end and one person pulling the foot end. If the loaded stretcher must be carried, it is best to use four people, one person at each corner. The use of four peo-

ple offers more stability and less strength is required to carry the stretcher. If the stretcher must be carried through a narrow area, only two people will be able to carry it. The two rescuers should face each other from opposite ends of the stretcher. Carrying the stretcher with two people requires that each person be strong enough to maintain the balance of the stretcher. As an EMR, you may also be asked to assist with loading a patient into the ambulance. Learn the method of loading ambulance stretchers that your EMS unit uses and practice this procedure with the EMS unit. It is important to lift as a team to avoid injury to yourself or to the other rescuers.

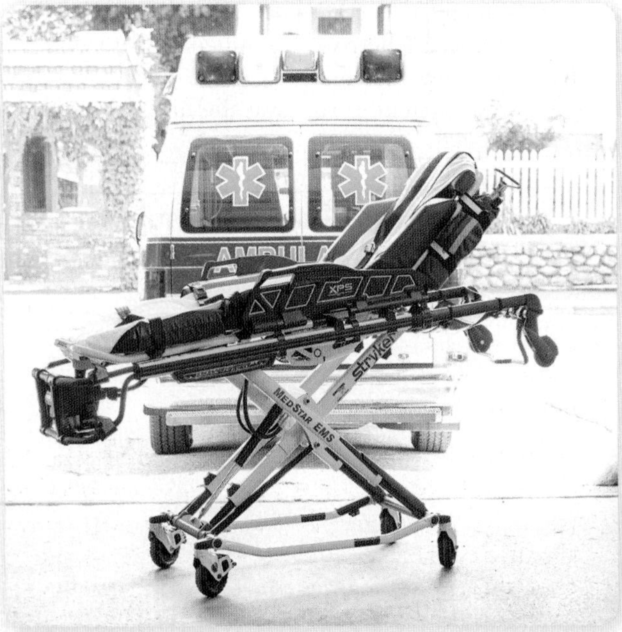

> **Words of Wisdom**
>
> Patient-moving equipment includes the following:
> - Wheeled ambulance stretcher
> - Portable stretcher
> - Stair chair
> - Long backboard
> - Short backboard (vest-type immobilizer)
> - Scoop stretcher

▶ Portable Stretchers

Use a **portable stretcher** when you cannot move the wheeled ambulance stretcher into a small space. They are smaller and lighter to carry than wheeled stretchers. You can carry a portable stretcher in the same ways that you carry a wheeled stretcher. An example of one type of portable stretcher is shown in **Figure 3-18**.

▶ Stair Chairs

A **stair chair** is a portable moving device that is used to carry a patient in a sitting position. The stair chair is useful for patients who are short of breath or who are more comfortable in a sitting position. They are small, lightweight, and easy to carry in narrow spaces. Do not use the stair chair with patients who have experienced any type of trauma. When carrying a stair chair, the rescuers face each other and lift on a set command. If you are going to assist your local EMS unit with this device, learn how to unfold it and how to assist with carrying it. One type of stair chair is shown in **Figure 3-19**.

▶ Immobilization Devices

Use backboards to immobilize patients who have neck or back injuries. You can also use such devices to assist in lifting patients and as an aide in immobilizing lower extremity injuries. This section discusses three types of backboard devices: long backboards, short backboard devices, and scoop stretchers.

Figure 3-17 A wheeled ambulance stretcher.
© Jones & Bartlett Learning.

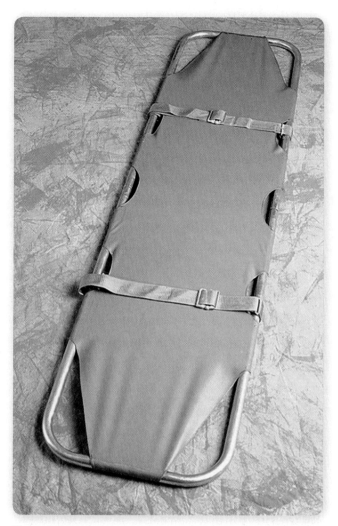

Figure 3-18 A portable stretcher.
© American Academy of Orthopaedic Surgeons.

Long Backboards

Use long backboards to move patients who have experienced trauma, especially if they may have neck or back injuries. You can also use long backboards for lifting and moving patients who are in small places or who need to be moved off the ground or floor. Long backboards make lifting a patient much easier for the rescuers. Most long backboards are made of plastic or fiberglass. Secure the patient with straps after he or she is placed on the long backboard; if the patient has sustained back or neck injuries, immobilize the head. Procedures for assisting EMS providers with these devices are covered later in this chapter. One type of long backboard is pictured in **Figure 3-20**.

Special Populations

When you move older patients, remember some of them have fragile bones that have been weakened by osteoporosis. Move older patients carefully to avoid further injuries.

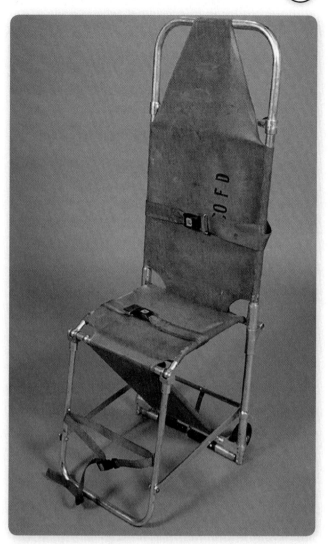

Figure 3-19 A stair chair.
© Jones & Bartlett Learning. Courtesy of MIEMSS.

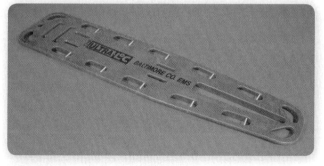

Figure 3-20 A long backboard.
© Jones & Bartlett Learning. Courtesy of MIEMSS.

Short Backboard Devices

Short backboard devices are used to immobilize the head and spine of patients found in a sitting position who may have sustained head or spine injuries. Short backboard devices are usually made of plastic. Some of these devices are in the form of a vest-like garment that wraps around the patient **Figure 3-21**. Procedures to help you assist other EMS providers in applying these devices are covered later in this chapter.

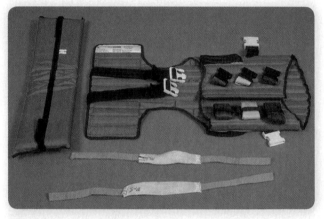

Figure 3-21 This vest-type immobilizer is one type of short backboard device. It is sometimes called a Kendrick Extrication Device or KED.
© Jones & Bartlett Learning. Courtesy of MIEMSS.

Scoop Stretchers

A **scoop stretcher** or orthopaedic stretcher is a rigid device that separates into a right half and a left half. Apply these devices by placing one half on each side of the patient and then attaching the two halves together. These devices are helpful when moving patients out of small spaces. Do not use a scoop stretcher if the patient has sustained head or spine injuries. One type of scoop stretcher is shown in Figure 3-22 .

If your EMS department uses scoop stretchers, practice using them. The steps for applying a scoop stretcher are shown in Skill Drill 3-2 .

1. With the scoop stretcher separated, measure the length of the scoop and adjust to the proper length Step 1 .
2. Position the stretcher, one side at a time. Lift the patient's side slightly by pulling on the far hip and upper arm, while your partner slides the stretcher into place Step 2 .
3. Lock the stretcher ends together by engaging its locking mechanisms one at a time and continue to lift the patient slightly as needed

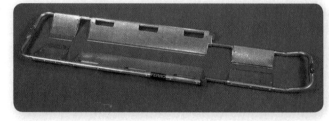

Figure 3-22 A scoop stretcher.
© Jones & Bartlett Learning. Courtesy of MIEMSS.

Skill Drill 3-2

Using a Scoop Stretcher

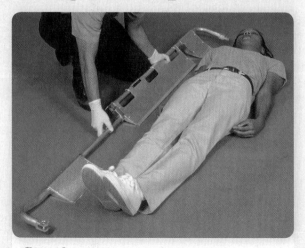

Step 1 Adjust the length of the stretcher.

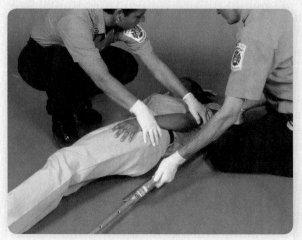

Step 2 Lift the patient slightly and slide the stretcher into place, one side at a time.

© Jones & Bartlett Learning. Courtesy of MIEMSS.

Skill Drill **3-2** *Continued*

Using a Scoop Stretcher

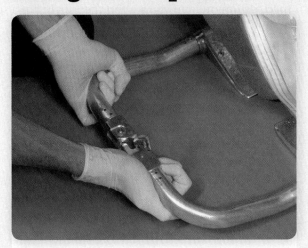

Step 3 Lock the stretcher ends together and avoid pinching both the patient and/or your fingers.

© Jones & Bartlett Learning. Courtesy of MIEMSS.

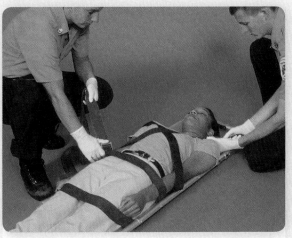

Step 4 Secure the patient to the scoop stretcher, and transfer it to the stretcher.

to avoid pinching the patient and/or your fingers. **Step 3**.

4. Apply and tighten the straps to secure the patient to the scoop stretcher before transferring it to the stretcher **Step 4**.

Words of Wisdom

In an emergency situation, you can use the following objects for improvised backboards:

- Wide, sturdy planks
- Doors
- Ironing boards
- Sturdy folding tables
- Full-length lawn chair recliners
- Surfboards
- Snowboards

■ Treatment of Patients With Suspected Head or Spine Injuries

Any time a patient has sustained a traumatic injury, you should suspect injury to the head, neck, or spine. Improper treatment can lead to permanent damage or paralysis. Immobilize the patient's head and neck in a neutral position using your hands (manual stabilization), a blanket roll, or foam blocks. It is also important that you be able to assist other EMS personnel in caring for patients who may have sustained head or spine injuries. The following sections show you how to immobilize a patient's head and neck and how to assist other EMS providers in placing a patient on a backboard. More information on spinal cord injuries is presented in Chapter 15, *Injuries to Muscles and Bones*.

▶ Applying a Cervical Collar

Use a **cervical collar** to minimize (but not completely prevent) movement of the patient's head and neck **Figure 3-23**. These collars do not totally prevent head and neck movement; rather, they minimize the movement. After you apply a cervical collar, it is still necessary for you to manually stabilize the patient's head and neck.

Soft cervical collars do not provide sufficient support for trauma patients. Many different types of rigid cervical collars for trauma patients are available. **Figure 3-24** shows how one common style of rigid cervical collar is applied. Apply the cervical collar before the patient is placed on a backboard.

▶ Movement of Patients Using Backboards

Placing a patient on a backboard is not your primary responsibility, but you may be required to assist other EMS personnel with this task. Therefore, be familiar with the proper handling of patients who must be moved on backboards. Any patient who has sustained spinal trauma in a motor vehicle crash or fall and any person who has sustained gunshot wounds to the trunk should be transported on a backboard.

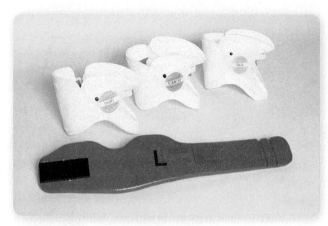

Figure 3-23 Types of cervical collars.
© Jones & Bartlett Learning. Courtesy of MIEMSS.

Although the specific technique you will use depends on the circumstances, the general principles described in the remainder of this chapter are relevant in nearly all cases.

The following principles of patient movement are especially important if you suspect the patient has a spinal injury:

1. Move the patient as a unit.
2. Transport the patient faceup (supine), the only position that provides adequate spinal immobilization. However, because patients secured to backboards often vomit, be prepared to turn the patient and backboard quickly as a unit to permit the vomitus to drain from the patient's mouth.
3. Keep the patient's head and neck in a neutral position.
4. Be sure all rescuers understand what is to be done before attempting any movement.
5. Be sure one rescuer is responsible for giving commands.

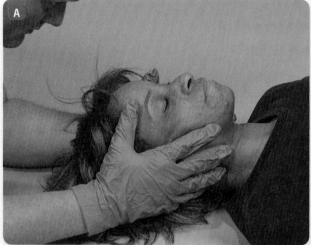

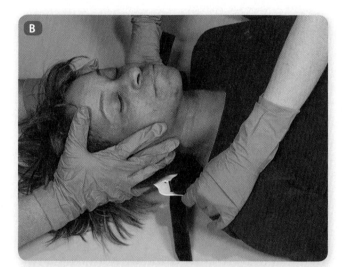

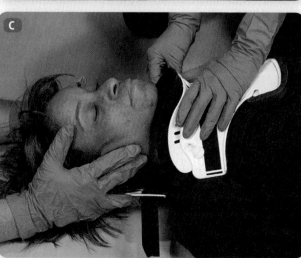

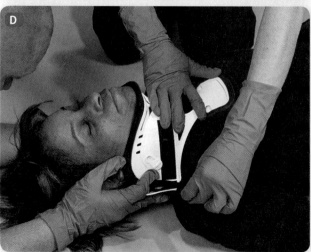

Figure 3-24 Applying a cervical collar. **A.** Stabilize head and neck. **B.** Insert back part of collar. **C.** Apply front part of collar. **D.** Secure collar together.
A, B, C, & D: © Jones & Bartlett Learning. Courtesy of MIEMSS.

application of this device. Skill Drill 3-3 illustrates how
one common type of short backboard device is applied.

1. Position Responder One behind the patient to stabilize the head. Responder Two then applies a cervical collar **Step 1**.
2. While maintaining neutral, in-line manual stabilization, Responder One leans the patient forward and Responder Two inserts the device behind the patient, starting with the head portion **Step 2**. Responder One then carefully eases the patient onto the backboard.
3. Responder Two fastens the middle strap of the device **Step 3** and then fastens the rest of the straps **Step 4**.
4. Responder Two then places the wings of the device around the patient's head **Step 5**.
5. Responder One maintains in-line manual stabilization until Responder Two has secured the head strap of the device **Step 6**.

Special Populations

Many older patients have irregular curves in their spine. When immobilizing these patients, you may need to add extra padding to conform to the unusual shape of their spine.

Words of Wisdom

In some EMS departments, there may be times when emergency medical technicians or paramedics evaluate a patient who has had his or her neck or back immobilized and are able to remove the immobilization from the patient by following a well-defined protocol. This is not something that you should consider. As an EMR, you should keep a patient immobilized until he or she has been evaluated by a more highly qualified medical person.

▶ Assisting With Short Backboard Devices

Short backboard devices are used to immobilize patients found in a sitting position who have sustained trauma to the head, neck, or spine. Short backboard devices allow rescuers to immobilize the patient before moving. After the short backboard device is applied, the patient is carefully placed on a long backboard. As an EMR, you will not be applying a short backboard device by yourself. However, you may need to assist with the

▶ Log Rolling

Log rolling is the primary technique you will use to move a patient onto a long backboard. It is usually easy to accomplish, but it requires a team of four rescuers for safety and effectiveness—three to move the patient and one to maneuver the backboard. Log rolling is the movement technique of choice in all patients with suspected spinal injury. Because log rolling requires

Skill Drill **3-3**

Applying a Short Backboard Device

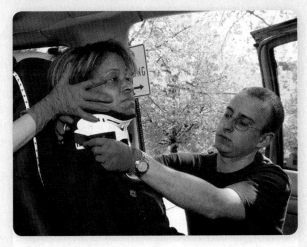

Step 1 Stabilize the head and apply a cervical collar.

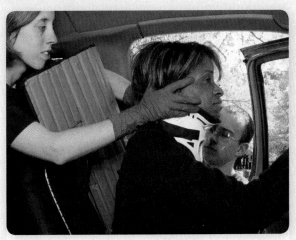

Step 2 Insert the device headfirst.

Skill Drill 3-3 Continued

Applying a Short Backboard Device

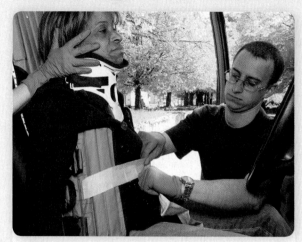

Step 3 Apply the middle strap.

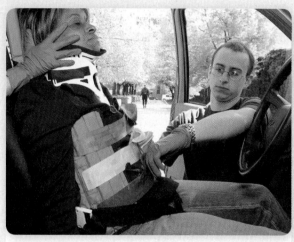

Step 4 Apply the other straps.

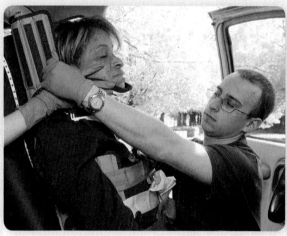

Step 5 Place wings around the head.

Step 6 Secure the head strap.

© Jones & Bartlett Learning. Courtesy of MIEMSS.

sufficient space for four rescuers, it is not always possible to perform it correctly. That is why the principles of movement, rather than specific rules, are stressed here. The procedure for the four-person log roll is shown in Skill Drill 3-4 :

1. All rescuers get into position to roll the patient Step 1 .
2. Once Rescuer One gives the command, rescuers roll the patient onto his or her side Step 2 .
3. The fourth person slides the backboard toward the patient Step 3 .
4. Once Rescuer One gives the command, rescuers roll the patient onto the backboard Step 4 .
5. Center the patient on the backboard. Secure the patient before moving Step 5 .

When using any patient movement technique, everyone must understand who is directing the maneuver, especially if you suspect the patient has a spinal injury. The rescuer holding the patient's head (Rescuer One) should always give the commands so all rescuers can better coordinate their actions. The specific wording of the command is not important, as long as every team member understands what the command is. Each member of the team must understand his or her specific position and function.

All patient movement commands have two parts: a question and the order for movement. Rescuer One says, "The command will be 'Ready? Roll!'" When everyone is ready to roll the patient, Rescuer One says, "Ready?" (This question is followed by a short pause to allow for response from the team.) Then Rescuer One says, "Roll!"

Skill Drill 3-4

Four-Person Log Roll

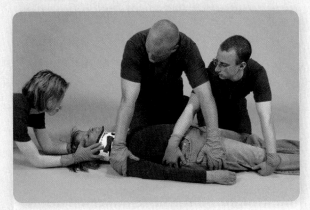

Step 1 Rescuers get into position to roll the patient.

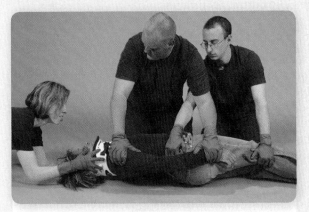

Step 2 Roll the patient onto his or her side.

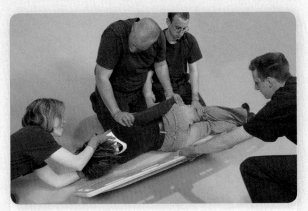

Step 3 The fourth rescuer slides the backboard toward the patient.

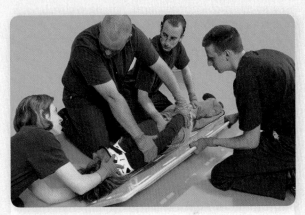

Step 4 Roll the patient onto the backboard.

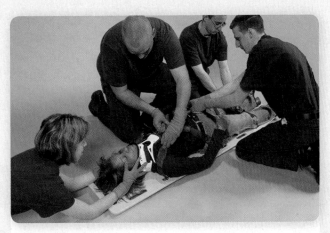

Step 5 Center the patient on the backboard and secure the patient before moving.

In any log-rolling technique, you must move the patient as a unit. Keep the patient's head in a neutral position at all times. Do not allow the head to rotate, move backward (extend), or move forward (flex). Sometimes this is simply stated as, "Keep the nose in line with the belly button at all times."

▶ Straddle Lift

Use the straddle lift to place a patient on a backboard if you do not have enough space to perform a log roll. Modified versions of the straddle lift are commonly used to remove patients from motor vehicles. The straddle lift requires five rescuers: one at the head and neck, one to straddle the shoulders and chest, one to straddle the hips and thighs, one to straddle the legs, and one to insert the backboard under the patient after the other four have lifted the patient 0.5 inch (1 cm) to 1 inch (3 cm) off the ground Figure 3-25 .

The most difficult part of the straddle lift technique is coordinating the lifting so the patient is raised just enough to slide the backboard under the patient. Because such team coordination can be difficult, it is important to practice this lift frequently.

▶ Straddle Slide

In the straddle slide, a modification of the straddle lift technique, the rescuers move the patient rather than the backboard Figure 3-26 . This technique may be useful when the patient is in an extremely narrow space and cannot otherwise be moved to a backboard. The rescuers' positions are the same as for the straddle lift. Each rescuer should have a firm grip on the patient (or the patient's clothing). Lift the patient as a unit just enough to be able to slide (break the resistance with the ground) him or her forward onto the waiting backboard. Slide the patient forward about 10 inches (25 cm) at a time. Trying to slide the patient a distance of greater than 10 inches to 12 inches (25 cm to 30 cm) at a time can cause coordination problems among the team.

Each rescuer should lean forward slightly and use a swinging motion to bring the patient onto the backboard. Rescuer One (who is at the patient's head) faces the other rescuers and moves backward during each movement. Rescuer One must not allow the patient's head to be driven into his or her knees!

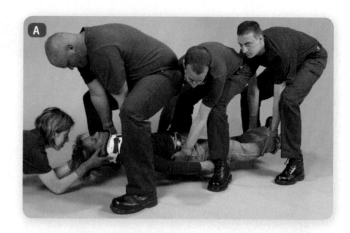

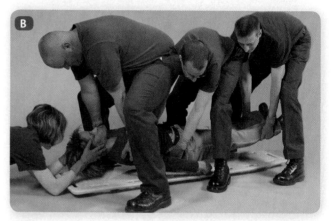

Figure 3-25 Straddle lift. **A.** Lift the patient as a unit. **B.** Slide the backboard under the patient.
A&B: © Jones & Bartlett Learning. Courtesy of MIEMSS.

Safety

When you are using the up-and-forward movement, make it a single, smooth action. Lifting the patient up and then forward can strain your muscles.

▶ Straps and Strapping Techniques

Secure every patient who is on a backboard with straps to avoid having him or her slide or slip off the backboard. There are many ways to strap a patient to a backboard. The straps should be long enough to go around

YOU are the Provider　　CASE 3

You are at the scene of a motor vehicle crash involving a vehicle that has collided with a tree. An EMS provider is sitting behind the driver and is holding manual cervical spine stabilization. As other team members gather and prepare to put the patient on a backboard, the EMS provider asks you to put a cervical collar on the patient.

1. What type of cervical collar should be placed on the patient?
2. Explain how you would apply a cervical collar to the patient.

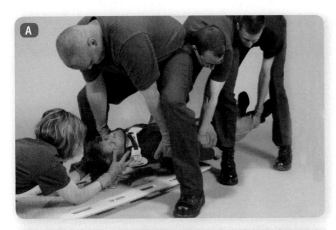

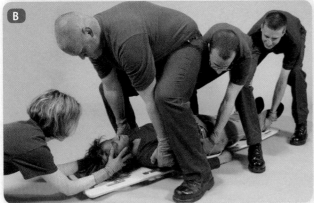

Figure 3-26 Straddle slide. **A.** Slide the patient about 10 inches (25 cm) at a time onto the backboard. **B.** Center the patient on the backboard.
A&B: © Jones & Bartlett Learning. Courtesy of MIEMSS.

the backboard and a large patient. Straps that are 6 feet to 9 feet (2 m to 3 m) long with seat belt-type buckles work well Figure 3-27 .

Once the patient is centered on the board, secure the upper torso with straps. Consider padding voids between the patient and the backboard. Next, secure the pelvis and upper legs, using padding as needed. To reduce the chance of head movement, secure the straps around the wrist and hip area and the knees before securing the head to the backboard. Strap placement is shown in Figure 3-28 . Different EMS systems use many different types of straps and strapping techniques. Learn and implement the method used by your EMS department.

▶ Head Immobilization

After a patient has been secured to the backboard, immobilize the head and neck using commercially available devices (such as foam blocks) or improvised devices (such as a blanket roll). The use of a blanket roll is explained here because it works well and because a blanket is almost always available. Assemble the blanket roll ahead of time. Fold and roll the blanket (with towels as bulk filler) as shown in Skill Drill 3-5 .

1. Fold the blanket into a long rectangular shape Step 1 .
2. Insert a rolled towel and roll the blanket from each end Step 2 .

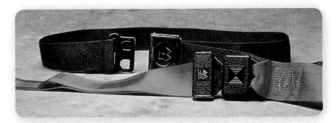

Figure 3-27 Seat belt-type straps.
© American Academy of Orthopaedic Surgeons.

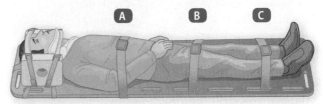

Figure 3-28 Strap placement for effective immobilization on a backboard. **A.** Arms. **B.** Upper legs. **C.** Below the knees.
© Jones & Bartlett Learning.

3. Roll the ends together Step 3 .
4. Place extra cravats in between the two rolled ends Step 4 .
5. Tie the rolled ends together with two cravats Step 5 and Step 6 .

To place the blanket roll under a patient's head, one rescuer unrolls it enough to fit around the patient's head as another rescuer maintains manual stabilization. The rescuer holding the patient's head (Rescuer One) carefully slides his or her hands out from between the blanket and immobilization is maintained by the blanket roll Skill Drill 3-6 .

1. Rescuer One stabilizes the patient's head Step 1 .
2. Both rescuers apply a cervical collar Step 2 .
3. Place straps around the backboard and the patient Step 3 .
4. Insert the blanket roll under the patient's head.
5. Roll the blanket snugly against the patient's neck and shoulders Step 4 .
6. Tie two cravats around the blanket roll.
7. Continue to stabilize the patient's head.
8. Tie two more cravats around the blanket roll and backboard Step 5 .
9. Assess sensory and motor function after immobilization.

Provide motion restriction throughout the entire procedure (first by manual stabilization of the patient's head, then by immobilization using the blanket roll). The blanket roll must be fitted securely against the patient's shoulders to widen the base of support for the patient's head. Secure the blanket roll to the head with two cravats tied around the blanket roll: one over the patient's forehead and the other under the chin. Use two more cravats in the same positions to bind the head and the blanket roll to the backboard. The patient's head and

Skill Drill 3-5

Preparing a Blanket Roll

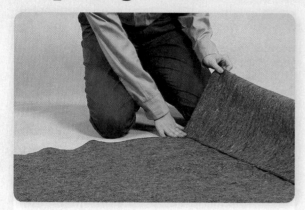

Step 1 Fold a blanket.

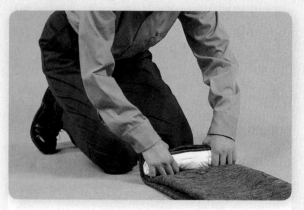

Step 2 Insert a rolled towel and roll the blanket from each end.

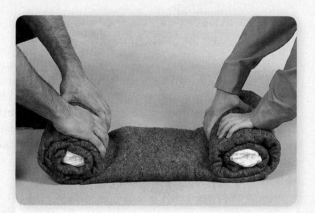

Step 3 Roll the ends together.

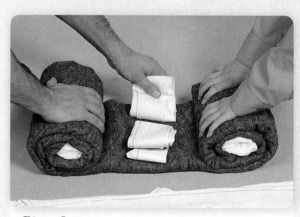

Step 4 Place extra cravats inside.

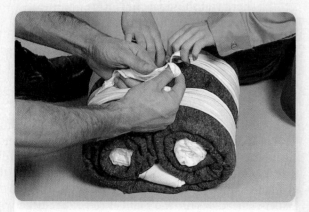

Step 5 Tie with two cravats.

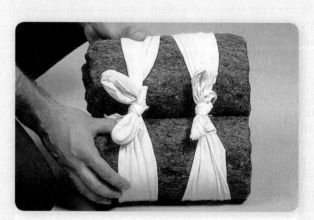

Step 6 The finished blanket roll.

Applying the Blanket Roll to Stabilize the Patient's Head and Neck

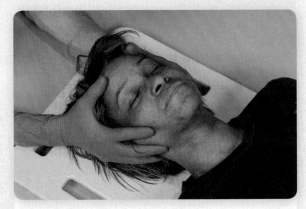

Step 1 Stabilize the head.

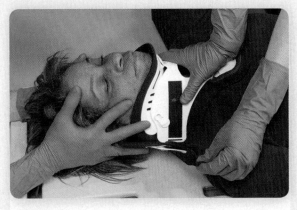

Step 2 Apply a cervical collar.

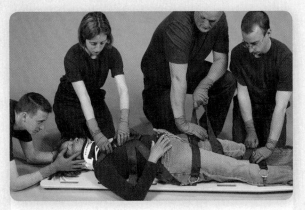

Step 3 Place the straps around the backboard and patient.

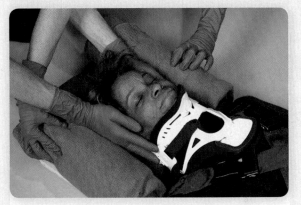

Step 4 Insert the blanket roll and roll each side of the blanket snugly against the neck and shoulders.

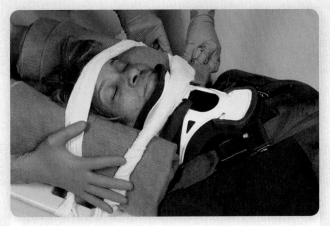

Step 5 Tie two cravats around the blanket roll, then two more around the blanket roll and backboard.

neck are now adequately stabilized against the backboard. This head immobilization technique, coupled with proper placement of straps around the backboard, adequately immobilizes the spine of an injured patient and packages the patient for movement as a unit. Foam blocks are quick to apply and provide good immobilization of the patient's head and neck. The use of one type of foam block is shown in Figure 3-29 .

In an extreme emergency where a patient must be moved from a dangerous environment and a commercially available backboard is unavailable, improvise. Make sure the improvised backboard is strong enough to hold the patient without breaking. Use improvised devices only when a patient must be moved to prevent further injury or death and when a commercially available backboard is not available.

Treatment

Carefully monitor all immobilized patients for airway problems.

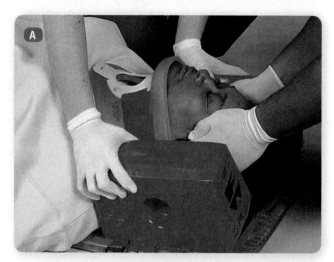

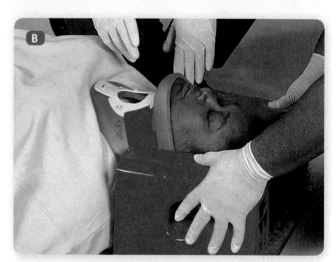

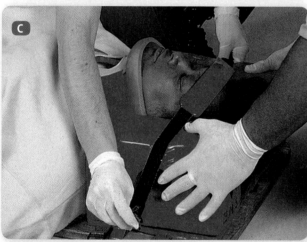

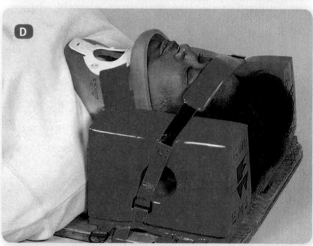

Figure 3-29 Application of a commercial device to immobilize a patient's head and neck. **A.** Apply the foam blocks. **B.** Secure the device. **C.** Apply the immobilization straps. **D.** The head is immobilized.
A, B, C, & D: © American Academy of Orthopaedic Surgeons.

YOU are the Provider   CASE 4

You are dispatched to a nearby apartment for a report of an unresponsive man. After a short drive, you arrive at the apartment and are directed to a bathroom by the man's wife. She appears to be about 70 years old. As you enter the very small bathroom, you find a man who appears to have been sitting on the toilet. He is now slumped against the wall. He does not respond to verbal stimuli. He does not appear to be breathing and you determine he has no carotid pulse.

1. How do you decide whether or not to move this patient before you begin further assessment and treatment?
2. If you decide you need to move this patient, what method would you use?

You are the Provider: CASE 1

1. Under what circumstances would it be necessary to move this patient before the EMS transport unit arrives?

One of the most important decisions facing you as an emergency medical responder (EMR) is whether to move a patient. Generally, you should not move a patient except in extreme emergency situations. These include fires, explosions, structural collapse, the presence of hazardous materials, unsafe vehicle crash scenes, and situations where you need to move a patient to perform cardiopulmonary resuscitation (CPR). In general, when an imminent threat to the patient's safety exists that can be eliminated by moving the patient, it is better to do so. Otherwise, it is usually better to wait for additional personnel before moving a patient. Place the patient in a comfortable position and cover her with a blanket to preserve body heat. Treat the injuries you are equipped to treat.

2. Why is it often better for EMRs to delay moving a patient until the arrival of an EMS transport unit?

There are several reasons why it is usually better to wait for additional emergency medical services (EMS) providers before moving a patient. Emergency medical technicians and paramedics have more training in lifting and moving patients. EMS transport units carry a variety of equipment for lifting and moving patients. The expression "Many hands make light work" is certainly true here. Injuries to rescuers are less likely and patient safety is enhanced when there are an adequate number of people to move a patient. Because EMRs usually do not transport patients, there is no hurry to move patients before the arrival of an EMS transport unit unless one of the emergency situations listed on the previous page is present.

You are the Provider: CASE 2

1. How can you quickly remove this patient from the burning vehicle?

First, decide if you can safely rescue the driver from this vehicle without risk of harm to you. If you determine a rescue attempt is feasible, approach the vehicle and try to open a door. Determine if the patient can assist with his own rescue. If the patient is unresponsive, you will need to grasp the patient under his arms.

Cradle the patient's head between your arms. Pull the patient down into a horizontal position as you ease him from the vehicle. Although there is no effective way to remove a patient from a vehicle by yourself without causing some movement, it is important to try to prevent excess movement of the patient's neck. Use this technique only if the patient is in danger and must be moved.

2. How do you determine where to place this patient after removal?

Move the patient only as far as you need to get him to a safe place. In this case, you need to get the patient far enough from the burning vehicle that the vehicle fire will not pose a danger to either you or the patient. You also need to consider traffic hazards. Place the patient in a place where distracted drivers will not cause further harm to the patient.

You are the Provider: CASE 3

1. What type of cervical collar should be placed on the patient?

A variety of cervical collars are available in the prehospital environment. Trauma patients should receive a rigid cervical collar. Although these devices are not designed to completely immobilize the cervical spine, they provide some degree of immobilization and serve as a reminder to the patient not to move his or her head and neck. Proper sizing of the collar is key. Most commercial cervical collars allow you to adjust the size of the collar; therefore, adjust the collar to create the best fit for the patient.

2. Explain how you would apply a cervical collar to the patient.

Begin by selecting the appropriate cervical collar and size. Make sure someone is maintaining manual in-line cervical spine stabilization during this procedure and remind this person to continue providing stabilization even after the collar is in place. Then, slide the back portion of the collar along the posterior portion of the patient's neck. Wrap the front portion of the collar around the anterior aspect of the neck, making sure the chin is properly seated in the chin-groove of the collar. Finally, secure the collar in place using the straps.

YOU are the Provider   SUMMARY *Continued*

You are the Provider: CASE 4

1. How do you decide whether or not to move this patient before you begin further assessment and treatment?

It is not unusual to discover a patient in cardiac arrest in a small bathroom. This patient will require a lot of care to give him the best chance for recovery. If the bathroom is too small for all the necessary providers to enter and provide adequate treatment, then it is better to quickly move the patient to a larger room. It is easier to move this patient before you begin treatment than to start treatment in a small place and then try to move the patient.

2. If you decide you need to move this patient, what method would you use?

If the patient is wearing sufficient clothing, then grasp the patient's clothing in the neck and shoulder area, rest the patient's head on your arms, and quickly drag the patient from the tight space to a larger room that has space to perform CPR and advanced life support skills. You may also need to move furniture out of the way to provide enough space. You can accomplish these actions in a short time.

Prep Kit

▶ Ready for Review

- In most situations, you can treat the patient in the position found and later assist other emergency medical services (EMS) personnel in moving the patient. In some situations, however, the patient's survival may depend on your knowledge of emergency movement techniques.
- Every time you move a patient, keep the following general guidelines in mind:
  - Do no further harm to the patient.
  - Move the patient only when necessary.
  - Move the patient as few times as possible.
  - Move the patient's body as a unit.
  - Use proper lifting and moving techniques to ensure your own safety.
  - Have one rescuer give commands when moving a patient.
- Always use good body mechanics when you move patients, including:
  - Know your own physical limitations and capabilities.
  - Keep yourself balanced when lifting or moving a patient.
  - Maintain a firm footing.
  - Lift and lower the patient by bending your legs, not your back. Keep your back as straight as possible at all times and use your leg muscles to do the work.
  - Try to keep your arms close to your body for strength and balance.

- Place unconscious patients who have not sustained trauma in the recovery position.
- If a patient is lying on the floor or ground during an emergency situation, you may have to drag the person away from the scene instead of trying to lift and carry the person. Make every effort to pull the patient in the direction of the long axis of the body to protect the patient's spine.
- Do not lift or move a patient if you suspect a spinal injury, unless it is necessary to remove the patient from a life-threatening situation.
- EMS departments typically use wheeled ambulance stretchers, portable stretchers, stair chairs, long backboards, short backboards, and scoop stretchers to immobilize and move patients.
- Any time a patient has sustained a traumatic injury, you should suspect injury to the head, neck, or spine. Keep the patient's head in a neutral position and immobilized. Use a cervical collar to prevent excessive movement of the head and neck.
- Log rolling is the primary technique you will use to move a patient onto a backboard. Secure every patient who is on a backboard with straps to avoid having him or her slide or slip off the backboard.
- After you secure a patient to the backboard, immobilize the head and neck using commercially available devices or improvised devices.

▶ Vital Vocabulary

arm-to-arm drag An emergency move that consists of the rescuer grasping the patient's arms from behind; used to remove a patient from a hazardous environment.

Prep Kit *Continued*

blanket drag An emergency move in which a rescuer encloses a patient in a blanket and drags the patient to safety.

cervical collar A neck brace that partially immobilizes the neck following injury.

clothes drag An emergency move used to remove a patient from a hazardous environment; performed by grasping the patient's clothes and moving the patient head first from the unsafe area.

cradle-in-arms carry A one-rescuer patient movement technique used primarily for children; the patient is cradled in the hollow formed by the rescuer's arms and chest.

extremities The arms and legs.

firefighter drag A method of moving a patient without lifting or carrying him or her; used when the patient is heavier than the rescuer.

log rolling A technique used to move a patient onto a long backboard.

one-person walking assist A method used if the patient is able to bear his or her own weight.

pack-strap carry A one-person carry that allows the rescuer to carry a patient while keeping one hand free.

portable stretcher A lightweight, nonwheeled device for transporting a patient; used in small spaces where the wheeled ambulance stretcher cannot be used.

recovery position A sidelying position that helps an unconscious patient maintain an open airway.

scoop stretcher A firm device used to carry a patient; can be split into halves and applied to the patient from both sides.

stair chair A small portable device used for transporting a patient in a sitting position.

straddle lift A method used to place a patient on a backboard if there is not enough space to perform a log roll.

straddle slide A method of placing a patient on a long backboard by straddling both the board and patient and sliding the patient onto the board.

two-person chair carry A method of carrying a patient in which two rescuers use a chair to support the weight of the patient.

two-person extremity carry A method of carrying a patient out of tight quarters using two rescuers and no equipment.

two-person seat carry A method of carrying a patient in which two rescuers link arms behind the patient's back and under the patient's knees; requires no equipment.

two-person walking assist A method used when a patient cannot bear his or her own weight; two rescuers completely support the patient.

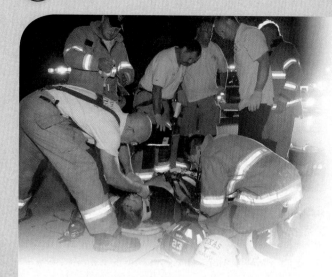

Assessment
in Action

You and your partner have been called to an assisted-living facility to help evacuate patients because floodwaters caused by a hurricane are threatening to cut off the access road to the facility. The officer in charge assigns you and your partner to one wing that has four patients. He asks you to bring the patients to the front lobby where they will be assigned to vehicles for evacuation.

1. Which of the following techniques is NOT an example of good body mechanics when moving patients?

   A. Lift and lower by bending your legs, not your back.
   B. Do not try to lift too heavy a load.
   C. Try to keep your arms away from your body for strength and balance.
   D. Move the patient as few times as possible.

2. Which of the following situations is NOT a reason for using an emergency drag to move a patient?

   A. To begin cardiopulmonary resuscitation on a patient who has experienced cardiac arrest
   B. To remove the patient from a scene that cannot be protected
   C. To remove the patient from inclement weather
   D. To remove the patient from the scene of an explosion, fire, or structural collapse

3. The first gentleman tells you he can walk slowly, but he is weak. Which technique would you use to move this man to the lobby?

   A. Straddle slide
   B. One-person walking assist
   C. Two-person extremity carry
   D. Pack-strap carry

4. The second room is occupied by a woman who has a brace on her ankle. She is not supposed to put weight on her sprained ankle. Which of the following carries would you consider using for this patient?

   A. Two-person extremity carry
   B. Pack-strap carry
   C. Two-person chair carry
   D. Direct ground lift

5. On the third floor, you find an 82-year-old woman who says she has a heart condition and gets short of breath if she walks very far. The elevator is not working. How would you move this person, assuming the following equipment is available?

   A. Scoop stretcher
   B. Long backboard
   C. Stair chair
   D. Portable stretcher

6. The fourth person is confined to bed because she experienced a stroke 2 years ago. A nurse brings you a stretcher and asks you to use it to move the patient. How would you move this woman to the stretcher?

   A. Draw sheet method
   B. Log roll
   C. Clothes drag
   D. Direct ground lift

7. If a backboard were available to move the fourth person, what technique would you use to get the patient on the backboard?

   A. Straddle slide
   B. Log roll
   C. Straddle lift
   D. Direct ground lift

8. Why is it important for you and your partner to communicate when lifting and moving patients?

9. You are assigned to assist with getting patients from the front lobby into emergency medical services vehicles for evacuation. What type of devices can be used for patients who are supine?

10. When you are moving a patient on a portable stretcher, what are some important lifting techniques to keep in mind?

Medical, Legal, and Ethical Issues

National EMS Education Standard Competencies

Preparatory

Uses simple knowledge of the emergency medical services (EMS) system, safety/well-being of the emergency medical responder (EMR), medical/legal issues at the scene of an emergency while awaiting a higher level of care.

Medical/Legal and Ethics

> Consent/refusal of care (pp 63–64)
> Confidentiality (p 67)
> Advance directives (p 64)
> Tort and criminal actions (p 62)
> Evidence preservation (p 68)
> Statutory responsibilities (pp 62–65; pp 67–69)
> Mandatory reporting (pp 68–69)
> Ethical principles/moral obligations (p 63)
> End-of-life issues (pp 64–65)

Knowledge Objectives

1. Describe the legal duty to act for an emergency medical responder (EMR). (p 62)
2. Explain how to comply with the standard of care. (p 62)
3. Discuss the ethical responsibilities of an EMR. (p 63)

4. Define consent, and include how it relates to decision making. (p 63)
5. Differentiate between expressed consent and implied consent. (p 63)
6. Discuss consent as it relates to minors who require treatment or transport. (p 63)
7. Discuss consent as it relates to patients with a mental illness. (pp 63–64)
8. Discuss the EMR's role and obligations if a patient refuses treatment or transport. (p 64)
9. Discuss the three types of advance directives and how they impact patient care. (p 64)
10. Explain the legal concepts of abandonment, people dead at the scene, negligence, and confidentiality. (p 65; p 67)
11. Recognize that most patient information is confidential and protected by the Health Insurance Portability and Accountability Act (HIPAA). (p 67)
12. Describe the role of Good Samaritan laws. (p 68)
13. Explain the requirements for reportable events, including crimes and certain infectious diseases. (p 68)
14. Explain the reasons for documentation. (pp 68–69)

Skills Objectives

There are no skills objectives for this chapter.

Introduction

As an emergency medical responder (EMR), you need to know some basic legal principles that guide how you provide care to patients. Knowing these principles can help you provide the best possible care for your patients and prevent situations that could result in legal difficulties for you, your public service agency, or your department. Because some laws differ from one location to another, you will need to learn the specific laws of your state and your local jurisdiction (the area in which you work). It is easy to become concerned about the legal consequences of providing emergency medical care or immediate care or treatment. Remember the following concepts when providing patient care:

- Above all else, do no harm.
- Provide all your care in good faith, keeping the patient's best interest uppermost in your mind.
- Provide proper, consistent care; be compassionate; and maintain your composure.

These concepts can help prevent many of the legal issues that are discussed in this chapter.

Duty to Act

The first legal principle to consider is the **duty to act**. An uninvolved citizen (bystander) who arrives on the scene of a motor vehicle crash is not required by law to stop and give emergency care to injured people. However, if you are employed by an agency that has designated you as an EMR and you are dispatched to the scene of an injury or illness, then you do have a duty to act. You must proceed quickly to the scene and provide emergency medical care within the limits of your training and available equipment **Figure 4-1**. Any failure to respond or provide necessary emergency medical care leaves both you and your agency vulnerable to legal action.

Standard of Care

What level of care are you expected to give to a patient? As a trained EMR, you cannot provide the same level of care as a physician, but you are responsible for

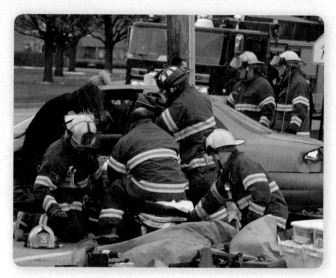

Figure 4-1 EMRs dispatched to an emergency scene.
Courtesy of Captain David Jackson, Saginaw Township Fire Department.

providing the level of care that a person with similar training would provide under similar circumstances. You are expected to use your knowledge and skills to the best of your ability under the circumstances. The circumstances under which you must provide care may affect the standard of care. The **standard of care** is the manner in which you must act or behave. To comply with the standard of care, you must meet two criteria: (1) You must treat the patient to the best of your ability and (2) you must provide care that a reasonable, prudent person with similar training would provide under similar circumstances. It is important to know your local standards of care and what statutes affect your community. Failure to provide proper care because of a wrongful act could result in legal action being taken against your public safety agency or against you as an individual health care provider. A wrongful act is called a tort by the legal community.

Scope of Care

The scope of care you give as an EMR is defined on several levels. The *Emergency Medical Responder Education Standards*, originally developed by the US Department of Transportation, specify the skills taught in this course and the way those skills should be performed. These standards

YOU are the Provider

CASE 1

As a new EMR, you have mastered the knowledge and skills covered in your course. However, you are concerned about the possibility of making a mistake that might result in legal action against you or your department.

1. How does the concept of a standard of care protect you?
2. Why is the concept of confidentiality so important for you to follow?

have evolved into the current *National Emergency Medical Services (EMS) Education Standards*. States also have scope of care laws that may modify the specifications in the education standards. In most states, a law outlines the roles and responsibilities of EMRs. You may be required to operate under the license of your medical director. The medical director for your department may use medical protocols or **standing orders** to specify your scope of care. In some cases, online medical direction is provided by radio or a wireless communication device. Your state gives you the responsibility to practice within the limits specified within the law. You have a professional responsibility to your patients, to your medical director, and to the public you serve.

Ethical Responsibilities and Competence

Your community and your department have entrusted you, as an EMR, with certain moral and ethical responsibilities. This moral responsibility means that the community expects you to follow the established codes of what is right and wrong. It is your ethical responsibility as an EMR to follow these codes. Treating a patient ethically means doing so in a manner that conforms to accepted professional standards of conduct. These standards include staying up to date on the EMR skills and knowledge you need to provide good patient care. You are also responsible for reviewing your performance and assessing the techniques you use. Evaluate your response times and try to follow up patient care outcomes with your medical director or hospital personnel. Always look for ways to improve your performance. Continuing education classes and refresher courses are designed to keep your knowledge and skills current. It is in your best interest to make the most of these opportunities. It is also a good idea to participate in quality improvement activities within your department.

Ethical behavior requires honesty. Your reports should accurately reflect the conditions found at the scene. Always provide complete and correct reports to other EMS providers. If you make a mistake on the report or document information incorrectly, then do not try to cover it up. Never change a report except to correct an error. (See Chapter 5, *Communications and Documentation*, for more information about reporting.) Remember, the actions you take in the first few minutes of an emergency may make the difference between life and death for a patient. Your ethical behavior and competence will be invaluable to both you and your patient.

Consent for Treatment

Consent simply means giving approval or permission. Legally, however, several types of consent exist. In **expressed consent**, the patient actually lets you know—verbally or nonverbally—that he or she is willing to accept the treatment you provide. Expressed consent is

based on the idea that the patient has the right to determine what will be done to his or her body. The patient must be of legal age (in most states, older than 18 years) and able to make a rational decision. As you approach a patient, be sure the patient understands who you are, tell him or her what you are going to do, and be sure he or she agrees to treatment. For example, if you say, "You have a cut on your arm. I need to bandage it to stop the bleeding," and the response is "OK," then the patient has given you expressed consent. Expressed consent is sometimes called actual consent or informed consent. In situations in which a patient is under the influence of alcohol or other drugs, has a mental impairment, or has a medical condition that affects his or her mental status, it may be hard to determine whether the patient is capable of making decisions about his or her health care. In these situations, carefully explain to the patient what needs to be done and try to provide the care the patient needs.

Any patient who does not specifically refuse emergency medical care can be treated under the principle of **implied consent**. The principle of implied consent is best understood in the situation of an unconscious patient. Because an unconscious patient is unable to communicate, the law assumes the patient would agree to treatment if he or she were able to do so. Therefore, never hesitate to treat an unconscious patient.

▶ Consent for Minors

A minor is a person who has not yet reached the legal age designated by a particular state. Under the law, minors (usually people younger than 18 years) are not considered capable of speaking for themselves. Many states have laws that permit a minor to have the rights of an adult if the minor is considered emancipated. Learn the laws of your state related to the issues surrounding emancipated minors. In most cases, emergency medical treatment of a minor by a physician must wait until a parent or legal guardian consents to the treatment. If a minor requires emergency medical care in the field (out of the hospital) and you cannot quickly get the permission of a parent or legal guardian, then do not hesitate to give appropriate emergency medical care. Never delay or withhold emergency medical treatment of a minor just to obtain permission from a parent or legal guardian **Figure 4-2**. Let hospital officials determine what treatment can be postponed until permission is obtained. Remember, good prehospital patient care is your first responsibility. By following the course of action that is best for the patient, you will stand on firm legal ground.

▶ Consent of Patients With a Mental Illness

An adult who is conscious, alert, and mentally in control, or **competent**, may legally refuse to be treated—even if doing so may result in serious injury or death. The legal issues are more complicated if the patient who refuses to be treated appears to be out of touch with reality and is a

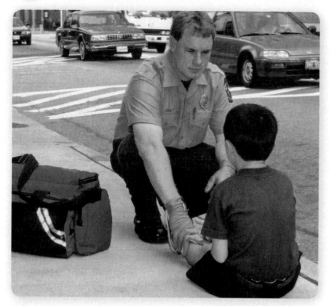

Figure 4-2 Do not delay or withhold emergency medical treatment from a patient who is a minor.
© Jones & Bartlett Learning. Courtesy of MIEMSS.

danger to himself or herself or others. The difficult part, even for highly trained medical personnel, is determining whether such a patient is rational. Generally, if the person appears to be a threat to himself or herself or others, then arrangements need to be made to place this person under medical care. The legal means by which these arrangements are made vary from state to state. You and other members of the EMS system should know your local policies for handling patients who refuse to be treated and who do not appear to be making rational and reasonable decisions. Do not hesitate to involve law enforcement agencies, because this process may require the issuance of a warrant or an order of protective custody.

Patient Refusal of Care

A competent adult has a legal right to refuse treatment from emergency medical personnel at any time. You can continue to talk with a person who refuses treatment and try to help him or her understand the consequences of this action. Explain the treatment to the person, why it is needed, the potential risks if treatment is not provided, and any alternative treatments that may help. Sometimes another EMS provider or a law enforcement officer may have more success in convincing a patient that he or she

needs to receive treatment. If the patient is firm in his or her refusal, then tell the patient that he or she should call EMS again if the patient changes his or her mind. Carefully document patient refusals on your patient care report according to your agency protocols. Many agencies require a second person to witness this refusal. Follow all local EMR protocols related to patient care refusal.

Advance Directives

An **advance directive** is a document that specifies what a person would like to be done if the person becomes unable to make his or her own medical decisions. Three kinds of advance directives exist. The first is called a **living will**. A living will is a written document drawn up by a patient, a physician, and a lawyer. A living will states the types of medical care a person wants or wants withheld if the person is unable to make his or her own treatment decisions. Living wills are often written when a patient has a terminal (incurable) condition. A living will does not let the person select someone to make decisions for them.

A second type of advance directive is a **durable power of attorney for health care** or medical power of attorney. A durable power of attorney for health care allows a patient to designate another person to make decisions about medical care for the patient if he or she is unable to make decisions for himself or herself. The person designated to be a patient's health care representative is often a family member. This representative may be referred to as the patient's health care agent or health care proxy.

A **do not resuscitate (DNR) order** is the third type of advance directive. It is a written request giving permission to medical personnel to withhold resuscitation in the event of cardiac arrest. Advance directives may include DNR orders but are not required to include them. DNR orders are most frequently used for patients who are in hospitals or nursing homes. DNR orders are most common in cases of terminal disease or medical futility (as discussed in the consensus statement from the International Liaison Committee on Resuscitation [ILCOR]).

If you are unable to determine whether an advance directive is legally valid, then begin appropriate medical care and leave the questions about advance directives to physicians. Some states have systems, such as bracelets, to identify patients with advance directives. Know your local policies and protocols.

YOU are the Provider   CASE 2

You are dispatched to a call for a 9-year-old boy who was bitten by a dog. When you arrive, the child is crying and holding his head. He is bleeding from a gash on the side of his cheek. He tells you his parents are not at home. A police officer is nearby, and she reports that she has also been unsuccessful in reaching the parents. The child says he has no other relatives in the area that he can call.

1. You ask the child if you can help and he says yes. What should you do next?
2. You have finished applying a bandage to the wound on the boy's cheek when the police officer tells you she still cannot reach the parents. What should you do now?

Legal Concepts

As an EMR, it is important for you to understand some legal concepts that relate to your work. These concepts include abandonment, people dead at the scene, negligence, and confidentiality. Each of them is explained in the following section.

▶ Abandonment

Abandonment occurs when a trained person begins emergency medical care and then leaves the patient before another trained person arrives to take over. After you have started treatment, you must continue that treatment until a person who has skills and/or training at the same or a higher level arrives on the scene and takes over or until you deliver the patient to another medical care provider at a medical facility. Never leave a patient without care after you begin treatment. The most common abandonment scenario occurs when an EMS provider responds to a call, examines the patient, assesses the patient's condition, fails to transport the patient to a hospital, and finds out later that the patient died. Emergency medical care began, but the patient was abandoned.

▶ People Dead at the Scene

If you see any signs that a person is alive when you arrive on the scene, then begin providing necessary care. People who are obviously dead should be handled according to the laws of your state and the protocols of your service. Generally, you cannot assume a person is dead unless one or more of the following conditions exist:

- **Decapitation.** Decapitation means that the head is separated from the body. When this occurs, there is obviously no chance of saving the patient.
- **Rigor mortis.** Rigor mortis is the temporary stiffening of muscles that occurs several hours after death. The presence of this stiffening indicates the patient is dead and cannot be resuscitated.

- **Tissue decomposition.** Body tissue begins to decompose and flesh begins to decay only after a person has been dead for more than 1 day.
- **Dependent lividity. Dependent lividity** is the red or purple color that occurs on the parts of the patient's body that are closest to the ground. It is caused by blood seeping into the tissues on the dependent, or lower, part of the person's body. Dependent lividity occurs after a person has been dead for several hours.

If one or more of these signs are present, then you can usually consider the patient to be dead. Know the protocol your department uses in dealing with patients who are dead on the scene � Figure 4-3 . Chapter 8, *Professional Rescuer CPR*, covers these criteria as they relate to starting CPR.

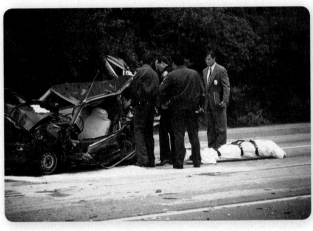

Figure 4-3 Learn the protocol for dealing with patients who are obviously dead at the scene.
© Corbis/Getty.

Words of Wisdom

Four legal concepts you should understand:

1. Abandonment
2. People dead at the scene
3. Negligence
4. Confidentiality

YOU are the Provider   CASE 3

You respond to a call for an unresponsive 85-year-old man who is not breathing. Over the phone, dispatch attempted to guide family members through the steps of cardiopulmonary resuscitation (CPR). The family members are not able to follow the dispatcher's instructions. On your arrival, family members say that they think the man has a do not resuscitate or DNR order; however, they are unable to provide you with the document.

1. What should you do in this situation?
2. What level of emergency medical care should you provide?

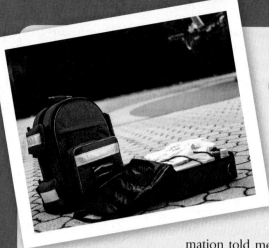

Voices *of* Experience

I was the attendant-in-charge dispatched to a rollover motor vehicle collision at about 0230 hours one dreary, rainy night. Dispatch information told me a sport utility vehicle (SUV) was involved and our county sheriff's department was already at the scene. We were sent to direct aid with an adjoining fire department engine that arrived on scene first. We arrived on scene a couple of minutes after the engine and discovered there were multiple patients. I made contact with the engine company lieutenant and became the medical group supervisor.

> **❝ I can recall thinking to myself that this was not what I had come into this profession to do. ❞**

The story was a sad one. The sheriff deputy already had taken the driver of the SUV into custody. He told me there were four occupants in the SUV who were taking methamphetamines and drinking alcohol. They were not wearing any vehicle restraints. When the sheriff had tried to pull the vehicle over, the driver evaded the pursuit and in the ensuing chase, the SUV rolled over and ejected three of the four occupants.

I began triage and found one passenger on the roadside, screaming in pain from an open femur fracture. There were already EMTs preparing her for transport. I immediately called for a second EMS unit. The other two occupants had been thrown from the vehicle in opposite directions. They were approximately 25 feet (8 m) from the vehicle, sustaining fatal injuries. These two patients were teenagers. To this day, I can recall thinking to myself that this was not what I had come into this profession to do. I didn't like the tremendous responsibility of declaring someone dead. I was there to save the lives of people. Look at this tragedy; these two young people had no futures ahead of them. Did their parents know where they were?

I persuaded the sheriff's department to release the driver into my care for evaluation at the emergency department. Due to the mechanism of injury and the deaths of the other occupants as risk factors, it was important to have the driver examined for any hidden injuries. As I transferred the patient to the bed in the emergency department, a vial of methamphetamines fell out of his pocket. He lay there laughing, displaying no remorse for the deaths of his "friends."

As an EMS provider, it is difficult to respond to situations like this one. Ethically, it can be a challenge to treat patients who act irresponsibly and put their own lives and the lives of others in unnecessary danger. However, we must put our own personal feelings aside and treat the patient regardless of our feelings. In situations like this one, it is helpful to have the assistance of a law enforcement officer to ensure scene safety while the patients are triaged and treated. Police assistance is especially important in cases where drug and alcohol use may affect the behavior of the patients.

T.J. Bishop, NREMT-P
Clinical Officer
North Country EMS
Yacolt, Washington

▶ Negligence

Negligence is the failure of a medical care provider at any level to meet the required standard of care in his or her treatment of a patient. Remember, the standard of care represents the manner in which a reasonable, similarly trained provider would have acted in a similar situation. For a legal claim for negligence to be sustained, four conditions must be present:

1. Duty to act
2. Breach of duty
3. Resulting injuries
4. Proximate cause

As an EMR who has been dispatched or otherwise called to the scene of an incident to provide patient care, you will have a duty to act to help the patient. This means that you have a duty to provide care within your scope of training and certification in a manner in which a reasonable similarly trained and certified provider would under similar circumstances. Failure to provide such care represents breach of duty. If the patient becomes injured as a result of your actions, then you may be considered negligent and therefore considered responsible for causing those injuries. The proximate cause element of the legal claim means that your act of negligence has to be directly responsible for the patient's resulting injury for you to be held responsible. For example, if you drag a patient with a neck injury out of a vehicle without properly immobilizing him or her and that patient becomes paralyzed as a direct result of your moving him or her, then you could be considered negligent and responsible for causing the spinal cord injury. If the patient later fell during physical therapy while recovering from the spinal cord injury and broke his or her leg as a result of the fall, then you would not be responsible for the broken leg because your action in dragging the patient from the vehicle was not the direct cause of the broken leg.

▶ Confidentiality

Most patient information is confidential. Confidential information includes the patient history, assessment findings, and treatment provided, as well as your communication with the patient. This information should be shared only with other medical personnel who are directly involved in the patient's care. Do not discuss this private information with your family or friends. Most departments have strict policies prohibiting the release of any patient information over social media.

In certain situations, you may release confidential information to designated people. In most states, records may be released when a legal subpoena is presented or the patient signs a written release. The patient must be mentally competent and fully understand the nature of the release.

Some information about a patient's care may be classified as public information. This information often includes the patient's name, address, and age and the hospital to which he or she was transported. Learn what patient information is considered public information in your state. Public information can be released to the news media through your department's approved process.

HIPAA

HIPAA is the acronym for the Health Insurance Portability and Accountability Act of 1996. Although this act had many aims, including improving the portability and continuity of health insurance coverage and combating waste and fraud in health insurance and in the provision of health care, the section of the act that most affects EMS relates to patient privacy. The aim of this section was to strengthen laws for the protection of the privacy of health care information and to safeguard patient confidentiality. It provides guidance on what type of information is protected, the responsibility of health care providers regarding that protection, and the penalties for breaching that protection.

Most personal health information is protected and should not be released without the patient's permission. If you are not sure, then do not give any information to anyone other than those directly involved in the care of the patient. For specific policies, each EMS service is required to have a manual and a privacy officer who can answer questions. You can expect to receive further training on how this act impacts your specific response agency and resource hospital.

Words of Wisdom

In this time of ever-present digital devices and cell phones with cameras, realize that patient confidentiality extends to photographs and videos. Do not take or send images of a patient without permission of both the patient and your supervisor.

YOU ▶ are the Provider   CASE 4

You and your partner are sent to the home of a 63-year-old woman who is reporting difficulty breathing and minor chest pain. She is in a part of the house that will require you to use a stair chair to get her to the street. While your partner is inside beginning to deliver emergency care to the woman, a neighbor stops you outside of the home. "Is Marie okay?" she asks.

1. How does HIPAA impact the way you respond to the neighbor?
2. Does this patient have the right to refuse treatment? If so, what should you do?

Good Samaritan Laws

Most states have adopted Good Samaritan laws, which protect citizens from liability for errors or omissions in giving good faith emergency medical care. These laws vary from state to state, and they may or may not apply to EMRs in your state. Recently, legal experts have noted that Good Samaritan laws may no longer be needed because they provide little or no legal protection for an EMS provider.

Any properly trained EMR who practices the skills and procedures learned in an EMR course should not be overly concerned about lack of protection under Good Samaritan statutes.

Regulations

As an EMR, you are subject to a variety of federal, state, local, and agency regulations. Become familiar with these regulations so you can follow them. The most important regulations guide your ability to work as an EMR. You may have to become registered or certified as an EMR through a state agency or you may have to register through the National Registry of Emergency Medical Technicians. It is your responsibility to keep any required certification or registration up to date.

Reportable Events

State and federal agencies have requirements for reporting certain events, including crimes and certain infectious diseases. Reportable crimes include knife wounds, gunshot wounds, motor vehicle crashes, suspected child abuse, domestic violence, elder abuse, dog bites, and rape. Learn which crimes are reportable in your area and know your agency's procedures for reporting these crimes. It is important that you learn how this process is handled in your agency and what you are required to do. Failure to notify proper authorities of reportable events may result in penalties against you or your agency.

Crime Scene Operations

Many emergency medical situations are also crime scenes. As an EMR, keep the following considerations in mind:

1. Protect yourself. Be sure the scene is safe before you try to enter.
2. If you determine that a crime scene is unsafe, then wait in a safe location until law enforcement personnel tell you the scene is safe for entry.
3. Your first priority is patient care. Nothing except your personal safety should interfere with that effort.
4. When you assess the scene, document anything you see that seems unusual.
5. Move the patient only if necessary, such as for rapid transport to the hospital, for administration of CPR, or for treatment of severe shock. If you must move the patient, then take a mental "snapshot" of the scene.
6. Touch only what you need to touch to gain access to the patient.
7. Preserve the crime scene for further investigation **Figure 4-4**. Do not move furniture or objects unless they interfere with your ability to provide care. If you must move anything out of the way, then move it no further than necessary to provide care.
8. Be careful not to cut through knife or bullet holes in the patient's clothing.
9. Be careful where you put your equipment to avoid changing or destroying evidence.
10. Keep nonessential people, such as curious bystanders, away from the scene.
11. Work with the appropriate law enforcement authorities on the scene to ensure that everyone has the information they need.
12. After you have attended to a patient at a crime scene, write a short report about the incident as soon as possible and make a sketch of the scene that shows how and where you found the patient. This may be useful information if you are required to recall the incident 2 or 3 years later.

Documentation

After you have finished treating the patient, record your observations about the scene, the patient's condition, and the treatment you provided. Complete your documentation according to the policies of your organization. These policies should follow appropriate local and state laws. Your documentation is important because it is the initial account describing the patient's condition and the care administered. You will not be able to remember the treatment you provide to each patient without documentation. It also serves as a legal record of your treatment, and it will be required in the event of a lawsuit.

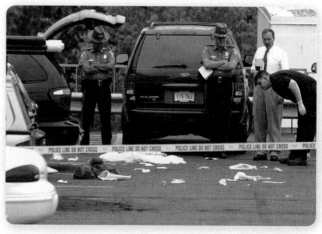

Figure 4-4 Crime scene operations require you to change the scene as little as possible.
© Bob Child/AP Photo.

Documentation also provides a basis for evaluating the quality of care you provided. Documentation should be clear, concise, accurate, and readable. Documentation may be completed using a paper form or an electronic device. More information on documentation is presented in Chapter 5, *Communications and Documentation*.

Documentation should include the following information:

1. The condition of the patient when found
2. The patient's description of the injury or illness
3. The patient's initial and repeat vital signs
4. The treatment you gave the patient
5. The agency and personnel who took over treatment of the patient
6. Any reportable conditions present
7. Any infectious disease exposure
8. Anything unusual regarding the situation

YOU are the Provider   SUMMARY

You are the Provider: CASE 1

1. How does the concept of a standard of care protect you?

The standard of care is the manner in which you act and behave when treating a patient. A standard of care requires that you treat all patients to the best of your ability and training. This concept takes into account your level of training and the conditions under which you provide care to the patient. It does not hold you to the standard of a person who has received more advanced training than you have.

2. Why is the concept of confidentiality so important for you to follow?

The concept of confidentiality is one of the cornerstones on which the health care system is based. Confidential patient information includes the patient history, assessment findings, and the treatment provided. The federal HIPAA law safeguards the right of patients to keep their personal and medical information private. Remember, this information can be shared only with other medical providers who are directly participating in the patient's care. Consider how you would want your private medical information to be safeguarded.

You are the Provider: CASE 2

1. You ask the child if you can help and he says yes. What should you do next?

Although the child has given you expressed consent to treat him, the child is considered a minor and the law requires that a parent or legal guardian give consent for treatment or transport. However, in this situation, the parents cannot be reached, so do not delay treatment because the child is an unaccompanied minor. Provide emergency care in the field and transport the patient to a local hospital.

2. You have finished applying a bandage to the wound on the boy's cheek when the police officer tells you she still cannot reach the parents. Because you treated the bite wound, can you now leave the child alone?

Leaving the child after you have begun treatment is abandonment and leaves you and your organization legally vulnerable. After you have started treatment, you must stay with the patient until he is delivered to a hospital or until someone of an equal or higher level of training arrives and takes over his care.

You are the Provider: CASE 3

1. What should you do in this situation?

Without a copy of a legally executed living will or DNR order in hand, you must begin to provide care for the patient. On arrival at the nearest hospital, inform the hospital staff about the patient's condition and the care provided and let them continue appropriate medical care.

2. What level of emergency medical care should you provide?

As with any patient, provide treatment that is in line with the scope of care as outlined by the *Emergency Medical Responder Education Standards* and those set by local medical protocols.

You are the Provider: CASE 4

1. How does HIPAA impact the way you respond to the neighbor?

HIPAA, which stands for the Health Insurance Portability and Accountability Act of 1996, prevents you from sharing any details about the patient with the neighbor.

2. Does this patient have the right to refuse treatment? If so, what should you do?

Yes, the patient has the right to refuse treatment even though it appears she is in need of immediate medical attention. If the patient is competent (mentally in control), then she can refuse treatment. As an EMR, it is your responsibility to try to convince the patient to consent to treatment and transport. If you are unsuccessful in convincing the patient, then follow your organization's guidelines for patients who refuse medical treatment and advise the woman to call EMS immediately if she changes her mind and decides she needs help. Carefully document patient refusals in your patient care report according to your agency's protocols. Many agencies require a second person to witness this refusal.

Prep Kit

▶ Ready for Review

- As an EMR, you have a duty to act when you are dispatched on a call as a part of your official duties.
- You are held to a certain standard of care, which is related to your level of training, and you are expected to perform to the level to which a similarly trained person would perform under similar circumstances.
- You should understand the differences among expressed consent, implied consent, consent for minors, consent of mentally ill persons, and the right to refuse care.
- Advance directives consist of living wills, durable powers of attorney, and do not resuscitate orders. They give a patient the right to have care withheld and to appoint someone to act for him or her if he or she is not able to act. If emergency medical responders cannot determine the validity of these documents, it is best to begin treatment for these patients.
- You should understand the concepts of abandonment, negligence, and confidentiality, as well as the purpose of Good Samaritan laws.
- You must understand the importance of federal and state regulations that govern your performance as an emergency medical responder. You must also understand your department's operational regulations. Certain events that deal with contagious diseases, abuse, or illegal acts must be reported to the proper authorities. You should know how to deal with these reportable events.
- Crime scene operations are complex environments. Follow proper procedures to ensure that the patient receives good medical care and that the crime scene is not compromised for the law enforcement investigation.
- Your job is not complete until the patient report is completed. Always document your findings and treatment. This provides good patient care and adequate legal documentation.
- By understanding and following these legal concepts, you will build the foundation for the skills you need to be an effective EMR.

▶ Vital Vocabulary

abandonment Failure of the emergency medical responder to continue emergency medical treatment until relieved by someone with the same or a higher level of training.

advance directive A legal document that indicates what a person wants done if he or she cannot make his or her own medical decisions. Advance directives include living wills, durable powers of attorney for health care, and do not resuscitate orders.

certification A process in which a person, institution, or a program is evaluated and recognized as meeting certain predetermined standards to provide safe and ethical patient care.

competent Able to make rational decisions about personal well-being.

consent In the context of emergency medical services, permission to provide care.

dependent lividity Blood settling to the lowest point of the body after death, causing discoloration of the skin.

do not resuscitate (DNR) order A written request giving permission to medical personnel not to attempt resuscitation in the event of cardiac arrest.

durable power of attorney for health care A legal document that allows a patient to designate another person to make medical decisions for him or her if the patient is unable to make his or her own treatment decisions.

duty to act An emergency medical responder's legal responsibility to respond quickly to an emergency scene and provide medical care (within the limits of training and available equipment).

expressed consent Consent actually given by a person, either verbally or nonverbally, authorizing the emergency medical responder to provide care or transportation.

Good Samaritan laws Laws that encourage citizens to voluntarily help an injured or suddenly ill person by minimizing the liability for any errors or omissions in providing good faith emergency care.

implied consent Consent to receive emergency medical care that is assumed because the individual is unconscious, underage, or so badly injured or ill that he or she cannot respond.

living will A legal document that states the types of medical care a person wants or wants withheld if he or she is unable to make his or her own treatment decisions. Living wills may include do not resuscitate orders.

negligence Deviation from the accepted standard of care resulting in further injury to the patient.

standard of care The manner in which an individual must act or behave when giving care.

standing orders Written documents, signed by the emergency medical service system's medical director, that outline specific directions, permissions, and sometimes prohibitions regarding patient care; also called protocols.

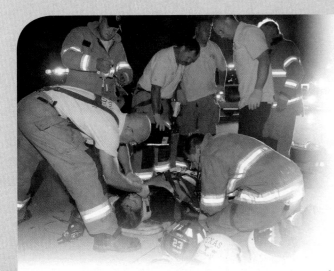

Assessment
in Action

On Saturday afternoon, just as you are finishing lunch, you and your partner are dispatched to a local park. When you arrive, you find an 11-year-old girl who was skateboarding and has fallen. She is crying, scared, and in pain. Her right wrist is noticeably deformed, and she has some blood seeping from scrapes on her right arm and right leg. When you ask her about her parents, she says she does not know where they are.

1. What should be your first action?

   A. Send your partner to locate her parents.
   B. Call for help in locating her parents.
   C. Treat the girl to the best of your ability.
   D. Withhold your treatment until her parents have been located.

2. What type of consent, if any, do you have to treat this patient?

   A. Expressed
   B. None
   C. Informed
   D. Implied

3. To what level must you provide care to this patient?

   A. You cannot treat this patient because a parent is not on scene to give you permission.
   B. You must treat the patient to the best of your ability, and provide care that a reasonable, prudent person with similar training would provide under similar circumstances.
   C. You should splint the wrist, bandage the wounds, and let the child return to the park.
   D. You should transport the child to the hospital but should not treat the injuries without parental consent.

4. If you were to treat this patient's injuries and let her 15-year-old brother take her home, then you would be guilty of:

   A. libel.
   B. abandonment.

   C. scope of care.
   D. duty to act.

5. Assume for a moment that the child's injuries were the result of a crime. In this case, you should:

   A. treat the child immediately without worrying about the scene.
   B. clean up the scene around the patient so it is easier to provide care.
   C. provide emergency care to the patient, write a short report about the incident, and make a sketch of the scene showing how and where you found the patient.
   D. enlist the help of bystanders to help you move the patient from the crime scene.

6. Another person at the park approached the child and began to assist her before you arrived on the scene. The bystander would be covered by what rules in terms of providing aid?

   A. Duty to act
   B. Advance directives
   C. Scope of practice
   D. Good Samaritan laws

7. For negligence to occur, what four conditions must be present?

   A. Duty to act, scope of care, abandonment, proximate cause
   B. Duty to act, breach of duty, resulting injuries, proximate cause
   C. Scope of care, rigor mortis, dependent lividity, standard of care
   D. Abandonment, resulting injuries, implied consent, standard of care

Assessment *in Action* Continued

8. When writing your report on the care of the child, your documentation should include all of the following information EXCEPT:

   A. your observations about the scene.
   B. the patient's condition.
   C. the treatment you provided.
   D. the amount of time you and your partner took for lunch.

9. To whom can you give information about the patient's illness or injury?

10. What are some circumstances that could make this situation a reportable event?

Communications and Documentation

National EMS Education Standard Competencies

Preparatory

Uses simple knowledge of the emergency medical services (EMS) system, safety/well-being of the emergency medical responder (EMR), medical/legal issues at the scene of an emergency while awaiting a higher level of care.

Documentation

> Recording patient findings (p 85)

EMS System Communication

Communication needed to

> Call for resources (pp 76–77)
> Transfer care of the patient (p 77)
> Interact within the team structure (pp 74–78)

Therapeutic Communication

Principles of communicating with patients in a manner that achieves a positive relationship

> Interviewing techniques (pp 78–83)

Medical Terminology

Uses simple medical and anatomic terms.

Knowledge Objectives

1. Describe the importance of communication and documentation for emergency medical responders (EMRs). (p 74)
2. Describe the different types of equipment used by EMRs in voice, radio, telephone, and data systems. (pp 74–76)
3. Summarize the functions of radio communications during the following phases of a response:
   a. Dispatch (p 76)
   b. Response to the scene (p 76)
   c. Arrival at the scene (p 76)
   d. Update of responding emergency medical services (EMS) units (pp 76–77)
   e. Transfer of patient care to other EMS personnel (p 77)
   f. Postrun activities (p 77)
4. Describe the guidelines for radio communications. (p 78)
5. Discuss the techniques of effective verbal communication. (pp 78–80)
6. Describe the guidelines for effective communication with patients. (p 78)
7. Explain the skills that will help EMRs communicate with:
   a. Patients who are hard of hearing or deaf (pp 80–81)
   b. Patients who are visually impaired (p 81)
   c. Non–English-speaking patients (pp 81–82)
   d. Geriatric patients (p 82)
   e. Pediatric patients (p 82)
   f. Patients with a developmental disability (p 82)
   g. Patients displaying disruptive behavior (pp 82–83)
8. Explain the role of medical terminology. (p 83)
9. Describe the legal significance of documentation. (p 85)
10. List the items that EMRs should include in a patient care report to ensure proper documentation. (p 85)

Skills Objectives

1. Demonstrate proper radio communications. (p 78)
2. Demonstrate an understanding of the rules of communication with colleagues, patients, and bystanders as an EMS professional. (pp 79–80)
3. Demonstrate the techniques of successful cross-cultural communication. (p 80)
4. Demonstrate completion of a patient care report. (p 85)

Introduction

A vital part of your role as an emergency medical responder (EMR) involves communication and documentation. **Communication** is the transmission of information to another person. Effective communication is important during every phase of a call. The dispatcher must communicate the location and type of call to designated responders. As an EMR, you need to communicate with patients, bystanders, family members, dispatchers, and other members of the public safety community. After you have completed a call, you must document the condition of the patient and the treatment given to the patient. **Documentation** is the written or electronically reported portion of a patient care interaction. This chapter describes a variety of communications systems and techniques and provides guidelines for creating written documentation for patient care.

Data and Communications Systems

The purpose of a communications system is to send information from one location to another when it is impossible to communicate face-to-face. The results of using a communications system will be only as accurate as the information that is put into the system. As an EMR, you should have a basic idea of how your department's communications system works. Communications systems can be divided into two categories: those that transmit voice communications and those that transmit data.

Words of Wisdom

It is important for different agencies that are working together to have the ability to communicate with one another. This concept is called *interoperability*.

▶ Voice Systems

Voice communications systems transmit the spoken word from one location to another. The two types of voice systems most commonly used in public safety agencies are radio systems and telephone systems.

Radio Systems

Most EMRs use some type of radio communications system. It is important that you have a working knowledge of the basics of a radio communications system and that you understand how to properly operate the radio system used by your department. Radio communications are regulated by the Federal Communications Commission (FCC). A **channel** is an assigned frequency or frequencies used to carry voice and/or data communications.

Frequencies are assigned according to the function of your organization. EMRs who are part of a law enforcement agency are usually assigned different frequencies than EMRs who are part of a fire department.

Many public safety agencies use a **trunked communications system**, a computer-controlled radio system that allows the sharing of a few radio frequencies among a large group of users. Each functional group using the trunked system is assigned to a specific "talk group." Trunked systems permit more efficient use of the limited radio frequencies available to public safety agencies. These systems can transmit voice communications as well as other forms of digital communications. If your agency uses a trunked radio system, then you need to learn how to use it.

Several different types of radios exist. A **base station** is a powerful two-way radio that is located in a fixed place and attached to one or more antennas. Dispatchers use base stations to send and receive messages to and from the service area. A base station may be attached to several different antennas to reach all parts of a geographic service area. Base stations may be designed to transmit and receive on multiple frequencies. Some systems are designed so that different frequencies are used for different functions of communications.

A **mobile radio** is mounted in a vehicle, such as a fire truck, and draws electricity from the electrical system of the vehicle. It has an external antenna, which is usually mounted on the roof or cab of the vehicle. The operating console is mounted so the driver or passenger of the vehicle can conveniently operate the radio. Mobile radios can be used to send and receive voice messages and data.

A **portable radio** is a handheld, self-contained unit that includes a two-way radio with a battery, a built-in microphone, and a built-in antenna 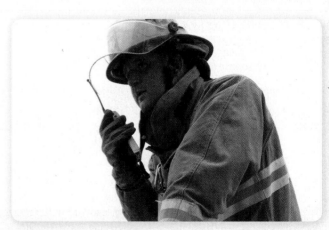 **Figure 5-1** . Most portable radios are capable of operating on multiple channels. One drawback of many portable radios is that the controls are small and hard to see in darkness; therefore, EMS providers who use these radios must become extremely familiar with the controls and operation. Portable radios are low-powered devices and are often

Figure 5-1 A portable radio.
© Jones & Bartlett Learning. Courtesy of MIEMSS.

used with a repeater system. A **repeater** is a device that receives a weak radio signal, strengthens that signal, and then automatically rebroadcasts it. Repeaters are used to cover geographic areas where radio signals are too weak for effective communications. These geographic areas are sometimes called *dead spots*.

Telephone Systems

Telephone systems primarily send voice communications. Public safety agencies may use phone systems to send dispatch information or to handle routine administrative communications. Landline phone systems are tied together through an above-ground or below-ground hardwired system. Mobile phones rely on radio waves between a mobile phone and a cellular tower to create and receive messages. Smartphones use advanced operating systems that combine the features of a cellular phone with those of a personal computer and global positioning systems (GPS).

▶ Data Systems

Communications systems are increasingly used to send and receive data through radios, phones, and the Internet. Many different types of data can be sent between EMS personnel and communications centers. Computer-generated routing information is an example of data that are useful for EMS personnel.

Paging systems can transmit text messages or voice communications. Pagers are radio receivers that are silent unless activated by a dispatcher. Some departments use paging systems to alert members to emergency incidents.

A **mobile data terminal (MDT)** transmits data messages through a radio system **Figure 5-2** and is frequently incorporated into a mobile radio system. MDTs reduce the amount of time the radio frequency is in use.

A **fax machine** is sometimes used to send written data or images over a phone or radio system. Some public safety providers use fax machines to transmit dispatch information. **Telemetry** is a process used by advanced life support providers to transmit electrocardiograms and other patient data to online medical control. Telemetry can operate through a phone system or through a radio system.

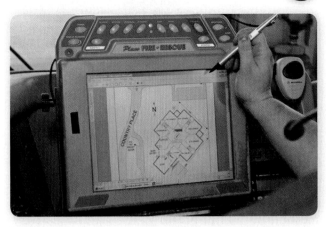

Figure 5-2 A mobile data terminal (MDT) can be used to display routing information transmitted from the dispatch center.
© Jones & Bartlett Learning. Courtesy of MIEMSS.

Digital messaging is technology that includes email, text messages, and social media, which are increasingly used by EMRs to send and receive information within public safety agencies. See your department for policies on the use of digital messaging. Remember, most patient information is confidential (see Chapter 4, *Medical, Legal, and Ethical Issues*, for more information).

As an EMR, you may not use all these types of communications in your department, but you should understand how various communications devices operate. It is more important for you to understand how to send and receive data than it is to understand how the system is built.

▶ The Functions of Radio Communications

Throughout the different phases of an EMS call, communications systems are used for different functions. Calls for medical assistance can be divided into six phases: dispatch, response to the scene, arrival at the scene, updating responding EMS units, transfer of patient care to other EMS personnel, and postrun activities. During these phases, it is important to communicate certain findings to other members of the EMS or public safety team.

YOU are the Provider   CASE 1

Soon after you start your shift at 0700 hours, you hear alert tones from the speaker and hear your dispatcher say, "Unit 433 respond to 85 Norwood Avenue for a 72-year-old woman who is experiencing severe chest pain." You acknowledge the call, verify the location, and begin to respond.

1. Why is it important to know how to operate your radio communications system?
2. Why is it important to use the patient's name, maintain eye contact with the patient, and use language the patient can understand?
3. Why is it important to learn how to communicate effectively with patients with special needs?

Dispatch

The function of dispatch can be accomplished using a phone system, a paging system, a fax, or a radio system. Dispatch may use voice, text messaging, or an MDT to alert you to an emergency. It is your responsibility to keep your equipment ready to receive a call whenever you are on duty. Listen carefully to voice messages to ensure that you receive the information correctly. If you are not sure that you have received all the dispatch information correctly, then ask the dispatcher to repeat it. If you receive dispatch information via an MDT, text message, or a fax, then you can refer to the message to verify the location and type of call.

Words of Wisdom

Phases of an EMS call:

1. Dispatch
2. Response to the scene
3. Arrival at the scene
4. Updating responding EMS units
5. Transfer of patient care to other EMS personnel
6. Postrun activities

Response to the Scene

To respond quickly and efficiently to the scene of an emergency, you need to know your response area. Learn how to use maps or GPS devices to help get you to the scene. Listen carefully to your dispatcher; he or she may be able to give you further information about the location of the call or the condition of the patient while you are en route. If you are delayed in responding to the incident (for example, because your vehicle will not start or you encounter traffic, a blocked railroad crossing, weather conditions, or other unexpected delays), then notify your dispatcher of the situation. Your message will enable the dispatcher to contact and send another unit to the same call if necessary 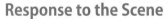 **Figure 5-3** .

Words of Wisdom

To ensure you take the fastest route, do not start responding to a call until you know where you are going.

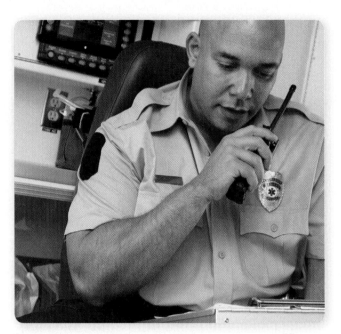

Figure 5-3 Notify your dispatcher if you encounter any problems while en route to the scene.
© Jones & Bartlett Learning. Courtesy of MIEMSS.

Arrival at the Scene

As you arrive at the scene, perform a scene size-up—which includes a visual survey or an overview of the incident and its surroundings (scene size-up is discussed further in Chapter 9, *Patient Assessment*). Your scene size-up of the entire incident gives you an impression of the overall situation, including the number of patients involved and the severity of their injuries. After you have performed a scene size-up, give the communications center a brief verbal description of the scene. For a simple call with one patient, your patient care report will be more concise than the report you deliver for a more complex call. Your report should verify the location of the incident, the type of incident, any hazards present, the number of patients, and any additional assistance required. Next, determine if you need to call for additional resources. It is better to request assistance and find you do not need it than to wait and then call for help after determining the need is urgent **Figure 5-4** .

▶ Update Responding EMS Units

In some EMS systems, you will be expected to update responding EMS units about the condition of your

YOU are the Provider CASE 2

You are dispatched to a middle school at 1117 hours on a Wednesday morning for a sick 12-year-old girl.

1. What additional information would be useful in helping you to get to the patient quickly?
2. List some ways that will help you to effectively assess and treat this patient.

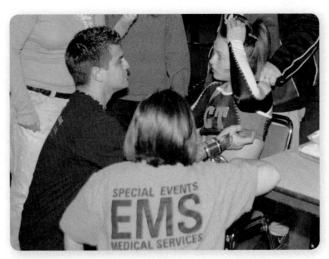

Figure 5-4 Arrival of an EMR at an emergency scene.
© Jones & Bartlett Learning. Courtesy of MIEMSS.

patient. Your report should include the age and sex of the patient; the chief complaint; the level of responsiveness; and the status of the patient's airway, breathing, and circulation. Let the responding EMS unit know what equipment you need brought in to the patient. By providing this update, you are helping other EMS units know what to expect when they arrive on the scene.

▶ Transfer of Patient Care to Other EMS Personnel

With many EMS incidents, you will be the first trained person to arrive on the scene. You will have performed a primary assessment and started some treatment before emergency medical technicians (EMTs) or paramedics arrive. When EMTs or paramedics arrive, it is important for you to provide them with a handoff report. Describe your findings concisely and accurately.

The easiest way to report your patient assessment results is to use the same systematic approach you follow during patient assessment (see Chapter 8, *Patient Assessment*, for more information):

1. Provide the age and sex of the patient.
2. Describe the history of the incident.
3. Describe the patient's chief complaint.
4. Describe the patient's level of responsiveness.
5. Describe how you found the patient.
6. Report the status of the patient's vital signs, airway, breathing, and circulation (including severe bleeding).
7. Describe the results of the physical examination.
8. Report any pertinent medical conditions using the SAMPLE (Signs and symptoms, Allergies, Medications, Pertinent past medical history, Last oral intake, and Events leading to injury or illness) format.
9. Report the interventions you provided and how the patient responded to them.

Working in a systematic manner as you assess the patient will help ensure that you do not overlook any significant symptoms, signs, or injuries. This process will help to make the handoff report complete and accurate.

EMTs and paramedics contact online medical control to secure permission to perform certain skills, to get direction regarding patient care, and to give the hospital their patient care reports. As an EMR, you may be present when other EMS providers contact the online medical control through their radio or cellular phone systems. In most EMS systems, EMRs are not required to contact medical control for the basic skills they are permitted to perform. If your EMS system uses online medical control for EMRs, then you will need to learn how and when to contact medical control.

▶ Postrun Activities

After you have turned over the care of the patient to other EMS providers, you need to report your status to your communications center. Let the communications center know how long it will take you to get your unit ready for service and when you will be available for another call. Providing a written report of a call is covered later in this chapter in the section on documentation.

The rules, or *protocols*, for communicating with others during each phase of an EMS call may vary from one system to another. Learn and follow the standard procedures and protocols of your department Table 5-1.

YOU are the Provider   CASE 3

After lunch, you are sent to a single motor vehicle crash. Dispatch reports that police officers are on the scene and only one patient requires medical attention. The driver was outside of the vehicle when police officers arrived. When you arrive on the scene, you park your vehicle in a safe position given the nature of the incident. As you are walking to the location of the crash, a second vehicle traveling down the road passes by you at a high rate of speed and collides with a tree. You see major damage to the front of the vehicle. Both front doors are damaged, and you are not sure if you can open them. Multiple air bags have deployed.

1. What should be your first action?
2. How many additional EMS units should you request?

Table 5-1	**Guidelines for Effective Radio Communications**

Monitor the channel before transmitting to avoid interfering with other radio traffic.

Plan your message before pushing the transmit switch. This step will keep your transmissions brief and precise. Use a standard format for your transmissions.

Press the push-to-talk (PTT) button on the radio, then wait for 1 second before starting your message. Otherwise, the first part of your message may be cut off before the transmitter is working at full power.

Hold the microphone about 2 to 3 inches (5 to 8 cm) from your mouth. Speak clearly and evenly, but never shout into the microphone. Speak at a moderate, understandable rate, in a clear, even voice.

Identify the person or unit you are calling first, then identify your unit as the sender. You will rarely work alone, so say "we" instead of "I" when describing yourself.

Acknowledge a transmission as soon as you can by saying "Go ahead" and then "Over and out" when you are finished (or whatever terminology is commonly used in your area). If you cannot take a long message, simply say "Stand by" until you are ready.

Use plain English. Avoid meaningless phrases ("Be advised"), slang, or complex codes. Avoid words that are difficult to hear, such as "yes" and "no." Use "affirmative" and "negative."

Be brief. If your message takes more than 30 seconds to send, pause after 30 seconds and say, "Do you copy?" The other party can then ask for clarification if needed. Also, the pause lets other EMS providers with emergency traffic to break through if necessary.

Avoid voicing negative emotions, such as anger or irritation, when transmitting. Courtesy is assumed, making it unnecessary to say "please" and "thank you," which wastes air time. Listen to other communications in your system to get a good idea of the common phrases and their uses.

When transmitting a number with two or more digits, say the entire number first and then each digit separately. For example, say "sixty-seven," followed by "six-seven."

Do not use profanity on the radio. It is a violation of FCC rules and can result in substantial fines and even loss of your organization's radio license.

Use EMS frequencies for EMS communications. Do not use these frequencies for any other type of communications.

Reduce background noise as much as possible. Move away from wind, noisy motors, or tools. Close the window if you are in a moving ambulance. When possible, shut off the siren during radio transmissions.

© Jones & Bartlett Learning.

Verbal Communication

As an EMS provider, you need to communicate effectively. Verbal communication is an essential part of providing high-quality patient care. Most verbal communication occurs through face-to-face conversations. Effective communication means that the person receiving the message understands exactly what the person who sent the message meant. This process requires feedback; the receiver needs to communicate to the sender that the message has been received and understood.

Both external and internal distractions can negatively affect your ability to communicate. External distractions include noise and the use of electronic devices. Internal distractions include letting yourself think about a personal matter while at the scene. Communication can also be affected if an EMR lacks empathy for a patient or shows prejudice against a certain type or group of people. Effective communication requires you to be patient and to think carefully about your interactions with others. To achieve effective patient communication, always maintain your composure, show empathy, and keep an open mind.

As an EMR, you should master certain communication skills that will enable you to communicate effectively with EMS personnel and other public safety providers, as well as the patient and his or her family. You must be able to determine what the patient needs and then explain this information to others. The following section includes guidelines for effective communication with patients. Most of these guidelines will also promote effective communication with other public safety personnel.

▶ Guidelines for Effective Communication With Patients

Your communication skills will be put to the test when you communicate with patients and/or family members in emergency situations. Remember that someone who is sick or injured is scared and might not understand what you are doing and saying. Therefore, your gestures, body movements, and attitude toward the patient are critically important in gaining the trust of both the patient and family. It cannot be stressed enough that maintaining your composure and showing that you care are a vital part of patient care during stressful situations. The following guidelines for communication will help you calm and reassure your patients.

Introduce Yourself

Introduce yourself by name and title. This gives the patient, family members, and bystanders an idea of who you are and lets them know your qualifications. Many citizens in your community may not understand that trained EMRs arrive in a variety of vehicles, including fire trucks, police vehicles, and private vehicles. Introducing yourself helps put the patient at ease and makes your job of assessing and treating the patient easier Figure 5-5 .

Ask the Patient's Name and Use It

Ask the patient what he or she wishes to be called. Knowing the patient's name helps you to establish contact with him or her. Use the patient's first name only if the patient is a child or the patient asks you to use his or her first name. For example, if a young man says his name is "Ron," then he probably wants to be called "Ron." Otherwise, use a courtesy title such as "Mrs. Smith" or "Mr. Jones." Avoid using terms such as "Pops" or "Dear;" these are disrespectful terms and many patients find them irritating.

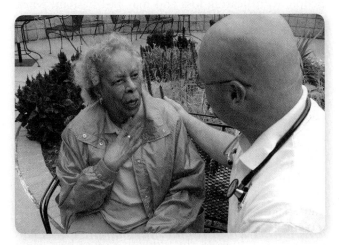

Figure 5-5 Introduce yourself by name and title.
© Jones & Bartlett Learning. Courtesy of MIEMSS.

Make and Keep Eye Contact

Look into the patient's eyes as you talk. Doing so shows the patient that you are focused on his or her needs and that you are speaking to the patient. Maintain eye contact as you listen to the patient. Emergency scenes can be noisy and confusing. By maintaining good eye contact, you help the patient focus on communicating with you.

Use Language the Patient Can Understand

Use language that is clear and accurate. Avoid using technical medical terms that may frighten or confuse the patient. It is disrespectful to talk down to a patient. Use feedback to determine whether the level of your language is appropriate for the patient.

Speak Slowly and Clearly

In the middle of an emergency call, it is easy for both you and patients to feel rushed. It is important for you to slow down and to speak in a clear voice. By slowing down and speaking clearly, you can avoid having to repeat questions and explanations. This will save you time in the long run and reduce communication errors.

Tell the Truth

It is important to tell patients the truth. Telling the truth helps build trust with a patient. If you fail to tell the truth, then the patient will not believe what you say in the future. There may be times when you do not need to tell the patient all the details in response to a question. There will also be times when you do not know the answer to a patient's question. In these cases, "I don't know" is an acceptable answer.

Allow Time for the Patient to Respond

Rushing a patient can negatively affect communication and delay the exchange of critical information. Because emergency situations can be hectic, use a calm approach. Patients who are sick or injured may be confused and may not be thinking clearly. Some patients may need time to answer even simple questions. Ask one question at a time and allow enough time for the patient to respond to each question.

Limit the Number of People Talking With the Patient

Designate one EMS provider to talk with the patient. This allows the patient to focus on the questions from one person. It avoids the confusion that results when multiple people are trying to question the patient at the same time. If other EMS providers have questions for the patient, then these questions can be addressed to the designated EMS provider.

Be Aware of Your Body Language

Your body language is a type of nonverbal communication. Do not talk down to a patient. If a patient is sitting or lying on the ground, then kneel down or position yourself to get close to the same level as the patient's face. Get close enough to the patient for comfortable conversation **Figure 5-6** . However, avoid getting so close that you invade the comfort zone of the patient. Pay attention to your stance. Crossing your arms in front of you may be interpreted by the patient as an uncaring attitude.

Act and Speak in a Calm, Confident Manner

Emergency scenes can be noisy, confusing, and frightening for patients. Remember that although the situation is not an emergency for you, the event taking place is an emergency for the patient. Your role is to give medical care that helps bring the emergency phase of this situation to an end. You need to convey a calm, caring, confident manner to the people present at the scene. Try to make the patient physically comfortable and relaxed.

Respect the Cultural Norms of the Patient

The actions that are considered respectful toward other people vary from one culture to another. Although it is impossible to learn the norms of all cultures, make an effort to learn the respectful actions toward the cultures that are represented within your community. Knowing which actions are acceptable and which actions are upsetting will enable you to give better care, make your job easier, and create a more positive relationship with these members of your community.

Use Open-Ended and Closed-Ended Questions Appropriately

When you must question patients to obtain information, structure your questions in one of two formats. The first type of question is an open-ended question, which

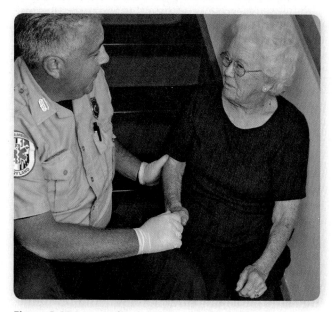

Figure 5-6 Be aware of body language. Get close enough to the patient to allow for comfortable yet respectful conversation.
© Jones & Bartlett Learning. Courtesy of MIEMSS.

allows a patient to answer in his or her own words. It helps you to get a sense of the patient's thoughts. An example of an open-ended question is, "Can you tell me what happened to you?"

The second type of question is a closed-ended question, which you can use when you are looking for specific information. Often, you will receive a "Yes" or "No" in response. An example of a closed-ended question is, "Does your arm hurt?"

Treat All Patients as if They Were Members of Your Family

Treat every patient the way you would like a member of your family to be treated. Remember that every patient you treat is someone's mother, father, sister, brother, daughter, or son. This guideline will help you communicate effectively with patients of all ages.

> **Treatment**
>
> Treat all patients as if they were members of your family.

▶ Communicating With Patients With Special Needs

Communicating with patients who have special needs requires additional considerations. Patients with special needs include patients who are hard of hearing or deaf, patients who are visually impaired, non–English-speaking patients, geriatric patients, pediatric patients, patients with a developmental disability, and patients displaying disruptive behavior.

Communicating With Patients Who Are Hearing Impaired

One of the major challenges you will face as an EMR is communicating with a person who is hard of hearing or deaf. Most people have few skills for interacting with people with hearing loss and may feel hesitant when asked to do so. A patient of any age may be unable to hear you for a variety of reasons: hereditary deafness; long-term hearing loss caused by illness, ear infections, or injury; or temporary deafness caused by an explosion or other loud noise. A patient with long-term hearing impairment usually develops skills to help compensate for the loss of hearing, such as the ability to read lips. A patient who is temporarily deaf does not have such skills.

In either case, your job is to address the medical needs of the patient. Ask, "Can you hear me?" A patient who is deaf may respond by pointing at his or her ear and shaking his or her head to suggest deafness. A patient who is temporarily deaf may feel anxious and panicky because he or she suddenly cannot hear. Help him or her focus on the issue by pointing at your ear and shaking your head to show the patient that you are trying to assess whether he or she can hear. Another option is to write out the question, "Can you hear?" on a piece of paper and show it to the patient.

After you determine the patient is hearing impaired or deaf, do not continue to rely on verbal communication; use other methods. A patient with long-term deafness may try to communicate with you by using sign language (using the hands and fingers to communicate). If you do not know sign language, then use writing and gestures to communicate.

As you examine the patient for injury, use your own body to show the patient how to inform you whether he or she has pain in a particular location. Touch a place on your body and make a face to show pain. Then look at the patient and repeat the step on the patient's body. Most people will understand what you are trying to do. Do a complete patient assessment on every patient, whether or not he or she can communicate with you.

Keep the patient informed by making gestures to show that certain things are happening (for example, when the ambulance arrives). Touching is an important part of communication and reassurance for patients who are hard of hearing or deaf, as well as for hearing patients. For example, hold the patient's hand so he or she knows you are there to help.

When working with patients who are hard of hearing or deaf, use the following techniques:

- Identify yourself by showing the patient your patch or badge.
- Touch the patient; a patient who is hard of hearing or deaf needs human contact just as much as a hearing patient.
- Face the patient when you speak so he or she can see your lips and facial expressions.
- Speak slowly and clearly; do not shout.
- Watch the patient's face for expressions of understanding or uncertainty.
- Repeat or rephrase your comments in clear, simple language.
- If all of these attempts at communication fail, then write down your questions and offer paper and a pencil to the patient to respond.
- Some people are both deaf and blind. This double loss may make it difficult for you to treat the patient. Take your time, be patient, and use touch as a way of communicating.

If the patient is a hearing child of parents who are deaf, then be sure to communicate with the parents about the child's condition and your actions. Like all parents in similar circumstances, parents who are deaf must consent for you to treat their child. They have a right to know what is being done and are just as upset as hearing parents would be. If the patient is a child who is deaf and has hearing parents, then you need to involve the parents even more than usual. They can assist you in communicating with the child.

If the patient is a parent who is deaf and has a hearing child, then resist the urge to use the child as an interpreter unless the child is obviously mature and capable. Young children cannot understand medical terminology, and misinterpretation can have serious results. Communicate directly with the patient, using whatever methods are most effective.

▶ Communicating With Patients Who Are Visually Impaired

During your initial overview of the scene, look for signs that suggest the patient may be visually impaired. These signs may include the presence of eyeglasses, a cane, or a service animal. As you approach, introduce yourself to the patient. If you think the patient is visually impaired, then ask, "Can you see?"

A patient who is visually impaired may feel vulnerable, especially during the chaos of an emergency scene. Explain what you are doing to the patient. Tell patients when they will feel movement or hear noise and explain any treatments they require. The patient may have learned to use other senses such as hearing, touch, and smell to compensate for the loss of sight. The sounds and smells of the scene may be disorienting. The patient may rely on you to make sense of everything. Tell the patient what is happening, identify noises, and describe the situation and surroundings, particularly if you must move the patient.

Learn the patient's name and use it throughout your examination and treatment, just as you would with a sighted patient. Touch the patient to provide emotional support. If the patient has a service animal such as a dog, then he or she may initially be more concerned about the dog than about his or her own injuries. Recognize that the dog and the patient are a unique team who depend on each other. Let the patient direct the dog or tell you how to handle the dog. Restate your question or redirect the patient's attention to the issue at hand. Service dogs are usually not aggressive; try to keep the patient and the dog together. If a patient who is visually impaired must be moved and can walk, then ask the patient to hold on to your elbow and stand slightly to your side and rear. Tell the patient about obstructions, steps, and curbs as you lead the way.

Do not make the mistake of talking louder when communicating with patients who are visually impaired. Visual impairment and hearing impairment are not related. When you have a patient who is visually impaired, it may be helpful to maintain physical or verbal contact with the person to let him or her know that you are still there.

▶ Communicating With Non–English-Speaking Patients

In many communities across the country, English is not the first or even the most common language. If your patient speaks a language other than English and you cannot understand each other, then you must find ways to communicate so you can meet your responsibility as an EMR to provide the appropriate standard of care. To achieve successful cross-cultural communication, you may be able to adapt some of the techniques recommended for communicating with a patient who is hard of hearing or deaf, such as hand gestures, finger-pointing, and facial expressions. Determine how much English the patient speaks and whether a family member or a friend can act as an interpreter.

If your jurisdiction has a large non–English-speaking population, then memorize common phrases and questions so you can use them when treating these patients. Your community may offer language assistance services that you can access by phone, an electronic device, or through the dispatcher.

> ### Special Populations
>
> If you encounter a non–English-speaking patient with whom you cannot communicate, then seek out a family member or friend to act as your interpreter.

▶ Communicating With Geriatric Patients

Older people tend to require EMS more frequently than younger people. As people age, they are more likely to experience both decreased vision and hearing. When you encounter older people who have hearing or visual impairment, use the same communication skills you would for any other patient with a similar condition. Do not assume all older patients have physical or mental impairments. Many older people are alert and healthy. Assess all patients carefully and give them time to respond to your questions. Be aware of how older patients respond to you; it may give you clues as to how best to communicate with them.

▶ Communicating With Pediatric Patients

Caring for ill or injured children is stressful for most EMS providers. Children are often frightened, anxious, and unable to communicate clearly; their parents or caregivers are usually frightened and anxious as well. Familiar objects and faces can help calm a child. Let a child keep a favorite doll, toy, or blanket to give the child some sense of comfort. Because children often take cues from their parents, use the parents to help you reassure and calm the child. Talk to both the parents and the child as much as possible and explain to them what is happening. Ask a parent to hold the child if the illness or injury permits.

Speak to the child in a professional yet friendly manner. Tell the child your first name and explain what you are doing. Try to reassure the child that you

are there to help in every possible way. Avoid standing over the child; instead, squat, kneel, or sit down so that you are on the child's level and establish eye contact Figure 5-7 . Ask the child simple questions about the pain, and ask for his or her help in pointing out any painful areas. Children can see through lies and deception, so be honest with them. You may be surprised at the remarkable level of understanding you can receive from an ill or injured child.

▶ Communicating With Patients With a Developmental Disability

You may find it difficult to communicate with patients who have a developmental disability. Ask the family or caregiver about the patient's typical level of communication. Speak slowly, using short sentences and simple words. You may need to repeat statements several times or to rephrase them until the patient understands what you want.

Again, offer emotional support by taking time to touch your patients. Because the chaos surrounding an injury or illness may confuse or frighten these patients, use extra care in dealing with patients with a developmental disability. You may be able to adapt many of the techniques recommended for communicating with children.

▶ Patients Displaying Disruptive Behavior

Disruptive behavior can present a danger to you, the patient, and other people at the scene and can cause delays in treatment. At some time in your career, you will encounter a person who challenges your patience and communication skills.

To manage any patient who acts in a disruptive way, take the following steps:

1. Assess the situation. Try to determine the cause of the patient's disruptive behavior.
2. Protect the patient and yourself.

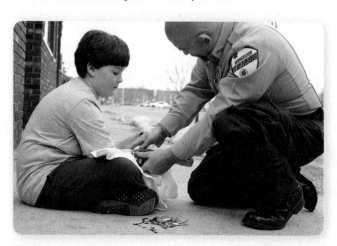

Figure 5-7 Squat, kneel, or sit when treating a pediatric patient.
© Jones & Bartlett Learning.

3. Stay between the patient and an exit whenever possible.
4. Do not take your eyes off the patient or turn your back.
5. If the patient has a weapon, then stay clear and wait for law enforcement personnel—no matter how badly injured the patient seems to be.
6. As soon as your personal safety is ensured, carry out the appropriate emergency medical care.

There may be times when you are unable to approach a patient; the person will not allow anyone to come near, despite all efforts to help. Sometimes family members or friends of the disruptive patient may insist that you take the person to the hospital, but EMS personnel cannot take a competent patient to the hospital against his or her expressed wishes (unless you are a law enforcement officer). Some frightened, agitated, drugged, or disruptive patients can cause serious injury to you, bystanders, or themselves. It is best to wait for assistance from law enforcement in these situations.

■ Medical Terminology

Medical terminology is a collection of technical terms used by medical personnel to identify anatomic parts of the body, specify illnesses and injuries, and indicate treatments. Medical terminology is intended to clarify language so that one person can communicate clearly to another. Using proper medical terminology allows you to communicate a clear message, avoid errors, and save time.

As an EMR, you are not expected to understand all the medical terminology used by a physician. Your job is to communicate your message to other medical providers as clearly as possible. Do not use medical terms if you are unsure of their meaning. It is much better to report that a patient is short of breath, gasping, and breathing at a rate of 32 breaths per minute than to try to remember the correct word for shortness of breath. Using the incorrect word will result in confusion.

The first few chapters have already introduced you to some medical terms. Chapter 6, *The Human Body*, will introduce you to many new terms. Note that a new word will be accompanied by a definition of the word.

As new terminology is introduced, look at the parts of each word. The center of a word contains the *stem* or *root*. There may be a *prefix* at the beginning of the word and a *suffix* at the end of the word. Each of these parts helps you to determine and remember the meaning of the word. By learning a few of these commonly occurring prefixes and suffixes, you will gain some insight into new words you encounter. For example, the prefix *hyper-* means above or excessive. *Hypertension* means excessive tension or pressure. Therefore, *hypertension* is the medical term for what we commonly call high blood pressure.

A list of some of the more commonly encountered prefixes is provided in **Table 5-2**. Learning these simple prefixes will help you to understand a significant number of medical terms. A list of additional medical terms and their definitions is available in Appendix A, *Medical Terminology*.

As you progress through the rest of this book, pay special attention to the medical terminology. When you see a new word, look for the root, the prefix, and the suffix. The medical terminology presented is designed to help you communicate more clearly. As you interview patients and relate information to other medical care providers, remember to communicate your thoughts as clearly as you can.

Table 5-2	Prefixes Commonly Used in Medical Terminology
Prefix	**Meaning**
Brady-	Slow
Tachy-	Rapid or swift
Therm-	In relation to quantities of heat
Hyper-	Above, excessive, or beyond
Hypo-	Below, underneath, or deficient
Naso-	Denoting the nose
Oro-	Denoting the mouth
Arterio-	Relationship to an artery
Cardio-	Heart
Hem-, hema-, hemo-	Blood
Neuro-	Denoting nerve, nervous system, or nervous tissue
Vaso-	Vessel, as in blood vessel

© Jones & Bartlett Learning.

YOU are the Provider   CASE 4

You are called to the home of an 85-year-old woman who reports chest pain. You arrive to find her sitting in a chair and leaning forward. She is sweating, struggling to breathe, and appears uncomfortable. You approach the patient, introduce yourself, and quickly realize she has hearing loss.

1. What techniques should you use to communicate with the woman?
2. As you gather information about her condition, the woman repeatedly asks, "Am I going to die?" How should you respond?

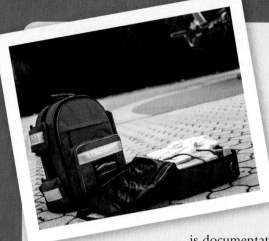

Voices *of* Experience

No matter what an EMR's public safety responsibilities are, documentation is one of his or her most important duties. Nowhere is documentation more important than when one responds to medical emergencies and renders patient care and/or transport.

My most humiliating moment in EMS was early in my career (over 30 years ago) when I was subpoenaed to our local state district court for a civil case concerning a motor vehicle crash that had happened several years earlier. Not only did I not remember anything about the incident, but my employer had lost the run report. Our testimony was brief and disappointing. My partner and I testified truthfully that we did not remember the case and that our run report had been lost. Everyone in the courtroom laughed at us. Everyone, that is, except the attorneys and the judge. We were quickly dismissed from the courtroom, after a serious scolding from the judge about our service's lack of professionalism.

> **" We were quickly dismissed from the courtroom, after a serious scolding from the judge about our service's lack of professionalism. "**

The courtroom is not the only place where documentation is important. First and foremost, the caregivers who receive the patient need to know the results of your assessments, your interventions, and how the patient responded. The trending of this information over a period of time is as important as the information itself.

In my current full-time position as EMS Licensing Program Manager for the State of Louisiana, I read a number of patient reports as part of complaint investigations. Every EMS complaint that my agency has investigated has been made or broken by the quality of documentation. Some seemingly insignificant fact is frequently omitted. I can't overemphasize the importance of completeness as well as accuracy and legibility. If something is missing in a patient contact report, then the legal assumption is that it was not done, *not* that you forgot to write it down. This is especially important when documenting patient assessments and interventions. If there is some legitimate reason that you deviated from protocol, or the standard of care, then it must be explained.

Therefore, I ask all EMRs to remember to document patient encounters accurately, completely, and legibly.

Steve Erwin, BS, NREMT-I/T, EMSI
Entergy Operations
River Bend Power Station
Louisiana

▪ Documentation

Documentation is the second major type of communication that you will use in your daily work as an EMR. Documentation is a process for verifying your actions using written records or computer-based (electronic) records ⟨**Figure 5-8**⟩. By recording the actions you took at an emergency incident, you provide a record for others and a document you can refer to in the future if necessary. Documentation is helpful to you because you will not be able to remember all the details of every call. It also provides a legal record for the actions you took. It is often said that if you did not document it, then it was not done. Documentation also provides a basis to evaluate the quality of care you gave. Remember, the call is not over until the paperwork is completed.

Proper documentation includes the following:

- The age and sex of the patient
- The history of the incident
- The condition of the patient when found
- The patient's description of the injury or illness
- The patient's chief complaint
- The patient's level of responsiveness
- The status of initial and subsequent vital signs: airway, breathing, and circulation (including severe bleeding)
- The results of the physical examination
- Pertinent medical conditions using the SAMPLE format (discussed in Chapter 8, *Patient Assessment*)
- The treatment you gave the patient
- Any change in the patient's condition after treatment
- The agency and personnel who took over treatment of the patient
- The following times: the time you were dispatched, the time you arrived on the scene, the time other EMS providers arrived on the scene, the time you departed the scene
- Any reportable conditions present
- Any infectious disease exposure
- Anything unusual about the situation
- Any other helpful facts

Include all these items in your handoff report. Complete your patient care report as soon as possible after each call. Your documentation should be clear, concise, and accurate. Follow the standards of your organization. Some agencies use a paper-based reporting system, whereas others use a computer-based (electronic) system. Each type of system works well, provided that you complete the reports accurately. If you make a mistake on the form, then draw a line through it and correct it.

Your organization may rely on patient care reports for documenting reportable events. As discussed in Chapter 4, *Medical, Legal, and Ethical Issues*, reportable events include certain infectious diseases and crimes such as knife wounds, gunshot wounds, motor vehicle collisions, suspected child abuse, domestic violence, elder abuse, dog bites, and rape. Learn which crimes are reportable in your area, your agency's procedures on reporting these crimes, and what you are required to do.

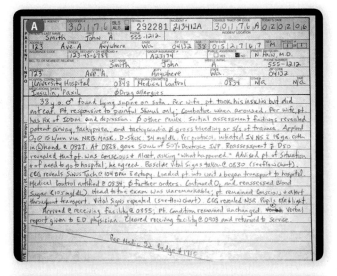

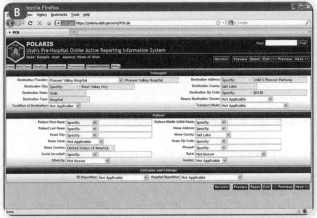

Figure 5-8 A. A paper-based run form. **B.** A wide variety of electronic equipment can also be used to document and maintain patient care records.

A: © Jones & Bartlett Learning. Courtesy of MIEMSS; B: Courtesy of the Utah Department of Health.

YOU are the Provider | SUMMARY

You are the Provider: CASE 1

1. Why is it important to know how to operate your radio communications system?

Your radio system is your primary way to communicate with your dispatcher, other public safety providers, and hospitals. You use it to direct you to emergency scenes, communicate your status to others, and call for additional help. It is important that you understand the day-to-day operations of your communications system and the special uses that are reserved for unusual circumstances. You cannot be an effective member of the EMS team without an efficient communications system.

2. Why is it important to use the patient's name, maintain eye contact with the patient, and use language the patient can understand?

In emergency situations, patients and family members are experiencing a high level of stress. Emergency scenes are often noisy and confusing and can be dark. These factors make effective communication difficult. Therefore, it is important to work hard to increase the effectiveness of your communication. Use the patient's name, maintain eye contact, and use language the patient can understand to enhance your communication and reduce the stress the patient is feeling.

3. Why is it important to learn how to communicate effectively with patients with special needs?

EMS personnel provide care to all the citizens of their community. It can be challenging to understand and communicate with patients with special needs. Therefore, it is helpful to learn how to handle the challenges presented by their special needs so you can provide the appropriate standard of care.

You are the Provider: CASE 2

1. What additional information would be useful in helping you to get to the patient quickly?

When responding to a large building that contains many rooms, it may be hard to locate a patient without further information. It is helpful to know which entrance to use when driving into a large complex, and you should know which building entrance is closest to the patient. Having someone at the front door to direct you to the patient can save valuable time. If this information is not given to you by the dispatcher, you can request the dispatcher to call back for further information.

2. List some ways that will help you to effectively assess and treat this patient.

This 12-year-old patient is a child who may think that she is approaching adulthood and may behave maturely for her age, or she may act as if she were a younger child. Remember to introduce yourself, ask the patient's name, and maintain good eye contact. Be sure to use clear language that the child can understand, but do not talk down to her. Let the patient know what you are going to do to prevent frightening her. Gather additional information about her illness from the patient and from the teacher or nurse who has been caring for her. Just as you would do with an adult patient, be aware of your body language and use open- and closed-ended questions appropriately.

You are the Provider: CASE 3

1. What should be your first action?

Your first action should be to call your dispatch center to report your initial assessment of the second collision and request sufficient EMS units to care for the number of patients needing care. In addition, evaluate the need for units to perform extrication, and make sure the scene of both collisions is being secured by law enforcement officers to prevent further accidents.

2. How many additional EMS units should you request?

In the early stages of an emergency, you may not know exactly how many resources will be needed. Therefore, give the dispatch center your best estimate of the number of injured patients and the severity of their injuries. It is better to err on the side of requesting more resources than you need, rather than not having enough emergency providers to treat and transport the patients. Responding units that are not needed can be canceled while en route to the scene.

You are the Provider: CASE 4

1. What techniques should you use to communicate with the woman?

Speak to the patient face-to-face so she can see your facial expressions and, perhaps, read your lips. Also, repeat your comments. If you are still having difficulty communicating, then use a sheet of paper to write questions.

2. As you gather information about her condition, the woman repeatedly asks, "Am I going to die?" How should you respond?

Always be honest and share relevant information with the patient. With this type of question, you should tell the woman you are doing everything you can to get her to the hospital safely.

Prep Kit

▶ Ready for Review

- Communications systems allow you to send information from one location to another when it is impossible to communicate face-to-face. Excellent communication skills are crucial during every phase of a call.
- It is important for you to have a basic idea of how your department's communications system works.
- The two types of voice communications systems are radio systems and telephone systems. As an EMR, you will use two-way radio communications, which include mobile and handheld portable radios. You must know when to use these devices and what type of information you can transmit.
- Throughout the different phases of an EMS call, communications systems are used for different functions. The six phases of an EMS call include dispatch, response to the scene, arrival at the scene, updating responding EMS units, transfer of patient care to other EMS personnel, and postrun activities.
- The protocols for communicating with others during each phase of an EMS call may vary from one system to another. Learn and follow the standard procedures and protocols of your department.
- In addition to radio and telephone communications, you must have excellent person-to-person communication skills. Be able to effectively interact with the patient and any family members, friends, or bystanders. Always maintain your composure, show empathy, and keep an open mind.
- Remember that people who are sick or injured may not understand what you are doing or saying. Therefore, your body language and attitude are important in gaining the trust of both the patient and the family. Take special care of patients such as children, geriatric patients, patients who are hearing impaired, patients who are visually impaired, non–English-speaking patients, patients with a developmental disability, and patients displaying disruptive behavior.
- Medical terminology is used to clarify language so that one provider can communicate to another the anatomic location of an injury, signs and symptoms of a disease, and treatment given. Do not use medical terms if you are unsure of their meaning.

- Along with your radio report and oral report, you must also complete a formal handoff report that will be given to other EMS professionals at the scene. Documentation provides a legal record of the actions you took and provides a basis to evaluate the quality of care given. Remember that the call is not over until the paperwork is completed.

▶ Vital Vocabulary

base station A powerful two-way radio that is permanently mounted in a communications center.

channel An assigned frequency or frequencies that are used to carry voice and/or data communications.

communication The transmission of information to another person.

digital messaging Technology that includes email, text messages, and social media, which are increasingly used by emergency medical responders to send and receive various types of information.

documentation The recorded portion of the emergency medical responder's patient interaction, either written or electronic.

fax machine A device used to send or receive printed text documents or images over a telephone or radio communications system.

mobile data terminal (MDT) A computer terminal mounted in a vehicle that sends and receives data through a radio communications system.

mobile radio A two-way radio that is permanently mounted in an emergency vehicle that draws electricity from the electrical system of the vehicle.

paging systems Communications systems used to send voice or text messages over a radio system to specially designed radio receivers.

portable radio A handheld, battery-operated, two-way radio.

repeater A radio system that automatically retransmits a radio signal on a different frequency.

telemetry A process in which electronic signals are transmitted and received by radio or telephone; commonly used for sending electrocardiogram tracings.

trunked communications system A computer-controlled radio system that allows the sharing of a few radio frequencies among a large group of users.

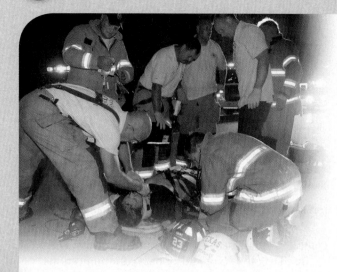

Assessment
in Action

At 2130 hours on a Thursday evening, you are dispatched to a residence for the report of a 2-year-old child who is having a seizure. The mother reports that the child seemed sick all day and is running a high fever. The residence is about 3 minutes from your location.

1. Which phase of an EMS call occurs immediately after an emergency call has been received at the dispatch center?

   A. Arrival at the scene
   B. Response to the scene
   C. Dispatch
   D. Transfer of patient care to other EMS personnel

2. Which of the following techniques will help you to communicate effectively with a pediatric patient?

   A. Stand up straight while talking to the patient.
   B. Use proper medical terminology.
   C. Kneel down to the level of the patient's face.
   D. Turn your back on the child while talking.

3. What should you do if you are unsure of the proper medical term used to describe your patient's illness or injury?

   A. Have the dispatcher look it up for you.
   B. Skip over that part of the transmission.
   C. Describe the illness or injury in plain English.
   D. Use slang terminology.

4. When you send patient information via a portable radio, communications should be:

   A. brief and concise.
   B. coded and scripted.
   C. spoken in a loud voice.
   D. unhurried, with long descriptions.

5. What agency has responsibility for regulating the use of your radio communications?

   A. Your state EMS agency
   B. Your local department
   C. Federal Communications Commission
   D. Department of Homeland Security

6. Your documentation of this call should include all of the following information EXCEPT:

   A. the age of the mother.
   B. the patient's chief complaint.
   C. the patient's level of consciousness.
   D. the results of the patient assessment.

7. Which of the following statements regarding your written documentation is true?

   A. It is a legal document.
   B. It cannot be used in a court of law.
   C. It must be destroyed after 1 year.
   D. It is used only for billing purposes.

8. Why is it important to introduce yourself to the patient using your name and title?

9. What are the six phases of an EMS call?

10. How might your communications change if the patient were a 78-year-old patient with hearing loss rather than a 2-year-old child?

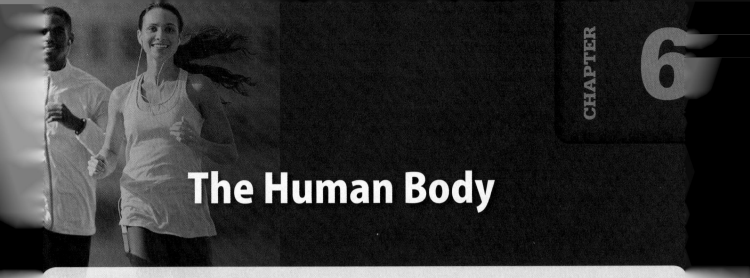

The Human Body

National EMS Education Standard Competencies

Anatomy and Physiology

Uses simple knowledge of the anatomy and function of the upper airway, heart, vessels, blood, lungs, skin, muscles, and bones as the foundation of emergency care.

Life Span Development

Uses simple knowledge of age-related differences to assess and care for patients.

Knowledge Objectives

1. Know the basic topographic anatomy terms to describe locations on the human body, including the anatomic position and the planes of the body. (p 90)
2. Discuss the anatomy and function of the respiratory system. (pp 91–92)
3. Discuss the anatomy and function of the circulatory system. (pp 92–93)
4. Identify the anatomy and function of the skeletal system. (pp 93–95)
5. Describe the anatomy and function of the muscular system. (pp 95–96)
6. Discuss the anatomy and function of the nervous system. (p 96)
7. Discuss the anatomy and function of the digestive system. (p 96)
8. Describe the anatomy and function of the genitourinary system. (p 97)
9. Name the three major functions of the skin. (p 97)
10. Describe the changes that occur during growth and development at different ages. (p 99)
11. Name the factors that can influence or change vital signs. (p 100)

Skills Objective

1. Identify selected topographic anatomy on a live or simulated patient. (p 90)

Introduction

To be an effective emergency medical responder (EMR), you must understand the basic structure and functions of the human body. This knowledge helps you better understand the specific location of symptoms the patient is experiencing, perform an adequate patient examination, communicate your findings to the other members of the emergency medical team, and provide proper emergency treatment for the patient's condition. This chapter discusses the human anatomy, the relationships among the eight body systems, and how the body changes as it ages.

Topographic Anatomy

The anatomic terms used in this section describe the location of injury or pain. You must know the basic anatomic terms for human body parts because all members of the emergency medical team must be able to speak the same language when treating a patient. However, if you cannot remember the proper anatomic term for a certain body location, you can use lay terms.

Visualize a person standing, facing you, with arms at the sides and thumbs pointing outward (palms toward you). This is the standard anatomic position; keep it in mind when describing a location on the body. **Figure 6-1** identifies **topographic anatomy**.

The first terms that should be clarified are left and right. These terms always refer to the patient's left and right, not yours. **Anterior** means front and **posterior** means back. The **midline** refers to an imaginary vertical line drawn from head to toe that divides the body into equal left and right sides.

Two other useful terms are medial and lateral. **Medial** means closer to the midline of the body; **lateral** means farther from the midline. In this context, the eyes are lateral to the nose.

The term **proximal** means close and **distal** means distant. On the body, proximal means close to the point where an arm or leg is attached. Distal means farther from the point of attachment. For example, if the thigh bone (femur) is broken, the break can be either

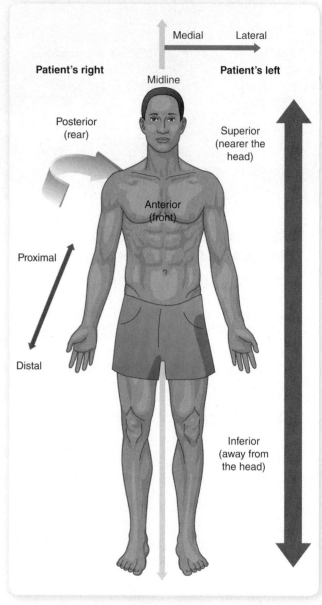

Figure 6-1 Topographic anatomy terms for describing a location on the body.
© Jones & Bartlett Learning.

proximal (the end closer to the hip) or distal (the end farther from the hip).

The term **superior** means closer to the head and **inferior** means closer to the feet. For example, the hips are inferior to the chest and the chest is superior to the hips.

YOU are the Provider   CASE 1

In the middle of the night you are dispatched to 114 Foster Center Road for a 69-year-old man reported as sick. As you arrive, the man's wife tells you her husband is having chest pains. As you begin to examine the patient, you notice a long scar down the middle of the man's chest. You ask him if he had a heart operation.

1. Why is some knowledge of anatomy and an understanding of the functions of body systems important in cases like this?

Body Systems

Body systems work together to perform common functions. By studying these body systems, you will have a better background for understanding and treating illnesses and injuries.

▶ The Respiratory System

Because airway maintenance is one of the most important skills you will learn as an EMR, the **respiratory system** is the first body system we will review.

The respiratory system consists of all the structures of the body that contribute to normal breathing **Figure 6-2**. The function of the respiratory system is to bring oxygen into the body and remove the waste gas, carbon dioxide.

The airway consists of the nose (nasopharynx), mouth (oropharynx), throat, **larynx** (voice box), trachea (windpipe), and the passages within the lungs **Figure 6-3**.

At the upper end of the larynx is a small flap of tissue called the **epiglottis**. The epiglottis keeps food from entering the larynx. The larger air passages of the lungs, or bronchi, branch into many narrower passages called bronchioles. The airway ends in tiny air sacs called alveoli. These air sacs are surrounded by tiny blood vessels called capillaries.

Oxygen in the inhaled air passes through the thin walls that separate the air sacs from the blood vessels and is absorbed by the blood. **Carbon dioxide**, a waste product of metabolism, passes from the blood across the same thin walls into the air sacs and is exhaled. This exchange of carbon dioxide for oxygen occurs 12 to 16 times per minute, 24 hours a day, without any conscious effort on your part **Figure 6-4**. The rate of breathing increases when the body needs more oxygen or when it generates additional carbon dioxide. Blood transports the inhaled oxygen to all parts of the body through the circulatory system.

Air is inhaled when the **diaphragm**, a large muscle that forms the bottom of the chest cavity, moves downward and the chest muscles contract to expand the size of the chest. Air is exhaled when these muscles relax, thus decreasing the size of the chest **Figure 6-5**.

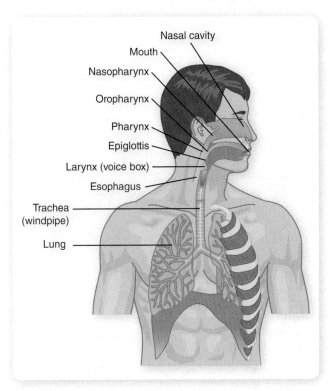

Figure 6-3 The airway.
© Jones & Bartlett Learning.

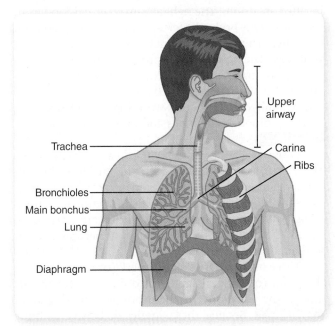

Figure 6-2 The respiratory system.
© Jones & Bartlett Learning.

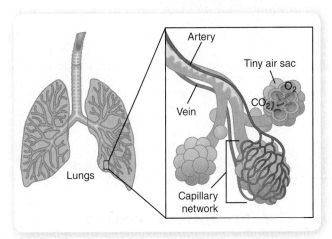

Figure 6-4 The exchange of carbon dioxide (CO_2) and oxygen (O_2) in the lungs.
© Jones & Bartlett Learning.

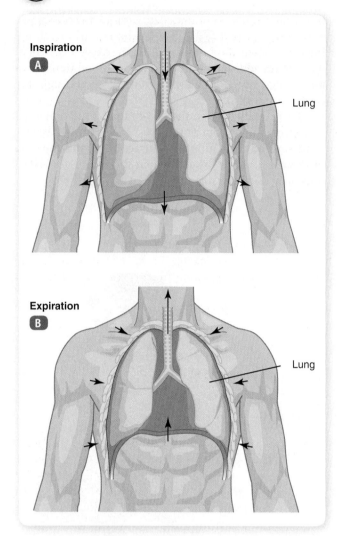

Figure 6-5 Mechanism of breathing. **A.** Diaphragm moves downward. **B.** Diaphragm relaxes.
A & B: © Jones & Bartlett Learning.

Special Populations

Infants and children have somewhat different respiratory systems than adults:

- A child's airway is smaller and more flexible. When you perform rescue breathing on a child, do not apply as much pressure as for an adult.
- Because a child's airway is smaller, it is more easily blocked by a foreign object.
- Infants can breathe only through their noses. Therefore, if an infant's nose becomes blocked, the infant will show signs of respiratory distress.

▶ The Circulatory System

The **circulatory system** is responsible for pumping and circulating blood through the body through a network of blood vessels. The circulatory system includes the heart, blood, and blood vessels Figure 6-6 .

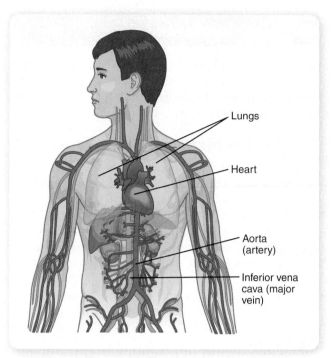

Figure 6-6 The circulatory system.
© Jones & Bartlett Learning.

After blood picks up oxygen from the lungs, it travels to the heart, which pumps it to the rest of the body. The cells of the body absorb oxygen and nutrients from the blood and release waste products (including carbon dioxide), which the blood carries back to the lungs and kidneys for removal. In the lungs, the blood exchanges the carbon dioxide for more oxygen, and the cycle begins again.

The human heart has four chambers: two on the right side and two on the left side. Each upper chamber is called an atrium. The right atrium receives blood from the veins of the body; the left atrium receives blood from the lungs. The bottom chambers are the right and left ventricles. The right ventricle pumps blood to the lungs; the left ventricle pumps blood throughout the body and is the most muscular chamber of the heart. The four chambers of the heart work together in sequence to pump blood to the lungs and to the rest of the body Figure 6-7 .

One-way check valves in the heart and the veins allow the blood to flow in only one direction through the circulatory system. The arteries carry blood away from the heart at high pressure and therefore have thick walls. The arteries closest to the heart are quite large (about 1 inch [2 cm] in diameter) but become smaller farther away from the heart.

Three major arteries are the neck (or carotid) artery, the groin (or femoral) artery, and the wrist (or radial) artery. The locations of these arteries are shown in Figure 6-8 . Because these arteries lie between a bony structure and the skin, they are used as locations to measure the patient's **pulse**, or the wave of pressure that is created by the heart as it forces blood into the arteries.

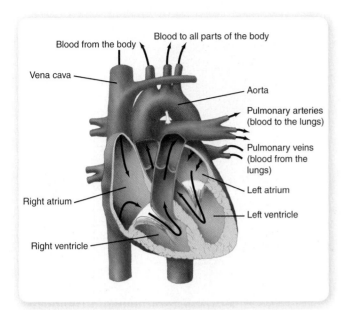

Figure 6-7 Schematic representation of the functions of the four chambers of the heart.
© Jones & Bartlett Learning.

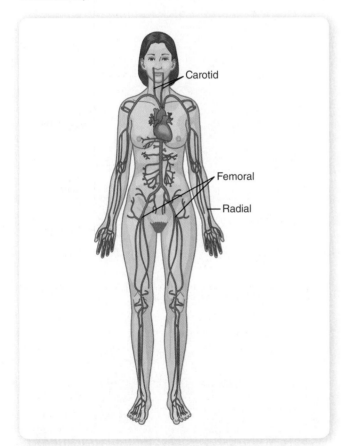

Figure 6-8 The location of the carotid, radial, and femoral pulses.
© Jones & Bartlett Learning.

The capillaries are the smallest vessels in the circulatory system. Some capillaries are so small that only one blood cell at a time can go through them. At the capillary level, oxygen and nutrients pass from the blood cells into the cells of body tissues, and carbon dioxide and other waste products pass from the tissue cells to the blood cells, which then return to the lungs.

Veins are the thin-walled vessels of the circulatory system that carry blood back to the heart.

Blood has several components: **plasma**, the clear, yellowish fluid part of the blood, red blood cells, white blood cells, and **platelets**, which are responsible for forming blood clots. Blood gets its red color from the red blood cells that carry oxygen from the lungs to the body tissue and bring carbon dioxide back to the lungs. The white blood cells are known as infection fighters because they devour bacteria and other disease-causing organisms.

▶ The Skeletal System

The skeletal system consists of bones and connective tissues that protect and support the framework for the body. The three main functions of the skeletal system are to:

1. Support the body.
2. Protect vital structures.
3. Produce red blood cells.

The skeletal system is divided into seven areas beginning with the skull **Figure 6-9** .

The Skull

The bones of the head include the **skull** and the lower jawbone. The skull consists of many bones fused together to form a hollow sphere that contains and protects the brain. The jawbone is a movable bone that is attached to the skull and completes the structure of the head.

The Spine

The spine consists of a series of 33 separate bones called **vertebrae**. The spinal vertebrae are stacked one on top of the other and are held together by muscles, **tendons** (cords that attach muscle to bone), disks, and **ligaments** (fibrous bands that connect bone to bone). The spinal cord, a group of nerves that carry messages to and from the brain, passes through the hole in the center of each spinal vertebra. The vertebrae provide excellent protection for the spinal cord. In addition to protecting the spinal cord, the spine is the primary support structure for the entire body. The spine has five sections **Figure 6-10** :

1. **Cervical spine** (neck)
2. **Thoracic spine** (upper back)
3. **Lumbar spine** (lower back)
4. **Sacrum** (base of spine)
5. **Coccyx** (tailbone)

The Shoulder Girdles

The **shoulder girdles** are the bones that connect the arms to the skeleton. Each shoulder girdle supports an arm and consists of the collarbone (clavicle), the shoulder blade (scapula), and the upper arm bone (humerus).

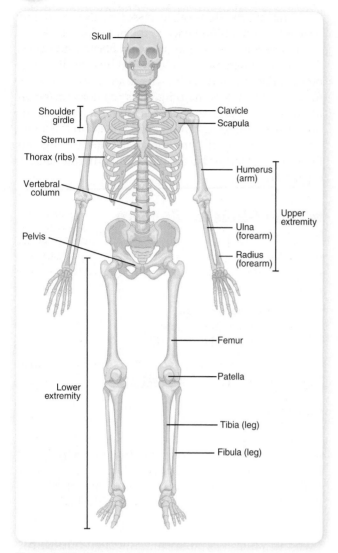

Figure 6-9 The human skeleton.
© Jones & Bartlett Learning.

The Upper Extremity

The upper extremity consists of three major bones. The upper arm has one bone (the **humerus**) and the forearm has two bones (the **ulna** and the **radius**). The radius is located on the thumb side of the arm, or lateral, and the ulna is located on the little-finger or medial side. The wrist and hand are part of the upper extremity and consist of several bones, whose names you do not need to learn at this time. You can consider these bones as one unit for the purposes of emergency medical treatment.

The Rib Cage

The fifth area of the skeletal system is the rib cage (chest). The twelve sets of **ribs** protect the heart, lungs, liver, and spleen. All of the ribs attach to the spine **Figure 6-11**. The upper five sets of ribs connect directly to the **sternum** (breastbone). The ends of the sixth through tenth rib sets are connected to each other and to the sternum by a bridge of **cartilage**. The eleventh and twelfth rib sets are attached to the spine but are not attached to the sternum in any way; they are called **floating ribs**.

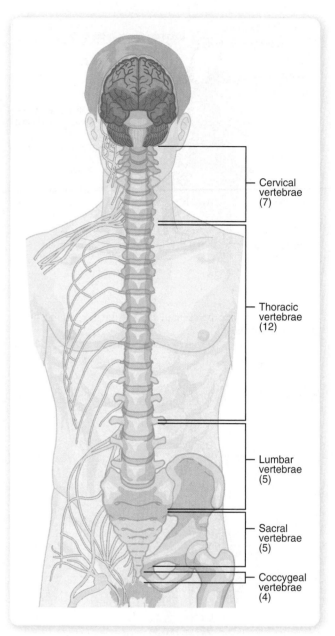

Figure 6-10 The five sections of the spine.
© Jones & Bartlett Learning.

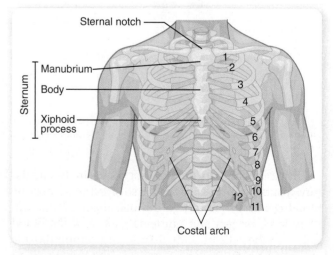

Figure 6-11 The rib cage.
© Jones & Bartlett Learning.

The sternum is located in the front of the chest. The pointed structure at the bottom of the sternum is called the **xiphoid process**.

The Pelvis

The **pelvis** is a closed bony ring that serves as the link between the body and the lower extremities. It protects the reproductive organs and the other organs located in the lower abdominal cavity.

You can see that a protective bony structure covers each of the essential organs of the body:

- The skull protects the brain.
- The vertebrae protect the spinal cord.
- The ribs protect the heart and lungs.
- The pelvis protects the lower abdominal and reproductive organs.

The Lower Extremity

The lower extremities consist of the thigh and the leg. The thighbone (femur) is the longest and strongest bone in the body. The leg has two bones, the tibia and fibula. The kneecap (patella) is a small, relatively flat bone that protects the front of the knee joint. Like the wrist and hand, the ankle and foot contain a large number of smaller bones that you can consider as one unit.

Words of Wisdom

When you describe the location of an injury or pain, it is more important that other EMS personnel clearly understand the site of the injury or pain than it is that you use exact anatomic terminology. Use the proper names when you can, but strive for accuracy over proper terminology.

Joints

At the point where two bones come in contact, a **joint** is formed. Supporting tissues called tendons and ligaments help to hold the joint together. Joints are lubricated by a thin fluid that is contained in a sac surrounding the joint.

There are three main types of joints. Fused joints do not permit any movement between the bone ends. The skull is an example of a fused joint. Hinge joints allow movement in one plane. The knee, elbow, and fingers are examples of hinge joints. Ball-and-socket joints allow movement in more than one plane. The shoulder and the hip are examples of ball-and-socket joints. **Figure 6-12** shows different types of joints.

Moveable joints are designed to permit a certain amount of movement. If movement occurs beyond these limits, injury and damage to the joint will occur.

▶ The Muscular System

The body contains three different types of muscles: skeletal, smooth, and cardiac. Skeletal muscle provides both support and movement. This muscle is attached to bone by tendons. This muscle causes movement by alternately contracting (shortening) and relaxing (lengthening). To move bones, skeletal muscles are

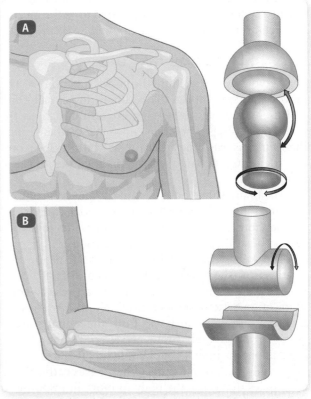

Figure 6-12 Different types of joints. **A.** The shoulder is a ball-and-socket joint. **B.** The elbow joints are hinge joints, which allow motion only in one plane.
A & B: © Jones & Bartlett Learning.

YOU are the Provider   CASE 2

At 1527 hours on a spring afternoon, you are dispatched to your local skateboard park for the report of an injured skateboarder. As you arrive, you find a 14-year-old boy sitting against a wall, cradling his right arm and moaning in pain. You notice that the lower part of his forearm is bent at an unnatural angle just above his wrist. As you examine the fingers on his right hand, he says they feel numb.

1. Given the location of the young man's injury, what body systems do you think may have been affected?
2. What purpose does the skeletal system serve?

usually paired in opposition: as one member of the pair contracts, the other relaxes. This mechanical opposition enables you to open and close your hand, turn your head, and bend and straighten your elbow. For example, when the biceps relaxes, an opposing muscle on the back of the arm contracts, straightening the elbow. Because skeletal muscles are under direct voluntary control of the brain and can be stimulated to contract or relax at will, they are also called *voluntary muscle*.

Smooth muscle carries out many of the automatic functions of the body, such as propelling food through the digestive system. You have no control over smooth muscle, so it is called *involuntary muscle*.

Cardiac muscle is found only in the heart, so this muscle is constantly working. It has a rich blood supply and can live only a few minutes without an adequate supply of oxygen.

The skeletal and muscular systems function together. The two systems combined are referred to as the musculoskeletal system.

▶ The Nervous System

The **nervous system** governs the body's functioning. The nervous system consists of the brain, the spinal cord, and the individual **nerves** that extend throughout the body Figure 6-13. The brain and spinal cord are called the *central nervous system*. The cables of nerve fibers outside the central nervous system are called the *peripheral nervous system*.

The brain is the body's central computer. It controls the functions of thinking, voluntary actions (things you do consciously), and involuntary (automatic) functions such as breathing, heartbeat, and digestion.

The spinal cord is a long, tube-like structure that extends from the base of the brain. It consists of a complex network of nerves that make up a two-way communication system between the brain and the rest of the body. Nerves branch out from the spinal cord to every part of the body. Some nerves send signals to the brain about the body—for example, whether it is feeling heat, cold, pain, or pleasure. Other nerves carry signals to muscles that cause the body to move in response to the sensory signals it has received. Without the nervous system, you would not have these sensations, nor would you be able to control the movement of your muscles.

▶ The Digestive System

The **digestive system** processes and breaks down food. It also absorbs the food's nutrients and carries them by the circulatory system to the cells of the body. Food that is not used is eliminated as solid waste from the body.

The major organs of the digestive system are located in the abdomen. The digestive tract is about 35 feet (11 m) long. It begins at the mouth and continues through the throat, esophagus (tube through which food passes), stomach, small intestine, large intestine, rectum, and anus. Besides the digestive tract, the digestive system also includes the liver, gallbladder, and pancreas Figure 6-14.

The liver performs several digestive functions, including the production of bile. Bile is stored in the gallbladder and released into the small intestine to help digest fats.

The pancreas also has several digestive functions. Probably its best-known function is the production of **insulin**. Insulin is released directly into the bloodstream and aids the body in its use of glucose. Diabetes mellitus is caused when insulin production is disrupted.

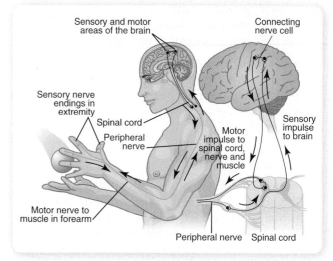

Figure 6-13 The nervous system.
© Jones & Bartlett Learning.

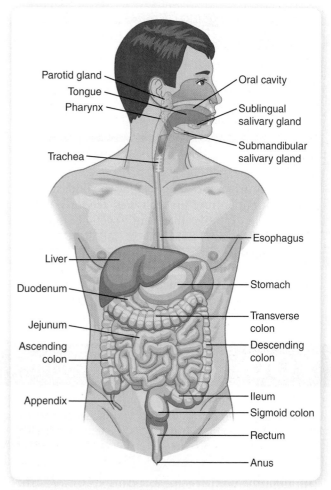

Figure 6-14 The digestive system.
© Jones & Bartlett Learning.

▶ The Genitourinary System

The **genitourinary system** includes the reproductive organs and the urinary system. It is responsible for sexual reproduction functions and for the removal of waste products from the bloodstream.

The major organs of the male reproductive system are the testes, which produce sperm, and the penis, which delivers sperm to fertilize the female egg. The major organs of the female reproductive system are the ovaries, which produce eggs, and the uterus, which holds the fertilized egg as it develops during pregnancy. The egg released by the ovaries travels to the uterus through the fallopian tubes. The external opening of the female reproductive system is called the birth canal (vagina).

The removal of waste products by the genitourinary system begins in the kidneys, which filter the blood to form urine. The urine flows down from the kidneys through tubes (ureters) into the bladder. The bladder collects and stores the urine before it passes out of the body through the urethra.

▶ Skin

Skin is the largest organ of the body. Skin covers all parts of the body and has three major functions:

1. Protects against harmful substances in the environment
2. Regulates body temperature
3. Transmits information from the outside environment to the brain

Figure 6-15 identifies the layers of the skin. The dermis is the deeper or inner layer of the skin. The prefix *epi-* means upon. Therefore the epidermis is the outer layer of skin that is located upon the dermis.

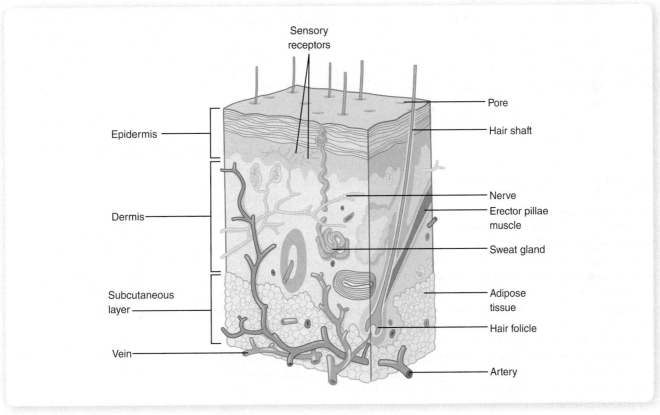

Figure 6-15 The skin.
© Jones & Bartlett Learning.

YOU are the Provider   CASE 3

Just before 1200 hours on an extremely hot summer day, you are sent to the home of a 74-year-old woman. She called 9-1-1 saying she was feeling weak. She tells you she was working in her garden for a couple of hours this morning, felt tired, and came back into her house about 2 hours ago. She states she felt weak and has not had much to eat or drink since she came back into her house. Her skin feels cool to your touch.

1. Why is it important to know how a person's body systems change in response to aging?
2. What part of the body helps regulate temperature?

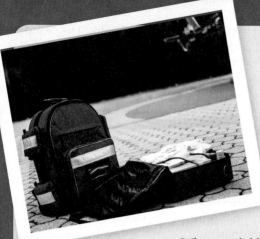

Voices *of* Experience

In 1982, when I completed my first responder course (now EMR), we did not learn a great deal about the human body. What we *did* learn, I thought was too much. I remember saying to a classmate, "Why do we have to learn all this stuff about the body? Who cares?" I only wanted to learn about how to fix the blood and gut injuries.

> **" As a young EMS provider eager to save the world, my first reaction was one of disappointment— he was *only* shot in the leg. "**

Not long after completing the course, my fire department was dispatched to a person who had been shot, and I then realized that everything I had learned about the human body was worth every minute of class time. We arrived to find a 20-something-year-old man on the ground, in a left lateral recumbent position. The patient was awake and alert, complaining of being shot in the leg. As a young EMS provider eager to save the world, my first reaction was one of disappointment—he was *only* shot in the leg. We completed our primary assessment and proceeded to our secondary assessment after we confirmed there were no obvious life threats. We were taught to look for entrance wounds and exit wounds when there was a penetrating injury. Our assessment revealed only an entrance wound behind (posterior) his left upper leg. We thought, "Hey, no big deal," except that this patient was quickly deteriorating and began to complain of left shoulder pain.

I remembered my instructor telling us that a gunshot entry wound without an exit wound means the bullet can be anywhere. Now we were thinking about the possible path of travel this bullet took and what organs might be affected. From its entrance point, we determined that the popliteal, femoral, or iliac artery may be damaged. If the bullet took an upward path, any organ in the abdominal cavity—especially the left lower and left upper quadrants—could be affected, yet the abdomen was soft and non-tender during the assessment. I remembered the diaphragm separated the abdominal and thoracic cavity, so the chest was our next thought. This patient was quickly becoming pale, his pulse was increasing, and his mental state was altered; all signs of shock (hypoperfusion). We decided the bullet could have injured the heart itself, the great vessels (aorta and vena cava), or the lungs. His breathing was rapid but he had equal chest rise.

Because we were unable to locate exactly what was affected, but we concluded that the patient was seriously injured, we placed him supine (flat on his back) on a long backboard and packaged him for transport as soon as the ambulance arrived. While awaiting the ambulance, we administered oxygen and maintained the patient's body temperature. When the ambulance arrived, they were able to leave immediately after our handoff report.

We later learned that the bullet had nicked the pericardial sac that surrounds the heart. The patient was taken into surgery and survived. Our knowledge of the human body, as little as it was, allowed us to quickly realize what the potential injuries might be and prepare this patient for immediate transport.

Guy Peifer, BS, NREMT-P, CIC, RF/PC
Paramedic Program Coordinator, Borough of Manhattan Community College
EMS Education Coordinator, Yonkers Fire Department
Yonkers, New York

Skin protects the body from the environment. Because skin provides an intact layer of cells that serves as a barrier to most foreign substances, it prevents harmful materials from getting into the body. The skin is an effective barrier to bacteria and viruses as long as it is not broken by injury.

Skin regulates the internal temperature of the body. If the body gets too hot, the small blood vessels close to the skin open up (dilate) and bring more body heat to the surface of the skin, where the heat is transferred to the air. Another source of cooling occurs when sweat released by the skin evaporates on the skin's surface. If the body becomes cold, the blood vessels near the skin surface constrict, transferring more body heat to the inside or core part of the body.

Skin receives information from the environment. The skin can perceive touch, pressure, and pain, and it can sense degrees of heat or cold. These perceptions are picked up by special sensors in the skin and transmitted through the nerves and the spinal cord to the brain. The brain serves as the computer to interpret these sensations.

■ Stages of Life—Growth and Development

The moment after birth, the body begins an ever-changing journey. As a person grows and develops, the body changes from being a tiny, fragile, totally dependent infant to a full-grown, independent adult. As the body then progresses through the natural aging process from adulthood to old age, there is a gradual decline in the functioning of all body systems.

Throughout a person's life, the body constantly changes. You need to know how these changes affect the treatment of your patients.

In an infant, the airway is very small and is easily obstructed by swelling or foreign bodies. At birth, infants can breathe only through their noses. Therefore, make sure their noses are not obstructed. Infants experience rapid heat loss, so keep them warm. Toddlers (aged 1 to 3 years) are unsteady and prone to explore. Their poor coordination and balance put them at a high risk for injuries from falls. School-aged children (6 to 12 years) lose their primary teeth, which are then replaced with permanent teeth. They are physically active and prone to injuries from bicycle riding and other athletic mishaps. Adolescents (13 to 18 years) test the limits of authority. They see themselves as invincible and do not fully understand the consequences of dangerous actions. During this period, most adolescents get their driving licenses. Inexperience and risk taking lead to higher incidences of motor vehicle crashes for young drivers.

Early adulthood (20 to 40 years) is the period when most body systems are fully developed. Most people enjoy good health during this period. Lifestyle issues such as drinking excess amounts of alcohol and drug abuse contribute to a higher incidence of injuries and illness. Middle adulthood (41 to 60 years) is generally the time when body systems start to decline. Vision and hearing become less acute. Cardiovascular and respiratory systems start to weaken. The incidence of a variety of cancers increases during this period. Women experience menopause during their late 40s and early 50s. Weight control becomes more difficult for most people during this period. During older adulthood (61 and older), the declines that started in middle adulthood become more pronounced. Respiratory and circulatory systems decline further. Most people in this age group experience some loss of bone strength, which makes them more prone to fractures. Many older people experience decreased sensation to heat and cold. Because of this, people in this age group are more prone to sustain burns. Many older adults have poor balance and decreased muscle tone. These factors contribute to a higher incidence of falls. The incidence of mental decline and senility increases in this age group.

Normal physiologic changes throughout a person's life result in an increased occurrence of certain illnesses and injuries at certain stages of life. By understanding these changes, you will be better prepared to provide quality care for your patients. Additional information about physiologic changes throughout life is presented in Chapter 9, *Patient Assessment*; Chapter 17, *Pediatric Emergencies*; and Chapter 18, *Geriatric Emergencies*.

YOU are the Provider   CASE 4

Early Saturday morning you are dispatched to a local soccer field for a 13-year-old boy injured during a soccer game. You can hear his screams as you are getting out of the ambulance. Family members are surrounding him on the field. You walk up and see that he is cradling his left arm with his right arm. His left shoulder is bruised and deformed.

1. What type of joint is involved and how does it work?
2. What impact would the child's injury have on his vital signs?

▶ Vital Signs

Measuring a patient's vital signs allows you to evaluate a variety of bodily functions. The most commonly measured vital signs are pulse (heart rate), respiration rate, and blood pressure. As an EMR, it is important for you to understand how to measure these vital signs. This skill will be covered in Chapter 9, *Patient Assessment*. It is also important for you to know the normal values for vital signs for infants (newborn to age 1 year), children (ages 1 to 12 years), and adults. The normal range of these vital signs is shown in Table 6-1.

Normal vital signs change with age. The normal pulse rate decreases with age. The normal pulse rate for infants is 90 to 180 beats/min. This rate drops to 60 to 100 beats/min for adults. Respiratory rates also decrease with age. The normal respiratory rate for infants is 25 to 60 breaths/min. This rate drops to 12 to 20 breaths/min for adults. The values for systolic blood pressure increase with age. The normal systolic blood pressure for infants is 50 mm Hg to 95 mm Hg. In adults, the blood pressure increases to 90 mm Hg to 140 mm Hg.

Significant variation in normal vital sign values exists within any age group. These variations are dependent on a person's size, his or her degree of physical conditioning, and the medications he or she takes. For example, the normal pulse rate for young adults is 60 to 100 beats/min. However, a long-distance runner or a competitive bicyclist in this age group may have a resting heart rate of 45 beats/min. A person of the same age who is out of shape and overweight may have a resting heart rate of 82 beats/min. Each of these values is normal for that person in his or her condition. Many factors can influence vital signs. Some factors increase certain vital signs and others decrease them. Table 6-2 lists some of the factors you should consider when assessing a patient's condition.

Words of Wisdom

Because it may be hard to remember the normal ranges of vital signs for each age group, many EMS agencies keep a list of these values available electronically or in their life support kits so their personnel can quickly refer to them when needed.

Table 6-1	Typical Vital Sign Values Based on Age		
Age	**Pulse Rate (Heart Rate) (beats/min)**	**Respirations (breaths/min)**	**Systolic Blood Pressure (mm Hg)**
Infants (newborn to age 1 year)	90–180	25–60	50–95
Children (ages 1 to 12 years)	70–150	15–30	80–110
Adults	60–100	12–20	90–140

Data from: American Heart Association. *2015 Guidelines for Cardiopulmonary Resuscitation and Emergency Cardiovascular Care*; Chameides L, Samson RA, Schexnayder SM, Hazinski MF, eds. *Pediatric Advanced Life Support Provider Manual*. Dallas, TX: American Heart Association; 2011.

Table 6-2	Factors That Can Change Certain Vital Signs	
Increase Pulse Rate, Respirations, and/or Systolic Blood Pressure	**Decrease Pulse Rate, Respirations, and/or Systolic Blood Pressure**
Exercise Fever Illness Pain Stress Excess body weight Abuse of illegal drugs	Athletic conditioning Blood pressure medications Abuse of illegal drugs

© Jones & Bartlett Learning.

YOU are the Provider

SUMMARY

You are the Provider: CASE 1

1. Why is some knowledge of anatomy and an understanding of the functions of body systems important in cases like this?

Having some knowledge of anatomy and the functions of body systems helps you better understand the source of an injury or illness and can improve the care you provide to the patient. Knowing the location of body organs and systems helps you to better determine the types of injuries or illnesses that are more likely to occur. Understanding anatomic terms and medical terminology helps you better communicate with other members of the medical care team. Using proper terminology will also help you avoid misunderstandings when sharing your assessment findings.

You are the Provider: CASE 2

1. Given the location of the young man's injury, what body systems do you think may have been affected?

Given the type of trauma the skateboarder experienced, the location of the injury, and your findings, you should suspect injury to his skeletal system, possible injury to his muscular system, possible injury to the nerves in his right forearm, and possible injury to some of the blood vessels around the injury site, even if there are no signs of external bleeding. In addition, it is important to examine the patient for additional injuries due to the type of trauma he suffered.

2. What purpose does the skeletal system serve?

The skeletal system protects vital structures, such as the spinal cord. It supports the body and produces red blood cells.

You are the Provider: CASE 3

1. Why is it important to know how a person's body systems change in response to aging?

When you are providing care for geriatric patients, it is important for you to know that as the body ages, its ability to sense heat and cold decreases. As a result, older adults tend to have difficulty maintaining a cool body temperature in hot weather, especially when they are exercising or are outside for a long period of time. In the winter time, older adults may have difficulty keeping warm and may wear more clothing than younger people.

2. What part of the body helps regulate temperature?

The skin regulates the internal temperature of the body. If the body gets too hot, blood vessels close to the skin dilate and bring body heat to the surface of the skin. The skin also releases sweat, which evaporates and promotes cooling. If older adults do not drink enough water, their body's cooling mechanism may not be able to keep their bodies cool. If the body becomes cold, blood vessels near the skin surface constrict, keeping heat in the body.

You are the Provider: CASE 4

1. What type of joint is involved and how does it work?

Joints are where two bones meet. The shoulder is a ball-and-socket joint, which allows movement in more than one plane. The hip is also a ball-and-socket joint.

2. What impact would the child's injury have on his vital signs?

Pain and stress are among the many factors that can influence a patient's vital signs. On the basis of the child's level of pain indicated by his screams, it would not be surprising if his blood pressure, pulse rate, and respiratory rate were higher than normal.

Prep Kit

▶ Ready for Review

- You need to know basic anatomic terms to understand the location of a patient's specific signs or symptoms and to better communicate with all members of the emergency medical team.
- The respiratory system consists of the lungs and the airway. This system functions to take in air through the airway and transport it to the lungs. In the lungs, red blood cells absorb the oxygen and release carbon dioxide so it can be expelled from the body.
- The circulatory system consists of the heart (the pump), the blood vessels (the pipes), and blood (the fluid). Its role is to transport oxygenated blood to all parts of the body and to remove waste products, including carbon dioxide.
- The skeletal system consists of the bones of the body. These bones function to provide support, to protect vital structures, and to produce red blood cells.
- The muscular system consists of three kinds of muscles: voluntary (skeletal) muscle, smooth (involuntary) muscle, and cardiac (heart) muscle. Muscles provide both support and movement. The skeletal system works with the muscular system to provide motion. These two systems together are called the musculoskeletal system.
- The nervous system consists of the brain, the spinal cord, and individual nerves. The brain serves as the central computer, and the nerves transmit messages between the brain and the body.
- The digestive system consists of the mouth, esophagus, stomach, intestines, liver, gallbladder, and pancreas. This system breaks down usable food for use by the body and eliminates solid waste.
- The genitourinary system consists of the organs of reproduction together with the organs involved in the production and excretion of urine.
- Skin covers the entire body. It protects the body from the environment, regulates the internal temperature of the body, and transmits sensations from the skin to the nervous system.
- You need a basic understanding of the body systems to treat the illnesses and injuries you will encounter as an emergency medical responder.
- An understanding of some of the changes that occur at different stages within the life cycle helps you to better treat the wide variety of patients you will encounter.
- Vital signs change at different stages of the life cycle. It is important for you to understand these changes so you understand the values you encounter in patients.

▶ Vital Vocabulary

anterior The front surface of the body.

carbon dioxide The gas formed as a waste product of metabolism and excreted through the respiratory system during exhalation.

cartilage A tough, elastic form of connective tissue that covers the ends of most bones to form joints; also found in some specific areas such as the nose and the ears.

cervical spine That section of the spinal column consisting of the seven vertebrae located in the neck.

circulatory system The heart and blood vessels, which together are responsible for the continuous flow of blood throughout the body.

coccyx The tailbone; the small bone at the base of the spinal column.

diaphragm A muscular dome that separates the chest from the abdominal cavity. Contraction of the diaphragm and the chest wall muscles brings air into the lungs; relaxation expels air from the lungs.

digestive system The gastrointestinal tract (stomach and intestines), mouth, salivary glands, pharynx, esophagus, liver, gallbladder, pancreas, rectum, and anus, which together are responsible for the absorption of food and the elimination of solid waste from the body.

distal Describing structures that are farther from the trunk (or torso) or nearer to the free end of an extremity. Opposite of proximal.

epiglottis The valve located at the upper end of the voice box that prevents food from entering the larynx.

floating ribs The eleventh and twelfth ribs, which do not connect to the sternum.

genitourinary system The organs of reproduction, together with the organs involved in the production and excretion of urine.

humerus The upper arm bone.

inferior Nearer to the feet than the head.

insulin A hormone produced by the pancreas that enables glucose in the blood to be used by the cells of the body; supplementary insulin is used in the treatment and control of diabetes mellitus.

joint The point where two bones come into contact.

larynx A structure composed of cartilage in the neck that guards the entrance to the windpipe and functions as the organ of voice; also called the voice box.

lateral Away from the midline of the body.

Prep Kit *Continued*

ligaments Fibrous bands that connect bones to bones and support and strengthen joints.

lumbar spine The lower part of the back formed by the lowest five nonfused vertebrae.

medial Closer to the midline of the body.

midline An imaginary vertical line drawn from the head to toe that divides the body into equal left and right sides.

nerves Fiber tracts or pathways that carry messages from the spinal cord and brain to all body parts and back; sensory, motor, or a combination of both.

nervous system The brain, spinal cord, and nerves.

pelvis The closed bony ring, consisting of the sacrum and the pelvic bones, that connects the trunk to the lower extremities.

plasma The clear, yellowish fluid of the blood that carries blood cells, transports nutrients, and removes cellular waste materials.

platelets Microscopic disk-shaped elements in the blood that are essential to the formation of a blood clot, the mechanism that stops bleeding.

posterior The back surface of the body.

proximal Closer to the trunk (or torso). Opposite of distal.

pulse The wave of pressure that is created by the heart when it contracts as a result of forcing the blood out and into the major arteries.

radius The bone on the thumb side of the forearm.

respiratory system All body structures that contribute to normal breathing.

ribs The paired arches of bone, 12 on either side, that extend from the thoracic vertebrae toward the anterior midline of the trunk.

sacrum One of three bones (sacrum and two pelvic bones) that makes up the pelvic ring; forms the base of the spine.

shoulder girdles The three bones of the upper extremity; each shoulder supports the clavicle, the scapula, and the humerus.

skull The bones of the head, collectively; the protective structure for the brain.

sternum The breastbone.

superior Closer to the head or above a body part.

tendons Tough, rope-like cords of fibrous tissue that attach muscle to bone.

thoracic spine The 12 vertebrae that attach to the 12 ribs; the upper part of the back.

topographic anatomy The superficial landmarks on the body that serve as location guides to the structures that lie beneath them.

ulna The bone on the little-finger side of the forearm.

vertebrae The 33 bones of the spinal column: 7 cervical, 12 thoracic, 5 lumbar, 5 sacral, and 4 coccygeal vertebrae.

xiphoid process The flexible cartilage at the lower tip of the sternum.

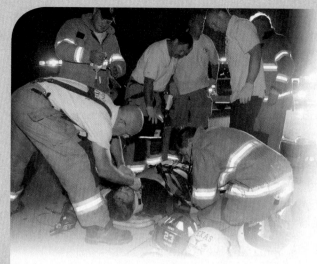

Assessment
in Action

You and your partner are dispatched to a downtown intersection where a 59-year-old woman has been struck by a school bus. As you examine the patient, you find bruising on the right side of her upper back and a small amount of blood coming from her hand. She is having difficulty breathing and reports pain in her abdomen. She also reports pain in her left leg just above her ankle. This area is discolored and appears deformed.

1. All of the following body system(s) may be affected from these injuries EXCEPT:

   A. respiratory system.
   B. circulatory system.
   C. digestive system.
   D. genitourinary system.

2. The blood from the patient's hand is most likely coming from the:

   A. arteries.
   B. veins.
   C. capillaries.
   D. aorta.

3. How would you describe the location of the injury to her lower extremity?

   A. Distal part of her thigh
   B. Proximal part of her thigh
   C. Proximal part of her leg
   D. Distal part of her leg

4. What part of the skeletal system is designed to protect the heart, lungs, and spleen?

   A. Spine
   B. Shoulder girdles
   C. Rib cage
   D. Vertebrae

5. The woman is now reporting numbness in her hands. What system may have been injured?

   A. Circulatory system
   B. Respiratory system
   C. Nervous system
   D. Genitourinary system

6. The normal respiratory rate for an adult is how many breaths per minute?

   A. 8 to 12
   B. 12 to 20
   C. 15 to 30
   D. 20 to 40

7. On the basis of the woman's injuries, what body system should you address first?

   A. Respiratory system
   B. Digestive system
   C. Nervous system
   D. Skeletal system

8. What is the significance of the patient's breathing difficulties?

9. What are the components that make up blood?

10. Why should you measure the patient's vital signs in this situation?

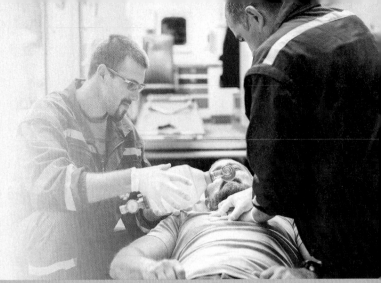

SECTION 2

Airway

Opener photo: © bluecinema/E+/Getty.

Airway Management

National EMS Education Standard Competencies

Airway Management, Respiration, and Artificial Ventilation

Applies knowledge (fundamental depth, foundational breadth) of general anatomy and physiology to assure a patent airway, adequate mechanical ventilation, and respiration while awaiting additional EMS response for patients of all ages.

Airway Management

Within the scope of practice of the EMR:

> Airway anatomy (pp 108–109)
> Airway assessment (p 111)
> Techniques of ensuring a patent airway (pp 111–114)

Respiration

> Anatomy of the respiratory system (pp 108–110)
> Physiology and pathophysiology of respiration (pp 108–110)
  • Pulmonary ventilation (pp 108–109)
  • Oxygenation (pp 108–110)
  • Respiration (pp 108–110)
    - External (pp 108–110)
    - Internal (pp 108–110)
    - Cellular (pp 108–110)
> Assessment and management of adequate and inadequate respiration (p 119)
> Supplemental oxygen therapy (pp 132–134)

Artificial Ventilation

Assessment and management of adequate and inadequate ventilation

> Artificial ventilation (pp 119–127)
> Minute ventilation (pp 108–109)
> Alveolar ventilation (pp 108–109)
> Effect of artificial ventilation on cardiac output (pp 108–109)

Pathophysiology

Uses simple knowledge of shock and respiratory compromise to respond to life threats.

Medicine

Recognizes and manages life threats based on assessment findings of a patient with a medical emergency while awaiting additional emergency response.

Respiratory

Anatomy, signs, symptoms, and management of respiratory emergencies including those that affect the:

> Upper airway (pp 119–132)
> Lower airway (pp 119–132)

Knowledge Objectives

1. Identify the anatomic structures of the respiratory system, including the function of each structure. (pp 108–110)
2. State the differences between the respiratory systems of infants, children, and adults. (p 110)
3. Explain how to check a patient's level of responsiveness. (p 111)
4. Describe how to perform the head tilt–chin lift maneuver. (p 111)
5. Describe how to perform the jaw-thrust maneuver. (pp 111–112)
6. Explain how to check for fluids, foreign bodies, or dentures in a patient's mouth. (p 112)
7. List the steps needed to clear a patient's airway using finger sweeps and suction. (pp 112–114)
8. Describe the steps required to maintain a patient's airway using the recovery position, oral airways, and nasal airways. (pp 114–117)
9. Describe the signs of adequate breathing, the signs of inadequate breathing, the causes of respiratory arrest, and the major signs of respiratory arrest. (p 119)
10. Describe how to check a patient for the presence of breathing. (p 119)
11. Describe how to perform rescue breathing using a mouth-to-mask device, a mouth-to-barrier device, mouth-to-mouth techniques, and a bag-valve mask. (pp 119–125)
12. List the steps for recognizing respiratory arrest and performing rescue breathing in infants, children, and adults. (pp 125–127)
13. Describe the differences between the signs and symptoms of a mild airway obstruction and those of a severe or complete airway obstruction. (pp 127–128)
14. List the steps in managing a foreign body airway obstruction in infants, children, and adults. (pp 128–132)
15. Describe the special considerations of airway care and rescue breathing in children and infants. (pp 126–127)
16. Describe the indications for using supplemental oxygen. (p 132)
17. Describe the equipment used to administer oxygen. (pp 132–133)

18. Describe the safety considerations and hazards of oxygen administration. (pp 133–134)
19. Explain the steps in administering supplemental oxygen to a patient. (pp 133–134)
20. Describe the function and operation of a pulse oximeter. (pp 134–135)
21. List the special considerations needed to perform rescue breathing in patients with stomas. (pp 135–136)
22. Define gastric distention. (p 136)
23. Describe the hazards that dental appliances present during the performance of airway skills. (p 136)
24. Describe the steps in providing airway care to a patient in a vehicle. (p 136)

Skills Objectives

1. Demonstrate how to check a patient's level of responsiveness. (p 111)
2. Demonstrate the head tilt–chin lift maneuver for opening blocked airways. (p 111)
3. Demonstrate the jaw-thrust maneuver for opening blocked airways. (pp 111–112)
4. Demonstrate how to check for fluids, solids, and dentures in a patient's airway. (p 112)
5. Demonstrate how to correct a blocked airway using finger sweeps and suction. (pp 112–114)
6. Demonstrate how to place a patient in the recovery position. (p 115)
7. Demonstrate the insertion of oral and nasal airways. (pp 115–117)
8. Demonstrate how to check for the presence of breathing. (p 119)
9. Demonstrate how to perform rescue breathing using a mouth-to-mask device, a mouth-to-barrier device, mouth-to-mouth, and a bag-valve mask. (pp 119–125)
10. Demonstrate the steps in recognizing respiratory arrest and performing rescue breathing on an adult, a child, and an infant. (pp 125–127)
11. Demonstrate the steps needed to remove a foreign body airway obstruction in an infant, a child, and an adult. (pp 128–132)
12. Demonstrate administration of supplemental oxygen using a nasal cannula and a nonrebreathing mask. (pp 133–134)
13. Demonstrate the operation of a pulse oximeter. (pp 134–135)
14. Demonstrate rescue breathing on a patient with a stoma. (pp 135–136)
15. Demonstrate airway management on a patient in a vehicle. (p 136)

■ Introduction

This chapter introduces the two most important lifesaving skills: airway care and rescue breathing. To survive, patients must have an open airway and must maintain adequate breathing. By learning and practicing the simple skills in this chapter, you can often make the difference between life and death for a patient.

This chapter begins with a review of the major structures of the respiratory system. After you learn the functions of these structures, you will have the base knowledge you need to become proficient in performing airway care and rescue breathing skills.

The skills of airway care and rescue breathing are as easy as A and B—the *A* stands for airway, and the *B* stands for breathing. Because you must assess and correct the airway before you turn your attention to the patient's breathing status, it is helpful to remember the AB sequence. (Note: In Chapter 8, *Professional Rescuer CPR*, the letter *C* will be added to this sequence for the assessment and correction of the patient's circulation. Airway, breathing, and circulation are known together as the ABCs. As you will learn, in the case of an unresponsive patient who may be in cardiac arrest, you should check the patient's circulation first before checking the airway and breathing. This CAB sequence minimizes the time to the beginning of compressions.)

A second mnemonic that will be used throughout both this chapter and Chapter 8 is "check and correct." This two-step sequence will help you remember the steps needed to check and correct problems involving the patient's airway, breathing, and circulation.

The *A*, or airway, section presents airway skills, including how to check a patient's level of consciousness (responsiveness) and manually correct a blocked airway by using the head tilt–chin lift and jaw-thrust maneuvers. You must check the patient's airway for foreign objects. If you find a foreign object blocking the airway, you must remove the object by using either a manual technique or a suction device. You will learn when and how to use oral and nasal airways to keep the patient's airway open.

The *B*, or breathing section, describes how to check patients to determine whether they are breathing adequately. You will learn how to correct breathing problems by using four rescue breathing techniques: mouth-to-mask, mouth-to-barrier device, bag-valve mask (BVM), and mouth-to-mouth. You will learn the indications for using supplemental oxygen and how to administer it using a nasal cannula and a nonrebreathing mask.

You will also learn how to check patients to determine whether they have an airway obstruction. Such respiratory blockages can cause death in only a few minutes. You will learn how to correct this condition using manual techniques that require no special equipment.

Remember that patients with airway problems will likely be extremely anxious during the episode. It is your responsibility as an emergency medical responder (EMR) to treat these patients and their families with compassion while you provide care.

As you study this chapter, remember the check-and-correct process for both airway and breathing skills. Do not forget that the airway and breathing skills presented in this chapter will be performed with circulation skills in Chapter 8. After you have learned the airway, breathing, and circulation skills, you will be able to perform **cardiopulmonary resuscitation (CPR)**. CPR is used to save the lives of people who are experiencing cardiac arrest (stoppage of the heart).

Anatomy and Function of the Respiratory System

To maintain life, all organisms must receive a constant supply of certain substances. In humans, these basic life-sustaining substances are food, water, and **oxygen**. A person can live several weeks without food because the body can use nutrients it has stored. Although the body does not store as much water, it is possible to live several days without fluid intake. However, lack of oxygen, even for a few minutes, can result in irreversible damage and death.

The most sensitive cells in the human body are located in the brain. If brain cells are deprived of oxygen and nutrients for 4 to 6 minutes, they begin to die. Brain death is followed by the death of the entire body. Brain cells cannot be replaced once they are destroyed, which is why it is important for you to understand the anatomy and function of the respiratory system and the critical role it plays in supporting life.

The main purpose of the respiratory system is to provide oxygen and to remove carbon dioxide from the red blood cells as they pass through the lungs. This action forms the basis for your study of the lifesaving skill of CPR.

The parts of the body used in breathing are shown in Figure 7-1 and include the mouth (**oropharynx**), the nose (**nasopharynx**), the throat (**pharynx**), the **trachea** (windpipe), the lungs, the diaphragm (the muscle between the chest and the abdomen), and numerous chest muscles (including the intercostal muscles). Air enters the body through the nose and mouth. In an unconscious patient lying on his or her back, the passage of air through both nose and mouth may be blocked by the tongue Figure 7-2 .

The tongue is attached to the lower jaw (**mandible**). When a person has a loss of consciousness, the jaw relaxes and the tongue falls backward into the rear of the mouth, effectively blocking the passage of air from both the nose and the mouth to the lungs. A partially blocked airway often produces a snoring sound. At the back of the throat are two passages: the **esophagus** (the tube through which food passes) and the trachea. The epiglottis is a thin flapper valve that allows air to enter the trachea but helps prevent food or water from entering the airway. Air passes from the throat to the larynx (voice box), which can be seen externally as the Adam's apple in the front of the neck. Below the trachea, the **airway** divides into the **bronchi** (two large tubes supported by cartilage). The bronchi branch into smaller and smaller airways in the **lungs**. The lungs are located on either side of the heart and are protected by the sternum at the front of the body and by the rib cage at the sides and back (Figure 7-1).

The smaller airways that branch from the bronchi are called bronchioles. The bronchioles end as tiny air sacs called **alveoli**. The alveoli are surrounded by very small blood vessels, the **capillaries**. The actual exchange of gases takes place across a thin membrane that separates the capillaries of the circulatory system from the alveoli of the lungs Figure 7-3 . The incoming oxygen passes from the alveoli into the blood, and the outgoing carbon dioxide passes from the blood into the alveoli. The exchange of oxygen and carbon dioxide that occurs in the alveoli is called **alveolar ventilation**. The amount of air pulled into the lungs and removed from the lungs in 1 minute is called **minute ventilation**.

When a patient is not breathing, artificial ventilation is necessary to supply oxygen to the heart and the rest of the body. During CPR, the blood being pushed out of the heart (cardiac output) depends on the oxygen supplied by artificial ventilation.

YOU are the Provider   CASE 1

At 1943 hours you are dispatched to an apartment complex for the report of a 67-year-old woman who is sick. While you are responding to the scene, your dispatcher informs you that the patient's husband states the woman is now unresponsive. When you arrive at the apartment, the patient's husband tells you his wife became dizzy shortly after taking a new medicine ordered by her physician. You approach the woman and ask if she can hear you. She does not respond. You gently shake the patient's shoulder and get no response.

1. What is the next step you should take to assess and treat this patient?
2. How would your method of opening the patient's airway change if the patient had fallen or blacked out?
3. What techniques can you use to maintain an open airway?

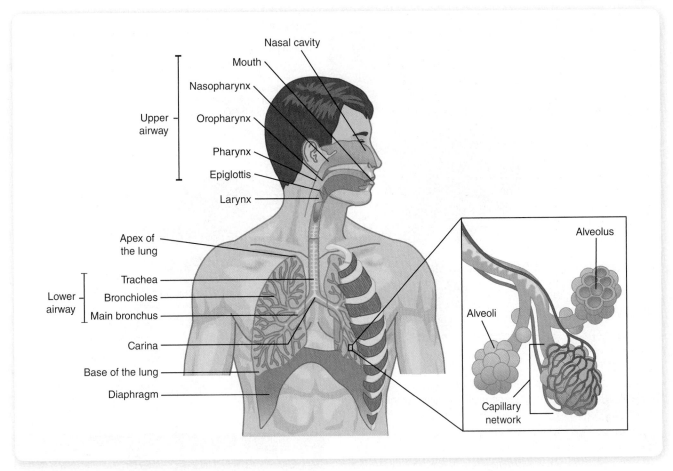

Figure 7-1 Anatomy of the respiratory system.
© Jones & Bartlett Learning.

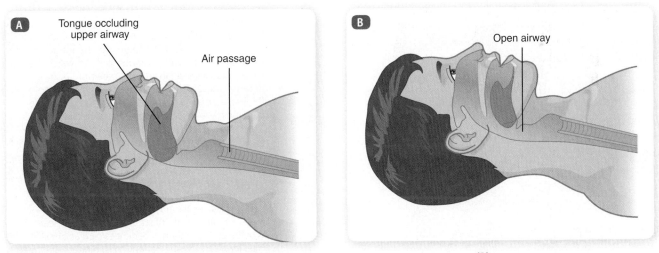

Figure 7-2 In an unconscious patient, the airway may be blocked by the tongue **(A)** or an open airway **(B)**.
A&B: © Jones & Bartlett Learning.

The lungs consist of soft, spongy tissue with no muscles. Therefore, movement of air into the lungs depends on movement of the rib cage and the diaphragm. As the rib cage expands, air is drawn into the lungs through the trachea. The diaphragm, a muscle that separates the abdominal cavity from the chest, is dome shaped when it is relaxed. When the diaphragm contracts during inhalation, it flattens and moves downward. This action increases the size of the chest cavity and helps draw air into the lungs through the trachea. On exhalation, the diaphragm relaxes and once again becomes dome shaped. In normal breathing, the combined actions of the diaphragm and the rib cage automatically produce adequate inhalation and exhalation **Figure 7-4** .

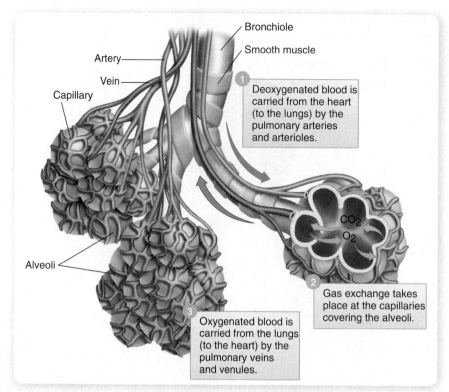

Figure 7-3 The exchange of gases occurs in the alveoli of the lungs.
© Jones & Bartlett Learning.

Labels in figure:
Bronchiole
Smooth muscle
Artery
Vein
Capillary
Alveoli
CO_2
O_2

1 Deoxygenated blood is carried from the heart (to the lungs) by the pulmonary arteries and arterioles.

2 Gas exchange takes place at the capillaries covering the alveoli.

3 Oxygenated blood is carried from the lungs (to the heart) by the pulmonary veins and venules.

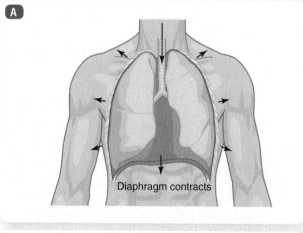

A Diaphragm contracts

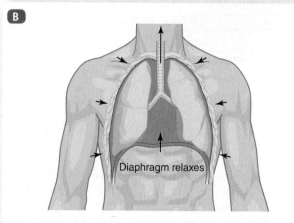

B Diaphragm relaxes

Figure 7-4 Normal mechanical act of breathing. **A.** Inhalation. **B.** Exhalation.
A&B: © Jones & Bartlett Learning.

Special Populations

- The structures of the respiratory system in children and infants are smaller than they are in adults. Therefore, the air passages of children and infants may be more easily blocked by secretions or by foreign objects.
- In children and infants, the tongue is proportionally larger than it is in adults. Therefore, the tongue of these smaller patients is more likely to block the airway than it would in an adult patient.
- Because the trachea of an infant or child is more flexible than that of an adult, it is more likely to become narrowed or blocked than that of an adult.
- The head of a child or an infant is proportionally larger than the head of an adult. You will learn slightly different techniques for opening the airways of children.
- Children and infants have smaller lungs than adults. You need to give them smaller breaths when you perform rescue breathing.
- Most children and infants have healthy hearts. When a child or infant experiences cardiac arrest, it is usually because the patient has a blocked airway or has stopped breathing, not because there is a problem with the heart.

■ A Is for Airway

The patient's airway is the pipeline that transports life-giving oxygen from the air to the lungs and transports the waste product, carbon dioxide, from the lungs to the air. In healthy people, the airway automatically stays open.

An injured or seriously ill person, however, may not be able to protect the airway and it may become blocked.

If a patient cannot protect his or her airway, you must take certain steps to check the condition of the patient's airway and correct the problem to keep the patient alive.

▶ Check for Responsiveness

The first step you will take in assessing a patient's airway is to check the patient's level of responsiveness. When you first approach a patient, you can immediately determine whether the patient is responsive (conscious) or unresponsive (unconscious) by asking, "Are you okay? Can you hear me?" **Figure 7-5** . If you get a response, you can assume the patient is conscious and has an open airway.

If you do not get a response, grasp the patient's shoulder and gently shake the patient. Then repeat your questions. If the patient still does not respond, you can assume the patient is unconscious and you will need more help. Before doing anything for the patient, call 9-1-1 if the emergency medical services (EMS) system has not already been activated, especially if you are the only rescuer. Position the patient by supporting the patient's head and neck and placing the patient on his or her back.

Treatment

The steps in airway assessment are as follows:

1. Check for responsiveness.
2. Correct the blocked airway using the head tilt–chin lift or jaw-thrust maneuver.
3. Check the airway for fluids, foreign bodies, or dentures.
4. Correct the airway using finger sweeps or suction if a foreign body is seen.
5. Manually maintain the airway with an oral or nasal airway, or place the patient in the recovery position (explained later in this chapter).

▶ Correct the Blocked Airway

An unconscious patient will not be able to keep his or her airway open. An unconscious patient's airway is often blocked (occluded) because the tongue has dropped back and is obstructing it. In this case, simply opening the airway with the head tilt–chin lift or jaw-thrust maneuver may enable the patient to breathe spontaneously.

Head Tilt–Chin Lift Maneuver

To open a patient's airway using the **head tilt–chin lift maneuver**, place one hand on the patient's forehead and place the fingers of your other hand under the bony part of the lower jaw near the chin. Push down on the forehead and lift up and forward on the chin **Figure 7-6** . Be certain you are not merely pushing the mouth closed when you use this maneuver.

Follow these steps to perform the head tilt–chin lift maneuver:

1. Place the patient on his or her back and kneel beside the patient.
2. Place one hand on the patient's forehead and apply firm pressure backward with your palm. Move the patient's head back as far as possible.
3. Place the tips of the fingers of your other hand under the bony part of the lower jaw near the chin.
4. Lift the chin forward to help tilt back the head.

Jaw-Thrust Maneuver

The **jaw-thrust maneuver** is another way to open a patient's airway. If a patient was injured in a fall, diving mishap, or motor vehicle crash and has a suspected neck injury, tilting the head may cause permanent paralysis. If you suspect a neck injury, first try to open the airway using the jaw-thrust maneuver. Open the airway by placing your fingers under the angles of the jaw and pushing upward. At the same time, use your

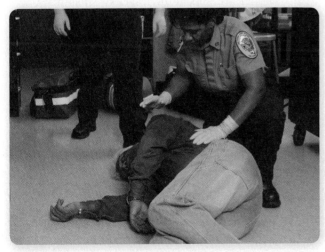

Figure 7-5 Establish the level of consciousness.
© Jones & Bartlett Learning. Courtesy of MIEMSS.

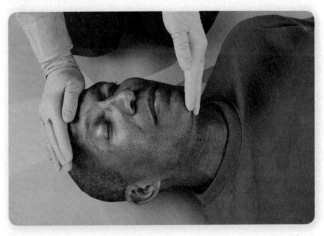

Figure 7-6 Open the patient's airway using the head tilt–chin lift maneuver.
© Jones & Bartlett Learning.

thumbs to open the mouth slightly. The jaw-thrust maneuver should open the airway without extending the neck **Figure 7-7**.

Follow these steps to perform the jaw-thrust maneuver:

1. Place the patient on his or her back and kneel at the top of the patient's head. Place your fingers behind the angles of the patient's lower jaw and move the jaw forward with firm pressure.
2. Tilt the head backward to a neutral or slight sniffing position. Do not extend the cervical spine in a patient who has sustained an injury to the head or neck.
3. Use your thumbs to pull down the patient's lower jaw, opening the mouth enough to allow breathing through the mouth and nose.

If you are unable to open the patient's airway using the jaw-thrust maneuver, try the head tilt–chin lift maneuver as a secondary attempt to open the patient's airway.

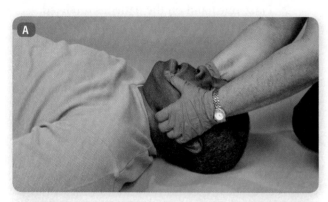

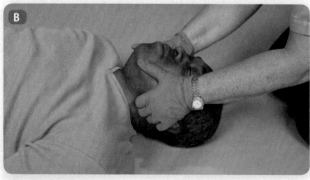

Figure 7-7 The jaw-thrust maneuver should open the patient's airway without extending the neck. **A.** Kneeling above the patient's head, place your fingers behind the angles of the lower jaw and move the jaw upward. Use your thumbs to help position the lower jaw. **B.** The completed maneuver should look like this.
A&B: © Jones & Bartlett Learning. Courtesy of MIEMSS.

Safety

Take standard precautions whenever you may be in contact with body secretions that might contain blood.

▶ Check for Fluids, Foreign Bodies, or Dentures

After you have opened the patient's airway by using either the head tilt–chin lift or the jaw-thrust maneuver, look in the patient's mouth to see if anything is blocking the patient's airway. Potential blocks include secretions, such as vomitus, mucus, or blood; foreign objects, such as candy, food, or dirt; and dentures or false teeth that may have become dislodged and are blocking the patient's airway. If you find anything in the patient's mouth, remove it by using one of the techniques noted in the following sections. If the patient's mouth is clear, consider using one of the devices described in the section on airway devices.

▶ Correct the Airway Using Finger Sweeps or Suction

You must clear vomitus, mucus, blood, and foreign objects from the patient's airway. You can accomplish this step by using finger sweeps, suctioning, or by placing the patient in the recovery position.

Finger Sweeps

Finger sweeps can be done quickly and require no special equipment except a set of medical gloves. Finger sweeps should be your first attempt at clearing the airway even if suction equipment is available. To perform a finger sweep, follow the steps in **Skill Drill 7-1**:

1. Turn the patient onto his or her side **Step 1**.
2. Insert your gloved fingers into the patient's mouth **Step 2**.
3. Curve your fingers into a C-shape and sweep them from one side of the back of the mouth to the other side **Step 3**. Scoop out as much of the foreign material as possible. A gauze pad wrapped around your gloved fingers may help remove the obstructing materials. Repeat the finger sweeps until you have removed all the foreign material in the patient's mouth.

Suctioning

Sometimes a finger sweep is not enough to clear the materials completely from the patient's mouth and upper airway. Suction machines can be helpful in removing secretions such as vomitus, blood, and mucus from the patient's mouth. Two types of suction devices are available: manual and mechanical. Suctioning the airway (either manually or mechanically) is a lifesaving technique. Although a gauze pad and your gloved fingers can do most of the work, the use of supplementary suction devices enables you to remove a greater amount of obstructing material from the patient's airway.

Skill Drill 7-1

Clearing the Airway Using Finger Sweeps

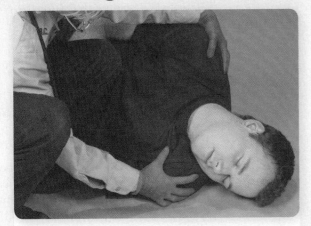

Step 1 Turn the patient onto his or her side.

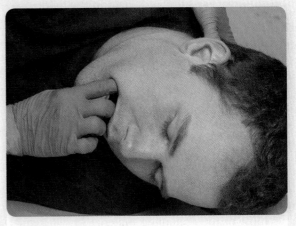

Step 2 Insert your fingers into the patient's mouth.

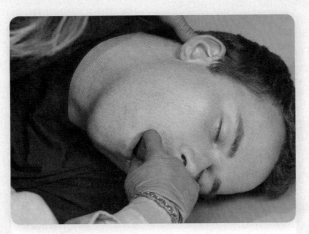

Step 3 Curve your fingers into a C-shape and sweep them from one side of the back of the mouth to the other side.

© Jones & Bartlett Learning. Courtesy of MIEMSS.

Safety

If the possibility of a spinal cord injury exists, log roll the patient onto his or her side and keep the head, neck, and spine aligned. Open the mouth and use your gloved fingers in the same manner to clean out the mouth.

Manual Suction Devices. Several manual suction devices are available to EMRs **Figure 7-8**. These devices are relatively inexpensive and are compact enough to fit into your life support kit. With most manual suction devices, you insert the end of the suction tip into the patient's mouth and squeeze or pump the hand-powered pump. Be sure that you do

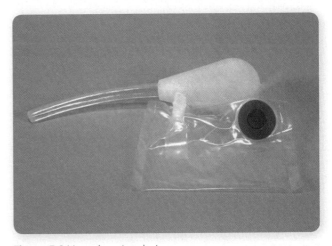

Figure 7-8 Manual suction device.
© Jones & Bartlett Learning. Courtesy of MIEMSS.

not insert the tip of the suction device farther than you can see. Manual suction devices are used in the same way as the mechanical suction devices described in the following section. The only difference is the power source. Follow local medical protocols on authorization to use suction devices in the field.

Mechanical Suction Devices. A **mechanical suction device** uses either a battery-powered pump or an oxygen-powered **aspirator** to create a vacuum that will draw the obstructing materials from the patient's airway **Figure 7-9** . Usually, both a rigid suction tip and a flexible whistle-tip catheter can be used with mechanical suction devices. To use this type of suction machine, you must first learn how to operate the device and control the force of the suction. When using mechanical suction, first clear the patient's mouth of large pieces of material with your gloved fingers. After the mouth is clear, turn on the suction device and use the rigid tip to remove most of the remaining material **Figure 7-10** . Do not suction for more than 15 seconds at a time because the suction draws air out of the patient's airway, as well as any obstructing material. If the rigid tip has a suction control port (a small hole located close to the tip's handle), place a finger over the hole to create the suction. Do not keep your finger over this control port for longer than 15 seconds at a time because you may rob the patient of oxygen.

Safety

Do not suction any deeper than you can see into the patient's mouth.

After you have cleared most of the obstructing material out of the patient's mouth and upper airway with the rigid tip, change to the flexible tip and clear out material from the deeper parts of the patient's throat **Figure 7-11** . Flexible whistle-tip catheters also have

suction control ports, which are located close to the end of the catheter that attaches to the suction machine. Again, place a finger over the control port to achieve suction.

Special Populations

- Do not suction a child's airway longer than 10 seconds at a time.
- Do not suction an infant's airway longer than 5 seconds at a time.

▶ Maintain the Airway

If your patient is unable to keep his or her airway open, you must open the airway manually by using the head tilt–chin lift or jaw-thrust maneuver. You can continue to keep the airway open by holding the patient's head to maintain the head tilt–chin lift or the jaw-thrust position.

If the patient is breathing adequately, you can keep the airway open by placing the patient in the recovery position. You can also insert an oral or nasal airway adjunct to maintain the patient's airway after you have opened it manually.

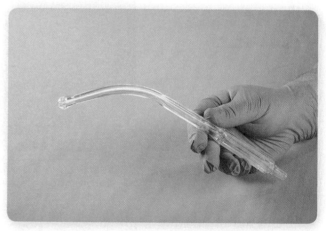

Figure 7-10 Rigid suction tip.
© Jones & Bartlett Learning.

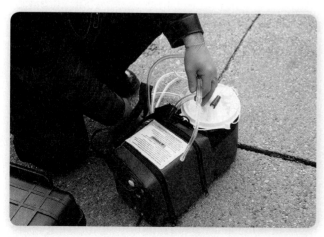

Figure 7-9 Battery-powered suction device.
© Jones & Bartlett Learning.

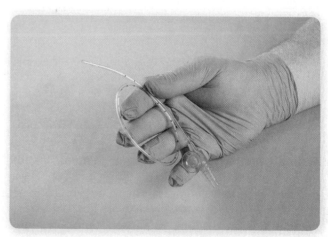

Figure 7-11 Flexible suction catheter.
© Jones & Bartlett Learning.

▶ Recovery Position

If an unconscious patient is breathing and has not sustained trauma, one way to keep the airway open is to place the patient in the recovery position **Figure 7-12**. The recovery position helps keep the patient's airway open by allowing secretions to drain out of the mouth instead of draining into the trachea. It also uses gravity to help keep the patient's tongue and lower jaw from blocking the airway.

To place a patient in the recovery position, carefully roll the patient onto one side, while you support the patient's head. Roll the patient as a unit without twisting the body. You can use the patient's hand to help hold his or her head in the proper position. Place the patient's face on its side so any secretions drain out of the mouth. The head should be in a position similar to the tilted-back position of the head tilt–chin lift maneuver.

▶ Airway Adjuncts

This section discusses the indications for the use of oral airways and nasal airways and the steps required for the proper insertion of each.

Oral Airway

An **oral airway**, also called an oropharyngeal airway, has two primary purposes: It maintains the patient's airway after you have manually opened the airway, and it functions as a pathway through which you can suction the patient **Figure 7-13**. You can use oral airways for unconscious patients who are breathing or who are in **respiratory arrest** (sudden stoppage of breathing). You can use an oral airway in any unconscious patient who does not have a **gag reflex**. You cannot use oral airways in conscious patients because they have a gag reflex. These airways can be used with mechanical breathing devices such as the **pocket mask** or a **bag-valve mask (BVM)**.

Two styles of oral airways are available: One style has an opening down the center, and the other has a slot (or opening) along each side. The slot permits the free flow of air and allows you to suction through the airway. Before you insert the oral airway, you need to select the proper size. Choose the proper size by measuring from the earlobe to the corner of the patient's mouth. When properly inserted, the airway will rest inside the mouth. The curve of the airway should follow the contour of the tongue. The flange should rest against the lips. The other end should be resting in the back of the throat.

Follow these steps to insert an oral airway **Skill Drill 7-2**:

1. Select the proper size airway by measuring from the patient's earlobe to the corner of the mouth **Step 1**.
2. Open the patient's mouth with one hand after manually opening the patient's airway with either a head tilt–chin lift or jaw-thrust maneuver.
3. Hold the airway upside down with your other hand. Insert the airway into the patient's mouth and guide the tip of the airway along the roof of the patient's mouth, advancing it until you feel resistance **Step 2**.
4. Rotate the airway 180° until the flange comes to rest on the patient's teeth or lips **Step 3**.

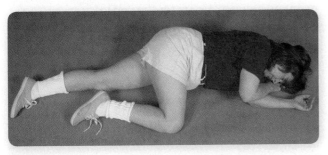

Figure 7-12 Recovery position for an unconscious patient.
© Jones & Bartlett Learning. Courtesy of MIEMSS.

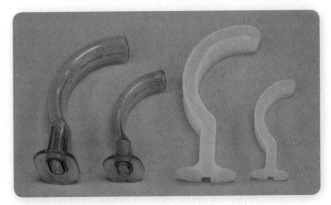

Figure 7-13 Oral airways.
© Jones & Bartlett Learning. Courtesy of MIEMSS.

Skill Drill 7-2

Inserting an Oral Airway

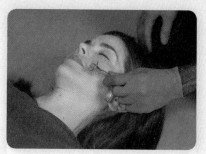

Step 1 Size the airway by measuring from the patient's earlobe to the corner of the mouth.

Step 2 Insert the oral airway upside down along the roof of the patient's mouth until you feel resistance.

Step 3 Rotate the airway 180° until the flange comes to rest on the patient's lips and teeth.

© Jones & Bartlett Learning. Courtesy of MIEMSS.

Be especially careful when you insert the airway. You could injure the roof of the patient's mouth by the rough insertion of an oral airway. Remember, an oral airway does not open the patient's airway. It will maintain the open airway after you have opened it with a manual technique.

Special Populations

The roof of a child's mouth is more fragile than that of an adult, so be especially careful to avoid injuring it as you insert the oral airway. The technique for inserting an oral airway in a child is almost the same as for an adult patient. However, to make it easier to insert the airway, use two or three stacked tongue blades and depress the tongue. This method will press the tongue forward and away from the roof of the mouth so you can insert the airway.

Nasal Airway

A second type of device you can use to keep the patient's airway open is a **nasal airway**, also called a nasopharyngeal airway [Figure 7-14]. This device is inserted into the patient's nose. You can use nasal airways in both unconscious and conscious patients who are unable to maintain an open airway. Usually a patient will tolerate a nasal airway better than an oral airway. It is not as likely to cause vomiting. One disadvantage of a nasal airway is that you cannot suction through it because the inside diameter of the airway is too small for the standard whistle-tip catheter suction tip.

You will have to select the proper size nasal airway for the patient. Measure from the earlobe to the tip of

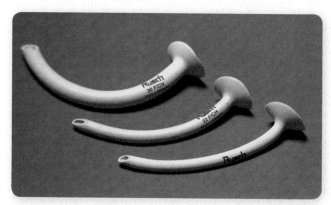

Figure 7-14 Nasal airways.
© Jones & Bartlett Learning. Courtesy of MIEMSS.

the patient's nose. Coat the airway with a water-soluble lubricant before inserting it. This step makes it easier for you to insert the airway and reduces the chance of causing trauma to the patient's airway. Insert the airway in the larger nostril. As you insert the airway, follow the curvature of the floor of the nose. The airway is fully inserted when the flange or trumpet rests against the patient's nostril. At this point, the other end of the airway will reach the back of the patient's throat and it will maintain an open airway for the patient.

Treatment

If a patient has sustained severe head trauma, it is possible that the insertion of a nasal airway may further damage the brain. Check with your local medical control to determine the protocol for using a nasal airway in patients with head trauma.

Follow these steps to insert a nasal airway Skill Drill 7-3:

1. Select the proper size airway by measuring from the earlobe to the tip of the patient's nose Step 1.
2. Coat the airway with a water-soluble lubricant.
3. Select the larger nostril.
4. Gently stretch the nostril open by using your thumb.
5. Gently insert the airway until the flange rests against the nose Step 2 and Step 3. Do not force the airway. If you feel any resistance, remove the airway and try to insert it in the other nostril.

Treatment

To open the patient's airway:

1. Perform the head tilt–chin lift maneuver, or
2. Perform the jaw-thrust maneuver.

To maintain the patient's airway:

3. Continue to apply the head tilt–chin lift or jaw-thrust maneuver, and
   - Insert an oral airway, or
   - Insert a nasal airway.
4. Place the patient in the recovery position.

After you open and maintain the patient's airway, continue to monitor the status of the patient's breathing.

Skill Drill 7-3

Inserting a Nasal Airway

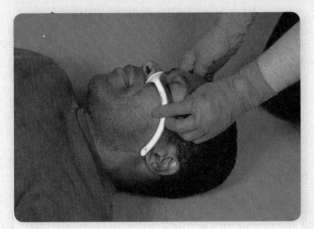

Step 1 Size the airway by measuring from the earlobe to the tip of the patient's nose.

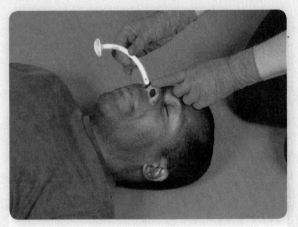

Step 2 Insert the lubricated airway into the larger nostril.

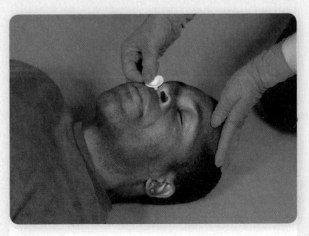

Step 3 Advance the airway until the flange rests against the nose.

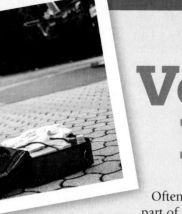

Voices *of* Experience

Often we forget that proper spinal immobilization is a critical part of airway control. Let me explain. I was nearly killed in a logging accident on December 13, 1983, while cutting large pine trees for a saw mill. I suffered multiple fractures and other injuries when a 65-foot (20-m) tree fell on me. I was transported by the ambulance being towed through the mud and snow with a log skidder and then driven a few miles on icy roads to the emergency department. This was just a few years before I was to become a paramedic—in fact, this accident is what sparked my interest in becoming an emergency medical responder.

To make a long story short, my chief complaint changed en route to the hospital from pain in my legs, arms, and chest to pain on the back of my head and difficulty breathing and swallowing. I couldn't keep the blood out of my airway. My face was badly lacerated and a couple of teeth had sheared off when the chainsaw came up into my face as the tree slammed me to the ground. Why did my head hurt so much after being put on a long backboard? Why was it so hard to breathe and swallow, making me feel like I was constantly choking? The way I was immobilized on the backboard was actually making my injuries worse.

> **"The way I was immobilized on the spine board was actually making my injuries worse."**

Tape was placed over my head, pulling the back of my skull tightly against the hard surface of the spine board, each jar and bump driving my head harder into the backboard. Imagine how much worse this would be for a trauma patient with gravel or broken glass embedded in his or her hair pushing into his or her skull as well. Not only does this position hurt, it also makes it hard to breathe and to control your own airway.

The standard of care where I work now is to pad the back of the patient's head to align the "hole in the ear," called the external meatus, with the anterior shoulder. For pediatric patients, we use the same alignment landmarks, but often the padding needs to be behind the body and not the head. Even then, some padding is added behind the head for comfort. When swallowing is easier, the patient's airway remains clear; breathing is easier and more effective. Pain and anxiety are decreased, lowering adrenaline release and decreasing both heart rate and oxygen demand. If advanced life support providers need to install an advanced airway later, it will be much easier with the trachea aligned properly.

By being a patient, I learned this valuable lesson. Hopefully you won't have to be a patient to learn it, too.

Kent Courtney, NREMT
EMS Instructor
Peabody Western Coal Company
Kayenta, Arizona

B Is for Breathing

After you have checked and corrected the patient's airway, you will next check and correct the patient's breathing. To do this, you must understand the signs of adequate breathing, the signs of inadequate breathing, and the signs and causes of respiratory arrest.

▶ Signs of Adequate Breathing

You will use the look, listen, and feel technique to assess if an unconscious patient is breathing adequately. In using this technique, you look for the rise and fall of the patient's chest, listen for the sounds of air passing into or out of the patient's nose and mouth, and feel the air moving on the side of your face. Place the side of your face close to the patient's nose and mouth and watch the patient's chest. By positioning yourself in this way, you can look for chest movements, listen for the sounds of air moving, and feel the air as it moves in and out of the patient's nose and mouth.

A normal adult has a resting breathing rate of approximately 12 to 20 breaths per minute. Remember, one breath includes both an inhalation and an exhalation.

▶ Signs of Inadequate Breathing

If a patient is breathing inadequately, you will detect signs of abnormal respirations. Sounds such as noisy respirations, wheezing, or gurgling indicate a partial blockage or constriction somewhere along the respiratory tract. Rapid or gasping respirations may indicate that the patient is not receiving an adequate amount of oxygen as a result of illness or injury. The patient's skin may be pale or even blue, especially around the lips or fingernail beds (cyanosis).

The most critical sign of inadequate breathing is respiratory arrest (total lack of respirations). As discussed previously, this critical state is characterized by a lack of chest movements, lack of breath sounds, and lack of air against the side of your face. In patients with severe hypothermia, respirations can be slowed (and/or shallow) to the point that the patient does not appear to be breathing.

Many causes of respiratory arrest exist. One common cause is heart disease, which claims 610,000 lives each year in the United States according to the Centers for Disease Control and Prevention. Other major causes of respiratory arrest include:

- Mechanical blockage or obstruction caused by the tongue
- Vomitus, particularly in a patient weakened by a condition such as a stroke
- Foreign objects such as broken teeth, dentures, balloons, marbles, pieces of food, or pieces of hard candy (especially in small children)
- Illness or disease
- Drug overdose
- Poisoning
- Severe loss of blood
- Electrocution by electrical current or lightning

▶ Check Breathing

As discussed previously, your assessment of any motionless patient begins by checking for responsiveness and assessing for breathing. If the patient is responsive (conscious) and breathing, assist him or her as needed. However, if the patient is unresponsive (unconscious), you need to determine if the patient requires assistance with breathing or other interventions. While checking to see if the patient is responsive, also check quickly to see if the patient is breathing. This step is accomplished by visualizing the patient's chest and observing for visible movement Figure 7-15 . If the patient is breathing adequately (about 12 to 20 breaths per minute with adequate depth), you can continue to maintain the airway and monitor the rate and depth of respirations to ensure that adequate breathing continues.

▶ Correct the Breathing

You must breathe for any patient who is not breathing adequately. As you perform **rescue breathing**, keep the patient's airway open by using the head tilt–chin lift maneuver (or the jaw-thrust maneuver for patients with suspected head or spinal injuries). To perform rescue breathing, pinch the patient's nose with your thumb and forefinger, take a deep breath, and blow slowly into the patient's mouth for 1 second Figure 7-16 . Use slow, gentle, sustained breathing and just enough breath

---

YOU are the Provider ⟩ CASE 2

At 0137 hours on a Saturday, you are dispatched to a local university dormitory for a report of a sick person. As you arrive at the student's room, you are met by a shocked-looking group of students. A young man is lying on his bed. He does not respond to verbal stimuli or to your shaking of his shoulder. He appears to be turning blue. One of the students says that Dan may have overdosed on drugs. He has a carotid pulse, so you look, listen, and feel for respirations. The patient has gurgling respirations only 2 to 3 times a minute.

1. What is the first action you should take?
2. How can you provide oxygen to this patient?
3. What methods do you have to keep his airway open?

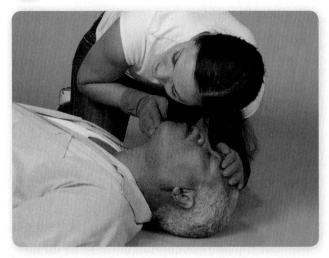

Figure 7-15 Determine responsiveness and check for breathing.
© Jones & Bartlett Learning. Courtesy of MIEMSS.

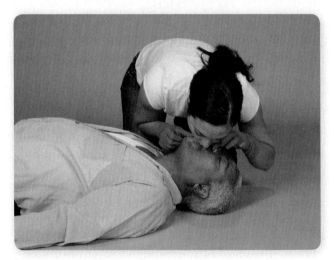

Figure 7-16 To perform rescue breathing, pinch the patient's nose with your thumb and forefinger.
© Jones & Bartlett Learning. Courtesy of MIEMSS.

to make the patient's chest rise to minimize the amount of air blown into the stomach. Remove your mouth and allow the patient's lungs to deflate. Breathe for the patient a second time. After these first two breaths, breathe once into the patient's mouth every 5 to 6 seconds. The rate of breaths should be 10 to 12 per minute for an adult. With an unresponsive patient, recall that you need to check for the presence of circulation before you correct the patient's breathing. These situations are described in Chapter 8, *Professional Rescuer CPR*.

You can perform rescue breathing by using a mouth-to-mask device, a barrier device, a BVM, or just your mouth. The skill of performing mouth-to-mouth ventilation is no longer recommended as a primary means of performing CPR but is presented here as a fallback method of performing ventilation if you have no equipment for performing other means of ventilation. The mouth-to-mask devices, barrier devices, and BVMs prevent you from putting your mouth directly on the patient's mouth. These devices should be available to you as an EMR. If a rescue breathing device is unavailable, you

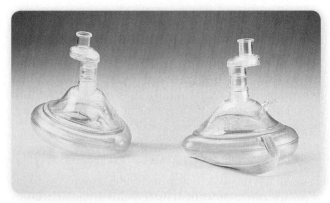

Figure 7-17 Types of mouth-to-mask ventilation devices.
© Jones & Bartlett Learning. Courtesy of MIEMSS.

must weigh the potential good to the patient against the limited chance that you will contract an infectious disease if you perform mouth-to-mouth rescue breathing.

Mouth-to-Mask Rescue Breathing

Your EMR life support kit should contain an artificial ventilation (breathing) device that enables you to perform rescue breathing without mouth-to-mouth contact with the patient. This simple piece of equipment is a mouth-to-mask ventilation device. A mouth-to-mask ventilation device consists of a mask that fits over the patient's face, a one-way valve, and a mouthpiece through which the rescuer breathes **Figure 7-17**. It may also have an inlet port for supplemental oxygen and a tube between the mouthpiece and the mask. Because mouth-to-mask devices prevent direct contact between you and the patient, they reduce the risk of transmitting infectious diseases.

To use a **mouth-to-mask ventilation device** for rescue breathing, follow the steps in **Skill Drill 7-4**:

1. Position yourself at the patient's head.
2. Use the head tilt–chin lift to open the patient's airway **Step 1**. Alternately, use the jaw-thrust maneuver for a patient with suspected head or spinal injuries **Step 2**.
3. Place the mask over the patient's mouth and nose. Make sure the mask's nose notch is on the nose and not the chin.
4. Grasp the mask and the patient's jaw, using both hands. Use the thumb and forefinger of each hand to hold the mask tightly against the face. Hook the other three fingers of each hand under the patient's face **Step 3**.
5. Maintain an airtight seal as you pull up on the jaw to maintain the proper head position.
6. Take a deep breath and then seal your mouth over the mouthpiece.
7. Breathe slowly into the mouthpiece for 1 second **Step 4**. Breathe until the patient's chest rises.
8. Monitor the patient for proper head position, air exchange, and vomiting.

Practice this technique frequently on a manikin until you can do it well.

Skill Drill 7-4

Performing Mouth-to-Mask Rescue Breathing

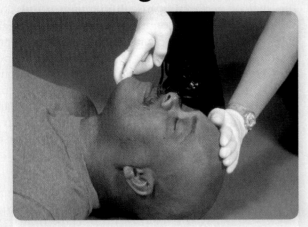

Step 1 Open the airway using the head tilt–chin lift maneuver.

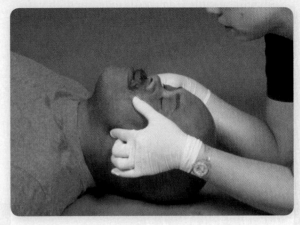

Step 2 Alternately, open the airway using the jaw-thrust technique.

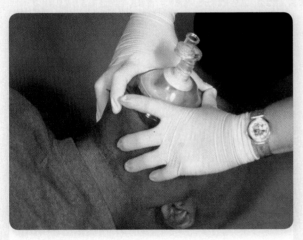

Step 3 Seal the mask against the patient's face.

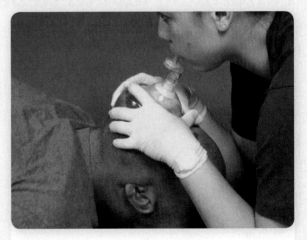

Step 4 Breathe through the mouthpiece.

© Jones & Bartlett Learning. Courtesy of MIEMSS.

Mouth-to-Barrier Rescue Breathing

Mouth-to-barrier devices also provide a barrier between the rescuer and the patient **Figure 7-18**. Some of these devices are small enough to carry in your pocket. Although a wide variety of devices is available, most of them consist of a port or hole that you breathe into and a mask or plastic film that covers the patient's face. Some also have a one-way valve that prevents backflow of secretions and gases. These devices provide variable degrees of infection control.

To perform mouth-to-barrier rescue breathing, follow the steps in **Skill Drill 7-5**:

1. Open the airway with the head tilt–chin lift maneuver. Press on the forehead to maintain the backward tilt of the head **Step 1**.

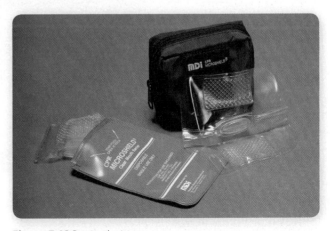

Figure 7-18 Barrier devices.
© Jones & Bartlett Learning. Courtesy of MIEMSS.

2. Keep the patient's mouth open with the thumb of whichever hand you are using to lift the patient's chin.
3. Place the barrier device over the patient's mouth **Step 2** .
4. Pinch the patient's nostrils together with your thumb and forefinger. Take a deep breath and then make a tight seal by placing your mouth on the barrier device around the patient's mouth.
5. Breathe slowly into the patient's mouth for 1 second. Breathe until the patient's chest rises **Step 3** .
6. Remove your mouth and allow the patient to exhale passively. Check to see that the patient's chest falls after each exhalation.

7. Repeat this rescue breathing sequence 10 to 12 times per minute (one breath every 5 to 6 seconds) for an adult.

Mouth-to-Mouth Rescue Breathing

The skill of performing mouth-to-mouth ventilation, although no longer recommended as a primary means of performing CPR, is presented here as a method of performing ventilation if you have no equipment for performing other means of ventilation. Mouth-to-mouth rescue breathing is an effective way of providing artificial ventilation for patients who are not breathing and requires no equipment except you. However, because there is a somewhat higher risk of contracting a disease when using this method, use a mask or barrier breathing device if available.

Skill Drill 7-5

Performing Mouth-to-Barrier Rescue Breathing

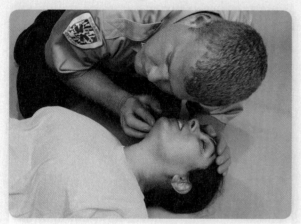

Step 1 Open the airway using the head tilt–chin lift maneuver.

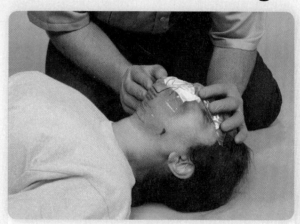

Step 2 Place the barrier device over the patient's mouth.

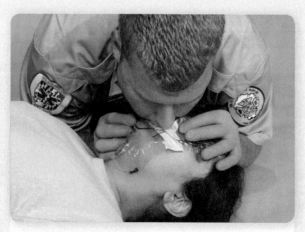

Step 3 Pinch the patient's nostrils together and perform rescue breathing.

To perform mouth-to-mouth rescue breathing, follow these steps:

1. Open the airway with the head tilt–chin lift maneuver. Press on the forehead to maintain the backward tilt of the head.
2. Pinch the patient's nostrils together with your thumb and forefinger.
3. Keep the patient's mouth open with the thumb of whichever hand you are using to lift the patient's chin.
4. Take a deep breath and then make a tight seal by placing your mouth over the patient's mouth.
5. Breathe slowly into the patient's mouth for 1 second. Breathe until the patient's chest rises.
6. Remove your mouth and allow the patient to exhale passively. Check to see that the patient's chest falls after each exhalation.
7. Repeat this rescue breathing sequence every 5 to 6 seconds or 10 to 12 times per minute for adult patients and every 3 to 5 seconds or 12 to 20 times per minute for children and infants.

Bag-Valve Mask

The BVM has three parts: a self-inflating bag, one-way valves, and a face mask **Figure 7-19** . To use this device, you place the mask over the face of the patient and make a tight seal. Squeezing the bag pushes air through a one-way valve, through the mask, and into the patient's mouth and nose. As the patient passively exhales, a second one-way valve near the mask releases the air.

The self-inflating bag refills with air when you release the pressure on it. The BVM delivers 21% oxygen (the percentage of oxygen in room air) without supplemental oxygen attached. However, supplemental oxygen is usually added to the BVM. A BVM can deliver up to 90% oxygen to a patient if 10 to 15 liters per minute (L/min) of oxygen is supplied into the reservoir bag. Many BVMs are designed to be discarded after a single use.

The BVM is used for the same purpose as a mouth-to-mask device—to ventilate a nonbreathing patient. Although the BVM can administer up to 90% oxygen when used with supplemental oxygen, there are two disadvantages to its use. As a single rescuer, you may find it difficult to maintain a seal between the patient's face and the mask with one hand. Additionally, the BVM may be difficult to use if you have small hands because you may not be able to squeeze the bag hard enough to get an adequate volume of air into the patient.

BVM Technique. To use a BVM, follow the same steps you use to perform rescue breathing. Determine whether the patient is unresponsive. Open the patient's airway using the head tilt–chin lift maneuver or the jaw-thrust maneuver for patients with suspected head or spinal injuries. Check to see if the patient is breathing by looking at the patient's chest, listening for the sound of air movement, and feeling for the movement of air on the side of your face and ear. If the patient is not breathing, consider using an oral or nasal airway.

> ## Treatment
>
> The three methods for performing rescue breathing are all potentially lifesaving. Use a mouth-to-mask device, a mouth-to-barrier device, or a BVM whenever possible. If a rescue breathing device is not available, you must weigh the potential good to the patient against the limited chance that you will contract an infectious disease from mouth-to-mouth breathing.

The specific steps for using a BVM are shown in Skill Drill 7-6 :

1. Kneel above the patient's head. This position will enable you to keep the airway open, make a tight seal on the mask, and squeeze the bag. Maintain the patient's neck in an extended position. The BVM does not maintain the patient's airway in an open position. You must continue to stabilize the head and maintain the head either in an extended position for the head tilt–chin lift maneuver or in a neutral position for the jaw-thrust maneuver.
2. Open the patient's mouth and check for fluids, foreign bodies, or dentures **Step 1** . Suction if needed. Consider the use of an oral or nasal airway.
3. Select the proper mask size **Step 2** . The mask should be large enough to seal over the bridge of the patient's nose and fit in the groove between the lower lip and the chin. A mask that is too small or too large may make it impossible to maintain a seal.
4. Place the mask over the patient's face. Start by putting the angled or grooved end of the mask over the bridge of the nose. Then bring the bottom of the mask against the groove between the lower lip and the chin **Step 3** .

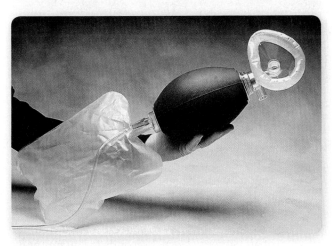

Figure 7-19 A bag-valve mask or BVM.
© Jones & Bartlett Learning. Courtesy of MIEMSS.

Skill Drill `7-6`

Using a BVM With One Rescuer

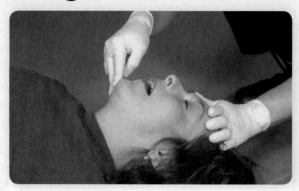

Step 1 Kneel at the patient's head and maintain an open airway. Check the patient's mouth for fluids, foreign bodies, and dentures.

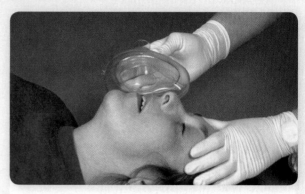

Step 2 Select the proper mask size.

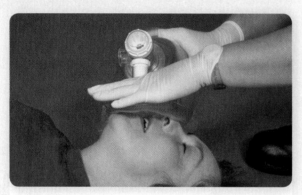

Step 3 Place the mask over the patient's face.

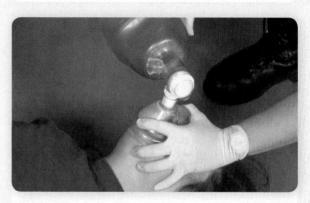

Step 4 Seal the mask.

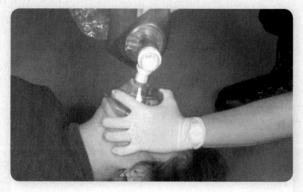

Step 5 Squeeze the bag with your other hand. Check for chest rise.

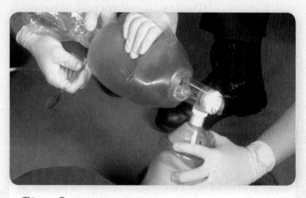

Step 6 Add supplemental oxygen.

© Jones & Bartlett Learning. Courtesy of MIEMSS.

5. Seal the mask. Place the middle, ring, and little fingers of one hand under the angle of the jaw. Lift up on the jaw. Make a C with the index finger and thumb of the same hand and place them over the mask. Clamp the mask by lifting the jaw and bringing the mask in contact with the jaw. Continue to hold the mask in position **Step 4**.

6. Using your other hand, squeeze the bag once every 5 seconds. Try to squeeze a large volume of air. Squeeze every 3 seconds for infants and children.

7. Check for chest rise **Step 5**. While you squeeze the bag, watch for a rise in the chest. If you do not see the chest rise, air is probably leaking around the mask or an obstruction is present in the airway. If air is leaking around the mask, try to make a better seal between the mask and the patient's jaw. If you suspect an airway obstruction, follow the steps already learned in this chapter regarding resolving airway obstructions.

8. Add supplemental oxygen **Step 6**. Using a BVM without supplemental oxygen supplies the patient with 21% oxygen. By adding 10 to 15 L/min of oxygen to the BVM, you can increase the oxygen concentration to 90%. Adjust the liter flow on the pressure regulator/flowmeter to deliver between 10 and 15 L/min and connect the oxygen tubing from the flowmeter outlet to the inlet nipple on the BVM. This higher percentage of oxygen is beneficial for a nonbreathing patient. The specific steps for using supplemental oxygen are explained later in this chapter.

With sufficient training and practice, a single rescuer can ventilate a patient using a BVM; however, it can be difficult to maintain a good seal and squeeze the bag. Use of a BVM is best accomplished as a two-person operation if additional rescuers are present **Figure 7-20**. With two rescuers, one person squeezes the bag and the other person uses both hands to seal the mask to the patient. Use the middle, ring, and little fingers of both hands under the angles of the jaw and use the index fingers and thumbs of both hands to form two C's around the face mask. Most people can seal the mask much more easily using both hands.

Using the BVM requires proper training and practice. The BVM can be a lifesaving tool. Your EMS agency may use BVMs for nonbreathing patients, or you may be asked to assist emergency medical technicians or paramedics in

ventilating nonbreathing patients so they can perform other needed skills. Check with your supervisor or medical director to learn the protocols for your service.

> ### Treatment
>
> If paramedics have inserted an endotracheal tube down the patient's windpipe (trachea), the BVM is connected directly to the end of the endotracheal tube. In this case, no face mask is needed. When you squeeze the BVM, you force air directly into the patient's lungs. You should receive instruction in this type of ventilation if you will be performing it.

■ Airway and Breathing Review

Assume that all patients may be in respiratory arrest until you can assess them and determine whether they are breathing adequately. A summary of the steps required to recognize respiratory arrest and perform rescue breathing in adults follows. Remember, you will learn the steps for checking and correcting circulation in Chapter 8, *Professional Rescuer CPR*.

▶ Airway

1. Check for responsiveness by shouting, "Are you okay?" and gently shaking the patient's shoulder. If the patient is unresponsive and has no pulse, place the patient on his or her back, activate the EMS system, and begin CPR as outlined in Chapter 8, *Professional Rescuer CPR*. If the patient has a pulse, continue with Step 2.
2. Correct a blocked airway by using the head tilt–chin lift maneuver or, if the patient has sustained any injury to the head or neck, use the jaw-thrust maneuver.
3. Check the mouth for any secretions, vomitus, or solid objects. If found, clear the mouth.
4. Correct a blocked airway, if needed, by using finger sweeps or suction to remove foreign substances.
5. Maintain the airway by manually holding it open or by using an oral or nasal airway.

▶ Breathing

1. Check that the patient is breathing adequately by looking for the rise and fall of the patient's chest and listening for the sound of air moving in and out of the patient's nose and mouth. If the patient is breathing adequately, place him or her in the recovery position. If the patient is not breathing, go to Step 2.
2. Correct the lack of breathing by performing rescue breathing using a mouth-to-mask or

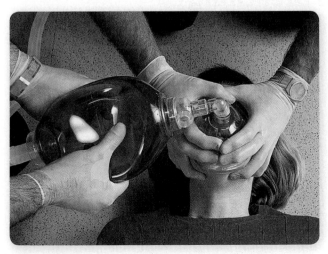

Figure 7-20 Using a BVM with two rescuers.
© Jones & Bartlett Learning. Courtesy of MIEMSS.

mouth-to-barrier device, if available. Blow slowly into the patient's mouth for 1 second, using slow, gentle, sustained breaths with enough force to make the chest rise. If using a BVM, slowly squeeze the bag for 1 second. Remove your mouth and allow the lungs to deflate. Breathe for the patient a second time. After these first two breaths, breathe once into the patient's mouth about every 5 to 6 seconds or 10 to 12 times per minute.

Often, when rescue breathing is necessary, **external cardiac compressions** are also required. External cardiac compressions are explained in Chapter 8, *Professional Rescuer CPR*.

▶ Performing Rescue Breathing on Children and Infants

The steps required to determine responsiveness and check and correct the patient's airway and breathing are similar for adults, children, and infants. However, some differences exist. You must learn and practice the different airway and breathing sequences for children and infants.

Rescue Breathing for Children

For the purposes of performing rescue breathing, a child is a person between age 1 year and the beginning of puberty (age 12 to 14 years). Keep the following differences between adult patients and children in mind:

1. Children are smaller and you will not have to use as much force to open their airways and tilt their heads.
2. The rate of rescue breathing is slightly faster for children. Give 1 rescue breath every 3 to 5 seconds (about 12 to 20 rescue breaths per

minute) instead of the adult rate of 1 rescue breath every 5 to 6 seconds (10 to 12 rescue breaths per minute).

Rescue Breathing for Infants

If the patient is an infant (younger than 1 year), you must vary rescue breathing techniques slightly. Remember, an infant is tiny and must be treated extremely gently. The steps in rescue breathing for an infant are shown in Skill Drill 7-7 :

Responsiveness

1. Check for responsiveness by gently shaking the infant's shoulder or tapping the bottom of the foot Step 1 . If the infant is unresponsive, place the infant on his or her back and shout for help or activate the emergency response system with a mobile phone. Proceed to Step 2.

Check Circulation and Breathing

2. Check the brachial pulse (located inside of the upper arm). Simultaneously check for the absence of breathing or only gasping breaths by looking for the rise and fall of the infant's chest and listening for the sound of air moving in and out of the infant's mouth and nose Step 2 . If the patient is not breathing and a pulse is present, proceed to Step 3.

Airway

3. Check the airway and open it by using the head tilt–chin lift maneuver. Do not tip the infant's head back too far because this may block the infant's airway. Tilt it only enough to open the airway Step 3 .

Skill Drill 7-7

Performing Infant Rescue Breathing

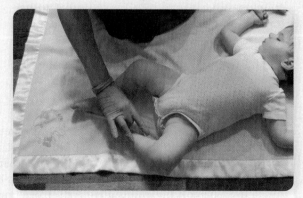

Step 1 Establish the patient's level of responsiveness.

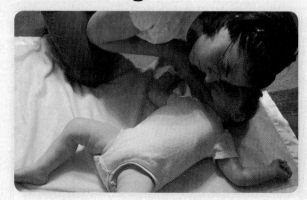

Step 2 Simultaneously check for circulation and breathing.

Courtesy of Jennifer and Marc Lemaire.

Skill Drill 7-7 Continued

Performing Infant Rescue Breathing

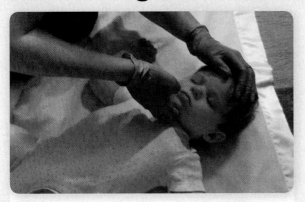

Step 3 Open the infant's airway using the head tilt–chin lift maneuver.

Courtesy of Jennifer and Marc Lemaire.

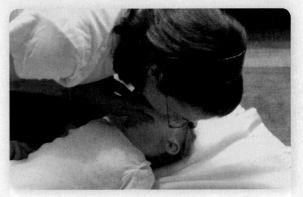

Step 4 Perform infant rescue breathing.

Breathing

4. Begin rescue breathing. Cover the infant's mouth and nose with your mouth. Blow gently into the infant's mouth and nose for 1 second **Step 4** . Watch the chest rise with each breath. Remove your mouth and allow the lungs to deflate.

5. Do not overinflate an infant's lungs. Use small puffs of air, enough to make the chest rise with each breath. After these first two breaths, give one rescue breath every 3 to 5 seconds, or 12 to 20 rescue breaths per minute.

The rate of rescue breathing for infants is the same as for children. If the patient is breathing adequately, place him or her in the recovery position. Often when rescue breathing is necessary, external cardiac compressions are also required. External cardiac compressions, the *C* part of the CABs, are explained in Chapter 8, *Professional Rescuer CPR*.

Foreign Body Airway Obstruction

The first part of this section discusses the causes and recognition of mild airway obstruction and severe airway obstruction. The second part of this section discusses the management of foreign body airway obstruction in adults, children, and infants.

▶ Causes of Airway Obstruction

Your attempt to perform rescue breathing on a patient may not be effective because of an **airway obstruction**. The most common airway obstruction is the tongue. If the tongue is blocking the airway, the head tilt–chin lift maneuver or jaw-thrust maneuver should open the airway. However, if a foreign body is lodged in the air passage, you must use other techniques.

Food is the most common foreign object that causes an airway obstruction. An adult may choke on a large piece of meat; a child may inhale candy, a peanut, or a piece of a hot dog. Children may put small objects in their mouths and inhale such things as tiny toys or balloons. Vomitus may obstruct the airway of a child or an adult **Figure 7-21** .

▶ Types of Airway Obstruction

Airway obstruction may be partial (a mild obstruction) or complete (a severe obstruction). The first step in caring for a conscious person who may have an obstructed airway is to ask, "Are you choking?" If the patient can reply to your question, the airway is not completely blocked. If the patient is unable to speak or cough, the airway is completely blocked.

Mild Airway Obstruction

In partial or mild airway obstruction, the patient coughs and gags. This indicates that some air is passing around the obstruction. The patient may even be able to speak, although with difficulty.

To treat a mildly obstructed airway, encourage the patient to cough. Coughing is the most effective way of expelling a foreign object. If the patient is unable to expel the object by coughing (if, for example, a bone is stuck in the throat), arrange for the patient's *prompt transport* to an appropriate medical facility. Such a patient must be monitored carefully while awaiting transport and during

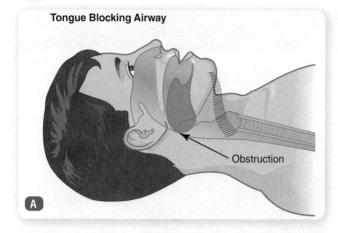

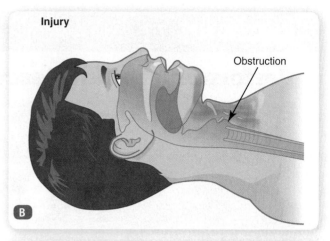

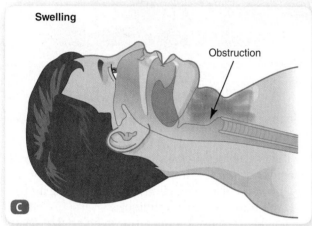

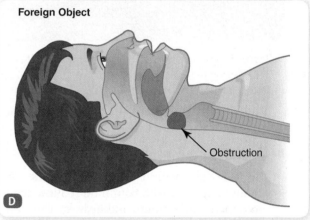

Figure 7-21 Common causes of airway obstruction.
A, B, C, & D: © Jones & Bartlett Learning.

transport because a mild obstruction can become a severe (complete) obstruction at any moment.

Severe Airway Obstruction

A patient with a severe (complete) airway obstruction will have different signs and symptoms than a patient with a mild airway obstruction. With no fresh oxygen entering the lungs, the body quickly uses all the oxygen breathed in with the last breath. The patient is unable to breathe in or out and, because he or she cannot exhale air, speech is impossible. Other symptoms of a severe airway obstruction may include poor air exchange, increased breathing difficulty, and a silent cough. If the airway is completely obstructed, the patient will become unconscious in 3 to 4 minutes.

The currently accepted treatment for a completely obstructed airway in an adult or child involves abdominal thrusts, also called the **Heimlich maneuver**. Abdominal thrusts compress the air that remains in the lungs, pushing it upward through the airway so that it exerts pressure against the foreign object. The pressure pops the object out, in much the same way that a cork pops out of a bottle after the bottle has been shaken to increase the pressure. Many rescuers report that abdominal thrusts can cause an obstructing piece of food to fly across the room. A person who has had an obstruction removed from his or her

airway by the Heimlich maneuver should be transported to a hospital for examination by a physician.

▶ Management of Foreign Body Airway Obstructions

Relieving a foreign body airway obstruction requires no special equipment. The following sections describe the steps that you need to learn to relieve foreign body airway obstructions in adults, children, and infants. Performing these steps can make the difference between life and death for these patients.

Airway Obstruction in an Adult

The steps to treat severe airway obstruction vary, depending on whether the patient is conscious or unconscious. If the patient is conscious, stand behind the patient and perform the abdominal thrusts while the patient is standing or seated in a chair.

Locate the xiphoid process (the bottom of the sternum) and the navel. Place one fist above the navel and well below the xiphoid process, thumb side against the patient's abdomen. Grasp your fist with your other hand. Then apply abdominal thrusts sharply and firmly, bringing your fist in and slightly upward. Do not give the patient a bear hug; rather, apply pressure at the point where your fist contacts the patient's abdomen.

Each thrust should be distinct and forceful. Repeat these abdominal thrusts until the foreign object is expelled or until the patient becomes unresponsive. Review the steps in **Skill Drill 7-8** until you can carry them out automatically. To assist a conscious patient with a complete airway obstruction, you must:

1. Ask, "Are you choking? Can you speak? Can I help you?" If there is no verbal response, assume the airway obstruction is complete **Step 1**.
2. Stand behind the patient and position the thumb side of your fist just above the patient's navel **Step 2**.
3. Press into the patient's abdomen with a quick, upward thrust **Step 3**. Repeat the abdominal thrusts until either the foreign body is expelled or the patient becomes unresponsive.
4. If the patient has obesity or is in the late stages of pregnancy, use chest thrusts instead of abdominal thrusts. Chest thrusts are done by standing behind the patient and placing your arms under the patient's armpits to encircle the patient's chest. Press with quick, backward thrusts.

   If the patient becomes unresponsive, continue with the following steps.
5. Ensure the EMS system has been activated.
6. Begin CPR:
   a. Perform chest compressions. (This part of the CPR sequence is covered in Chapter 8, *Professional Rescuer CPR*).
   b. Open the airway and look in the mouth. Remove the foreign body only if you can see it.

Skill Drill 7-8

Managing Airway Obstruction in a Conscious Patient

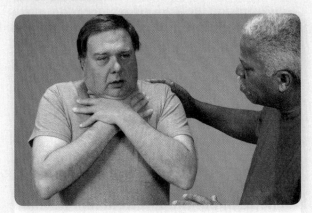

Step 1 Look for signs of choking.

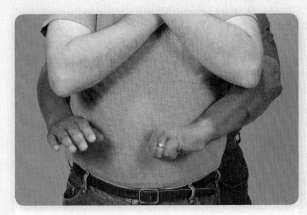

Step 2 Place your fist with the thumb side against the patient's abdomen, just above the navel.

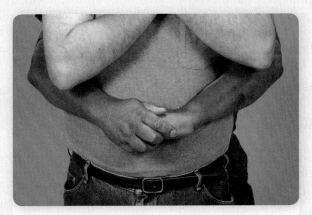

Step 3 Grasp the fist with your other hand and press into the abdomen with quick inward and upward thrusts.

c. Attempt to ventilate. If you are unable to ventilate, reposition the patient's head and reattempt ventilation. If both breaths do not produce visible chest rise, continue chest compressions.

7. Continue these steps of CPR until more advanced EMS personnel arrive.

Recent studies have shown that performing chest compressions on an unresponsive patient increases the pressure in the chest similar to performing abdominal thrusts and may relieve an airway obstruction. Therefore, performing CPR on a patient who has become unresponsive has the same effect as performing the Heimlich maneuver on a conscious patient.

A skill performance sheet titled Foreign Body Airway Obstruction in an Adult is shown in **Figure 7-22** for your review and practice.

Airway Obstruction in a Child

The steps for relieving an airway obstruction in a conscious child (age 1 year to the onset of puberty) are the same as for an adult patient. The anatomic differences between adults, children, and infants require that you make some adjustments in your technique. When opening the airway of a child or infant, tilt the head back just past the neutral position. Tilting the head too far back (hyperextending the neck) can actually obstruct the airway of a child or infant. If you are by yourself and a child with an airway obstruction becomes unresponsive, perform CPR for five cycles (about 2 minutes) before activating the EMS system.

A skill performance sheet titled Foreign Body Airway Obstruction in a Child is shown in **Figure 7-23** for your review and practice.

Airway Obstruction in an Infant

The process for relieving an airway obstruction in an infant (younger than 1 year) must take into consideration that an infant is extremely fragile. An infant's airway structures are very small, and they are more easily injured than those of an adult. If you suspect an airway obstruction, assess the infant to determine whether there is any air exchange. If the infant has an audible cry, the airway is not completely obstructed. Ask the person who was with the infant what was happening when the episode began. This person may have seen the infant put a foreign body into his or her mouth.

Suspect a severe airway obstruction if you observe no movement of air from the infant's mouth and nose, a sudden onset of severe breathing difficulty, a silent cough, or a silent cry. To relieve an airway obstruction in an infant, use a combination of back slaps and chest thrusts. You must have a good grasp of the infant to alternate the back slaps and the chest thrusts. Review the following sequence until you can carry it out automatically. To assist a conscious infant with a severe airway obstruction, you must:

1. Assess the infant's airway and breathing status. Determine that there is no air exchange.
2. Place the infant in a facedown position over one arm so you can deliver five back slaps. Support the infant's head and neck with one hand and place the infant facedown with the head lower than the trunk. Rest the infant on your forearm and support your forearm on your thigh. Use the heel of your hand and deliver up to five back slaps forcefully between the infant's shoulder blades.
3. Support the head and turn the infant faceup by sandwiching the infant between your hands and arms. Rest the infant on his or her back with the head lower than the trunk.
4. Deliver five chest thrusts in the middle of the sternum. Use two fingers to deliver the chest thrusts in a firm manner.
5. Repeat the series of back slaps and chest thrusts until the foreign object is expelled or until the infant becomes unresponsive.
6. If the infant becomes unresponsive, continue with the following steps:
7. Ensure the EMS system has been activated.
8. Begin CPR:
   - Perform chest compressions. (This part of the CPR sequence is covered in Chapter 8, *Professional Rescuer CPR*).
   - Open the airway and look in the mouth. Remove the foreign body only if you can see it.

YOU   are the Provider   CASE 3

You are enjoying a well-deserved day off. It is a mild and sunny day in spring, so you decide to go for a run in a local park. After a tiring but refreshing run, you are heading back to your vehicle when you notice an energetic group of young children from a daycare center. They seem to be enjoying an afternoon snack on the lawn. As you pass by, one of the caregivers begins to yell for help. You look over and see a boy about 9 years old, who is holding his neck and has a panicked look in his eyes. You run over and introduce yourself to the caregiver. She tells you the children were enjoying a snack and she thinks that Matt may have gotten something caught in his throat.

1. What is the first step you should take?
2. What else should you do for this patient?
3. How long should you continue your treatment?

Foreign Body Airway Obstruction in an Adult

Steps	Adequately Performed
1. Ask: "Are you choking?"	
2. Give abdominal thrusts (chest thrusts for pregnant patient or patient with obesity).	
3. Repeat thrusts until foreign body is dislodged or patient becomes unresponsive.	
If the patient becomes unresponsive:	
4. Ensure the EMS system has been activated.	
5. Perform chest compressions.	
6. Open the airway and look in the mouth. Remove the foreign body only if you can see it.	
7. Attempt to ventilate. If you are unable to ventilate, reposition the patient's head and reattempt ventilation. If both breaths do not produce visible chest rise, continue chest compressions.	
8. Continue these steps until more advanced EMS personnel arrive.	

Figure 7-22 Skill performance sheet: Foreign Body Airway Obstruction in an Adult.
© Jones & Bartlett Learning.

Foreign Body Airway Obstruction in a Child

Steps	Adequately Performed
1. Ask: "Are you choking?"	
2. Give abdominal thrusts.	
3. Repeat thrusts until foreign body is dislodged or patient becomes unresponsive.	
If the patient becomes unresponsive:	
4. If a second rescuer is available, have him or her activate the EMS system.	
5. Perform chest compressions.	
6. Open the airway and look in the mouth. Remove the foreign body only if you can see it.	
7. Attempt to ventilate. If you are unable to ventilate, reposition the patient's head and reattempt ventilation. If both breaths do not produce visible chest rise, continue chest compressions.	
8. Continue these steps until more advanced EMS personnel arrive.	
NOTE: If you are by yourself, perform CPR for 5 cycles (about 2 minutes) and then activate the EMS system.	

Figure 7-23 Skill performance sheet: Foreign Body Airway Obstruction in a Child.
© Jones & Bartlett Learning.

- Attempt to ventilate. If you are unable to ventilate, reposition the patient's head and reattempt ventilation. If both breaths do not produce visible chest rise, continue chest compressions.
9. Continue these CPR steps until more advanced EMS personnel arrive.

NOTE: If you are by yourself, perform CPR for five cycles (about 2 minutes) and then activate the EMS system.

Recent studies have shown that performing chest compressions on an unresponsive patient increases the pressure in the chest similar to performing chest thrusts and may relieve an airway obstruction. Therefore performing CPR

Foreign Body Airway Obstruction in an Infant	
Steps	**Adequately Performed**
1. Confirm severity of airway obstruction. Check for sudden onset of serious breathing difficulty, ineffective cough, silent cough or cry.	
2. Give up to 5 back slaps and up to 5 chest thrusts.	
3. Repeat Step 2 until the foreign body is dislodged or until the infant becomes unresponsive.	
If the infant becomes unresponsive:	
4. If a second rescuer if available, have him or her activate the EMS system.	
5. Perform chest compressions.	
6. Open the airway and look in the mouth. Remove the foreign body only if you can see it.	
7. Attempt to ventilate. If you are unable to ventilate, reposition the patient's head and reattempt ventilation. If both breaths do not produce visible chest rise, continue chest compressions.	
8. Continue these steps until more advanced EMS personnel arrive.	
NOTE: If you are by yourself, perform CPR for 5 cycles (about 2 minutes) and then activate the EMS system.	

Figure 7-24 Skill performance sheet: Foreign Body Airway Obstruction in an Infant.
© Jones & Bartlett Learning.

on an infant who has become unresponsive has the same effect as performing the chest thrusts on a conscious patient.

A skill performance sheet titled Foreign Body Airway Obstruction in an Infant is shown in **Figure 7-24** for your review and practice.

Oxygen Administration

Under normal conditions, the body can operate efficiently using the oxygen that is contained in the air, even though air contains only 21% oxygen. The amount of blood loss that occurs after a traumatic injury could mean that insufficient oxygen is delivered to the cells of the body. This results in shock. Administering supplemental oxygen to a patient showing signs and symptoms of shock increases the amount of oxygen delivered to the cells of the body and often makes a positive difference in the patient's outcome.

Patients who have experienced a heart attack or stroke or patients who have a chronic heart or lung disease may be unable to get sufficient oxygen from room air. These patients will also benefit from receiving supplemental oxygen.

Not all EMRs know how to administer oxygen; however, knowing this skill can help you when you are in a situation where EMS response may be delayed. By learning this skill, you will be able to assist other members of the EMS team. Administer oxygen only after receiving proper training and with the approval of your medical director.

▶ Oxygen Equipment

Several pieces of equipment are required to administer supplemental oxygen, including an oxygen cylinder, a pressure regulator/flowmeter, and a nasal cannula or face mask. The characteristics and operation of each piece of equipment are described in the following section.

Oxygen Cylinders

Oxygen is compressed to 2,000 pounds per square inch (psi) and stored in portable cylinders. The portable oxygen cylinders used by most EMS systems are either size D or E. D size cylinders hold 350 liters of oxygen, and E size cylinders hold 625 liters of oxygen. Oxygen cylinders must be marked with a green color and be labeled as medical oxygen. Depending on the flow rate, each cylinder lasts for at least 20 minutes. A valve at the top of the oxygen cylinder allows you to control the flow of oxygen from the cylinder. Oxygen administration equipment is shown in **Figure 7-25**.

Pressure Regulator/Flowmeter

Oxygen in the cylinder is stored at 2,000 psi. Oxygen can be used only when that pressure is regulated down to about 50 psi, which is done by using a pressure regulator. The pressure regulator and the **flowmeter** are a single unit attached to the outlet of the oxygen cylinder **Figure 7-26**. After the pressure has been reduced,

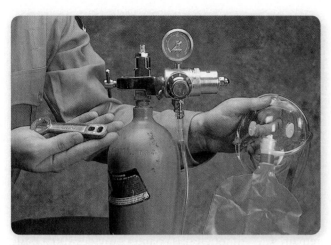

Figure 7-25 Oxygen administration equipment.
© Jones & Bartlett Learning. Courtesy of MIEMSS.

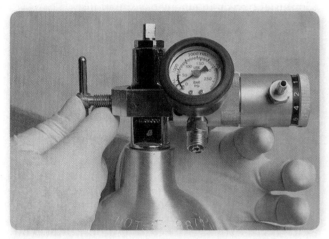

Figure 7-26 The regulator/flowmeter attaches to the outlet of the oxygen cylinder.
© American Academy of Orthopaedic Surgeons.

you can adjust the flowmeter to deliver oxygen at a rate of 2 to 15 L/min. Because patients with different medical conditions require different amounts of oxygen, the flowmeter lets you select the proper amount of oxygen to administer. A gasket between the cylinder and the pressure regulator/flowmeter ensures a tight seal and maintains the high pressure inside the cylinder. Always check for this gasket before attaching the regulator.

Nasal Cannulas and Face Masks

The third part of an oxygen-delivery system is a device that ensures the oxygen is delivered to the patient and is not lost in the air. A **nasal cannula** has two small holes, which fit into the patient's nostrils. At 1 to 6 L/min, the nasal cannula delivers between 24% and 44% oxygen. A **face mask** is placed over the patient's nose and mouth to deliver oxygen through the patient's mouth and nostrils. Nonrebreathing masks are most commonly used by EMRs. Nonrebreathing masks deliver high concentrations of oxygen (up to 90%). These two oxygen-delivery devices are discussed more fully in the section on administering supplemental oxygen.

Safety Considerations

Oxygen does not burn or explode by itself. However, it actively supports combustion and can quickly turn a small spark or flame into a serious fire. Therefore, keep all sparks, heat, flames, and oily substances away from oxygen equipment. Smoking is never safe around oxygen equipment.

The pressurized cylinders are also hazardous because the high pressure in an oxygen cylinder can cause an explosion if the cylinder is damaged. Secure the oxygen cylinder so that it will not fall. If the shut-off valve at the top of the cylinder is damaged, the cylinder can take off like a rocket. Oxygen cylinders should be kept inside sturdy carrying cases that protect the cylinder and regulator/flowmeter. Handle the cylinder carefully to guard against damage.

Administering Supplemental Oxygen

To administer supplemental oxygen, place the regulator/flowmeter over the stem of the oxygen cylinder and line up the pins on the pin-indexing system correctly **Figure 7-27** . Check for the mandatory gasket. Tighten the securing screw firmly by hand. With the special key or wrench provided, turn the cylinder valve two turns counterclockwise to allow oxygen from the cylinder to enter the regulator/flowmeter.

Check the gauge on the pressure regulator/flowmeter to see how much oxygen pressure remains in the cylinder. If the cylinder contains less than 500 psi, the amount of oxygen in the cylinder is too low for emergency use and should be replaced with a full cylinder (2,000 psi).

To administer oxygen, you will need to adjust the flowmeter to deliver the desired liter-per-minute flow of oxygen. The patient's condition and the type of oxygen delivery device you use (a mask or a nasal cannula) dictate the proper flow. When the oxygen flow begins, place the face mask or nasal cannula onto the patient's face.

Nasal Cannula

A nasal cannula is a simple oxygen-delivery device. As mentioned previously, it consists of two small prongs that fit into the patient's nostrils and a strap that holds the cannula on the patient's face **Figure 7-28** . A cannula delivers low-flow oxygen at 2 to 6 L/min and in concentrations of 35% to 50% oxygen. Low-flow oxygen can be used for fairly stable patients, such as those with slight chest pain or mild shortness of breath.

To use a nasal cannula, first adjust the liter flow to 2 to 6 L/min and then apply the cannula to the patient. The cannula should fit snugly but should not be tight.

Nonrebreathing Mask

A nonrebreathing mask consists of connecting tubing, a reservoir bag, one-way valves, and a face piece **Figure 7-29** . It is used to deliver a high flow of oxygen at 8 to 15 L/min. A nonrebreathing face mask can deliver concentrations of oxygen as high as 90%. The mask works by storing oxygen in the reservoir bag. When the

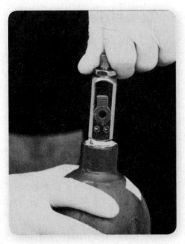

Figure 7-27 A valve stem with pin-index holes.
© Jones & Bartlett Learning. Courtesy of MIEMSS.

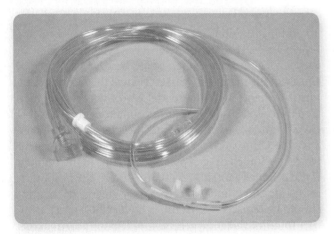

Figure 7-28 A nasal cannula.
© Jones & Bartlett Learning. Courtesy of MIEMSS.

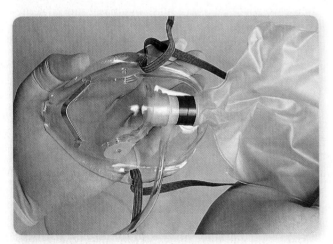

Figure 7-29 A nonrebreathing oxygen mask.
© Jones & Bartlett Learning. Courtesy of MIEMSS.

patient inhales, oxygen is drawn from the reservoir bag. When the patient exhales, the air is exhausted through the one-way valves on the side of the mask.

Use nonrebreathing face masks for patients who require higher flows of oxygen. These include patients experiencing serious shortness of breath, severe chest pain, carbon monoxide poisoning, and congestive heart failure. Patients who are showing signs and symptoms

of shock should also be treated with high-flow oxygen from a nonrebreathing face mask.

To use a nonrebreathing mask, first adjust the oxygen flow to 8 to 15 L/min to inflate the reservoir bag before putting it on the patient. After the bag inflates, place the mask over the patient's face. Adjust the straps to secure a snug fit. Adjust the liter flow to keep the bag at least partially inflated while the patient inhales.

▶ Hazards of Supplemental Oxygen

Supplemental oxygen can be lifesaving, but you must use it carefully so that you, your team, and the patient remain safe. Although this chapter provides you a basic outline on setting up oxygen equipment, you will need additional class work and practical training before you administer oxygen in emergency situations.

Safety

Avoid using oxygen around fire or flames. Secure oxygen cylinders to minimize the danger of explosion.

Words of Wisdom

Some patients who suffer from respiratory conditions such as asthma or emphysema may use a **metered dose inhaler (MDI)** to administer medications to help them breathe. An MDI is a miniature spray container used to direct medications through the mouth and into the lungs. MDIs deliver the same amount of medication each time they are used. MDIs should be shaken before medications administered to ensure the patient receives a uniform amount of medicine each time he or she uses the inhaler. Many patients will use their inhaler before they call for EMS assistance. If your local protocols permit you to assist patients with using their MDIs, you need to have special training in the proper use of these devices.

■ Pulse Oximetry

Pulse oximetry is used to assess the amount of oxygen saturated in the red blood cells. It does this through the use of a photoelectric cell that measures the light that passes through a fingertip or an earlobe. The machine that performs this function is called a pulse oximeter. A **pulse oximeter** consists of a sensing probe and a monitor. The sensing probe attaches to the patient's fingertip or earlobe by means of a spring-loaded clip. The sensing probe contains a light source and a receiving chamber. The sensing probe attaches to the monitor of the pulse oximeter by means of a cable. The pulse oximeter monitor contains an on-and-off switch and a screen for displaying the percent of oxygen saturation Figure 7-30 .

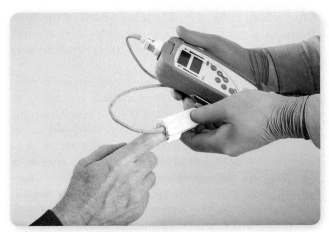

Figure 7-30 A pulse oximeter, which consists of a sensing probe and a monitor, is used to measure the percentage of oxygen saturation in the blood.
© Jones & Bartlett Learning.

To operate the pulse oximeter, turn on the monitor. Most pulse oximeters perform a self-check to ensure the machine is operating correctly. This self-check will vary depending on the brand of the oximeter. After you confirm the monitor is operating correctly, place the sensing probe over the patient's fingertip or earlobe. The monitor should then display the percent of saturation of the patient's blood. In a healthy patient, the oxygen saturation should be between 95% and 100% when breathing room air.

If a patient has difficulty breathing as a result of injury or a disease process, the percent of oxygen saturation may be much lower than 95%. The pulse oximeter cannot tell you what is wrong with the patient. You must perform a thorough patient assessment, including a good medical history. The pulse oximeter can help you to recognize that the patient is having a problem. It can also help you to determine whether your treatment is helping the patient. If the steps you are taking to treat the patient coincide with an increased percentage of oxygen saturation, you can take that as a positive sign.

Like any other device, a pulse oximeter has certain limitations. It will not give you an accurate reading if the patient is wearing nail polish or if the patient's fingers are very dirty. Also, if the patient is cold and the blood vessels in the fingertips or earlobes are constricted, the pulse oximeter reading will be inaccurate. Patients who have sustained considerable blood loss will also have an inaccurate pulse oximetry reading. Patients who have experienced carbon monoxide poisoning will have false readings because their red blood cells are saturated with carbon monoxide instead of with oxygen. It is important to understand that the pulse oximeter is a valuable tool to help you assess a patient's condition. However, like any tool, it has certain limitations that you must consider. Remember, no machine can replace a careful patient assessment, including a good medical history.

Special Considerations

As an EMR, you will encounter some situations that require a slight modification in your CPR technique. These situations include rescue breathing for patients with stomas, gastric distention, patients with dental appliances, and airway management in a vehicle. By adapting to these situations you can achieve effective CPR on these patients.

▶ Rescue Breathing for Patients With Stomas

Some people have had surgery that removed part or all of the larynx. In these patients, the upper airway has been rerouted to open through a **stoma** (hole) in the neck. These patients are called neck breathers. Therefore, you must give rescue breathing through the stoma in the patient's neck. The technique is called **mouth-to-stoma breathing**.

The steps in performing mouth-to-stoma breathing are as follows:

1. Check every patient for the presence of a stoma.
2. If you locate a stoma, keep the patient's neck straight; do not hyperextend the patient's head and neck.
3. Examine the stoma and clean away any mucus in it.
4. If you observe a breathing tube in the opening, remove it to be sure the opening is clear. Clean the breathing tube rapidly and replace it into the stoma. Moistening the tube will make it easier to insert the tube.
5. Place your mouth directly over the stoma and use the same procedures as in mouth-to-mouth

YOU ⟩ are the Provider   CASE 4

It is 2300 hours and you are dispatched to an unknown medical emergency at the home of a 54-year-old man. As you enter the home, the man's wife says he woke up out of a sound sleep reporting crushing chest pains. The patient is in bed. The man has difficulty speaking in full sentences and he is gasping. Your partner returns to the ambulance to get the stretcher. Your primary assessment shows a pulse oximetry reading of 80%.

1. What would be the most effective way to deliver oxygen to the man?
2. Suddenly, the man starts vomiting. What should you do?

breathing. It is not necessary to seal the mouth and nose of most people who have a stoma.

6. If the patient's chest does not rise, he or she may be a partial neck breather. In these patients, seal the mouth and nose with one hand and then breathe through the stoma. You can also use a BVM or pocket-mask device to ventilate a patient with a stoma Figure 7-31 .

▶ Gastric Distention

Gastric distention occurs when air is forced into the stomach instead of the lungs. This condition makes it harder to get an adequate amount of air into the patient's lungs, and it increases the chance that the patient will vomit. Breathe slowly into the patient's mouth just enough to make the chest rise.

Remember, the lungs of children and infants are smaller and require smaller, gentler breaths during rescue breathing. The excess air may enter the stomach and cause gastric distention. Preventing gastric distention is much better than trying to correct it later after it has occurred.

▶ Dental Appliances

Do not remove dental appliances that are firmly attached. They may help keep the patient's mouth full so you can make a better seal between the patient's mouth and your mouth or a breathing device. Loose dental appliances, however, may cause difficulties. Partial dentures may become dislodged during trauma or while you perform airway care and rescue breathing. If you discover loose dental appliances during your exam of the patient's airway, remove the dentures to prevent them from occluding the airway. Put them in a safe place so they will not get damaged or lost.

▶ Airway Management in a Vehicle

If you arrive on the scene of a motor vehicle crash and find that the patient has an airway problem, how can you best assist the patient and maintain an open airway?

If the patient is lying on the seat or floor of the vehicle, you can apply the jaw-thrust maneuver. Use the jaw-thrust maneuver if you suspect the crash could have caused a head or spine injury.

If the patient is in a sitting or semireclining position, approach him or her from the side by leaning in through the window or across the front seat. Grasp the patient's head with both hands. Put one hand under the patient's chin and the other hand on the back of the patient's head just above the neck, as shown in Figure 7-32 . Maintain a slight upward pressure to support the head and cervical spine and to ensure the airway remains open. This technique will often enable you to maintain an open airway without moving the patient. This technique has several advantages:

1. You do not have to enter the vehicle.
2. You can easily monitor the patient's carotid pulse and breathing patterns by using your fingers.
3. It stabilizes the patient's cervical spine.
4. It opens the patient's airway.

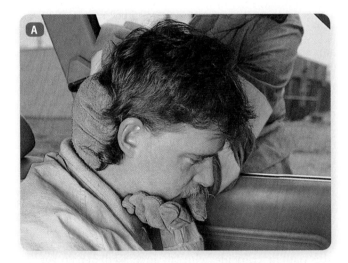

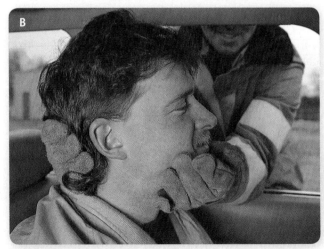

Figure 7-32 Airway management in a vehicle. **A.** To open the airway, place one hand under the chin and the other hand on the back of the patient's head. **B.** Raise the head to a neutral position to open the airway.
A&B: © Jones & Bartlett Learning. Courtesy of MIEMSS.

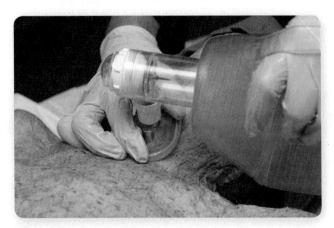

Figure 7-31 You can use a BVM to ventilate a patient with a stoma.
© Jones & Bartlett Learning. Courtesy of MIEMSS.

YOU are the Provider   SUMMARY

You are the Provider: CASE 1

1. What is the next step you should take to assess and treat this patient?

By asking the woman if she can hear you and by gently shaking her shoulder, you have checked for responsiveness. Because she is unresponsive, your next step is to open the woman's airway by using the head tilt–chin lift maneuver or the jaw-thrust maneuver.

2. How would your method of opening the patient's airway change if the patient had fallen or blacked out?

The method for opening the patient's airway depends on the patient's condition. If the patient has fallen or may have sustained an injury to the head or spine, first use the jaw-thrust maneuver to try to open the airway. For patients who have not been injured, use the head tilt–chin lift maneuver to open the airway.

3. What techniques can you use to maintain an open airway?

After opening a patient's airway, you can use the head tilt–chin lift maneuver or the jaw-thrust maneuver to maintain the airway. Other ways of maintaining the patient's airway include inserting an oral airway, inserting a nasal airway, or placing the patient in the recovery position.

You are the Provider: CASE 2

1. What is the first action you should take?

First, open the patient's airway by performing either the head tilt–chin lift maneuver or the jaw-thrust maneuver. This step may enable the patient to start breathing again. If the patient starts to breathe again, ensure he is breathing at a rate of 12 to 20 times a minute. If the patient does not begin to breathe adequately, then perform rescue breathing.

2. How can you provide oxygen to this patient?

To provide oxygen to this patient, begin rescue breathing. You can use a mouth-to-mask device, a mouth-to-barrier device, or a bag-valve mask. Ensure adequate chest rise with each rescue breath, and provide one breath every 5 to 6 seconds, or about 10 to 12 breaths per minute.

3. What methods do you have to keep his airway open?

You can maintain the airway in several different ways. One method to keep the airway open is to continue to apply the head tilt–chin lift maneuver. Another method is to insert either an oral airway or a nasal airway. A third method is to place the patient in the recovery position if he is breathing adequately.

You are the Provider: CASE 3

1. What is the first step you should take?

First, ask the boy whether he is choking. If he nods yes and cannot talk, assume he has a severe (complete) airway obstruction. At the same time, if a second person is present on the scene, instruct him or her to call 9-1-1. Patients who have sustained a severe airway obstruction must be evaluated by a physician.

2. What else should you do for this patient?

After you have determined that Matt has a severe airway obstruction, begin abdominal thrusts (the Heimlich maneuver). Stand behind the patient and position the thumb side of your fist just above the patient's navel. Press into the patient's abdomen with quick, upward thrusts.

3. How long should you continue your treatment?

Repeat the abdominal thrusts until either the foreign body is expelled or until the patient becomes unresponsive.

You are the Provider: CASE 4

1. What would be the most effective way to deliver oxygen to the man?

Given the man's inability to speak in full sentences and obvious difficulty breathing, your best choice is to use a nonrebreathing mask. A nonrebreathing face mask can deliver oxygen concentrations as high as 90%.

2. Suddenly the man starts vomiting. What should you do?

Use either a manual or mechanical suctioning device to clear out the man's mouth, being careful not to suction for more than 15 seconds at a time.

Prep Kit

▶ Ready for Review

- The main purpose of the respiratory system is to provide oxygen and to remove carbon dioxide from the red blood cells as they pass through the lungs. The structures of the respiratory system in children and infants are smaller than they are in adults. Thus, the air passages of children and infants may be more easily blocked by secretions or by foreign objects.

- When a patient experiences possible respiratory arrest, check for responsiveness; open the blocked airway using either the head tilt–chin lift or jaw-thrust maneuver; check for fluids, solids, or dentures in the mouth; and correct the airway, if needed, using finger sweeps or suction.

- Maintain the airway by continuing to manually hold the airway open, by placing the patient in the recovery position, or by inserting an oral or a nasal airway. Check the chest for signs of breathing and correct any problems by using a mouth-to-mask or mouth-to-barrier device, bag-valve mask, or by performing mouth-to-mouth rescue breathing. It is important to use the correct sequence for adults, children, and infants.

- If the airway is obstructed in a conscious adult or child, kneel or stand behind the patient and perform the Heimlich maneuver. Give abdominal thrusts until the obstruction is relieved or the patient becomes unconscious. For an unconscious adult or child with an airway obstruction, perform chest compressions. Move to the head, open the airway, and look in the patient's mouth. Do not perform a finger sweep—regardless of the patient's age—unless you can see the object. Attempt rescue breathing again. If the airway is still obstructed, repeat chest compressions, visualization of the mouth, and ventilation attempts until the obstruction is relieved.

- Administering supplemental oxygen to patients showing signs and symptoms of shock increases the amount of oxygen delivered to the cells of the body and often makes a positive difference in the patient's outcome. Patients who have experienced a heart attack or stroke or patients who have chronic heart or lung disease may also benefit from receiving supplemental oxygen.

- Use pulse oximetry to assess the amount of oxygen saturated in the red blood cells.

▶ Vital Vocabulary

airway The passages from the openings of the mouth and nose to the air sacs in the lungs through which air enters and leaves the lungs.

airway obstruction Partial (mild) or complete (severe) obstruction of the respiratory passages resulting from blockage by food, small objects, or vomitus.

alveolar ventilation The exchange of oxygen and carbon dioxide that occurs in the alveoli.

alveoli The air sacs of the lungs where the exchange of oxygen and carbon dioxide takes place.

aspirator A suction device.

bag-valve mask (BVM) A patient ventilation device that consists of a bag, one-way valves, and a face mask.

bronchi The two main branches of the trachea that lead into the right and left lungs. Within the lungs, they branch into smaller airways.

capillaries The smallest blood vessels that connect small arteries and small veins. Capillary walls serve as the membrane to exchange oxygen and carbon dioxide.

cardiopulmonary resuscitation (CPR) The artificial circulation of the blood and movement of air into and out of the lungs in a pulseless, nonbreathing patient.

esophagus The tube through which food passes. It starts at the throat and ends at the stomach.

external cardiac compressions A means of applying artificial circulation by applying rhythmic pressure and relaxation on the lower half of the sternum; also called chest compressions.

face mask A clear plastic mask used for oxygen administration that covers the mouth and nose.

flowmeter A device on oxygen cylinders used to control and measure the flow of oxygen.

gag reflex A strong involuntary effort to vomit caused by something being placed or caught in the throat.

gastric distention Inflation of the stomach caused when excessive pressures are used during artificial ventilation and air is directed into the stomach rather than the lungs.

head tilt–chin lift maneuver A method of opening the airway by tilting the patient's head backward and lifting the chin forward, bringing the entire lower jaw with it.

Heimlich maneuver A series of manual thrusts to the abdomen to relieve an upper airway obstruction.

Prep Kit *Continued*

jaw-thrust maneuver A method of opening the airway by bringing the patient's jaw forward without extending the neck.

lungs The organs that supply the body with oxygen and eliminate carbon dioxide from the blood.

mandible The lower jaw.

manual suction devices Hand-powered devices used for clearing the upper airway of mucus, blood, or vomitus.

mechanical suction device A battery-powered pump or an oxygen-powered aspirator used for clearing the upper airway of mucus, blood, or vomitus.

metered dose inhaler (MDI) A miniature spray container used to direct medications through the mouth and into the lungs.

minute ventilation The amount of air pulled into the lungs and removed from the lungs in 1 minute.

mouth-to-mask ventilation device A piece of equipment that consists of a mask, a one-way valve, and a mouthpiece. Rescue breathing is performed by breathing into the mouthpiece after placing the mask over the patient's mouth and nose.

mouth-to-stoma breathing Rescue breathing for patients who, because of surgical removal of the larynx, have a stoma.

nasal airway An airway adjunct that is inserted into the nostril of a patient who is unable to maintain a natural airway; also called a nasopharyngeal airway.

nasal cannula A clear plastic tube, used to deliver oxygen, that fits onto the patient's nose.

nasopharynx The posterior part of the nose.

oral airway An airway adjunct that is inserted into the mouth to keep the tongue from blocking the upper airway; also called an oropharyngeal airway.

oropharynx The posterior part of the mouth.

oxygen A colorless, odorless gas that is essential for life.

pharynx The throat.

pocket mask A mechanical breathing device used to administer mouth-to-mask rescue breathing.

pulse oximeter A machine that consists of a monitor and a sensing probe that measures the oxygen saturation in the capillary beds.

pulse oximetry An assessment tool that measures oxygen saturation in the capillary beds.

rescue breathing Artificial means of breathing for a patient.

respiratory arrest Sudden stoppage of breathing.

stoma A surgical opening in the neck that connects the windpipe (trachea) to the skin.

trachea The windpipe.

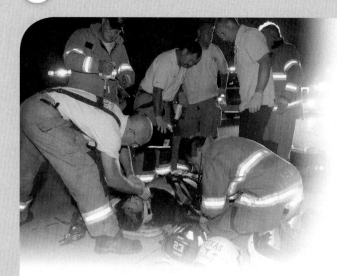

Assessment *in Action*

You are dispatched to a local park for a report of a woman who ran into a tree while roller skating. She was wearing a helmet. You can see she is bleeding heavily from a laceration on her knee. She is unresponsive. A friend skating with her says she tried to wake the woman up, but she was unable to rouse her.

1. Your first step in assessing this patient should be to:

   A. shake her shoulder.
   B. check her pulse.
   C. check for breathing.
   D. establish her level of responsiveness.

2. If you are unable to get oxygen into the patient the first time, what should be your next step?

   A. Log roll her onto her side.
   B. Attempt the jaw-thrust maneuver again and try to ventilate.
   C. Give a bigger rescue breath.
   D. Give abdominal thrusts.

3. From what you have learned about the respiratory system, what is the normal breathing rate for an adult?

   A. 4 to 10 breaths per minute
   B. 12 to 20 breaths per minute
   C. 22 to 30 breaths per minute
   D. 31 to 50 breaths per minute

4. The woman starts to vomit. You need to place her on her side to ensure she does not choke. How should you do that?

   A. Grab her arms and pull her over.
   B. Log roll her onto her side while making sure her head, neck, and spine are aligned.
   C. Turn her head to the side.
   D. Lift her to a semireclining position and start suctioning.

5. Supplemental oxygen is kept in cylinders and stored at 2,000 psi. Which device reduces the pressure for emergency use in the field?

   A. Gas gauge
   B. Nasopharynx airway
   C. Pressure regulator/flowmeter
   D. Nasal cannula

6. How do you open the airway in a patient who has suffered significant trauma?

7. The woman is breathing at a rate of 3 to 4 times a minute. What should you do next?

8. Which parts of the body are used in breathing?

9. The recovery position is used for:

   A. patients who need an open airway while rescue breathing is performed.
   B. patients who are breathing but unconscious and unable to maintain an open airway.
   C. patients who are not breathing at least 10 to 12 times per minute.
   D. draining secretions while cardiopulmonary resuscitation is performed.

10. What is a stoma?

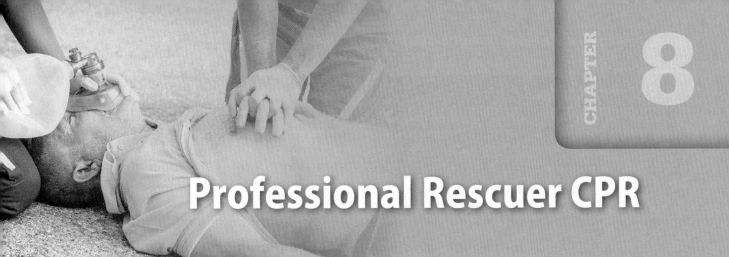

Professional Rescuer CPR

National EMS Education Standard Competencies

Shock and Resuscitation

Uses assessment information to recognize shock, respiratory failure or arrest, and cardiac arrest based on assessment findings and manages the emergency while awaiting additional emergency response.

Assessment

Uses scene information and simple patient assessment findings to identify and manage immediate life threats and injuries within the scope of practice of the EMR.

Primary Assessment

> Primary assessment for all patient situations (p 144)
> • Level of consciousness (p 146; p 149)
> • ABCs (pp 144–145)
> • Identifying life threats (p 144)
> Assessment of vital functions (pp 144–145)
> Begin interventions needed to preserve life (p 144)

Anatomy and Physiology

Uses simple knowledge of the anatomy and function of the upper airway, heart, vessels, blood, lungs, skin, muscles, and bones as the foundation of emergency care.

Pathophysiology

Uses simple knowledge of shock and respiratory compromise to respond to life threats.

Knowledge Objectives

1. Describe the anatomy and function of the circulatory system. (pp 142–144)
2. Describe some of the causes of cardiac arrest. (p 144)
3. Describe the components of cardiopulmonary resuscitation (CPR). (pp 144–145)
4. List the five links in the cardiac chain of survival. (p 145)
5. Describe the conditions under which emergency medical responders (EMRs) should start and stop CPR. (pp 145–146)

6. Describe how to perform external chest compressions on the following patients:
   • Adults (pp 144–148)
   • Infants (p 148)
   • Children (p 149)
7. Explain the steps in performing one-rescuer adult CPR. (pp 149–151)
8. Explain the steps in performing two-rescuer adult CPR. (pp 151–153)
9. Describe how to switch rescuer positions during two-rescuer adult CPR. (p 153)
10. Explain the steps in performing one-rescuer infant CPR. (pp 153–154)
11. Explain the steps in performing two-rescuer infant CPR. (p 155)
12. Explain the steps of child CPR. (pp 155–156)
13. List the four signs of effective CPR. (p 156)
14. Describe the complications of performing CPR. (pp 156–157)
15. Explain the importance of creating sufficient space to perform CPR. (p 157; p 159)
16. Describe the indications for the use of automated external defibrillation by EMRs. (p 159)
17. Explain the steps in performing automated external defibrillation. (pp 159–161)
18. Explain the importance of CPR training. (p 162)
19. Discuss the legal implications of performing CPR. (p 162)

Skills Objectives

1. Demonstrate chest compressions on an adult. (pp 146–148)
2. Demonstrate chest compressions on an infant. (p 148)
3. Demonstrate chest compressions on a child. (p 149)
4. Demonstrate one-rescuer adult CPR. (pp 149–151)
5. Demonstrate two-rescuer adult CPR. (pp 151–153)
6. Demonstrate how to switch rescuer positions during two-rescuer adult CPR. (p 153)
7. Demonstrate one-rescuer infant CPR. (pp 153–154)
8. Demonstrate two-rescuer infant CPR. (p 155)
9. Demonstrate child CPR. (pp 156–157)
10. Demonstrate creating sufficient space to perform CPR. (p 157; p 159)
11. Demonstrate automated external defibrillation. (pp 159–161)

Introduction

The purpose of this chapter is to teach you the remaining skills to perform cardiopulmonary resuscitation (CPR). CPR consists of three major skills: the C (circulation) skills, the A (airway) skills, and the B (breathing) skills. In Chapter 7, *Airway Management*, you learned the airway and breathing skills. These airway and breathing procedures may be lifesaving for a patient who has stopped breathing and whose heart is still beating. In most cases, however, by the time you arrive on the scene, the patient has not only stopped breathing, but the heart has stopped beating as well. If the patient has no heartbeat and is not breathing or only gasping, rescue breathing alone will not save the patient's life. Forcing air into the lungs is useless unless the circulatory system can carry the oxygen in the lungs to all parts of the body.

In this chapter, you will learn the C (circulation) skills. If the patient's heart has stopped, you can maintain or restore circulation manually through the use of **chest compressions** (closed-chest cardiac massage). According to recent studies, it is important to restore circulation before starting rescue breathing. Therefore, in this chapter you will learn to perform the circulation skills before you perform the airway and breathing skills (a CAB sequence). To maintain both a heartbeat and ventilation, chest compressions and rescue breathing must be done together. By combining the circulation, airway, and breathing skills, you will be able to perform CPR. Statistics show that about 70% of the patients who experience cardiac arrest are in a state of ventricular fibrillation—a condition in which the heart muscle is quivering and not effectively pumping blood. Therefore, this chapter covers the theory and the steps you need to learn to use an automated external defibrillator to defibrillate these patients.

Anatomy and Function of the Circulatory System

The **circulatory system** consists of a pump (the heart), a network of pipes (the blood vessels), and fluid (blood). After blood picks up oxygen in the lungs, it travels to the heart, which in turn pumps the oxygenated blood to the rest of the body.

In Chapter 6, *The Human Body*, you learned how the heart functions as a pump. The heart, which is about the size of your fist, is located in the chest between the lungs. The cells of the body absorb oxygen and nutrients (glucose) from the blood and produce waste products (including carbon dioxide) that the blood carries back to the lungs. In the lungs, the blood exchanges the carbon dioxide for more oxygen. Blood then returns to the heart to be pumped out again. Other metabolic waste products are removed by the kidneys and liver.

The human heart consists of four chambers, two on the right side of the heart and two on the left side. Each upper chamber is called an atrium. The right atrium receives blood from the veins of the body; the left atrium receives highly oxygenated blood from the lungs. The bottom chambers are known as the ventricles. The right ventricle pumps deoxygenated blood to the lungs; the left ventricle pumps highly oxygenated blood throughout the body. The most muscular chamber of the heart is the left ventricle, which needs the most power because it must force blood to all parts of the body. The four chambers of the heart work together in a well-ordered sequence to pump blood to the lungs and to the rest of the body **Figure 8-1**.

One-way valves in the heart and veins allow the blood to flow in only one direction through the

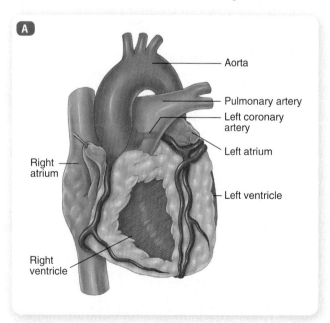

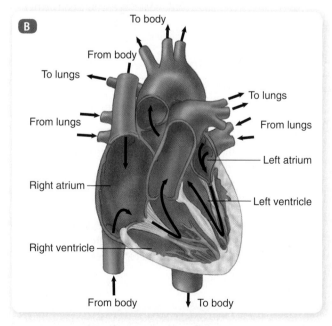

Figure 8-1 The heart functions as the pump of the human circulatory system. **A.** External view. **B.** Cross-sectional view.
A&B: © Jones & Bartlett Learning.

circulatory system. The arteries carry blood away from the heart at high pressure; therefore, the walls of arteries are thick. The main artery carrying blood away from the heart, the aorta, is quite large (about 1 inch [2.5 cm] in diameter), but arteries become smaller in diameter farther away from the heart. These smaller arteries eventually branch into the capillaries, the smallest pipes in the circulatory system. Some capillaries are so small that only one blood cell at a time can go through them. At the capillary level, oxygen passes from the blood cells into the cells of body tissues, and carbon dioxide and other waste products pass from the tissue cells to the blood cells, which then return to the lungs. Veins are the thin-walled pipes of the circulatory system that carry blood back to the heart.

The four major artery locations are as follows: the neck (carotid arteries); the wrist (radial arteries); the arm (brachial arteries); and the groin (femoral arteries). The locations of these arteries are shown in **Figure 8-2**. Because these arteries lie between a bony structure and the skin, you can use them to measure the patient's **pulse**. A pulse is generated when the heart contracts and sends a pressure wave through the artery. The **carotid pulse** is measured on either side of

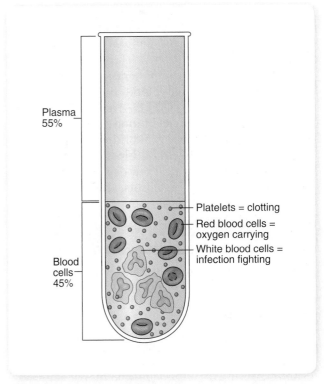

Figure 8-3 The components of blood.
© Jones & Bartlett Learning.

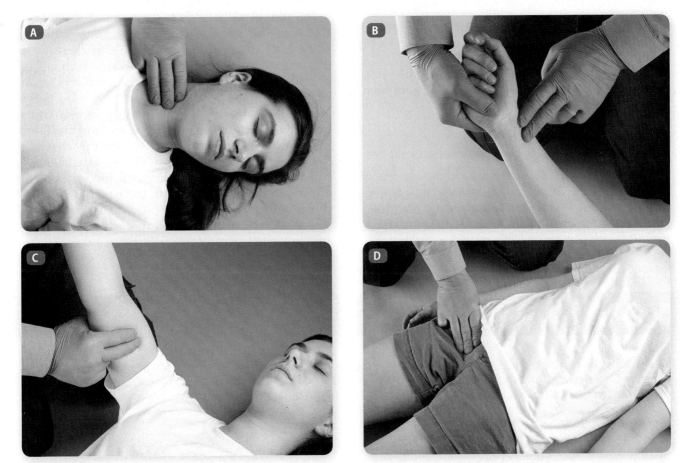

Figure 8-2 Locations for assessing the patient's pulse. **A.** Neck (carotid pulse). **B.** Wrist (radial pulse). **C.** Arm (brachial pulse). **D.** Groin (femoral pulse).
A, B, C, & D: © Jones & Bartlett Learning.

the neck, the **radial pulse** is taken at the thumb side of the wrist, the **brachial pulse** is taken on the inside of the upper arm, and the **femoral pulse** is taken at the groin.

Blood has several components: **plasma** (a clear, straw-colored fluid), red blood cells, white blood cells, and **platelets** Figure 8-3 . The red blood cells give blood its red color. Red blood cells carry oxygen from the lungs to the body and bring carbon dioxide back to the lungs. The white blood cells are called infection fighters because they devour bacteria and other disease-causing organisms. Platelets start the blood-clotting process.

■ Cardiac Arrest

Cardiac arrest occurs when the heart stops contracting and no blood is pumped through the blood vessels. Without a supply of blood, the cells of the body will die because they cannot get any oxygen or nutrients and they cannot eliminate waste products. As the cells die, organ damage occurs. Some organs are more sensitive to low oxygen levels than others. Brain damage begins within 4 to 6 minutes after the patient has gone into cardiac arrest. Within 8 to 10 minutes, the damage to the brain may become irreversible. Cardiac arrest may have many different causes, including the following:

1. Heart and blood vessel diseases such as heart attack and stroke
2. Respiratory arrest, if untreated
3. Medical emergencies such as epilepsy, diabetes, allergic reactions, electric shock, and poisoning
4. Drug overdose
5. Drowning
6. Suffocation
7. Trauma and shock caused by massive blood loss

A patient who has experienced cardiac arrest is unconscious and is not breathing or only gasping. You cannot feel a pulse and the patient looks dead. Regardless of the cause of cardiac arrest, the initial treatment is the same: provide CPR.

■ Components of CPR

The technique of CPR requires three types of skills: *C* (circulation) skills, *A* (airway) skills, and *B* (breathing) skills. From the airway and breathing skills that were detailed in Chapter 7, *Airway Management*, you learned how to check patients to determine whether the airway is open and to correct a blocked airway by using the head tilt–chin lift or jaw-thrust maneuver. You learned how to check patients to determine whether they are breathing. You also learned to correct the absence of breathing by performing rescue breathing.

To perform CPR, you combine the *A* (airway) and *B* (breathing) skills with *C* (circulation) skills in a CAB sequence. You begin by checking for the patient's pulse. With practice, you will be able to check for a pulse at the same time you are checking for signs of breathing. This helps to reduce the time it takes to begin treating the patient. If the patient has no pulse, you must restore the patient's circulation by starting external chest compressions. The airway and breathing techniques you learned previously will then be used to push oxygen into the patient's lungs. External chest compressions move the oxygenated blood throughout the body. By compressing the patient's sternum (breastbone), you change the pressure in the patient's chest and force enough blood through the system to sustain life for a short period of time.

YOU ▸ are the Provider   CASE 1

You have just finished the morning report. You and your partner are in the middle of checking your equipment when you are dispatched for a report of a sick woman. As you arrive at the residence, you are met by the patient's husband. He informs you that his wife has been reporting indigestion since 0430 hours. She is sitting on the living room couch and has taken several antacids without relief. As you begin to question the woman, she suddenly stops breathing and her head falls forward. She does not respond to your questions, to shouting, or to gentle shaking of her shoulder.

1. On the basis of the patient's unresponsiveness, what should you do now for the patient?
2. What are the chances for a successful resuscitation on this call?
3. What role does your automated external defibrillator (AED) play in this call?

CPR by itself cannot sustain life indefinitely. However, once it is recognized that the patient is pulseless and is not breathing or only gasping, start CPR as soon as possible to give the patient the best chance for survival. By performing all three parts of the CPR sequence, you can keep the patient alive until an AED is available and more advanced medical care can be delivered. In many cases, the patient will need defibrillation and medication to be successfully resuscitated from cardiac arrest.

Words of Wisdom

Patients who are experiencing cardiac events—as well as their family members and friends—will usually be fearful and anxious about the episode. It is important for you to demonstrate a caring attitude and to acknowledge those feelings. Although your primary goal is to ensure that the patient receives appropriate and timely care, you should understand that compassion is an important part of your care for patients experiencing a cardiac event.

The Cardiac Chain of Survival

In most cases of cardiac arrest, CPR alone is not enough to save lives, but it is the first treatment in the out-of-hospital chain of survival presented by the American Heart Association (AHA). The five links in the chain include:

1. Recognition of cardiac arrest and activation of the emergency response system
2. Immediate CPR with emphasis on high-quality chest compressions
3. Rapid defibrillation
4. Basic and advanced emergency medical services (EMS) care
5. Advanced life support (ALS) and postarrest care

As an emergency medical responder (EMR), you can help the patient by providing early CPR with an emphasis on high-quality chest compressions and by making sure that the EMS system has been activated.

Some EMRs are trained in the use of automated external defibrillators. By keeping these links of the chain strong, you will help keep the patient alive until early ALS care can be administered by paramedics and hospital personnel. Just as an actual chain is only as strong as its weakest link, the chain of survival is only as good as its weakest link. Your actions in performing early CPR are vital to giving cardiac arrest patients their best chance for survival **Figure 8-4** .

Words of Wisdom

Patients with chest pain are often in denial as to the reason for their chest pain. Many people will try to deny that their pain could be caused by a cardiac event. They may tell you that they are experiencing indigestion or that they have a cold. This denial often results in long delays before the patient decides to call 9-1-1. Treat any patient with chest pain as if his or her pain could be caused by a significant heart problem.

When to Start CPR

CPR should be started on all nonbreathing, pulseless patients, unless they are obviously dead or they have a do not resuscitate (DNR) order that is valid in your jurisdiction. (DNR orders are discussed more fully later in this chapter.) Few reliable criteria exist to determine death immediately.

As discussed in Chapter 4, *Medical, Legal, and Ethical Issues*, the following criteria are reliable signs of death and indicate that CPR should not be started:

1. **Decapitation.** Decapitation occurs when the head is separated from the rest of the body. When this occurs, there is obviously no chance of saving the patient.
2. **Rigor mortis.** This is the temporary stiffening of muscles that occurs several hours after death. Rigor mortis indicates the patient has been dead for a prolonged period of time and cannot be resuscitated.

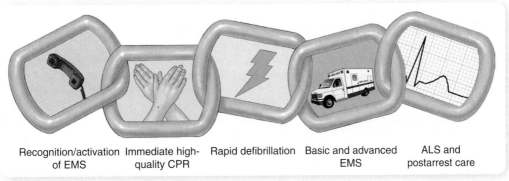

Recognition/activation of EMS   Immediate high-quality CPR   Rapid defibrillation   Basic and advanced EMS   ALS and postarrest care

Figure 8-4 The five links of the cardiac chain of survival.
© Jones & Bartlett Learning. Data from American Heart Association.

3. **Evidence of tissue decomposition.** Tissue decomposition or actual flesh decay occurs only after a person has been dead for more than 1 day.

4. **Dependent lividity.** Dependent lividity is the red or purple color that appears on the parts of the patient's body that are closest to the ground. It is caused by blood seeping into the tissues on the dependent, or lower, part of the person's body. Dependent lividity occurs after a person has been dead for several hours.

If any of the preceding signs of death are present in a pulseless, nonbreathing person, do not begin CPR. If none of these signs is present, you should activate the EMS system and then begin CPR. It is far better to start CPR on a person who is later declared dead by a physician than to withhold CPR from a patient whose life might have been saved.

When to Stop CPR

You should discontinue CPR only when:

1. Effective spontaneous circulation and ventilation are restored or the patient begins to move.
2. Resuscitation efforts are transferred to another person with an equal or higher level of training who continues CPR.
3. A physician orders you to stop.
4. The patient is transferred to properly trained EMS personnel.
5. Reliable criteria for death (as previously listed) are recognized.
6. You are too exhausted to continue resuscitation, environmental hazards endanger your safety, or continued resuscitation would place the lives of others at risk.

External Cardiac Compression

▶ External Chest Compressions on an Adult

An adult patient in cardiac arrest is unconscious, has no carotid pulse, and is not breathing or only gasping. If you suspect that the patient has experienced cardiac arrest, check the carotid pulse and look for no breathing or only gasping. To check the carotid pulse, place your index and middle fingers on the larynx (Adam's apple). Slide your fingers into the groove between the larynx and the muscles at the side of the neck ▐ Figure 8-5 ▌. Keep your fingers there for at least 5 seconds but no more than 10 seconds to be sure the pulse is absent and not just slow. At the same time, look for signs of chest movement and feel for air exchange.

If there is no carotid pulse in an unresponsive, nonbreathing patient, you must begin chest compressions. For chest compressions to be effective, the patient must

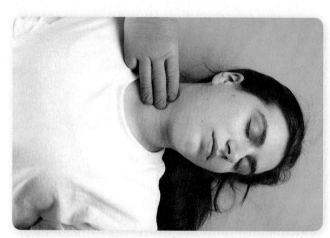

Figure 8-5 Check the patient's carotid pulse.
© Jones & Bartlett Learning.

YOU ▶ are the Provider   CASE 2

You have just finished your morning equipment check and you are thinking about a cup of coffee when your alert tones break the calm of your station. You are dispatched to 2739 Bliss Avenue, Apartment 208, for a report of an unresponsive woman. You recognize the address, which is located in a retirement community for senior citizens. After a 7-minute response, you and your partner arrive at the address and are met by an excited woman. She tells you that she arrived a few minutes earlier to clean Mrs. Ward's apartment and let herself in with her key. When she was unable to awaken Mrs. Ward, she immediately called 9-1-1. You hurry into the bedroom and see an older woman dressed in night clothes, lying in her bed. She is unresponsive to your voice and to gentle shaking. While you check for a carotid pulse and look for signs of breathing, you note that she feels very cool to your touch. Neither you nor your partner can detect any signs of a pulse, gasping, or breathing. As you start to move her arm away from her chest, you realize it is amazingly stiff.

1. What are the next steps you should take?

be lying on a firm, horizontal surface. If the patient is on a soft surface, such as a bed, it is impossible to compress the chest. Immediately place all patients needing CPR on a firm, level surface.

To position yourself so that you can perform chest compressions effectively, stand or kneel beside the patient's chest and face the patient. Place the heel of one hand in the center of the patient's chest, on the lower half of the sternum. Place the heel of your other hand on top of the hand on the chest and interlock your fingers Skill Drill 8-1 .

1. Locate the top and bottom of the sternum.
2. Place the heel of your hand in the center of the chest, on the lower half of the sternum Step 1 .
3. Place your other hand on top of your first hand and interlock your fingers Step 2 .
4. It is important to locate and maintain the proper hand position while applying chest compressions. If your hands are too high, the

Skill Drill 8-1

Performing Adult Chest Compressions

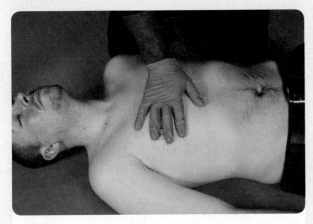

Step 1 Place the heel of your hand in the center of the chest, on the lower half of the sternum.

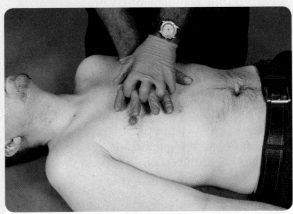

Step 2 Place your other hand on top of your first hand and interlock your fingers.

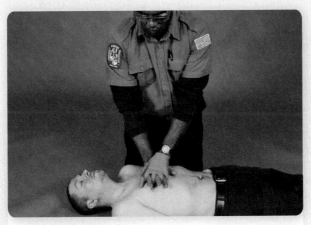

Step 3 Compress the chest of an adult at least 2 inches (5 cm) straight down.

force you apply will not produce adequate chest compressions. If your hands are too low, the force you apply may damage the liver. If your hands slip sideways off the sternum and onto the ribs, the compressions will not be effective and you may damage the ribs and lungs.

5. After you have both hands in the proper position, compress the chest of an adult at least 2 inches (5 cm) straight down **Step 3** . For compressions to be effective, stay close to the patient's side and lean forward so that your arms are directly over the patient. Keep your back straight and your elbows stiff so you can apply the force of your whole body to each compression, not just your arm muscles. Between compressions, make sure you completely release pressure on the chest to allow maximum filling of the patient's heart. Never lean on the chest during compressions. Compressions must be rhythmic and continuous. Each compression cycle consists of one downward push followed by a rest so that the heart can refill with blood. Push hard and push fast. Compressions should be at the rate of 100 to 120 compressions per minute in all patients—adults, children, and infants. After every 30 chest compressions, give two rescue breaths (1 second per breath). Practice on a manikin until you can compress the chest smoothly and rhythmically.

Treatment

Do not let your fingers touch the chest wall; your fingers could dig into the patient, causing injury. Interlocking your fingers will help avoid this.

▶ External Chest Compressions on an Infant

Infants (children younger than 1 year) who have experienced cardiac arrest will be unconscious, not breathing or only gasping, and will have no pulse. To check for cardiac arrest, begin by checking responsiveness. If the infant is unresponsive, check the brachial pulse and look, listen, and feel for signs of breathing. If a pulse is absent and there are no signs of breathing, begin CPR starting with chest compressions.

To check an infant's circulation, feel for the brachial pulse on the inside of the upper arm **Figure 8-6** . Use two fingers of one hand to feel for

the pulse and use your other hand to maintain the head tilt. If the infant has no pulse and is not breathing or only gasping, begin CPR starting with chest compressions. Draw an imaginary horizontal line between the two nipples and place your index finger just below the imaginary line in the center of the chest. Place your middle and ring fingers next to your index finger. Use your middle and ring fingers to compress the sternum at least one-third the depth of the chest (about 1.5 inches [4 cm]). Compress the sternum at a rate of 100 to 120 times per minute. If you are the only rescuer, give two rescue breaths (1 second per breath) after every 30 chest compressions. If two rescuers are present, give two rescue breaths after every 15 chest compressions.

When you perform chest compressions, place the infant on a solid surface such as a table or cradle the infant in your arm, as shown in **Figure 8-7** . You do not need to use much force to achieve adequate compressions on infants because they are so small and their chests are so flexible.

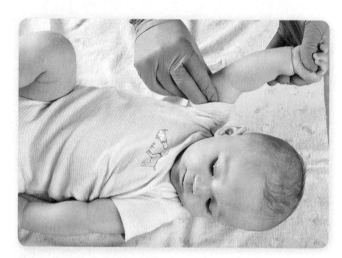

Figure 8-6 Check the brachial pulse on the inside of the infant's arm.
© Jones & Bartlett Learning.

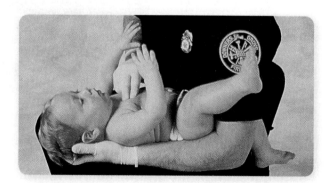

Figure 8-7 Positioning the infant patient for proper CPR.
© American Academy of Orthopaedic Surgeons.

External Chest Compressions on a Child

The signs of cardiac arrest in a **child** (from age 1 year to the onset of puberty [age 12 to 14 years]) are the same as those for an adult. Determine if the child is responsive. If the child is unresponsive, simultaneously check the carotid pulse and for no breathing and for gasping. If there is no pulse, no breathing, and only gasping, the patient is in cardiac arrest. Check the carotid pulse by placing two or three fingers on the larynx. Slide your fingers into the groove between the Adam's apple and the muscle. Feel for the carotid pulse with one hand.

To perform chest compressions on a small child, place the heel of one hand in the center of the chest, on the lower half of the sternum. In larger children, perform chest compressions with two hands, as with the adult. Compress the sternum at least one-third the depth of the chest (about 2 inches [5 cm]). Compress the chest at a rate of at 100 to 120 times per minute. If you are the only rescuer present, give two rescue breaths after every 30 chest compressions. If two rescuers are present, give two rescue breaths after every 15 compressions.

Adult CPR

One-Rescuer Adult CPR

In Chapter 7, *Airway Management*, you learned how to open the airway and perform rescue breathing. Now that you have learned how to check for circulation and do chest compressions, you are ready to put all your skills together to perform CPR. If you are the only trained person at the scene, you must perform **one-rescuer CPR**. Follow the steps in Skill Drill 8-2 :

1. Establish unresponsiveness Step 1 . Ask the patient, "Are you okay?" Gently shake the patient's shoulder. If you do not get a response, call for additional help, activate the EMS system, and send someone to get an AED if one is available.
2. Position the patient so he or she is flat on his or her back on a hard surface. Position yourself so that your knees are alongside the patient's chest.
3. Determine pulselessness by checking the carotid pulse and simultaneously checking for no breathing or only gasping. Check the pulse and breathing for no more than 10 seconds Step 2 .
4. If the patient has no pulse and is not breathing or only gasping, begin chest compressions. Place the heel of one hand in the center of the chest, on the lower half of the sternum. Place

your other hand on top of the first. Lock your fingers together and pull upward so that the only thing touching the patient's chest is the heel of your hand Step 3 .

5. Lean forward so your shoulders are directly over your hands and the patient's sternum. Keep your arms straight and compress the sternum at least 2 inches (5 cm), using the weight of your body. Relax between compressions, allowing the chest to fully recoil. Give 30 compressions at a rate of 100 to 120 compressions per minute, and count each one out loud as follows: "One and two and three and…." Each set of 30 compressions should take between 15 and 18 seconds to complete.
6. After 30 chest compressions, open the airway using a head tilt–chin lift or a jaw-thrust maneuver if you suspect a head or spinal injury Step 4 . Give two rescue breaths (1 second each). Ensure that each breath produces visible chest rise Step 5 .
7. Continue the cycles of 30 chest compressions and two breaths until additional personnel arrive, an AED arrives, or the patient starts to move.

Words of Wisdom

If you do not have a partner with you to help perform CPR, do not wait for another rescuer to arrive. Call 9-1-1 to activate EMS and then begin one-rescuer CPR immediately!

When performing one-rescuer CPR—whether the patient is an adult, child, or infant—deliver chest compressions and rescue breathing at a ratio of 30 compressions to two breaths. Immediately give two rescue breaths after each set of 30 chest compressions. Because you must interrupt chest compressions to ventilate, you should perform each series of 30 chest compressions in approximately 18 seconds (a rate of 100 to 120 compressions per minute).

A skill performance sheet titled One-Rescuer Adult CPR is shown in Figure 8-8 for your review and practice.

Although one-rescuer CPR can keep the patient alive, two-rescuer CPR is preferable because it is less exhausting for the rescuers. Whenever possible, CPR for an adult should be performed by two rescuers.

Two-Rescuer Adult CPR

In many cases, a second trained person will be on the scene to help you perform CPR. Two-rescuer CPR is more effective than one-rescuer CPR. One rescuer

Skill Drill 8-2

Performing One-Rescuer Adult CPR

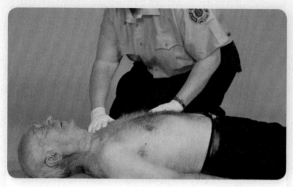

Step 1 Establish unresponsiveness by shouting and gently shaking the shoulder.

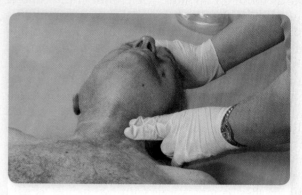

Step 2 If the patient is unresponsive, simultaneously check the carotid pulse and check for signs of breathing. Take no more than 10 seconds to do this. If the patient is unresponsive, activate the EMS system.

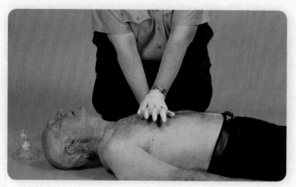

Step 3 If breathing and pulse are absent, begin a cycle of 30 chest compressions at a rate of 100 to 120 compressions per minute. Compress the chest at least 2 inches (5 cm) and release the pressure on the chest after each compression.

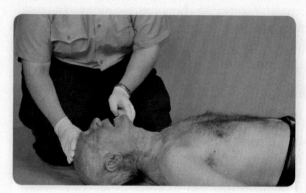

Step 4 After 30 compressions, open the airway with a head tilt–chin lift or a jaw-thrust maneuver if you suspect a head or spinal injury.

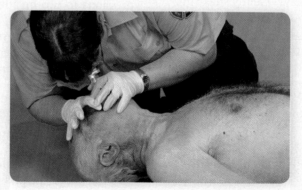

Step 5 Give two rescue breaths over 1 second. Watch for chest rise to ensure air is going into the lungs. Continue cycles of 30 compressions and two rescue breaths until an AED arrives, patient care is assumed by other providers, or the patient starts to move.

One-Rescuer Adult CPR	
Steps	**Adequately Performed**
1. Establish unresponsiveness by shouting and gently shaking the patient. If unresponsive and lack of breathing, activate the EMS system.	
2. Check for signs of circulation and breathing at the same time by checking the carotid pulse and watching for chest rise (within 10 seconds).	
3. If the patient has no pulse and is not breathing or only gasping, give cycles of 30 chest compressions at a rate of 100 to 120 compressions per minute.	
4. Open the airway using the head tilt–chin lift maneuver. (If trauma is present or you suspect a head or spinal injury, use the jaw-thrust maneuver.)	
5. Give 2 slow breaths (1 second per breath). If the chest does not rise, reposition the head and try to ventilate again. Watch for chest rise; allow for exhalation between breaths.	
6. Continue cycles of 30 chest compressions and 2 breaths until additional personnel arrive, an AED arrives, or the patient starts to move.	

Figure 8-8 Skill performance sheet: One-Rescuer Adult CPR.
© Jones & Bartlett Learning.

delivers chest compressions while the other performs rescue breathing. Chest compressions and ventilations can be given more regularly and without interruption. However, to avoid rescuer fatigue—which may result in less effective chest compressions—the two rescuers should switch roles after every five cycles of CPR (about every 2 minutes). Two rescuers should be able to switch roles quickly, interrupting CPR for 5 seconds or less. In any circumstance, CPR should not be interrupted for longer than 10 seconds.

In **two-rescuer CPR**, one rescuer delivers ventilations (mouth-to-mouth, bag-mask, or mouth-to-mask breathing) and the other gives chest compressions. If possible, position yourselves on opposite sides of the patient—one rescuer near the head and the other near the chest. The sequence of steps is the same as for one-rescuer CPR, but the tasks are divided Skill Drill 8-3 :

1. Rescuer One establishes unresponsiveness. Rescuer Two moves to the patient's side to be ready to deliver chest compressions. Rescuer One activates the EMS system Step 1 .

2. If the patient is unresponsive, Rescuer One determines pulselessness. Rescuer One simultaneously checks for signs of circulation and breathing by checking the carotid pulse and watching for chest rise for no more than 10 seconds Step 2 . If the patient has no pulse and is not breathing or only gasping, continue to Step 3.

3. The rescuers begin CPR, starting with chest compressions. Rescuer Two performs 30 chest compressions at a rate of 100 to 120 compressions per minute Step 3 .

4. Rescuer One opens the airway with a head tilt–chin lift or, in the case of a trauma or if a head or spinal injury is suspected, a jaw-thrust maneuver Step 4 .

5. Rescuer One gives two ventilations of 1 second each and observes for visible chest rise Step 5 .

6. Continue CPR for five cycles of 30 compressions and two ventilations (about 2 minutes). After 2 minutes of CPR, the rescuers switch positions. The switch time should take no longer than 5 seconds.

7. Continue cycles of 30 chest compressions and two ventilations until an AED arrives, ALS personnel take over, or the patient starts to move.

Compressions and ventilations should remain rhythmic and uninterrupted. By counting out loud, Rescuer Two can continue to deliver compressions at the rate of 100 to 120 compressions per minute, briefly pausing as Rescuer One delivers two rescue breaths. Once you and your partner establish a smooth pattern of CPR, you should limit interruptions in CPR to 10 seconds or less, such as when reassessing or moving the patient. A skill performance sheet titled Two-Rescuer Adult CPR is shown in Figure 8-9 for your review and practice.

Skill Drill 8-3

Performing Two-Rescuer Adult CPR

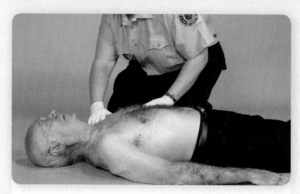

Step 1 Establish responsiveness and lack of breathing.

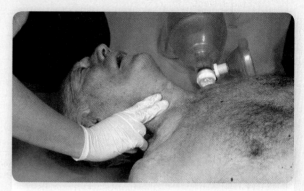

Step 2 If the patient is unresponsive, simultaneously check the carotid pulse and check for no breathing and only gasping. This should take no more than 10 seconds.

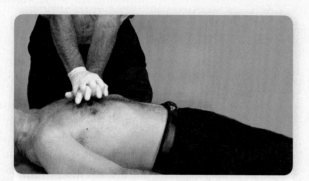

Step 3 Perform 30 chest compressions.

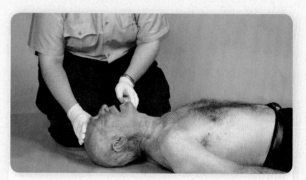

Step 4 Open the airway using the head tilt–chin lift or jaw-thrust maneuver.

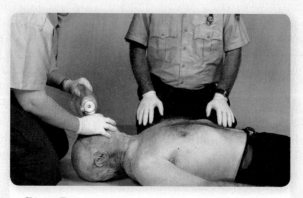

Step 5 Perform rescue breathing; give two breaths. Continue cycles of 30 compressions and two rescue breaths until an AED arrives, care is assumed by other providers, or the patient starts to move.

Two-Rescuer Adult CPR	
Steps	**Adequately Performed**
1. Rescuer One checks for responsiveness by shouting and gently shaking the patient's shoulder.	
2. If the patient is unresponsive, Rescuer One simultaneously checks the carotid pulse and looks for signs of no breathing or only gasping (within 10 seconds). Activate the EMS system.	
3. If the patient has no pulse and is not breathing or only gasping, Rescuer One instructs Rescuer Two to begin compressions.	
4. Rescuer Two begins chest compressions at the rate of 100 to 120 compressions per minute.	
5. After 30 compressions, Rescuer One opens the airway and gives two rescue breaths.	
6. The rescuers continue for 5 cycles of CPR.	
7. After 5 cycles of CPR are completed, the rescuers switch positions. Rescuer One begins compressions and Rescuer Two takes over rescue breathing.	
8. As soon as an AED is available it is placed in operation.	
9. Continue cycles of CPR until the patient moves or other rescuers arrive to take over the care of the patient.	

Figure 8-9 Skill performance sheet: Two-Rescuer Adult CPR.
© Jones & Bartlett Learning.

Words of Wisdom

When you have a patient who is in cardiac arrest, always be prepared for vomiting. It is a frequent event, and your preparation for it can be lifesaving.

▶ Switching Positions During CPR

If you and your partner must continue to perform two-rescuer CPR for any length of time, the rescuer performing chest compressions will become tired. Once a rescuer gets tired, the effectiveness of chest compressions decreases. Therefore rescuers should switch positions after every five cycles of CPR (about every 2 minutes). This will improve the quality of chest compressions and give the patient the best chance for survival.

A switch allows the person giving compressions (Rescuer Two) to rest his or her arms. Switching positions should be accomplished as smoothly and quickly (5 seconds or less) as possible to minimize the break in rate and regularity of compressions and ventilations. There are many orderly ways to switch positions. Learn the method practiced in your EMS system. One method is as follows:

1. As Rescuer Two tires, he or she says the following out loud (instead of counting): "We—will—switch—this—time." One word is spoken as each compression is done. These words replace the counting sequence for the first five compressions.

2. After 25 more chest compressions (a total of 30 compressions), Rescuer One completes two ventilations and moves to the chest to perform compressions.
3. Rescuer Two moves to the head of the patient to maintain the airway and ventilation.
4. Rescuer One then begins chest compressions.

Practice switching positions until you can do it smoothly and quickly. Switching positions is much easier if the rescuers work on opposite sides of the patient.

■ Infant CPR

▶ One-Rescuer Infant CPR

An infant is defined as anyone younger than 1 year. The principles of CPR are the same for adults and infants. In actual practice, however, you must use slightly different techniques for an infant. Follow these steps for one-rescuer infant CPR:

1. Position the infant faceup on a firm, flat surface.
2. Establish the infant's level of responsiveness. An unresponsive infant is limp. Gently shake or tap the infant to determine whether he or she is unconscious. Call for additional help if the patient is unconscious. Active the EMS system.
3. If the infant is unresponsive, simultaneously check the brachial pulse and check for signs of no breathing or only gasping. The brachial pulse is on the inside of the arm. You can

feel it by placing your index and middle fingers on the inside of the infant's arm, halfway between the shoulder and the elbow. Check for at least 5 seconds but no more than 10 seconds. Assess for breathing by looking at the infant's chest and abdomen.

4. If the infant has no pulse and is not breathing or only gasping, begin chest compressions. An infant's heart is located relatively higher in the chest than an adult's heart. Imagine a horizontal line drawn between the infant's nipples. To correctly position your fingers for chest compressions, imagine a line between the infant's nipples. Place your index finger in the middle of the sternum and just below the nipple line and your middle and ring fingers next to your index finger. Raise your index finger so that your middle finger and ring fingers remain in contact with the chest Figure 8-10.

5. With your fingers in the correct location, compress the chest 30 times with the pads of your fingertips. Compress the chest at least one-third the depth of the chest (about 1.5 inches [4 cm]) at a rate of 100 to 120 compressions per minute.

6. Open the infant's airway. This step is best done by the head tilt–chin lift maneuver. Gently tilt the infant's head to a neutral or slight sniffing position. Tilting it too far can obstruct the airway.

7. Give two breaths, each lasting 1 second. To breathe for an infant, place your mouth over the infant's mouth and nose. Because an infant has very small lungs, you should give only very small puffs of air, just enough to make the chest rise. Do not use large or forceful breaths.

8. Continue compressions and ventilations. If you are alone, give 30 compressions and two breaths. Continue to give 30 compressions followed by two rescue breaths until other providers arrive to take over the care of the infant or the infant begins to move.

A skill performance sheet titled One-Rescuer Infant CPR is shown in Figure 8-11 for your review and practice.

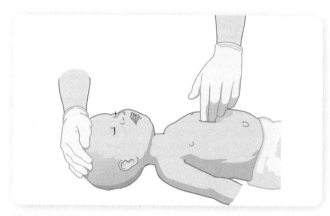

Figure 8-10 Perform chest compressions on an infant using two fingers in the middle of the chest just below the nipple line. Compress the chest at least one-third the depth of the chest (about 1.5 [4 cm] inches) at a rate of 100 to 120 compressions per minute.
© Jones & Bartlett Learning.

One-Rescuer Infant CPR	
Steps	**Adequately Performed**
1. Establish unresponsiveness by shouting and gently shaking the infant	
2. If unresponsive, simultaneously check the brachial pulse and look for movement of the chest and stomach for signs or breathing. Call for help if anyone else is around or if you have a mobile phone.	
3. If there is no pulse and no signs of breathing, begin chest compressions. Give 30 chest compressions by using 2 fingers in the middle of the chest just below the nipple line. Maintain a rate of 100 to 120 compressions per minute. Compress the chest 1.5 inches (4 cm).	
4. Open airway using the head tilt–chin lift maneuver to open the airway to a neutral or slight sniffing position. (If trauma is present, use the jaw-thrust maneuver.)	
5. Give 2 slow breaths (1 second per breath). If the chest does not rise, reposition the head and try to ventilate again. Watch for chest rise; allow for exhalation between breaths.	
6. Continue cycles of 30 chest compressions and two rescue breaths until the infant moves or until other EMS providers arrive to take over the care of the patient. If you are by yourself with no communications device, perform 2 minutes of CPR before leaving the victim to activate the EMS system.	

Figure 8-11 Skill performance sheet: One-Rescuer Infant CPR.
© Jones & Bartlett Learning.

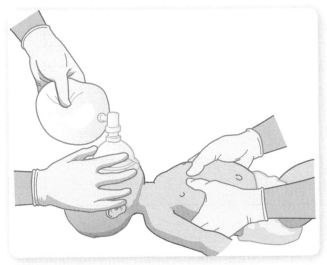

Figure 8-12 When performing two-rescuer infant CPR, use the two-thumb/encircling hands technique for chest compressions. Place both thumbs side by side over the lower half of the infant's sternum and encircle the infant's chest with your hands.
© Jones & Bartlett Learning.

▶ Two-Rescuer Infant CPR

If you are performing two-rescuer infant CPR, use the two-thumb/encircling hands technique for chest compressions Figure 8-12 . This technique is done by placing both thumbs side by side over the lower half of the infant's sternum and encircling the infant's chest with your hands. Compress the sternum at a rate of 100 to 120 compressions per minute. When you are performing two-rescuer infant CPR, perform a compression-to-ventilation ratio of 15 to 2. Rescuers should switch roles after 10 cycles of CPR (about 2 minutes) when using a compression to ventilation ratio of 15:2.

■ Child CPR

▶ One-Rescuer and Two-Rescuer Child CPR

A child is defined as a person between age 1 year and the onset of puberty (age 12 to 14 years). The steps for child CPR are essentially the same as for an adult; however, some steps may require modification for a child. These variations are as follows:

1. Use less force to compress the child's chest.
2. In small children, use only one hand to depress the sternum at least one-third the depth of the chest (about 2 inches [5 cm]). Use two hands in larger children.
3. Use less force to ventilate the child. Ventilate only until the child's chest rises.

Follow these steps to administer CPR to a child:

1. Establish the child's level of responsiveness. Tap and gently shake the shoulder and shout,

"Are you okay?" If a second rescuer is available, have him or her activate the EMS system and get an AED if available.
2. Place the child faceup on a firm, flat surface.
3. Check for circulation and simultaneously check for signs of no breathing or only gasping. Locate the larynx with your index and middle fingers. Slide your fingers into the groove between the larynx and the muscles at the side of the neck to feel for the carotid pulse. Check for at least 5 seconds but no more than 10 seconds.
4. If the child has no pulse and is not breathing or only gasping, begin chest compressions.
5. Begin a cycle of 30 chest compressions. Compress the chest at least one-third the diameter of the chest (approximately 2 inches [5 cm] in most children) at a rate of 100 to 120 compressions per minute Figure 8-13 . Count the compressions out loud: "One and two and three and…." In between compressions, allow the chest to fully recoil.
6. After 30 compressions, open the airway. Use the head tilt–chin lift maneuver or, if the child is injured, use the jaw-thrust maneuver. Maintain an open airway.
7. Give two rescue breaths. Blow slowly for 1 second, using just enough force to make the chest visibly rise. Allow the lungs to deflate between breaths.
8. Coordinate chest compressions and ventilations in a 30:2 ratio for one rescuer and 15:2 for two rescuers, making sure the chest rises with each ventilation.
9. After five cycles (about 2 minutes) of CPR, assess for signs of breathing or a pulse. If the child has no pulse and you have an AED, apply it now.
10. If you are alone with no communications device, perform 2 minutes of CPR before leaving the patient to activate the EMS system.

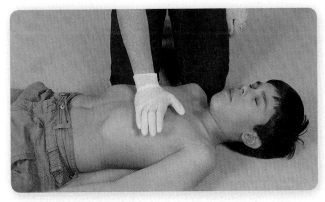

Figure 8-13 When performing chest compressions on a child, place the heel of your hand in the center of the chest, in between the nipples.
© Jones & Bartlett Learning. Courtesy of MIEMSS.

One-Rescuer Child CPR	
Steps	**Adequately Performed**
1. Establish unresponsiveness by shaking the child. If a second rescuer is available, have him or her activate the EMS system.	
2. Check for signs of circulation by checking the carotid pulse and simultaneously checking for no breathing and only gasping.	
3. If the child has no pulse and is not breathing or only gasping, give cycles of 30 chest compressions at a rate of 100 to 120 compressions per minute.	
4. Open the airway using the head tilt–chin lift maneuver. (If trauma is present or you suspect a head or spinal injury, use the jaw-thrust maneuver.)	
5. Give 2 effective breaths (1 second per breath). If the airway is obstructed, reposition the head and try to ventilate again. Watch for chest rise; allow for exhalation between breaths.	
6. Continue cycles of 30 chest compressions and 2 ventilations until additional personnel arrive or the patient starts to move. If you are alone with no communications device, perform 2 minutes of CPR before leaving the patient to activate the EMS system.	

Figure 8-14 Skill performance sheet: One-Rescuer Child CPR.
© Jones & Bartlett Learning.

11. Continue until other EMS providers arrive to take over the care of the patient or the patient starts to move.

A skill performance sheet titled One-Rescuer Child CPR is shown in **Figure 8-14** for your review and practice. In large children, remember that you may need to use two hands to achieve an adequate depth of compression. When you are performing two-rescuer CPR on a child, administer 15 compressions followed by two rescue breaths.

Signs of Effective CPR

It is important to know the signs of effective CPR so you can assess your efforts to resuscitate the patient. The signs of effective CPR are as follows:

1. A second rescuer feels a carotid pulse while you are compressing the chest.
2. The patient's skin color improves (from blue to pink).
3. The chest visibly rises during ventilations.
4. Compressions and ventilations are delivered at the appropriate rate and depth.

If some of these signs are not present, evaluate and alter your technique to try and achieve these signs.

Complications of CPR

A discussion of CPR is not complete without mentioning its complications, but you can minimize these complications by using proper technique.

▶ Broken Ribs

If your hands slip to the side of the sternum during chest compressions or if your fingers rest on the ribs, you may break a patient's ribs while delivering a compression. To prevent this complication, use proper hand positioning and do not let your fingers come in contact with the ribs. If you hear a cracking sound while performing CPR, check and correct your hand position but continue CPR. Sometimes you may break bones or cartilage even when using proper CPR technique.

▶ Gastric Distention

Bloating of the stomach is called **gastric distention**. It is caused when too much air is blown too fast and too forcefully into the stomach. A partially obstructed airway, which allows some of the air you breathe into the patient's airway to go into the stomach rather than into the lungs, can also cause gastric distention.

Gastric distention causes the abdomen to increase in size. A distended abdomen pushes on the diaphragm and prevents the lungs from inflating fully. Gastric distention also often causes regurgitation. If regurgitation occurs, quickly turn the patient to the side, wipe out the mouth with your gloved fingers, and then return the patient to a supine position.

You can prevent gastric distention by making sure you have opened the airway completely. Do not blow excessive amounts of air into the patient (deliver each breath over a period of 1 second). Be especially careful if you are a large person with a large lung capacity and the patient is smaller than you.

▶ Regurgitation

Regurgitation (passive vomiting) is a common occurrence during CPR, so you must be prepared to manage this complication. You can minimize the risk of regurgitation by minimizing the amount of air that enters the patient's stomach. Regurgitation commonly occurs if the patient has experienced cardiac arrest. When cardiac arrest occurs, the muscle that keeps food in the stomach relaxes. If there is any food in the stomach, it backs up, causing the patient to vomit.

If the patient regurgitates as you are performing CPR, immediately turn the patient onto his or her side to allow the vomitus to drain from the mouth. Clear the patient's mouth of remaining vomitus, first with your fingers and then with a clean cloth (if one is handy). Use suction if it is available.

The patient may experience frequent episodes of regurgitation, so you must be prepared to take these actions repeatedly. EMS units carry a mechanical suction machine that can clear the patient's mouth. However, you cannot wait until the mechanical suction machine arrives before beginning or resuming CPR. You must manage the regurgitation as it occurs so that CPR is not delayed.

Do your best to clear any vomitus from the patient's airway. If the airway is not cleared, two complications may arise:

1. The patient may breathe in (aspirate) the vomitus into the lungs.
2. You may force vomitus into the lungs with the next artificial ventilation.

It takes a strong stomach and the realization that you are trying to save the patient's life to continue with resuscitation after the patient has regurgitated—but you must continue. Remove the vomitus from the patient's mouth with a towel, the patient's shirt, your gloved fingers, or a manual suction unit if available. As soon as you have cleared away the vomitus, continue rescue breathing.

■ Creating Sufficient Space for CPR

As an EMR, you will frequently find yourself alone with a patient in cardiac arrest. One of the first steps you must take is to create or find a space where you can perform CPR. Ask yourself, "Is there enough room in this location to perform effective CPR?" To perform CPR effectively, you need 3 to 4 feet (approximately 1 m) of space on all sides of the patient. This will provide you with enough space so that rescuers can change places, advanced life support procedures can be implemented, and an ambulance stretcher can be brought in. If there is not enough space around the patient, you have two options:

1. Quickly rearrange the furniture in the room or arrange objects at the scene to make space.
2. Quickly drag the patient into an area that has more space; for instance, out of the bathroom and into the living room but not into a hallway Figure 8-15 .

YOU are the Provider   CASE 3

On your way back from getting fuel, you are suddenly dispatched for the report of an unknown emergency. As you arrive at the address, you are led to a basement workshop in a suburban home. A 12-year-old girl tells you that her father went down into his woodworking shop to work on a project. The girl tells you that she was upstairs doing homework when she heard her father yell for help. She ran downstairs and found him slumped over his band saw. As you approach the scene, you notice your patient seems to be grasping the power switch in one hand.

1. What should you do first?
2. What steps should you take to assess this patient?
3. Do you think an AED is important in this situation?

Voices *of* Experience

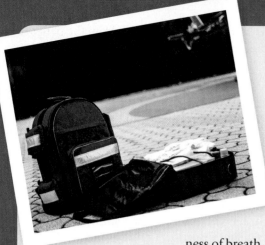

Paul, my friend of 10 years, was 70 years old and very physically fit. One day, while mowing the lawn, he began experiencing shortness of breath. He went inside to rest and felt better. Later that day, he had the same problem when he walked up the stairs. Paul called his doctor and made an appointment to be seen in his office the next week.

The following day, while eating breakfast, he began to complain of chest pain. Paul's wife, Donna, called 9-1-1 and help was on the way, but before they arrived, Paul's wife says, "He turned green and that was it."

> **"When emergency medical responders arrived, they found Paul unconscious and unresponsive."**

When emergency medical responders arrived, they found Paul unconscious and unresponsive. With the ambulance still on the way, they immediately began to administer professional rescuer CPR. A pulse check was done and they opened his airway, but Paul had no pulse and was not breathing. The team initiated compressions and an AED was attached, "*Shock advised, stand clear of patient.*" A shock was delivered. Paul had been in cardiac arrest for 4 minutes and 30 seconds.

Two weeks after Paul's incident, I sat at a local restaurant listening to this story. As Paul's wife spoke, it sent chills up my spine. Paul was in cardiac arrest for over 4 minutes. Yet, due to rapid implementation of the cardiac chain of survival and the actions of the EMRs, my friend sat beside his wife with tears in his eyes that day thanking me for teaching others the lifesaving skills that had saved his life.

As you study the material in this textbook, consider the following: Will you someday be the Paul whose life is saved by someone, or will you be a lifesaver yourself and save someone's Paul?

Charles Dixon
President, American Heritage Training
Training Officer, American Heritage Ambulance
Ladson, South Carolina

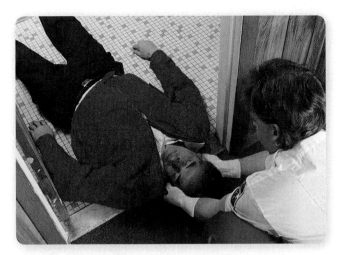

Figure 8-15 Create sufficient space for CPR.
© American Academy of Orthopaedic Surgeons.

Space is essential to a smooth rescue operation for a cardiac arrest patient. It takes a minimal amount of time to either clear a space around the patient or move the patient into a larger area.

Early Defibrillation by EMRs

According to the AHA, about 424,000 people in the United States die each year of coronary heart disease in an out-of-hospital setting. As mentioned previously, more than 70% of all out-of-hospital cardiac arrest patients have an irregular heart electrical rhythm called **ventricular fibrillation**. This condition, often referred to as V-fib, is the rapid, disorganized, and ineffective vibration of the heart. An electric shock applied to the heart will defibrillate it and reorganize the vibrations into effective heartbeats. A patient in cardiac arrest stands the greatest chance for survival when early defibrillation is available.

As an EMR, you are often the first emergency health care provider to reach a patient who has collapsed in cardiac arrest. When you perform effective CPR, you are helping to keep the patient's brain and heart supplied with oxygen until a defibrillator and advanced life support (ALS) providers arrive at the scene.

To get defibrillators to cardiac arrest patients more quickly, increasing numbers of EMS systems are equipping EMRs with **automated external defibrillators (AEDs)** Figure 8-16 . These machines accurately identify ventricular fibrillation and advise you to deliver a shock if needed. Such equipment allows you to combine effective CPR with early defibrillation to restore an organized heartbeat in a patient.

AEDs may be appropriate for your community if you work to strengthen all links of the cardiac chain of survival (see Figure 8-4). The links of the chain of survival include the following:

- Recognition of cardiac arrest and activation of the EMS system

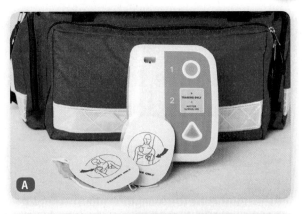

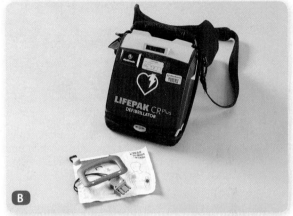

Figure 8-16 Automated external defibrillators can vary in their design, features, and operation.
A: © Photographee.eu/Shutterstock. B: © Jones & Bartlett Learning.

- Immediate CPR with emphasis on high-quality chest compressions
- Rapid defibrillation
- Basic and advanced EMS care
- Advanced life support and post arrest care

▶ Performing Automated External Defibrillation

The steps for using an AED are listed in Skill Drill 8-4 :

1. If CPR is in progress when you arrive, check the effectiveness of the chest compressions by checking for a pulse Step 1 . It is important to limit the amount of time compressions are interrupted. If the patient is responsive, do not apply the AED.

2. If the patient is unresponsive, begin providing chest compressions as soon as possible Step 2 . Perform compressions and rescue breaths at a ratio of 30 compressions to two breaths, continuing until an AED arrives and is ready for use. It is important to start chest compressions and use the AED as soon as possible. Compressions provide vital blood flow to the heart and brain, improving the patient's

Skill Drill 8-4

Procedure for Automated External Defibrillation

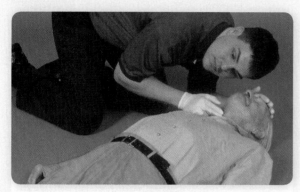

Step 1 Check for responsiveness by shouting and gently shaking the shoulder. If the patient is unresponsive, simultaneously check the carotid pulse and check for signs of breathing or only gasping. If pulse is absent and there are no signs of breathing, proceed to Step 2.

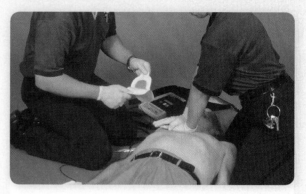

Step 2 Begin cycles of 30 compressions and two breaths. Use the AED as soon as it is available. If cardiac arrest is witnessed, proceed to Step 3.

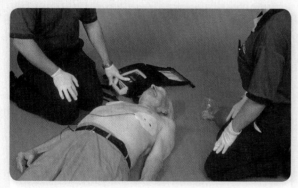

Step 3 Turn on the AED. Apply the adhesive pads and connect them to the AED. Press the analyze button. If your AED has voice prompts, follow the verbal instructions. Do not touch the patient. Allow the AED to analyze the rhythm.

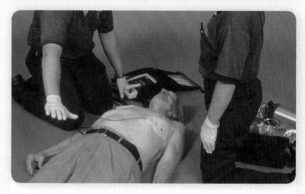

Step 4 If a shock is advised, press the button to defibrillate the patient. If no shock is advised, perform five cycles of CPR.

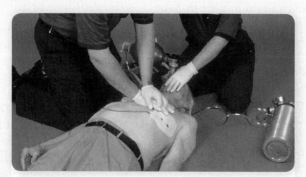

Step 5 As soon as the shock is delivered, begin CPR starting with chest compressions. Perform five cycles of CPR (about 2 minutes). After 2 minutes of CPR, go back to Step 3 to reanalyze the cardiac rhythm.

chance of survival. If the cardiac arrest is witnessed, attach the AED as soon as it is available.

3. Turn on the AED. Remove clothing from the patient's chest area. Apply the pads to the chest: one just to the right of the breastbone (sternum) just below the collarbone (clavicle), the other on the left lower chest area with the top of the pad 2 to 3 inches (5 cm to 8 cm) below the armpit. Be sure that the pads are attached to the patient cables (and that they are attached to the AED in some models). Plug in the pads connector to the AED **Step 3**.

4. Stop CPR.

5. State aloud, "Clear the patient," and ensure that no one is touching the patient.

6. Push the analyze button, if there is one, and wait for the AED to determine if a shockable rhythm is present.

7. If a shock is not advised, perform five cycles (about 2 minutes) of CPR beginning with chest compressions. Then reassess the patient's pulse and reanalyze the cardiac rhythm. If a shock is advised, reconfirm that no one is touching the patient and push the shock button. After the shock is delivered, immediately resume CPR, beginning with chest compressions **Step 4**.

8. After five cycles (about 2 minutes) of CPR, reanalyze the patient's cardiac rhythm. Do not interrupt chest compressions for more than 10 seconds **Step 5**.

9. Repeat the cycle of 2 minutes of CPR, one shock (if indicated), and 2 minutes of CPR.

10. Arrange for transport, and contact medical control as needed.

AEDs vary in design and operation, so learn how to use your specific AED. You must have the training required by your medical director to practice automated external defibrillation. Practice until you can perform the procedure quickly and safely. Because the recommended guidelines for using the AED change, always follow the most current CPR and Emergency Cardiac Care (ECC) guidelines.

Special Populations

You can safely use AEDs in pediatric patients using the pediatric-sized pads and a dose-attenuating system (energy reducer). However, if these items are unavailable, use an adult AED. During CPR, the AED should be applied to infants or children after the first five cycles of CPR have been completed. Cardiac arrest in children is usually the result of respiratory failure; therefore, oxygenation and ventilation are vitally important. After the first five cycles of CPR, use the AED to deliver shocks in the same manner as with an adult patient.

If the child is between 1 month and 1 year of age (an infant), a manual defibrillator is preferred to an AED; however, manual defibrillation is a paramedic-level skill. Therefore, call for paramedic backup immediately if you suspect an infant may be in cardiac arrest. If paramedic backup with a manual defibrillator is not available, an AED equipped with a pediatric dose attenuator is preferred. If neither is available, an AED without a pediatric dose attenuator may be used. Follow the manufacturer's instructions for use of the AED for pediatric patients.

Treatment

When preparing to defibrillate a patient, be alert for the following situations:

- If the patient is wet, dry the patient before initiating defibrillation. This will ensure that the defibrillation pads stick to the patient's chest and that the full shock is delivered safely.
- If the patient has excessive hair on his chest and a razor is available, quickly shave the area where the pads will be placed.
- If the patient has a pacemaker, you may need to reposition one of the defibrillation pads so that it is not placed directly over the pacemaker.
- If the patient has a transdermal medication patch on his or her chest, remove the patch and wipe the skin before defibrillating the patient.

YOU are the Provider   CASE 4

You are en route to the station when you are dispatched for a man reporting shortness of breath and jaw pain. On arrival at the scene, you find a 60-year-old man leaning over in a chair; he is diaphoretic, breathing rapidly, and he reports severe pain in his jaw. As you begin your primary assessment, he clutches his chest and falls forward. After positioning the patient on the ground, your partner applies the AED while you begin the steps of CPR. You stop CPR to allow the AED to analyze the patient's rhythm. The AED indicates that no shock is advised and to continue CPR.

1. Why should you stop providing CPR while the AED is analyzing the patient's rhythm?
2. Which heart rhythms are considered to be shockable rhythms?

CPR Training

As an EMR, you should successfully complete a CPR course through a recognized agency such as the Emergency Care and Safety Institute or the AHA. You should also regularly update your skills by successfully completing a recognized recertification course. You cannot achieve proficiency in CPR unless you have adequate practice on adult, child, and infant manikins. Your department should schedule periodic reviews of CPR theory and practice for all EMRs.

Legal Implications of CPR

Advance directives, living wills, and durable powers of attorney for health care are legal documents that specify the patient's wishes regarding specified medical procedures. These documents are explained in Chapter 4, *Medical, Legal, and Ethical Issues.* You may sometimes wonder whether you should start CPR on a person who has an advance directive or a living will. Because you are not in a position to determine whether the advance directive or living will is valid, CPR should be started on all patients unless signs of obvious death are present (such as rigor mortis, tissue decay, or decapitation) or a resuscitation attempt would put you in harm's way. If a patient has an advance directive or living will, the physician at the hospital will determine whether you should stop CPR. Follow your department's protocols regarding advance directives, living wills, and do not resuscitate (DNR) orders.

Do not hesitate to begin CPR on a pulseless, nonbreathing patient. Without your help, the patient will certainly die. Make sure you perform a careful assessment of the patient before beginning CPR.

Another potential legal pitfall is abandonment—the discontinuation of CPR without the order of a licensed physician or without turning the patient over to someone who is at least as qualified as you are. If you avoid these pitfalls, you need not be overly concerned about the legal implications of performing CPR. Your most important protection against a possible lawsuit is to become thoroughly skilled in the theory and practice of CPR.

YOU are the Provider   SUMMARY

You are the Provider: CASE 1

1. On the basis of the patient's unresponsiveness, what should you do now for the patient?

Because your patient does not respond to verbal stimuli or to gentle shaking of her shoulder, you need to simultaneously check for signs of circulation and breathing by checking the carotid pulse and watching for chest rise and movement. If the patient has no pulse and is not breathing or only gasping, move the patient from the couch to the floor and begin cardiopulmonary resuscitation (CPR). Perform cycles of 30 compressions and two breaths. Use the automated external defibrillator (AED) as soon as it is available. Make sure additional help has been dispatched. Give compressions at a rate of 100 to 120 compressions per minute at a depth of at least 2 inches (5 cm). Allow full chest recoil between compressions and minimize interruptions when switching between compressions and ventilations.

2. What are the chances for a successful resuscitation on this call?

A witnessed cardiac arrest has a higher probability for a successful resuscitation than an unwitnessed cardiac arrest. The sooner you are able to start CPR and apply the automated external defibrillation device to the patient, the greater the chance for a successful outcome.

3. What role does your AED play in this call?

Having an AED available greatly increases the possibility that you can successfully resuscitate this patient. If you have an AED available, apply it as soon as possible. Allow the AED to analyze the cardiac rhythm. If a shock is indicated, shock the patient. During the resuscitation, avoid interruptions in chest compressions as much as possible. During a witnessed cardiac arrest, immediate defibrillation will sometimes result in spontaneous return to a normal heart rhythm.

You are the Provider: CASE 2

1. What are the next steps you should take?

You have an unresponsive, pulseless, and nonbreathing patient. You do not have any way of determining when the patient went into cardiac arrest. The patient is cool and has rigid muscles. If you were to look under her clothing at her back, you would likely find dependent lividity. All are signs of a patient who has been dead for some time and cannot be resuscitated. When reliable signs of death are present—as in this case—do not start CPR. Know your local protocols regarding when to start and stop CPR and who you need to notify in cases of obvious death. In such situations, realize that you may still have other patients who need your understanding: the friends and family members who are grieving the loss of their loved one.

You are the Provider: CASE 3

1. **What should you do first?**

Your first step is to ensure the scene is safe. In this case, it appears there might be an electric problem associated with the band saw. Before you assess the patient, ensure that the power to the saw has been disconnected. This step may involve pulling the plug from an outlet or disconnecting the main power switch. Do not come into direct contact or otherwise touch the patient until you have made sure the scene is safe. If you become a patient yourself, you cannot provide any further emergency care.

2. **What steps should you take to assess this patient?**

Begin by establishing unresponsiveness. If the patient is responsive, ask him what happened, determine what signs and symptoms he has, and assess his breathing and circulation. If he is unresponsive, quickly assess his carotid pulse and breathing simultaneously. If the patient has no pulse and is not breathing or only gasping, begin chest compressions followed by rescue breathing. Make sure that additional help has been dispatched.

3. **Do you think an AED is important in this situation?**

If the patient is in cardiac arrest from contact with an electrical source, he may be in ventricular fibrillation. In this case, an AED may be able to convert his heart rhythm to a normal pattern and increase his chance for survival. Begin CPR with cycles of 30 compressions and two breaths. Use the AED as soon as it is available.

You are the Provider: CASE 4

1. **Why should you stop providing CPR while the AED is analyzing the patient's rhythm?**

It is important to clear the patient while the AED is analyzing the heart rhythm. Touching the patient while the AED is analyzing the heart rhythm may affect the accuracy of the rhythm being analyzed. It is also important to clear the patient before delivering a shock because the person who is touching the patient may also get shocked.

2. **Which heart rhythms are considered to be shockable rhythms?**

The AED will automatically analyze the heart rhythm of a pulseless patient. If the patient's heart rhythm is ventricular tachycardia (V-tach) or ventricular fibrillation (V-fib), the AED will indicate that a shock is advised. The AED will not advise delivering a shock and instruct you to continue CPR if the patient is not in V-tach or V-fib.

Prep Kit

▶ Ready for Review

- The circulatory system transports oxygenated blood from the lungs to the rest of the body. Each beat of the heart produces a pulse, which can be felt at various sites on the body, such as the inside of the wrist (radial), the neck (carotid), the inside of the upper arm (brachial), and the groin (femoral).
- Cardiac arrest occurs when the heart stops contracting and no blood is pumped through the blood vessels. Brain damage begins within 4 to 6 minutes after the patient has experienced cardiac arrest. Within 8 to 10 minutes, the damage to the brain may become irreversible.
- The chain of survival includes five links that are essential to successful emergency cardiac care: (1) recognition of cardiac arrest and activation of the emergency response system; (2) immediate high-quality CPR; (3) rapid defibrillation; (4) basic and advanced emergency medical services (EMS); and (5) advanced life support (ALS) and post cardiac arrest care.
- When you arrive at an emergency scene, first assess the area for potential safety hazards. If the scene is unsafe, make it as safe as possible for yourself and the patient. As you approach the patient, look for possible causes of illness or injury. Next, establish unresponsiveness. If he or she is unresponsive, simultaneously check for signs of circulation and breathing by checking the pulse and watching for chest rise. If the patient has no pulse and is not breathing or only gasping, begin cardiopulmonary

Prep Kit *Continued*

resuscitation (CPR) with chest compressions, followed by rescue breathing.

- Basic life support for adults and children follows the same general steps: Check responsiveness, circulation, airway, and breathing. Intervene at any point if the patient's airway is obstructed, the patient is not breathing or only gasping, or the patient has no pulse.
- Use the jaw-thrust maneuver to open the airway if you suspect a head or spinal injury and the head tilt–chin lift maneuver if you do not suspect a head or spinal injury.
- Rescue breathing should be performed at a rate of one breath every 5 to 6 seconds (10 to 12 breaths per minute) for adults and one breath every 3 to 5 seconds (12 to 20 breaths per minute) for children and infants.
- Chest compressions should be performed at a rate of 100 to 120 compressions per minute for adults and children. Perform 30 compressions and two breaths for adults and for one-rescuer CPR. Perform 15 compressions and two breaths for two-rescuer child and infant CPR.
- Basic life support for infants is similar to that provided for adults and children. The techniques may vary somewhat, but the same general steps apply: check responsiveness, simultaneously check circulation and for the absence of breathing or just gasping. Intervene at any point if the infant's airway is obstructed, the infant is not breathing or only gasping, or the infant has no pulse.

- Open an infant's airway by using the head tilt–chin lift maneuver if you do not suspect a spinal injury. Be careful not to hyperextend the neck, which could obstruct the airway.
- If the infant has no pulse, begin CPR. If you are alone, use two fingers to compress the chest 30 times, at a rate of 100 to 120 compressions per minute, to a depth equal to at least one-third the depth of the chest. After 30 compressions, give two breaths. If two rescuers are present, use the two-thumb/encircling hands technique and provide 15 compressions to two breaths.
- The single most important cardiac arrest survival factor is early defibrillation. The indications for using an automated external defibrillator (AED) are that the patient is unresponsive, pulseless, and not breathing or only gasping. After determining that a patient is in cardiac arrest, begin immediate CPR and apply the AED as soon as possible.
- Once you turn on the AED and attach it to the patient's bare chest, the AED will analyze the heart rhythm and advise whether a shock is indicated. If a shock is advised, ensure that no one is touching the patient, deliver the shock, and immediately perform CPR for 2 minutes before reanalyzing the patient's rhythm. If no shock is advised, perform CPR for 2 minutes and then reanalyze the patient's rhythm. Continue CPR and rhythm analysis until advanced life support personnel arrive.

Prep Kit *Continued*

▶ Vital Vocabulary

automated external defibrillator (AED) A portable, battery-powered device that recognizes ventricular fibrillation and advises when a countershock is indicated. The device delivers an electric shock to patients with ventricular fibrillation.

brachial pulse The pulse on the inside of the upper arm.

cardiac arrest Cessation of breathing and a heartbeat.

carotid pulse The pulse taken on either side of the neck.

chest compression A means of applying artificial circulation by applying rhythmic pressure and relaxation on the lower half of the sternum; also called external cardiac compressions.

child A person between the age of 1 year and the onset of puberty (age 12 to 14 years).

circulatory system The heart and blood vessels, which together are responsible for the continuous flow of blood throughout the body.

femoral pulse The pulse taken at the groin.

gastric distention Inflation of the stomach caused when excessive pressures are used during artificial ventilation and air is directed into the stomach rather than the lungs.

infant A person younger than 1 year.

one-rescuer CPR Cardiopulmonary resuscitation performed by one rescuer.

plasma The fluid part of the blood that carries blood cells, transports nutrients, and removes cellular waste materials.

platelets Microscopic disc-shaped elements in the blood that are essential to the process of blood clot formation, the mechanism that stops bleeding.

pulse The wave of pressure created by the heart as it contracts and forces blood out into the major arteries.

radial pulse The pulse taken at the thumb side of the wrist.

two-rescuer CPR Cardiopulmonary resuscitation performed by two rescuers.

ventilation The movement of air in and out of the lungs.

ventricular fibrillation An uncoordinated muscular quivering of the heart; the most common abnormal rhythm causing cardiac arrest; also called V-fib.

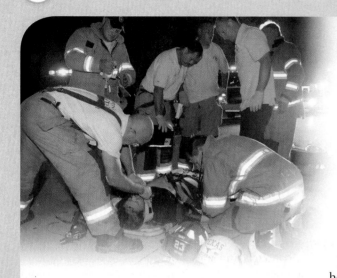

Assessment
in Action

At 1147 hours on a Sunday, you are dispatched to the First Community Church for a report of a 72-year-old man with severe chest pain. On arrival, you find an older man lying on the floor. His skin appears to be blue in color. He is unresponsive to your questions and does not respond when you shake his shoulder. Bystanders tell you that when they first noticed the man, he was clutching his chest. Several minutes after they called 9-1-1, he collapsed and fell to the floor.

1. Which is your first step in providing emergency care for this patient?

A. Check for a pulse.
B. Check for breathing.
C. Perform chest compressions.
D. Establish unresponsiveness.

2. Which of the following signs would indicate that cardiopulmonary resuscitation (CPR) is needed?

A. Shallow breathing
B. Dilated pupils
C. Absence of a pulse and breathing
D. Shortness of breath

3. Knowing when to start CPR is important. Which of the following criteria is NOT a reliable sign of death?

A. Evidence of tissue decomposition
B. Rigor mortis
C. Decapitation
D. Dilated pupils

4. What is the appropriate depth of chest compressions for an adult patient?

A. 0.25 inch (6 mm) to 0.5 inch (1 cm)
B. 0.5 inch (1 cm) to 1 inch (3 cm)
C. At least 2 inches (5 cm)
D. One-half the depth of the chest

5. When CPR is performed on this patient, what is the correct ratio of chest compressions to rescue breaths?

A. 5 to 1
B. 15 to 2
C. 30 to 2
D. 50 to 2

6. What is the rate at which you should compress the chest during adult CPR?

A. At least 100 times a minute
B. Exactly 100 times a minute
C. 100 to 120 times a minute
D. More than 110 times a minute

7. Which of the following is considered an acceptable reason to stop providing CPR?

A. You are too physically exhausted to continue.
B. Your partner orders you to stop.
C. You cannot feel a pulse.
D. You determine CPR is not working.

8. Why is it important to ensure your hands are off the chest between compressions?

9. At what point in this scenario should the automated external defibrillator be applied to the patient?

10. Why is it important to minimize interruptions of chest compressions when switching positions during two-rescuer CPR?

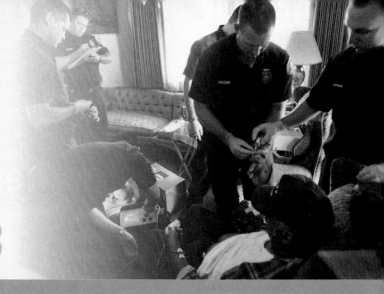

SECTION 3

Patient Assessment

Patient Assessment

National EMS Education Standard Competencies

Assessment

Use scene information and simple patient assessment findings to identify and manage immediate life threats and injuries within the scope and practice of the emergency medical responder (EMR).

Scene Size-up

❭ Scene safety (p 172)
❭ Scene management (pp 172–173)
- Impact of the environment on patient care (p 172)
- Addressing hazards (pp 172–173)
- Violence (p 172)
- Need for additional or specialized resources (p 173)
- Standard precautions (p 173)

Primary Assessment

❭ Primary assessment for all patient situations (pp 174–177)
- Level of consciousness (p 175)
- ABCs (pp 175–177)
- Identifying life threats (pp 175–177)
- Assessment of vital functions (pp 176–177)
❭ Begin interventions needed to preserve life (pp 176–177)

History Taking

❭ Determining the chief complaint (pp 178–179)
❭ Mechanism of injury/nature of illness (pp 172–173)
❭ Associated signs and symptoms (pp 178–180)

Secondary Assessment

❭ Performing a rapid full-body scan (pp 181–187)
❭ Focused assessment of pain (p 187)
❭ Assessment of vital signs (pp 187–191)

Reassessment

❭ How and when to reassess patients (pp 192–193)

Knowledge Objectives

1. Discuss the importance of each of the following five steps in the patient assessment sequence:
   - Step 1. Scene size-up (pp 171–173)
   - Step 2. Primary assessment (pp 174–177)
   - Step 3. History taking (pp 178–180)
   - Step 4. Secondary assessment (pp 181–191)
   - Step 5. Reassessment (pp 192–193)
2. Discuss the components of a scene size-up. (pp 171–173)
3. Explain why it is important to get an idea of the number of patients at an emergency scene as soon as possible. (p 173)
4. List and describe the importance of the following steps of the primary assessment:
   - Forming a general impression of the patient (p 174)
   - Determining the patient's level of responsiveness (p 175)

- Performing a rapid exam to identify life threats, including:
  - Assessing the patient's airway (p 176)
  - Assessing the patient's breathing (p 176)
  - Assessing the patient's circulation (pp 176–177)
- Updating responding EMS units (p 177)
5. Describe the differences in checking airway, breathing, and circulation when the patient is an adult, a child, or an infant. (pp 176–177)
6. Explain the purpose for obtaining a patient's medical history. (p 178)
7. Discuss the SAMPLE approach to obtaining a patient's medical history. (pp 179–180)
8. Explain the difference between a sign and a symptom. (p 181)
9. Describe the sequence used to perform a secondary assessment of the entire body. (p 182)
10. List the areas of the body that should be examined during the secondary assessment. (pp 182–187)
11. Explain the significance of the following signs: respiration, circulation, blood pressure, skin condition, pupil size and reactivity, and level of consciousness. (pp 187–191)
12. List the information that should be obtained during reassessment. (pp 192–193)
13. List the information about the patient's condition that should be addressed in your handoff report. (p 193)
14. Explain the differences between performing a patient assessment on a medical patient and performing one on a trauma patient. (p 195)

Skills Objectives

1. Demonstrate the following five steps of the patient assessment sequence:
   - Step 1. Scene size-up (pp 171–173)
   - Step 2. Primary assessment, including:
     - Forming a general impression of the patient (p 174)
     - Assessing the patient's level of responsiveness (p 175)
     - Assessing the patient's airway (p 176)
     - Assessing the patient's breathing (p 176)
     - Assessing the patient's circulation (including severe bleeding) (pp 176–177)
     - Updating responding EMS units (p 177)
   - Step 3. Obtaining the patient's medical history using the SAMPLE format (pp 179–180)
   - Step 4. Performing a secondary assessment, including:
     - Performing a secondary assessment of the entire body (pp 182–187)
     - Identifying and measuring a patient's vital signs (pp 187–191)
   - Step 5. Performing an ongoing reassessment (pp 192–193)

Patient Assessment

Scene Size-up

Ensure scene safety
Determine mechanism of injury/nature of illness
Take standard precautions
Determine number of patients
Consider additional resources

Primary Assessment

Form a general impression
Assess level of responsiveness
Perform a rapid exam to identify life threats
- Assess the airway
- Assess breathing
- Assess circulation
Update responding EMS units

History Taking

Investigate the chief complaint (SAMPLE history)

Secondary Assessment

Systematically assess the patient
Assess vital signs

Reassessment

Repeat the primary assessment
Reassess vital signs
Reassess the chief complaint
Recheck the effectiveness of the treatment
Identify and treat changes in the patient's condition
Reassess patient
- Unstable patients: every 5 minutes
- Stable patients: every 15 minutes
Provide a handoff report

Introduction

As an emergency medical responder (EMR), you will often be the first trained emergency medical services (EMS) provider at the incident scene. Your initial actions will affect not only you but also the patient and other responders. Your assessment of the scene and the patient will affect the level of care requested for the patient.

It is important that you are able to perform a systematic patient assessment to determine whether your patient has a medical condition or has sustained injuries from trauma. The patient assessment sequence consists of the following five steps:

Step 1. Perform a scene size-up.
Step 2. Perform a primary assessment.
Step 3. Obtain the patient's medical history.
Step 4. Perform a secondary assessment.
Step 5. Perform a reassessment.

By performing these five steps, you can systematically gather the information you need. After you have learned these steps, you will discover that you can modify the order in which you perform them to gather needed information about a patient who is experiencing a medical problem as opposed to a patient who has sustained trauma (a wound or injury).

The skills and knowledge presented in this chapter follow an **assessment-based care** model. With assessment-based care, the treatment rendered is based on the patient's symptoms. Assessment-based care requires you to conduct a careful and thorough evaluation of the patient so that you can provide appropriate care. If a given condition has already been diagnosed by a physician and is known to the patient, you will sometimes know the patient's diagnosis. Other times, you will have to respond to the signs and symptoms you find during the assessment process.

Throughout this text, you will learn about the signs and symptoms of various medical conditions. Careful and thorough study of the skills and knowledge related to patient assessment will go a long way in helping you perform as a valuable member of the EMS team in your community.

Patient Assessment Sequence

The patient assessment sequence is designed to provide you with a framework so you can safely approach an emergency scene, determine the need for additional resources, examine the patient to determine whether injuries or illnesses are present, obtain the patient's medical history, and report the results of your assessment to other EMS personnel. Recall that a complete patient assessment consists of the following five steps: Step 1, Scene size-up; Step 2, Primary assessment; Step 3, History taking; Step 4, Secondary assessment; and Step 5, Reassessment.

YOU are the Provider   CASE 1

You are dispatched to a rural section of highway for the report of a crash involving a single vehicle. As you arrive on the scene, you observe that the vehicle left the road and collided with a tree, resulting in moderate damage to the front end of the vehicle. As you are preparing to get out of your vehicle, you note an older man slumped over the steering wheel.

1. Why is it so important to follow the five steps in the patient assessment sequence as you evaluate this scene and this patient?
2. Why is it important to complete all of the steps of the patient assessment before you determine what is wrong with this patient?

Patient Assessment

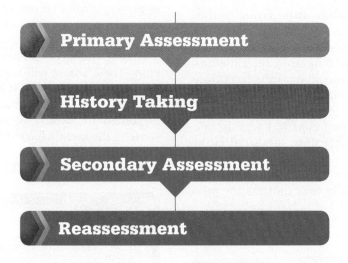

Scene Size-up

Ensure scene safety
Determine mechanism of injury/nature of illness
Take standard precautions
Determine the number of patients
Consider additional resources

Primary Assessment

History Taking

Secondary Assessment

Reassessment

Scene Size-up

The **scene size-up** is best defined as a general overview of the incident and its surroundings. On the basis of this information, you can determine the safety of the scene, the type of incident, any mechanism of injury, and the need for additional resources.

Review Dispatch Information

Your scene size-up actually begins before you arrive at the scene of the emergency. When you are alerted for an emergency call, you can anticipate possible conditions by reviewing and understanding the information received from the dispatcher. Your dispatcher should have obtained the following information: the location of the incident, the main problem or type of incident, the number of people involved, and any safety issues at the scene. As you receive the dispatcher's information, you should begin to assess it **Figure 9-1**.

In addition to the information obtained from the dispatcher, other factors can affect your actions. Consider, for example, factors such as the time of day, the day of the week, and weather conditions. A call from a school during school hours may require a different response than a call during the weekend. Finally, think

about the resources that may be needed and mentally prepare for other situations you may find when you arrive on the scene.

If you come across a medical emergency, notify the emergency medical dispatch center by using your two-way radio. If you do not have a two-way radio, use a cellular phone or send someone to call for help. Relay the following information: the location of the incident, the

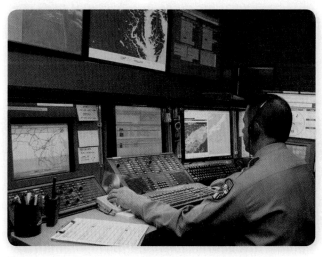

Figure 9-1 Begin your scene size-up by reviewing dispatch information.
© Jones & Bartlett Learning. Courtesy of MIEMSS.

Scene Size-up

main problem or type of incident, the number of people involved, and any safety issues at the scene.

Ensure Scene Safety

When you arrive at the scene, remember to park your vehicle so it helps to secure the scene and to minimize traffic blockage. As you approach the scene, scan the area to determine the extent of the incident, the possible number of people injured, and the presence of possible hazards **Figure 9-2**. It is important to scan the scene to ensure that you are not putting yourself in danger.

Hazards can be visible or invisible. Visible hazards include downed electrical wires, traffic, spilled gasoline, unstable buildings, a crime scene, weather, and crowds. Unstable surfaces such as slopes, ice, and water also pose potential hazards. Invisible hazards include electricity, biologic hazards, hazardous materials, and poisonous fumes. Downed electrical wires or broken poles may indicate an electrical hazard. Never assume a downed electrical wire is safe. Confined spaces such as farm silos, industrial tanks, and below-ground pits often contain poisonous gases or lack enough oxygen to support life. Hazardous materials placards on vehicles may indicate the presence of a chemical hazard.

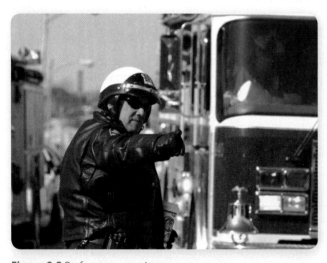

Figure 9-2 Perform a scene size-up.
© Dale A. Stork/Shutterstock.

As you take note of the hazards, consider your ability to manage them and decide whether to call for assistance. This assistance may include the fire department, additional EMS units, law enforcement officers, heavy-rescue equipment, hazardous materials teams, electric or gas company personnel, or other specialized resources. If a hazardous condition exists, make every effort to ensure that bystanders, rescuers, and patients are not exposed to it unnecessarily. If possible, see to it that any hazardous conditions are corrected or minimized as soon as possible. Noting such conditions early keeps them from becoming part of the problem later. Sometimes the first action needed at an incident scene is to prevent it from becoming worse. For example, it may be necessary to control traffic to prevent further crashes before it is safe to begin caring for injured patients.

Some emergency scenes will not be safe for you to enter. These scenes will require personnel with special training and equipment. If a scene is unsafe, keep people away until specially trained teams arrive. It is also important to identify potential exit routes from the scene in the event a hazard becomes life threatening to you or your patients and to wear appropriate personal protective equipment (PPE).

Safety

Never enter an enclosed space unless you have received proper training and are equipped with self-contained breathing apparatus (SCBA).

Determine the Mechanism of Injury or Nature of Illness

As you approach the scene, look for clues that may indicate how the incident happened **Figure 9-3**. This is called the mechanism of injury (MOI). If you can determine the MOI or the nature of the illness (NOI), you can sometimes predict the patient's injuries. For example, a ladder lying on the ground next to a spilled bucket of paint most likely indicates that the patient fell from the ladder and may have sustained bone fractures or a spinal injury. If the incident is a vehicle crash, knowing what type of crash occurred makes it possible to anticipate

YOU are the Provider   CASE 2

It is a cold day in February when you are dispatched to a two-story house for a report of a sick child. As you and your partner enter the front door, you detect a slight odor. The boy's mother appears to be about 35 years old. She tells you that her 9-year-old son has been feeling sick. He has a headache and has been sleeping a lot. She tells you she was going to take the child to see a physician, but she developed a headache and has been feeling increasingly sick. She thinks she needs to see a physician also. She also tells you that she has been feeling light-headed in the last few minutes.

1. What are the first actions that you should take?
2. What additional resources do you need?

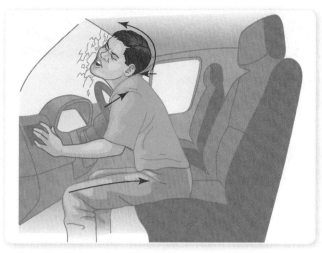

Figure 9-3 Determine the mechanism of injury or MOI.
© Jones & Bartlett Learning.

the types of injuries that may be present. For example, a rollover crash results in different injuries than a vehicle that has collided with a tree. It is also possible to anticipate injuries by examining the extent of damage to a vehicle. If the windshield is broken, look for head and spine injuries; if the steering wheel is bent, check for a chest injury. (See Chapter 15, *Injuries to Muscles and Bones*, for more information on MOIs that result in musculoskeletal injuries.)

Ask the patient (if conscious), family members, or bystanders for additional information about the MOI or the NOI. This may provide you with important trauma or medical information that you can use to assist the patient. You can use the same type of overview that gives you information at the scene of an incident to help provide you with information about a patient's condition. Do not, however, rule out any injury without conducting a secondary assessment of the entire body of the patient. The mechanism of the accident may provide clues, but it cannot be used to determine what injuries are present in a particular patient. Using the previous example, the house painter may have fallen from the ladder because he had a heart attack.

Take Standard Precautions

Before arriving at the scene, prepare yourself by anticipating the types of standard precautions for infectious diseases that may be required. You should always have gloves readily available and use them. Consider whether the use of additional protection, such as eye protection, gowns, or masks, may be necessary. Try to anticipate your needs for equipment to ensure that you and your patients are well protected from exposure to infectious diseases. Regardless of the standard precautions you take, wash your hands thoroughly after contact with a patient or contaminated materials. See Chapter 2, *Workforce Safety and Wellness*, for more information on standard precautions.

Determine the Number of Patients

Check to see if there is more than one patient. Then determine the total number of patients who need emergency care. Call for additional assistance if you think you might need help. It may be necessary to sort patients into groups according to the severity of their injuries to determine which patients should be treated and transported first. The topic of triage, or patient sorting, is covered more thoroughly in Chapter 21, *Incident Management*.

Consider Additional Resources

Many kinds of resources may be needed at the scene of an emergency. These resources include additional EMS units for treatment and transport; law enforcement personnel for traffic control or crowd control; fire department units for spilled fuel, fire, or extrication; utility company personnel for damaged utility lines; and wrecker operators for vehicle removal. As you prepare to make your initial report to the dispatcher, you may find it easier to report on the need for additional resources at the same time you report on the number of patients. Remember that your dispatcher cannot see the emergency scene. The only information the dispatcher has is the information you see and then communicate to the dispatcher.

Words of Wisdom

If you determine that additional resources are required, call for further assistance before beginning to treat the patient(s). It will take time for more help to arrive, so the sooner you request aid, the better. In addition, you are less likely to call for help if you are already involved in patient care, which can be detrimental to the patient's chance for recovery.

YOU are the Provider   CASE 3

You are riding third for station 403 as part of your required clinical rotation hours. Your team is dispatched to a vehicle versus pedestrian collision in the parking lot of the local supermarket. On arrival, your team ensures that the scene is safe. The paramedic in charge requests that you hold the patient's head to manually stabilize the patient's spine.

1. Identify scene safety issues that you should consider when you arrive at the scene of a vehicle crash.
2. Why do you think manual stabilization of the spine is necessary for the patient in this incident?

Patient Assessment

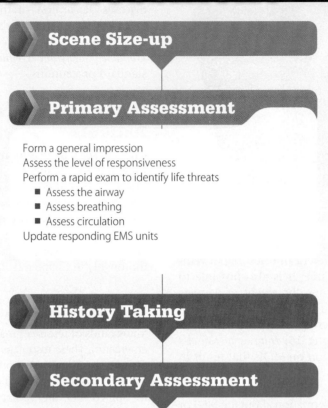

Scene Size-up

Primary Assessment

Form a general impression
Assess the level of responsiveness
Perform a rapid exam to identify life threats
- Assess the airway
- Assess breathing
- Assess circulation
Update responding EMS units

History Taking

Secondary Assessment

Reassessment

 Primary Assessment

The second part of the patient assessment sequence is the **primary assessment**. This is sometimes called the primary patient assessment or the initial patient assessment. The purpose of the primary assessment is to identify life threats to the patient. Life threats are defined as problems with the patient's airway, breathing, and circulation (the ABCs). It is important to quickly identify any life-threatening conditions so you can take immediate actions to correct these conditions. Notice that the primary assessment consists of evaluating the same functions that you evaluate when you are beginning to perform cardiopulmonary resuscitation (CPR).

The first step of the primary assessment is to form a general impression of the patient. You can do this as you approach the patient. The second step of the primary assessment is to determine the patient's level of responsiveness. The third step of the primary assessment consists of three parts: checking and correcting life-threatening problems connected to the airway, breathing, and

circulation. These three parts taken together comprise a rapid exam to identify life threats. The fourth and final step of the primary assessment is to update responding EMS units about the patient's condition.

Form a General Impression

As you approach the patient, form a general impression. Note the sex and the approximate age of the patient. Your scene size-up and general impression may help determine whether the patient has experienced trauma or illness. (If you cannot determine whether the patient is experiencing an illness or has sustained an injury, treat the patient as a trauma patient.) The patient's position or the sounds he or she is making may also help indicate to you the nature of the emergency. As you address the patient, you may gain some insight into the patient's level of consciousness. A quick look at the patient's face will often give you an idea of the level of pain he or she is experiencing. Although your first impression is valuable, keep an open mind and do not let it block out later information that may lead you in another direction (tunnel vision).

Assess the Level of Responsiveness

The first part of determining the patient's level of responsiveness is to introduce yourself. Many patients will be conscious and able to interact with you. As you approach the patient, tell the patient your name and function Figure 9-4 . For example, say: "I'm Jesse Phillips from the sheriff's department, and I'm here to help you." This simple introduction helps establish:

- Your reason for being at the scene
- The fact that you will be helping the patient
- The level of consciousness of the patient

The introduction is your first contact with the patient. You should be able to put the patient at ease by conveying that you are a trained person ready to help. Next, ask the patient's name and then use it when talking with the patient, family, or friends. The patient's response helps you determine the patient's level of responsiveness (consciousness). Avoid telling the patient that everything will be all right.

> ### Safety
>
> Remember, performing a patient assessment may bring you in contact with the patient's blood and other body fluids, waste products, and mucous membranes. You need to wear approved gloves and PPE and take other standard precautions to prevent any exposure to infected body fluids. Follow the latest standards from the Centers for Disease Control and Prevention and Occupational Safety and Health Administration.

Even if the patient appears to be unconscious, introduce yourself and talk with the patient as you conduct the rest of the patient assessment. Many patients who appear to be unconscious can hear your voice and need the reassurance it carries. Do not say anything you do not want the patient to hear!

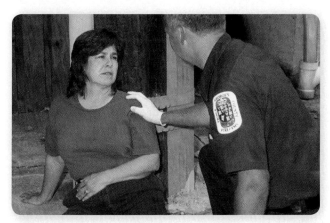

Figure 9-4 As you approach the patient, introduce yourself. If a patient appears unconscious, gently touch or shake the patient's shoulder to get a response.
© Jones & Bartlett Learning.

If a patient appears to be unresponsive (unconscious), speak to the patient in a tone of voice that is loud enough for the patient to hear. If the patient does not respond to the sound of your voice, gently touch the patient or shake the patient's shoulder to see if you can generate a response from the patient.

The patient's level of consciousness can range from fully conscious to unconscious. Describe the patient's level of consciousness using the four-level **AVPU scale**:

A **Alert.** An alert patient is able to answer the following questions accurately and appropriately: What is your name? Where are you? What is today's date? A patient who can answer these questions is said to be "alert and oriented."

V **Verbal.** A patient is said to be "responsive to verbal stimuli" even if the patient reacts only to loud sounds.

P **Pain.** A patient who is responsive to pain will not respond to a verbal stimulus but will move or cry out in response to pain. Response to pain is tested by pinching the patient's earlobe or pinching the patient's skin over the collarbone. If the patient withdraws from the painful stimulus, he or she is said to be "responsive to painful stimuli."

U **Unresponsive.** An unresponsive patient will not respond to either a verbal or a painful stimulus. This patient's condition is described as "unresponsive."

If the patient has sustained any type of major trauma, provide manual stabilization of the patient's neck as soon as possible. This step will prevent any further injury to the neck and spinal column.

> ### Special Populations
>
> Infants and children may not have the verbal skills to answer the questions used to assess responsiveness in adults. Therefore, you should assess how the children and infants interact with their environment and with their parents or caregivers.

Perform a Rapid Exam to Identify Life Threats

The rapid exam to identify life threats consists of three steps. The first step is to check the airway and correct any serious airway problems, such as a blocked airway. The second step is to check for breathing and correct any serious breathing problems, such as a lack of breathing or open chest injuries that interfere with adequate breathing. The third step of the rapid exam to identify life threats is to check the status of circulation and correct any life-threatening circulation problems. These problems include a lack of circulation because of cardiac arrest and control of serious external bleeding. In most cases, identifying and correcting life-threatening issues begins with the airway, followed by breathing and circulation (ABC). However, when a patient is in cardiac arrest, you must first check for circulation followed by airway and breathing (CAB). This sequence minimizes the time to the beginning of chest compressions. With practice, you will learn to check the patient's circulation and breathing at the same time.

Assess the Airway

The third part of the primary assessment starts with checking the patient's airway. If the patient is alert and able to answer questions without difficulty, then the airway is open. If the patient is unresponsive to verbal stimuli, then assume the airway may be closed. If the patient is unconscious, open the airway by using the head tilt–chin lift maneuver for patients with medical problems and use the jaw-thrust maneuver (without tilting the patient's head) for patients who have sustained trauma. After the airway is open, inspect it for foreign bodies or secretions. Clear the airway as needed, using finger sweeps or suction. You may need to insert an airway adjunct to keep the airway open. (See Chapter 7, *Airway Management*, for information about airway adjuncts.)

Assess Breathing

If the patient is conscious, assess the rate and quality of the patient's breathing. Does the chest rise and fall with each breath or does the patient appear to be short of breath? If the patient is unconscious, check for breathing by placing the side of your face next to the patient's nose and mouth. You should be able to hear the sounds of breathing, see the chest rise and fall, and even feel the movement of air on your cheek Figure 9-5 . If the patient is having difficulty breathing or if you hear unusual breath sounds, check for an object in the patient's mouth, such as food, vomitus, dentures, gum, chewing tobacco, or broken teeth, and remove it.

If you cannot detect any movement of the chest and no sounds of air are coming from the nose and mouth, breathing is absent. Take immediate steps to

check the patient's carotid pulse to assess whether there is any circulation. This step is described in the next section. If a carotid pulse is present but the patient is not breathing or only gasping, perform rescue breathing. If you suspect trauma, protect the cervical spine by keeping the patient's head in a neutral position and using the jaw-thrust maneuver to open the airway. Maintain manual cervical stabilization until the head and neck are fully immobilized. (These procedures are covered in Chapter 7, *Airway Management*.)

Assess Circulation

Next, check the patient's circulation (heartbeat). If the patient is unconscious, check the carotid pulse Figure 9-6 . Place your index and middle fingers together and touch the larynx (Adam's apple) in the patient's neck. Then slide your two fingers off the larynx toward the patient's ear until you feel a slight notch. Practice this maneuver until you are able to find a carotid pulse within 5 seconds of touching the patient's larynx. If you cannot feel the carotid pulse with your fingers in 5 to 10 seconds, begin CPR, which is covered in Chapter 8, *Professional Rescuer CPR*.

If the patient is conscious, assess the radial pulse rather than the carotid pulse Figure 9-7 . Place your index and middle fingers on the patient's wrist at the

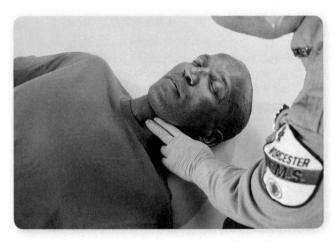

Figure 9-6 Check an unconscious patient's circulation by checking the carotid pulse.
© Jones & Bartlett Learning.

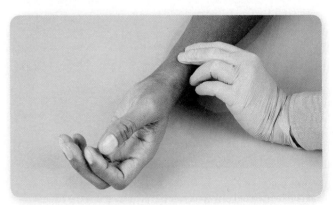

Figure 9-7 Take the radial pulse if the patient is conscious.
© Jones & Bartlett Learning.

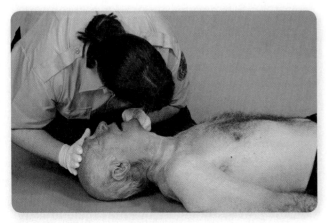

Figure 9-5 Check the patient's breathing.
© Jones & Bartlett Learning. Courtesy of MIEMSS.

thumb side. Practice taking the radial pulse often to develop this skill.

Special Populations

To assess circulation in an infant, check the brachial pulse, located on the inside of the upper arm. You can feel the brachial pulse by placing your index and middle fingers on the inside of the infant's arm halfway between the shoulder and the elbow **Figure 9-8**. Check for 5 to 10 seconds.

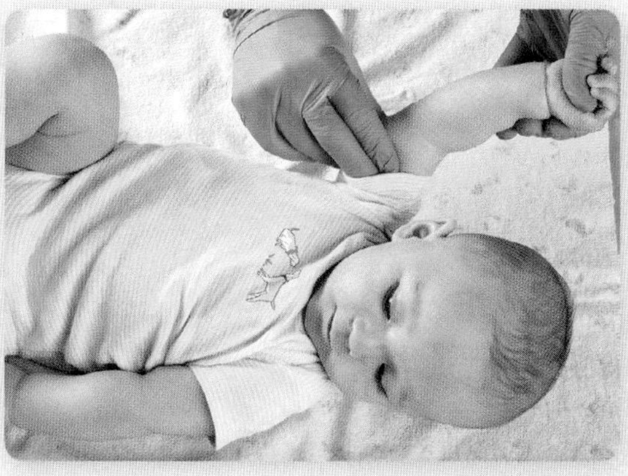

Figure 9-8 Take the brachial pulse if the patient is an infant.

© Jones & Bartlett Learning.

Next, quickly check the patient for any severe external bleeding. If you discover severe bleeding, you must take immediate action to control it by applying direct pressure over the wound or by applying a tourniquet. These procedures are covered in Chapter 14, *Bleeding, Shock, and Soft-Tissue Injuries*.

Quickly assess the patient's skin color and temperature. This assessment will help you determine whether the patient is experiencing internal bleeding and shock. It is important to check the color of the patient's skin when you arrive at the scene so that you can monitor the patient's skin for color changes as time goes on.

Skin color is described as:

- **Pale.** White or light in color, indicating decreased circulation to that part of the body or to all of the body. This could be caused by blood loss, poor blood flow, or low body temperature.
- **Flushed.** Red in color, indicating excess circulation to that part of the body
- **Blue.** Also called cyanosis, indicating lack of oxygen and possible airway problems
- **Yellow.** Also called jaundice, indicating liver problems
- **Normal.**

Patients with deeply pigmented skin may show color changes in the fingernail beds, in the whites of the eyes, on the palm of the hand, or inside the mouth.

Safety

Remember to wear gloves to avoid contact with body fluids that may contain blood.

Update Responding EMS Units

In some EMS systems, you will be expected to update responding EMS units about the condition of your patient. This report should include the age and sex of the patient; the chief complaint; the level of responsiveness; and the status of airway, breathing, and circulation. This update helps other responders know what to expect when they arrive at the scene.

Because many conditions present an immediate threat to life, you should try to perform all four steps of the primary assessment quickly as you make contact with the patient.

Patient Assessment

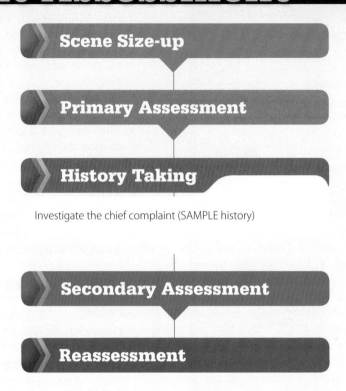

> **Scene Size-up**
>
> **Primary Assessment**
>
> **History Taking**
> Investigate the chief complaint (SAMPLE history)
>
> **Secondary Assessment**
>
> **Reassessment**

History Taking

Investigate the Chief Complaint

As you perform the primary assessment, you will often form an impression of the patient's **chief complaint**. It is important to acknowledge the patient's primary or chief complaint and provide reassurance **Figure 9-9**. A conscious patient will often report an injury that is causing him or her great pain or direct you to an injury that has obvious bleeding. However, keep in mind that this injury may not be the most serious injury the patient has sustained. Do not allow a conscious patient's comments to distract you from completing the patient assessment sequence. Acknowledge the patient's chief complaint by saying something like, "Yes, I can see that your arm appears to be broken, but let me finish checking you completely in case there are any other injuries. I will then treat your injured arm." In an unconscious patient, the primary "complaint" is unconsciousness.

The purpose of obtaining a medical history is to gather a systematic account of the patient's past medical conditions, illnesses, and injuries to determine the events leading up to the present medical

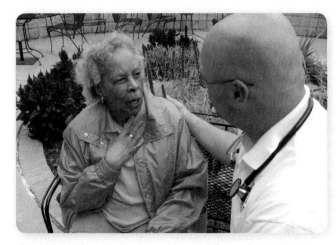

Figure 9-9 Acknowledge the patient's chief complaint.
© Jones & Bartlett Learning.

situation and to determine the signs and symptoms of the current condition **Figure 9-10**. It is important to question the patient in a clear and systematic manner to gain as much information as possible. Do not underestimate the importance of a good medical history. Physicians are taught that they can diagnose a patient's condition about 80% of the time after

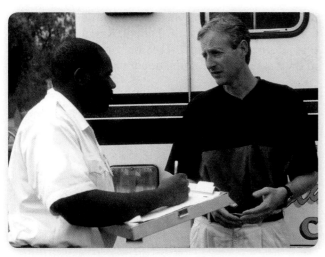

Figure 9-10 Obtain the patient's medical history.
© Jones & Bartlett Learning. Courtesy of MIEMSS.

completing a thorough medical history. You are not expected to have the knowledge and training of a physician, but you should be able to obtain a thorough medical history from a patient. Performing a medical history is an important part of the patient assessment sequence for injured patients and for ill patients, and it will help tie together your findings from the primary assessment.

Learn the relevant facts about the patient's past medical history. Ask the patient about any serious injuries, illnesses, or surgeries. Ask the patient what medications he or she is currently taking, including prescription, over-the-counter (OTC), and herbal medications. Find out if the patient is allergic to any medications, foods, or seasonal allergens such as ragweed.

Obtain SAMPLE History

To obtain a patient medical history in a consistent and thorough manner, remember the acronym SAMPLE. By using this easy-to-remember acronym, you can gain the information you need about past medical history as well as the events leading to the current episode of illness or injury.

It is important to use a systematic approach when obtaining a patient's medical history. The **SAMPLE history** provides a framework to ask needed questions of the patient. Remember to ask the patient one question at a time. Give the patient time to answer before you ask the next question. Listen carefully and maintain eye contact to let the patient know you are listening to the response. Designate one EMS provider to ask questions to avoid confusing the patient. Use the mnemonic SAMPLE to obtain the following information:

S **Signs and symptoms.** These should be the reasons that caused the patient to call 9-1-1. Ask the patient what signs and symptoms occurred at the beginning of the event. Ask the patient what signs and symptoms he or she is experiencing now. Ask the patient if he or she is feeling any pain. If the patient is experiencing pain, ask him or her to describe the pain.

A **Allergies.** Ask whether the patient is allergic to any medications or foods or has seasonal allergies. Ask the patient to describe his or her reactions to any allergies. If the patient states that he or she has no allergies, communicate this to other EMS personnel.

M **Medications.** Ask the patient if he or she is taking any medications prescribed by a physician. If the patient is taking prescription medications, ask the patient the purpose of these medications. Ask the patient if he or she is taking OTC supplements or herbal remedies.

P **Pertinent past medical history.** Ask if the patient is currently under the care of a physician. Ask the patient if he or she has any existing medical conditions, such as diabetes or a heart condition. Ask the patient if he or she has had a serious illness or a serious injury. Ask the patient if he or she has been hospitalized recently. Try to keep this part of the history relevant to the current condition. A cardiac bypass operation is probably very relevant to a patient experiencing chest pains because it indicates cardiovascular disease. An operation to remove an inflamed appendix 10 years ago, however, is most likely not relevant to an illness today.

L **Last oral intake.** Ask when the patient last had something to eat or drink. If the patient is experiencing abdominal pain, ask the patient what he or she had to eat and drink in the last few hours and how much he or she consumed.

E **Events leading up to this illness or injury.** Ask the patient to describe what he or she was doing when the symptoms of this event started or when the injury occurred. Ask the patient if he or she noticed anything unusual in the hours before this event started or if the patient was doing anything unusual just prior to the start of the illness or when the injury happened.

Table 9-1 summarizes the SAMPLE acronym.

If the patient is unconscious or senile, a family member, friend, or coworker may be able to answer your questions. Look for important information on a medical identification necklace, bracelet, or card. The

Table 9-1 — SAMPLE Medical History

S Signs and symptoms of the injury or illness. These should be the reasons that caused the patient to call for emergency medical services. Patients should describe signs and symptoms in their own words.

A Allergies. Patients may be allergic to medications, food, or airborne particles.

M Medications. What medications is the patient taking? Ask about medications prescribed by the patient's physician, over-the-counter (nonprescription) medications, and herbal remedies.

P Pertinent past medical history. What events or symptoms might be related to the patient's current illness? For example, it would be important to know whether a patient experiencing severe chest pain had a previous heart attack.

L Last oral intake. When was the last time the patient had anything to eat or drink? Find out what the patient last ate or drank and how much he or she consumed.

E Events associated with or leading up to this illness or injury. Knowing these events will help you put together the pieces of the medical history puzzle. Let patients describe these events in their own words.

© Jones & Bartlett Learning.

information you gain will help determine what steps you need to take to treat the patient. Next, communicate this information to other EMS personnel to help them in their assessment and treatment of the patient.

Words of Wisdom

Pay particular attention to patients who tell you their pain feels just like the kidney stone episode they had last year or their pain feels just like the heart attack they had 2 years ago. Patients who have experienced a certain kind of pain before are often correct in identifying that pain if it recurs.

YOU are the Provider — CASE 4

You are working as an EMR for an outdoor summer camp. You receive a radio call that one of the campers is feeling sick and weak about a half mile (less than 1 km) from the camp. You and your partner respond to the scene. You note the scene is stable. An 11-year-old girl is sitting on a log. The camp counselor tells you that they were returning from a 3-mile (5-km) hike around the lake when one of the campers, Mattie, started to lag behind the group. The counselor encouraged her to sit down on the log. Mattie states that she feels weak. You note that her pulse is slightly rapid and weak and that she is sweating.

1. What is Mattie's chief complaint?
2. Why is the SAMPLE history important when caring for a patient like this who has a vague chief complaint?

Patient Assessment

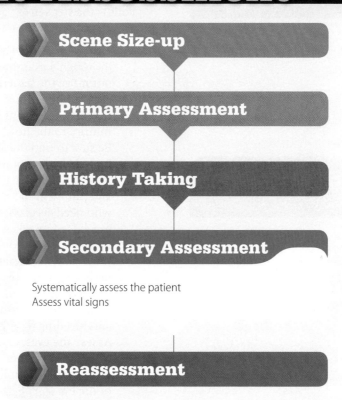

Scene Size-up

Primary Assessment

History Taking

Secondary Assessment

Systematically assess the patient
Assess vital signs

Reassessment

Secondary Assessment

After you have completed the primary assessment and stabilized any life-threatening conditions, perform a **secondary assessment** (the physical examination) of the patient from head to toe to assess non–life-threatening conditions. Vital signs are taken as part of the secondary assessment. They may be obtained before the physical examination is completed or after the examination is done. They can also be obtained by a second person while other parts of the patient assessment are being completed.

Information on signs and symptoms and vital signs is being presented here in this section because you need to understand how to measure some of these vital signs to provide a complete secondary assessment. The physical examination you conduct during the secondary assessment helps you to locate and begin initial management of the signs and symptoms of illness or injury. After you complete the secondary assessment, review any positive signs and symptoms of injury or illness. This review will help you get a better picture of the patient's overall condition.

Signs and Symptoms

In a careful and systematic patient assessment, you need to understand the difference between a **sign** and a **symptom**. Simply put, a sign is something about the patient you can see or feel for yourself. A symptom is something the patient tells you about his or her condition, such as, "My back hurts" or "I think I am going to vomit." You need to be able to assess selected signs and report them systematically when you transfer care. You also need to be able to understand and report the symptoms that the patient reports.

Systematically Assess the Patient

As you perform the secondary assessment, look and feel for the following signs of injury: deformities, open injuries, tenderness, and swelling. Use the mnemonic DOTS to remember these signs Table 9-2 . Alternately, some EMS providers find it helpful to use the mnemonic DCAP-BTLS when performing a full body examination to help them remember the patient's injuries. This acronym is presented in Table 9-3 . It is another option you can use for remembering the signs of injury.

Secondary Assessment of the Entire Body

Conduct a thorough, hands-on, secondary assessment of the entire body in a logical, head-to-toe, systematic manner. It is important to conduct the examination the same way each time to be sure you inspect all areas of

Table 9-2	Signs of Injury

D	Deformities
O	Open injuries
T	Tenderness
S	Swelling

© Jones & Bartlett Learning.

Table 9-3	DCAP-BTLS

D	Deformities
C	Contusions (bruises)
A	Abrasions
P	Punctures or Penetrations
B	Burns
T	Tenderness
L	Lacerations
S	Swelling

© Jones & Bartlett Learning.

the body for injuries. Use a clear, concise format to communicate your findings to other medical personnel.

The secondary assessment of the entire body can be done whether the patient is conscious or unconscious. Watch the reactions of a conscious patient during your examination. If you detect signs of discomfort, you may want to ask what the patient is feeling as you proceed with your examination. Remember that your secondary assessment of the entire body is the main focus of this part of the patient assessment. It is permissible to question the patient during your assessment, but do not let the questions distract you from completing a thorough assessment.

If the patient is unconscious, it is vitally important that you assess the airway, breathing, and circulation during the primary assessment. After you have addressed any problems with the patient's breathing and pulse, begin a secondary assessment of the entire body of the unconscious patient. Assessing an unconscious patient is difficult because the patient cannot cooperate or tell you where something hurts—although your assessment often will elicit grimaces or moans from an unconscious patient.

Assume all unconscious, injured patients have spinal injuries. Manually stabilize the head and spine to minimize movement during the patient examination. It is essential to immobilize all injured, unconscious

patients on a **backboard** before transporting them (see Chapter 3, *Lifting and Moving Patients*). Be cautious when treating a patient who is unconscious because of illness.

Follow the steps in **Skill Drill 9-1** to perform a secondary assessment of the entire body.

1. **Assess the head.** Use both hands to thoroughly examine all areas of the scalp. Do not move the patient's head! This precaution is especially important if the patient is unconscious or has sustained a spinal injury. Injuries to the head tend to bleed excessively. Be sure to find the actual wound; do not be fooled by areas of matted, bloody hair. If necessary, remove the patient's eyeglasses and put them in a safe place. Many patients who need eyeglasses become upset if their eyeglasses are taken away. Use your judgment in each case. Be considerate of the patient. If the patient is wearing a wig, it may be necessary to remove the hairpiece to complete the head examination. Be sure to check the entire head for bumps, areas of tenderness, and bleeding **Step 1**.

2. **Assess the eyes.** Cover one of the patient's eyes for 5 seconds. Then quickly open the eyelid and watch the pupil, the dark part at the center of the eye **Step 2**. The normal reaction of the pupil is to constrict (get smaller) within about 1 second. If you are examining a patient's eyes at night or in the dark, use a flashlight and aim the light at the closed eye. A pupil that fails to react to light or pupils that are unequal in size may be important diagnostic signs; report this information to personnel at the next level of medical care.

3. **Assess the nose.** Assess the nose for tenderness or deformity, which may indicate a broken nose. Check to see if there is any blood or fluid coming from the nose **Step 3**.

4. **Assess the mouth.** Your first assessment of the mouth should have taken place when you checked to see whether the patient was breathing. Now recheck the mouth for foreign objects such as food, vomitus, dentures, gum, chewing tobacco, and loose teeth **Step 4**. Be sure to carefully clear away any material that obstructs the patient's airway. In addition, be ready to manage any vomiting. It is important to prevent **aspiration** (inhalation) of vomitus into the lungs. Use your sense of smell to determine whether any unusual odors are present **Step 5**. A patient who has diabetes may have a fruity breath odor. Do not allow the presence of alcohol on the patient's breath to change the way you treat the patient. In fact, if you detect the smell of alcohol, you should conduct an especially careful physical examination,

particularly if the patient appears to be severely injured. Remember to place any unconscious patient who has not sustained trauma in the recovery position. This position helps keep the patient's airway open and prevents aspiration of vomitus into the airway or lungs.

5. **Assess the neck.** Assess the neck carefully using both hands, one on each side of the patient's neck. Be sure to touch the vertebrae (the bony part of the back of the neck) to see whether gentle pressure produces pain. Check the neck veins. Swollen (distended) neck veins may indicate heart conditions or major trauma to the chest **Step 6** ▸. Examine the neck for a stoma (opening), which indicates that the patient is a "neck breather." A neck breather is a person who has undergone a surgical procedure in which the airway above the stoma has been removed. The stoma may be the patient's only means of breathing, and the patient may not be able to speak normally. The stoma is often concealed behind an article of clothing or a bib.

Words of Wisdom

As your hands move down the patient's scalp and onto the neck, check for the presence of an emergency medical identification neck chain. Look for medical identification (MedicAlert) emblems as an indication of the patient's medical history. The internationally recognized symbol shown in **Figure 9-11** is found on necklaces, arm bracelets, ankle bracelets, watches, rings, and wallet cards and is carried by people who have a medical condition that warrants special attention if they become ill or injured. This is a patient directive that allows EMS personnel to access the patient's stored medical information by calling the MedicAlert Foundation. Each MedicAlert member has a unique, secure patient identifier engraved at the bottom of his or her emblem. By wearing this emblem, the patient has consented to the release of information to attending medical personnel. The stored patient history can include conditions, allergies, medications and dosages, and implanted devices. If you find such a warning on a patient, it is your responsibility to give this information to the next person in the EMS system.

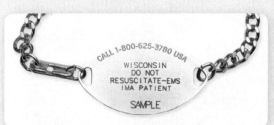

Figure 9-11 Medical identification is found on wrist and ankle bracelets, necklaces, watches, rings, and wallet cards.

Courtesy of the MedicAlert Foundation®. © 2006, All Rights Reserved. MedicAlert® is a federally registered trademark and service mark.

6. **Assess the face.** While you are performing the hands-on assessment of the head and neck, be sure to note the color of the facial skin, its temperature, and whether it is moist or dry **Table 9-4**. After you have completed the head examination, be sure to note any bumps, bruises, cuts, or other abnormalities.

Treatment

Be careful not to move the neck or head!

7. **Assess the chest.** If the patient is conscious, ask him or her to take a deep breath and tell you whether he or she feels any pain on **inhalation** or **exhalation**. Note whether the patient breathes with difficulty **Step 7** ▸. Look and listen for signs of difficult breathing such as coughing, wheezing, or foaming at the mouth. It is important to look at both sides of the chest completely, noting any injuries, bleeding, or sections of the chest that move abnormally, unequally, or painfully. Unequal motion of one side or section of the chest may be a sign of a serious condition, called a **flail chest**, which can result from multiple rib **fractures** (breaks). Be sure to run your hands over all parts of the chest. Like the head and neck examinations, try to move the patient as little as possible while you assess the chest.

Apply firm but gentle pressure to the collarbone (**clavicle**) to check for fractures. Check the chest for fractured ribs by placing your hands on the chest and pushing down gently but firmly. Then put your hands on each side of the chest and push inward, squeezing the chest **Step 8** ▸.

8. **Assess the abdomen.** Continue your assessment downward to the **abdomen** (stomach and groin). Look for any signs of

Table 9-4	Skin Color	
Color	**Term**	**Indicates**
Red	Flushed	Fever or sunburn
White or light in color	Pale	Shock
Blue	Cyanotic	Airway obstruction
Yellow	Jaundiced	Liver disease

© Jones & Bartlett Learning.

Skill Drill 9-1

Performing a Secondary Assessment

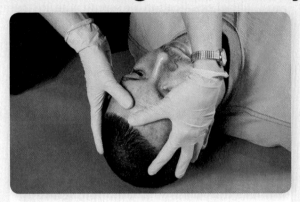

Step 1 Observe and palpate the head.

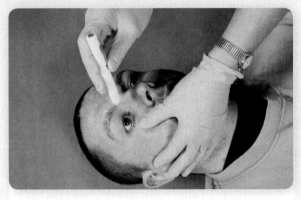

Step 2 Assess the eyes.

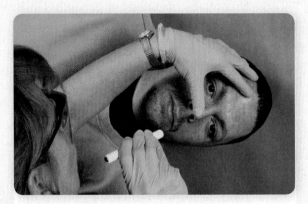

Step 3 Check the nose for blood and drainage.

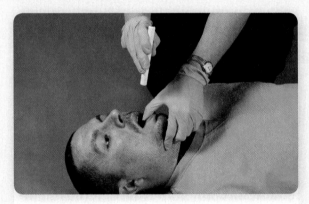

Step 4 Assess the mouth.

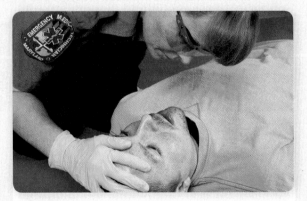

Step 5 Check for unusual breath odors.

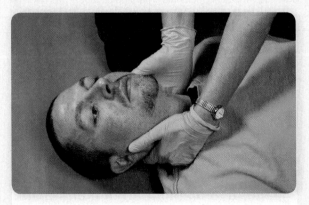

Step 6 Assess the neck.

Skill Drill 9-1 *Continued*

Performing a Secondary Assessment

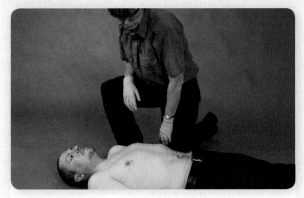

Step 7 Inspect the chest and observe breathing motion.

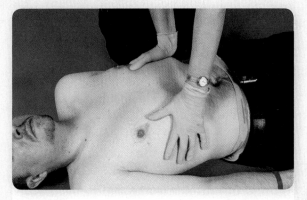

Step 8 Gently palpate the chest.

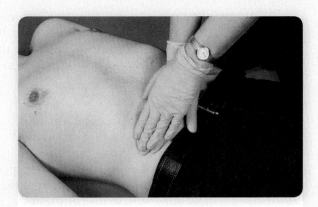

Step 9 Assess the abdomen.

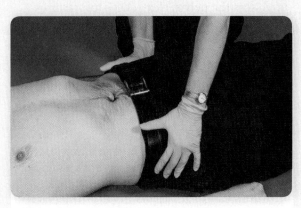

Step 10 Gently press on the pelvic bones.

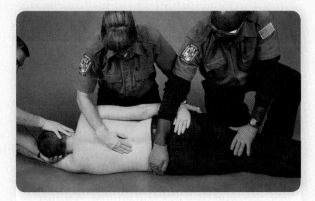

Step 11 Log roll the patient and assess the back.

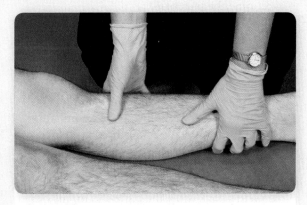

Step 12 Inspect the extremities.

external bleeding, penetrating injuries, or protruding parts, such as intestines **Step 9**. Ask the patient to relax the stomach muscles and observe whether the stomach remains rigid. Rigidity is often a sign of abdominal injury. Swelling is also a sign of abdominal injury.

Note whether the clothing has been soiled with urine or feces. This finding may be an important diagnostic sign for certain illnesses or injuries, such as stroke. Make sure you check the genital area for external injuries. Although both the patient and you may be socially uncomfortable during this examination, it must be done if there is any suspicion of injury.

Treatment

Continue talking to the patient throughout the entire patient assessment. Tell the patient what you are doing and why.

9. **Assess the pelvis.** Next, check for fractures of the pelvis. First check for signs of obvious bruising, bleeding, or swelling. If no pain is reported by the patient, then gently press on the pelvic bones **Step 10**. If the patient reports pain or tenderness or if you note any movement, a severe injury may be present in this region.

10. **Assess the back.** The patient's back should be checked one side of the back at a time. Use one hand to gently lift the patient's shoulder and then, using your other hand, slide it down the patient's back as you inspect the surface **Step 11**. In cases where a patient has been injured, move the patient as a unit, taking care to support the head and spine to keep them in proper alignment. Continue to stabilize the head and neck to prevent movement while you examine the patient.

    As you check each side of the back, be sure that your hands go all the way to the midline of the patient's body so you can feel the spinal column. Check half the back from one side, then switch sides and check the other side in the same manner. This ensures that no part of the back is missed during the examination. If the patient is lying on his or her side or stomach, it will be much easier to examine the patient's back. If the patient must be rolled onto a backboard, you can examine the patient's back while the patient is on his or her side. Do not wait for a backboard if this will delay your examination of the patient.

11. **Assess the extremities.** Do a systematic assessment of each extremity to determine whether there are any injuries. This examination consists of the following five steps:

    a. Observe the extremity to determine whether there is any visible injury. Look for bleeding and deformity.

    b. Examine for tenderness in each extremity by encircling it with both hands and gently, but firmly, squeezing each part of the limb **Step 12**. Watch the patient's face and listen to see if the patient shows any signs of pain.

    c. Ask the patient to move the extremity. Check for normal movement. Determine whether there is any pain when the patient moves the extremity.

    d. Check for sensation by touching the bare skin of each extremity. See if the patient can feel your touch.

    e. Assess the circulatory status of each extremity by checking for the presence of a pulse in that extremity and by checking for capillary refill (discussed later in this chapter).

    Each **upper extremity** consists of the **arm**, the forearm, the wrist, and the hand. The arm extends from the shoulder to the elbow; the forearm extends from the elbow to the wrist. Examine one upper extremity at a time as follows:

    a. Observe the extremity. Start by looking at its position. Is it in a normal or an abnormal position? Does it look broken (deformed) to you?

    b. Examine for tenderness. Encircle the upper extremity with your hands. Work from the shoulder downward to the hand. Firmly squeeze the limb to locate any possible fractures.

    c. Check for movement. Take the patient's hand in yours and ask the patient to squeeze your hand. Squeezing is usually painful for the patient if he or she has a fracture or other injury. If a conscious patient cannot squeeze your hand, assume the extremity is seriously injured or paralyzed.

    d. Check for sensation. Ask the patient if he or she feels any tingling or numbness in the extremity. Sensations such as tingling or numbness may be a sign of a spinal injury. Check for sensation by touching the palm of the patient's hand. See if the patient can feel your touch.

    e. Assess the circulatory status. Check the patient's radial pulse. Absence of a radial pulse indicates blood vessel damage. Check the fingers for capillary refill. Check the color, temperature, and moisture of the hand.

Treatment

Do not ask the patient to move an extremity if you find any deformity or tenderness during your examination.

Each **lower extremity** consists of the thigh, the **leg**, the ankle, and the foot. The thigh extends from the hip to the knee. The leg extends from the knee to the ankle. Examine one lower extremity at a time, as follows:

a. Observe the extremity. Look at the position and shape of the lower extremity. Is it deformed? Is the foot rotated inward or outward?

b. Examine for tenderness. Encircle the lower extremity with your hands, as you did with the upper extremities. Move from the groin to the foot. Be sure to make contact with all surfaces of the limb. Use firm but gentle pressure to identify tender (injured) areas.

c. Check for movement. Ask the patient to move the limb only if you have found no signs of injury in the first two steps. If there is a significant injury, movement most likely will be painful. If a conscious patient cannot move the foot or toes, the limb is seriously injured or paralyzed.

d. Check for sensation. Ask the patient whether he or she can feel your touch as you examine the extremity. Tingling or numbness in a limb is a sign of spinal injury.

e. Assess circulatory status. Check the posterior tibial pulse, located just behind the ankle bone on the medial (inner) side of the ankle. Absence of this pulse indicates blood vessel damage, which is sometimes caused by fractures. Check the toes for capillary refill. Check the skin color, temperature, and moisture of the extremity.

Exam of a Specific Area of the Body

An exam of a specific area of the body is generally performed on patients who have sustained nonsignificant MOIs or on responsive medical patients. This type of examination is based on the chief complaint. For example, in a person reporting a headache, you should carefully and systematically assess the head and/or neurologic system. A person with a laceration to the arm may need to have only that arm evaluated. The goal of the exam of a specific area of the body is to focus your attention on the immediate problem.

Words of Wisdom

While you are examining patients, it is important to preserve patient privacy and to maintain body temperature. Patients who are in public places need to be covered with a sheet or blanket to maintain their privacy. It is often necessary to cover patients to preserve their body temperature. Ill or injured patients will often be cold even when it does not feel cold to you.

Assess Vital Signs

The patient's **vital signs** consist of respiration, pulse, blood pressure, and skin condition.

Respiration

The **respiratory rate** is a vital sign that indicates how fast the patient is breathing. It is measured as breaths per minute. In a normal adult, the resting respiratory rate is between 12 and 20 breaths per minute. One cycle of inhaling (breathing in) and exhaling (breathing out) is counted as one breath (respiration). Count the patient's breaths for 1 minute to determine the respiratory rate.

Respirations may be rapid and shallow (characteristic of shock) or slow (characteristic of a stroke or drug overdose). Respirations may also be described as deep, wheezing, gasping, panting, snoring, noisy, or labored. If the patient is not breathing, respiration is described as absent, a condition that would have been addressed during the primary assessment.

When you are checking the rate or noting the quality of respirations, make sure that your face or hand is close enough to the patient's face to feel the exhaled air on your skin. Also watch for the rise and fall of the chest. When counting respirations in a conscious patient, try not to let the patient know that you are counting. If the patient knows you are counting respirations, you may not get an accurate count.

Pulse

The second vital sign is the **pulse**, which indicates the speed and force of the heartbeat. A pulse can be felt anywhere on the body where an artery passes over a hard structure such as a bone. Although there are many such places on the body, the four most common pulse points are the radial (wrist), the carotid (neck), the brachial (arm), and the posterior tibial (ankle).

The most commonly taken pulse is the **radial pulse**, located at the wrist where the radial artery passes over one of the forearm bones, the radius (see Figure 9-7). The **carotid pulse** is taken over a **carotid artery**, located on either side of the patient's neck, just under the jawbone (see Figure 9-6). The **brachial pulse** is taken on the inside of the arm, halfway between the shoulder and the elbow (see Figure 9-8). The **posterior tibial pulse** is located on the inner aspect of the ankle, just behind the ankle bone **Figure 9-12** .

In general, take the radial pulse of a conscious patient and the carotid pulse of an unconscious patient. When examining an infant, use the brachial pulse. The posterior tibial pulse is used to assess the circulatory status of a leg. When checking a patient's pulse, determine three things: rate, rhythm, and quality. To determine the pulse rate (heartbeats per minute), find the patient's pulse with your fingers, count the beats for 30 seconds, and multiply by two. In a normal adult, the resting pulse rate is about 60 to 100 beats per minute, although in a physically fit person (such as a jogger) the resting rate may be lower (about 40 to 60 beats per minute). In children, the pulse rate is normally faster (about 70 to 150 beats per minute; see Chapter 17, *Pediatric Emergencies*). A very slow pulse (fewer than 40 beats per minute) can be the result of a serious illness, whereas a very fast pulse (more than 120 beats per minute) can indicate that the patient is in shock. Remember, however, that a person who is in excellent physical condition may have a pulse rate of less than 50 beats per minute, and a person who is simply anxious or worried could have a fast pulse rate (more than 110 beats per minute).

You should also be able to determine the rhythm and describe the quality of the pulse. Note whether the pulse is regular or irregular. A strong pulse is often referred to as a **bounding pulse**. This is similar to the heart rate that follows physical exertion such as running or lifting heavy objects. The beats are very strong and well defined. A weak pulse is often called a **thready pulse**. The pulse is present, but the beats are not easily detected. A thready pulse is a more dangerous sign than a bounding pulse. A bounding pulse can be dangerous if the patient has high blood pressure and is at risk for a stroke. A more detailed explanation of where each pulse point is located was presented in the section on primary assessment.

Capillary Refill

Capillary refill is the ability of the circulatory system to return blood to the capillary vessels after the blood has been squeezed out. The capillary refill test is done on the patient's fingernails or toenails. To perform this test, squeeze the patient's nail bed firmly between your thumb and forefinger **Figure 9-13** . The patient's nail bed will look pale. Release the pressure. Count 2 seconds by saying "capillary refill." The patient's nail bed should become pink. This indicates a normal capillary refill time.

If the patient has lost a significant amount of blood and is in shock, or if the blood vessels supplying that limb have been damaged, the capillary refill will be delayed or entirely absent. Capillary refill will be delayed in a cold environment and should not be used as the sole means for assessing the circulatory status of an extremity. Check with your medical director to determine whether you should use the capillary refill test.

Blood Pressure

Blood pressure is another way to measure the condition of a patient's circulatory system. High blood pressure may indicate that the patient is susceptible to a stroke. Low blood pressure generally indicates one of the various types of shock (see Chapter 14, *Bleeding, Shock, and Soft-Tissue Injuries*).

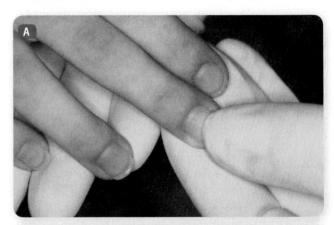

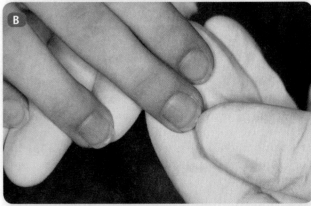

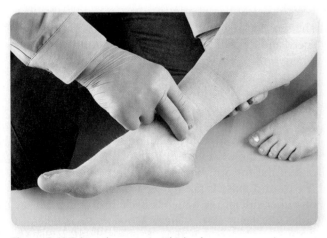

Figure 9-12 Taking the posterior tibial pulse.
© Jones & Bartlett Learning.

Figure 9-13 Checking capillary refill time. **A.** Squeeze the nail bed between your thumb and forefinger. **B.** Release the pressure.
A&B: © Jones & Bartlett Learning. Courtesy of MIEMSS.

The blood pressure measurement consists of a reading of two numbers (for example, 120 over 80, or 120/80). These numbers represent the pressures found in the arteries as the heart contracts and relaxes. The numbers are determined by the pressure exerted in millimeters of mercury (mm Hg), as shown on the dial. The higher number (120 mm Hg in the example of 120 over 80) is called the **systolic pressure**. The systolic pressure is the force exerted on the walls of the arteries as the heart contracts. The lower number (80 mm Hg in the example of 120 over 80) is known as the **diastolic pressure**. The diastolic pressure represents the arterial pressure during the relaxation phase of the heart.

Normal Blood Pressure. Blood pressure ranges may vary greatly. Excitement or stress may raise a person's blood pressure. **Hypertension** (high blood pressure) exists when the blood pressure remains greater than 140/90 mm Hg after repeated examinations over several weeks. Hypertension is a serious medical condition that requires treatment by a physician.

Hypotension (low blood pressure) exists when the systolic pressure (the higher number) falls to 90 mm Hg or below. A patient with this condition is usually in serious trouble. Immediately start treatment of shock if the patient is also experiencing other signs of shock (for example, cold, clammy, pale skin or dizziness) or if repeat measurements of blood pressure are decreasing.

Checking Blood Pressure by Palpation. To take a patient's blood pressure by **palpation** (by feeling it), apply the blood pressure cuff to the uninjured (or less injured) arm. Wrap the cuff around the upper arm. The bottom of the cuff should be 1 to 2 inches (3 cm to 5 cm) above the crease of the elbow. The arrow should point to the brachial artery, which is located on the medial side of the arm at the crease of the elbow **Figure 9-14**.

Blood pressure cuffs come in different sizes for adults, children, and infants. Be sure to use the appropriate size for your patient, such as a narrow cuff for a child and an extra-large cuff for an adult with obesity. Cuffs that are too small may give falsely high readings, and cuffs that are too large may give falsely low readings. Place the indicator dial in a position where you can easily see the movement of the indicator needle. Turn the control knob on the blood pressure inflator bulb clockwise to close the valve. Do not tighten it too much. With the fingers of your other hand, locate the radial pulse at the patient's wrist. Slowly pump up the blood pressure cuff until you can no longer feel the radial pulse. Continue to pump up the cuff for another 30 mm beyond the disappearing point of the radial pulse. Slowly release the pressure in the cuff (at 2 to 4 mm per second), by turning the valve counterclockwise **Figure 9-15**. Continue to feel for the radial pulse and when you first feel the pulse return, carefully note the position of the indicator needle on the dial. This number is the systolic pressure.

The palpation method of taking blood pressure does not give you a diastolic pressure. You will have only one number, the systolic pressure, instead of the two numbers. Report the results as "the blood pressure by palpation is 90."

Checking Blood Pressure by Auscultation. To take blood pressure by **auscultation** (by hearing it), you need both a blood pressure cuff and a stethoscope **Figure 9-16**. Apply the blood pressure cuff in the same manner and position as in the palpation method. After you apply the cuff, locate the brachial artery pulse on the medial side of the arm at the crease of the elbow.

Put the earpieces of the stethoscope in your ears with the earpieces pointing forward. Place the diaphragm of the stethoscope over the site of the brachial pulse. Using your index and middle fingers, hold the diaphragm snugly against the patient's arm. Do not use your thumb! If you use your thumb, you may hear your own heartbeat in the stethoscope.

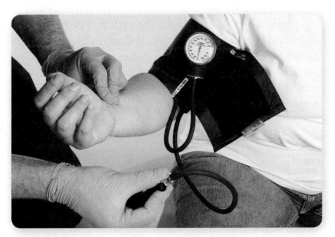

Figure 9-14 When using the palpation method, place your fingertips on the radial artery so you can feel the radial pulse.
© Jones & Bartlett Learning.

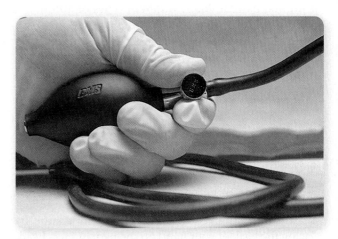

Figure 9-15 Slowly release pressure on the blood pressure cuff by turning the valve counterclockwise.
© American Academy of Orthopaedic Surgeons.

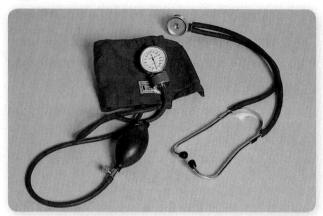

Figure 9-16 Blood pressure cuff and stethoscope.
© Jones & Bartlett Learning. Courtesy of MIEMSS.

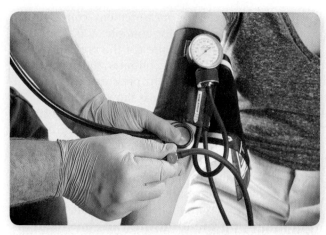

Figure 9-17 Taking blood pressure by auscultation.
© Jones & Bartlett Learning.

Listen as you inflate the blood pressure cuff. When you can no longer hear the sound of the brachial pulse, note the pressure on the dial. Continue to inflate the cuff for another 30 mm over the pressure at which the brachial pulse disappeared. Then slowly and smoothly release air from the cuff by opening the control valve at a rate of 2 to 4 mm per second. Carefully watch the indicator needle, listen for the pulse to return, and note the pressure reading when you first hear the pulse return. This is the systolic pressure. As the cuff pressure continues to fall (at 2 to 4 mm per second), listen for the moment when the pulse disappears. Note the number when you can no longer hear the pulse; this is the diastolic pressure.

Blood pressure taken by auscultation **Figure 9-17** is reported as systolic pressure over diastolic pressure (the larger number over the smaller number) and is always given in even numbers (for example, 120/84, 90/40, or 186/98).

It takes practice to become skilled in taking blood pressures. Take every opportunity to practice on as many healthy, uninjured people as possible. Practice on children and older people as well as on your friends and coworkers. This will help prepare you to measure the blood pressure of a seriously ill or injured patient. Many different types of automatic blood pressure devices are available today. Some EMS departments use these devices to measure blood pressure. If your department uses an automatic blood pressure machine, you need to become proficient in its operation.

Table 9-5 presents a table of typical vital sign values based on age.

Skin Condition

Check the patient's skin for color, temperature, and moisture. Normal body temperature is about 98.6°F (37°C). Precise body temperature is taken with a thermometer, but you can estimate a patient's body temperature by placing the back of your hand on the patient's forehead. The patient's skin temperature is judged, in relation to your skin temperature, as hot or cold.

Table 9-5	Typical Vital Sign Values Based on Age		
Age	**Pulse Rate (Heart Rate) (beats/min)**	**Respirations (breaths/min)**	**Systolic Blood Pressure (mm Hg)**
Infants (newborn to age 1 year)	90–180	25–60	50–95
Children (ages 1 to 12 years)	70–150	15–30	80–110
Adults	60–100	12–20	90–140

Data from: American Heart Association. *2015 Guidelines for Cardiopulmonary Resuscitation and Emergency Cardiovascular Care;* Chameides L, Samson RA, Schexnayder SM, Hazinski MF, eds. *Pediatric Advanced Life Support Provider Manual.* Dallas, TX: American Heart Association; 2011.

Some illnesses can cause the skin to become excessively moist or excessively dry. Therefore, together with its relative temperature, the patient's skin might be described as hot and dry, hot and moist, cold and dry, or cold and moist. Normal skin conditions are described as warm, pink, and dry.

After determining the patient's vital signs, you should also be able to identify and measure these other important signs: pupil size and reactivity and level of consciousness.

Pupil Size and Reactivity

It is important to examine each eye to detect signs of head injury, stroke, or drug overdose. Look to see whether the **pupils** (the circular openings in the middle of the eyes) are of equal size and whether they both react (constrict)

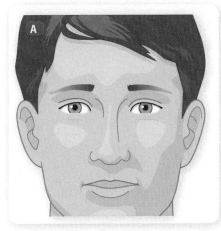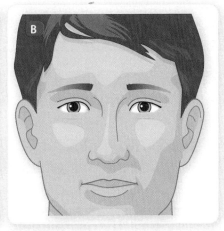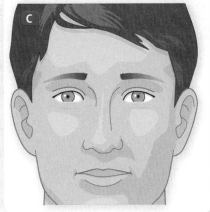

Figure 9-18 Normal pupils (**A**), dilated pupils (**B**), and constricted pupils (**C**).
A, B, & C: © Jones & Bartlett Learning.

when you shine a light into them [Figure 9-18]. The following findings are abnormal:

- **Pupils of unequal size.** Unequal pupils can indicate a stroke or injury to the brain [Figure 9-19]. A small percentage of people normally have unequal pupils, but in an unconscious patient, unequal pupils are often a sign of serious illness or injury.
- **Pupils that remain constricted.** Constricted pupils are often present in a person who is taking narcotics. They are also a sign of certain central nervous system diseases.
- **Pupils that remain dilated (enlarged).** Dilated pupils indicate a relaxed or unconscious state. Pupils will dilate within 30 to 60 seconds of cardiac arrest. Head injuries and the use of certain drugs, such as barbiturates or sleeping pills, can also cause dilated pupils.

Level of Responsiveness

You will usually assess the patient's level of responsiveness (consciousness) as part of your primary assessment. However, it is important to observe and note any changes that occur between the time of your arrival and the time you turn over the patient's care to personnel at the next level of the EMS system. Report any changes from one level of consciousness to another, using the AVPU scale.

Signs Review

Signs are indicators of illness or injury that you can observe in a patient. They help you determine what is wrong with the patient and the severity of the patient's condition. Vital signs include the patient's respirations (respiratory status),

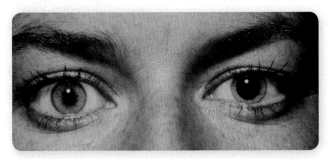

Figure 9-19 Unequal pupils may indicate a stroke or injury to the brain.
© American Academy of Orthopaedic Surgeons.

pulse, capillary refill, blood pressure (circulatory status), skin condition, and temperature. Other signs include pupil size and reactivity and level of consciousness.

To assess a patient's respiratory status, determine the patient's breathing rate and determine whether breaths are rapid or slow, shallow or deep, noisy or quiet. In assessing a patient's circulatory status, determine the rate, rhythm, and quality of the patient's pulse. You can also determine whether the patient's capillary refill is normal, slow, or absent. Determine the patient's blood pressure. Although you may not be able to determine the patient's exact temperature, you will be able to state whether the patient is hot or cold. Skin condition is measured by color and moisture and can be described as pale, flushed, blue, yellow, normal, dry, or moist. To assess the patient's pupils, check to see whether the pupils are equal or unequal in size and whether they remain constricted or dilated. Use the AVPU scale to assess the patient's level of consciousness: awake and alert, responsive to verbal stimuli, responsive to pain, or unresponsive.

Patient Assessment

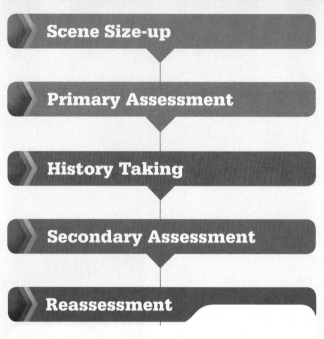

Scene Size-up

Primary Assessment

History Taking

Secondary Assessment

Reassessment

Repeat the primary assessment
Reassess vital signs
Reassess the chief complaint
Recheck the effectiveness of the treatment
Identify and treat changes in the patient's condition
Reassess patient
  ■ Unstable patients every 5 minutes
  ■ Stable patients every 15 minutes
Provide a handoff report

Reassessment

The first four steps of the patient assessment sequence help you determine the patient's initial condition. If other EMS personnel arrive to take over the care of the patient at any point, all you need to do is provide them with a report of your findings in the form of a hand-off report. However, if you need to continue to care for the patient, it is necessary to regularly repeat some parts of the patient assessment. This is the process of reassessment.

Repeat the Primary Assessment

The first step is to repeat the primary assessment. Recheck the patient's level of responsiveness and recheck the patient's airway, breathing, and circulation. Continue to maintain an open airway and to monitor breathing and the pulse for rate and quality.

Reassess Vital Signs

The second step is to reassess the patient's vital signs. Observe the patient's skin color and temperature. Reassess the patient's blood pressure.

Reassess the Chief Complaint

The third step is to reassess the chief complaint to see if there is any change.

Recheck the Effectiveness of the Treatment

Check to see if the interventions you took were effective. When there is a change, determine whether you need to alter your care of the patient.

Identify and Treat Changes in the Patient's Condition

The next step is to identify and treat changes you have noticed in the patient's condition.

Reassess Patient

Patients who appear stable can become unstable quickly. Therefore, it is essential that you reassess all patients carefully for changes in status. Reassess all stable patients every 15 minutes. If the patient is unstable, repeat the reassessment every 5 minutes.

Provide a Handoff Report

It is important that you describe your findings concisely and accurately to the EMS personnel who take over the care of your patients in a handoff report **Figure 9-20**.

The easiest way to report your patient assessment results is to use the same systematic approach you followed during the patient assessment:

1. Provide the age and sex of the patient.
2. Describe the history of the incident.
3. Describe the patient's primary or chief complaint.
4. Describe the patient's level of responsiveness.
5. Describe how you found the patient.
6. Report the status of the vital signs: airway, breathing, and circulation (including severe bleeding).
7. Describe the results of the secondary patient assessment.
8. Report any pertinent medical conditions using the SAMPLE format.
9. Report the interventions you provided and how the patient responded to them.

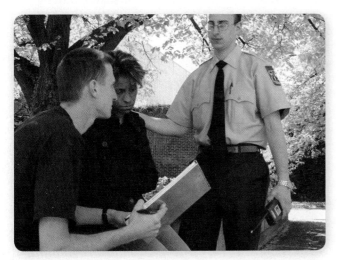

Figure 9-20 Communicate your findings in a handoff report.
© Jones & Bartlett Learning.

Working in a systematic manner will help ensure that you do not overlook any significant symptoms, signs, or injuries and will help to make the handoff report complete and accurate. For example, a handoff report on a 23-year-old man injured in a motor vehicle crash might include the following information:

1. The patient is a 23-year-old man.
2. He was involved in a two-vehicle, head-on collision.
3. He is reporting stomach pain and has a 2-inch (5-cm) cut on his forehead.
4. He is conscious and alert.
5. His pulse rate is 78 beats per minute and strong. His blood pressure is 128/82 mm Hg. His respirations are 16 breaths per minute and are regular and deep.
6. Examination revealed a 2-inch (5-cm) cut on his forehead, marks on his stomach, and moderate pain midway between his right knee and ankle.
7. He has no known medical conditions.
8. The patient is on his back, covered with a blanket to preserve his body heat. We have bandaged his laceration and immobilized his leg with an inflatable splint.

More information on the handoff report is included in Chapter 5, *Communications and Documentation*.

Remember that the purpose of the patient assessment sequence is to:

- Assist in finding the patient's injuries so you can treat them.
- Obtain information about the patient's condition, which you provide to the EMS personnel at the next level of medical care.

With practice, you can complete the entire patient assessment sequence in about 2 minutes. This is not a complete medical examination, but it allows you to perform a systematic patient assessment to determine what injuries or illnesses the patient may have. Remember that there are times when you may need to perform some of the steps of the patient assessment sequence in a slightly different order. Each step is numbered only to help you keep track of where you are in the patient assessment sequence.

Examine every patient involved in an incident before you begin major treatment of any single patient. The exceptions to this rule are patients with airway, breathing, and circulatory problems (severe bleeding or shock). These emergencies must be treated as you encounter them during patient assessment. Except for these life-threatening conditions, do not begin treatment until you have examined all patients to determine the extent and severity of injuries and to make sure that you treat injuries in the order of severity.

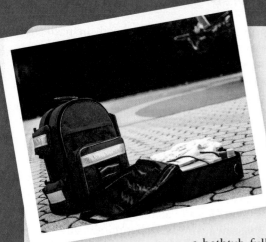

Voices Experience

We were called to respond to a report of a 50-year-old man who had attempted suicide. On arrival, we found the patient naked in a bathtub full of water, unconscious (responsive to pain only) but breathing. The patient had lacerated both wrists and was bleeding. The bath water was discolored by blood and feces. My team dressed and bandaged the wounds. We then lifted him out of the tub, put him on an ambulance blanket, which we used to quickly dry him, then transferred him to the gurney and covered him with another blanket. While this was happening, I took his pulse, respirations, listened to breath sounds, and checked his pupils. Each of these vital signs was unremarkable.

"What is a guy who has lost enough blood to be unconscious doing with a pulse of 68 and respirations of 14? What else did he do to himself?" I thought out loud. A rapid trauma exam revealed nothing more than the lacerations already noted.

> **" What is a guy who has lost enough blood to be unconscious doing with a pulse of 68 and respirations of 14? "**

We started an intravenous line, drew blood samples, and checked his blood glucose; it was 67 mg/dL; again, unremarkable. There was no smell of alcohol on his breath; his pupils were normal size, equal, and only slightly sluggish in response to light. His blood pressure was 110/68 mm Hg.

People who were at the scene said that he had had financial and legal troubles and had been despondent for several days. None of them knew of any medications that he might be taking and no bottles were found at the scene.

The next set of vital signs showed his heart rate had slowed to 58 beats per minute and his respirations had decreased to 9 breaths per minute! We were missing something. While reviewing everything we knew about the patient and the scene, I remembered thinking that when we pulled him out of the bathtub, the water was cold. A quick gloved hand placed under the blanket on the patient's belly confirmed what I should have already known. What we needed to be treating was hypothermia.

With 40 minutes left in our transport, we began aggressive reheating—hot packs, more blankets, turning up the heat in the ambulance, and so on. Within minutes, the patient's level of consciousness improved to the point where he would momentarily open his eyes when his name was called. By the time we arrived at the hospital he was able to ask where he was and complain about our treatment.

After 40 minutes of rewarming en route, his core temperature taken in the emergency room was a little over 85°F (29.6°C).

Focusing on the suicide attempt caused us to miss the incidental and accidental severe hypothermia that ultimately was the patient's only life-threatening problem.

Stephen Lance
Training Officer, Ouray County EMS
Medical Officer, Ouray Mountain Rescue Team
Ouray, Colorado

A Word About Medical and Trauma Patients

Patients generally can be divided into two main categories: those who have a sudden illness and those who sustain trauma. Examples of sudden illnesses include heart attacks, strokes, asthma, and gallbladder conditions. Trauma is the term used for an injury to a patient. The injury may be major or minor. Some incidents that cause trauma include falls, motor vehicle crashes, and sports-related injuries. The patient assessment sequence you have learned can be used to examine patients who have experienced illnesses, trauma, or both.

When you examine medical patients, follow the patient assessment sequence as you learned it:

1. Complete a scene size-up.
2. Perform a primary assessment.
3. Obtain the patient's medical history (SAMPLE).
4. Perform a secondary assessment.
5. Perform reassessment.

This sequence gives the information about the medical patient in a logical order. It allows you to assess the most critical factors first. Although you may have to vary the order of the steps somewhat for certain patients, you should generally try to follow this order. When caring for a trauma patient, modify the preceding sequence slightly. Perform the scene size-up and the primary assessment just like you do for a medical patient. However, when examining a trauma patient, perform the secondary assessment before taking the patient's medical history. By performing the secondary assessment of the entire body before the medical history, you gain information about the patient's injuries. In trauma situations, this is often more important than obtaining the medical history.

Although it is often helpful to consider whether the patient's problem is caused by trauma or sudden illness, avoid jumping to conclusions. Some patients need to be treated for both trauma and sudden illness. (For example, a person who has a heart attack while driving a vehicle needs to be treated for the heart attack and for any trauma sustained in the motor vehicle crash.) The most important factor to remember is to follow a system of patient assessment that will gather all the information needed.

YOU are the Provider   SUMMARY

You are the Provider: CASE 1

1. Why is it so important to follow the five steps in the patient assessment sequence as you evaluate this scene and this patient?

The five steps in the patient assessment sequence are designed to protect you, the patient, and the bystanders. The steps help you focus on the most important factors—responsiveness, airway, breathing, circulation, and shock—before evaluating additional factors. This sequence helps you to determine the need for additional resources so you can call for them as soon as possible. It assists you in performing a systematic examination of the patient so you do not miss signs and symptoms of illness and injury. Finally, it provides a framework for you to report your findings to other health care providers. By following the patient assessment sequence, you have a framework to provide appropriate care to your patients. It helps you perform these tasks in a systematic manner so you do not forget any parts of this important fact-gathering sequence.

2. Why is it important to complete all of the steps of the patient assessment before you determine what is wrong with this patient?

Often the injuries and symptoms that are most visible initially are not the most serious conditions. Complete the patient examination and the patient history before determining a course of action unless the patient has a problem with his or her airway, breathing, or circulation. Conditions are usually best treated if you acknowledge them as discovered, but perform the complete patient examination before attempting to determine the order in which you should treat various injuries or conditions. Remember that a patient who is injured may also have medical conditions, and a patient with medical conditions may also be injured. Keep an open mind. Do not get tunnel vision when assessing a patient.

You are the Provider: CASE 2

1. What are the first actions that you should take?

Your first responsibility at any scene is to ensure that the scene is safe. At different incident scenes, this may require different types of actions. In this situation you have two patients who have the same symptoms along with the suspicion of an odor in the house. Also, this situation is occurring in the middle of the winter when the house is closed tightly and the heating unit is in operation. All these factors should lead you to suspect that there may be a high level of a poisonous gas such as carbon monoxide. If you suspect that the environment may contain a poisonous gas, you need to make sure that you do not become a patient yourself, and you

YOU are the Provider   SUMMARY Continued

need to protect the occupants of the building from further potential harm. This process may involve removing them from the house and placing them in your vehicle or in a nearby house. These actions may be necessary to ensure scene safety for you and for the building occupants before you are able to determine the nature of the illness. In some situations, it may be necessary to request personnel with self-contained breathing apparatus to remove patients from a building.

2. What additional resources do you need?

Additional resources are needed to determine if there is carbon monoxide or another poisonous gas in the house, to assess the patients for poisoning, and to provide proper treatment and transportation for these patients. Most fire departments are equipped with meters to access the levels of carbon monoxide in the house. Many advanced life support providers carry equipment to evaluate the level of carbon monoxide in a patient's blood. In addition, you need to ensure that there are adequate transport units to care for and transport these patients to an appropriate medical facility for treatment. Your most important role at this scene is to carefully evaluate the information available to you and develop a plan. It is important to remove the patients from a potentially hazardous environment and to call for additional resources to evaluate the situation and to provide care and transport for these patients.

You are the Provider: CASE 3

1. Identify scene safety issues that you should consider when you arrive at the scene of a vehicle crash.

Vehicle crashes involve many safety hazards that should be considered as you begin providing patient care. Some of the considerations include: Is the scene safe so that additional crashes do not occur? Are the vehicles stable? Is there a fuel leak or threat of fire? Is there a chance another vehicle could become involved? In this case, where a vehicle traveling at a low speed hit a pedestrian, your primary concern should be for the safety of the pedestrian. Make sure the scene is protected with your vehicle or by diverting traffic. Ensure that the vehicle that struck the pedestrian is stabilized and will not move. Place the vehicle in park, apply the parking brake, and shut off the engine. Chock the wheels if you have a wheel chock. In an incident such as this, there is little chance for a fuel leak. Be certain that your vehicle or some other object is blocking traffic in a way that is likely to prevent you or your patient from

being struck by another vehicle. Once these steps have been taken, take standard precautions for infectious diseases and begin the other steps in the patient assessment sequence.

2. Why do you think manual stabilization of the spine is necessary for the patient in this incident?

After completing a primary assessment and forming a general impression of the patient, the paramedic had determined that spinal precautions are necessary. The mechanism of injury, a motor vehicle hitting a pedestrian, makes it likely that a spinal injury may be present. Stabilization of the spine should be initiated on patients who have sustained trauma. Follow your local protocols.

You are the Provider: CASE 4

1. What is Mattie's chief complaint?

The patient's chief complaint in this scenario is weakness. At this point in your patient assessment, you do not know what is causing this weakness, but you know that you need to complete all five steps of the patient assessment process to get as much information as possible. Focusing on the patient's chief complaint helps you to listen carefully to the patient to gain additional information and to be alert as you examine the patient.

2. Why is the SAMPLE history important when caring for a patient like this who has a vague chief complaint?

The SAMPLE history is a means to systematically obtain information about the patient's current illness or injury and to learn more about his or her past medical history. In this case, you learn the following about this patient: Mattie started to feel weak about 20 minutes earlier. She is not allergic to any foods or medications. She takes insulin twice a day for her diabetes. She has had diabetes for 4 years but does not have any other illnesses or medical conditions. Because she woke up late that morning, she only had a glass of milk and one piece of toast for breakfast 3 hours earlier. She took her regular insulin shot this morning before breakfast. By completing a SAMPLE history on this patient, you are able to gather a lot of additional information that helps you to determine what the patient's problem is and then you are able to determine what steps you can take in this situation to care for this patient. In this case, you may be able to give the patient some food or juice that contains sugar to help alleviate her weakness.

Prep Kit

Ready for Review

- A complete patient assessment consists of five steps: Step 1, perform a scene size-up; Step 2, perform a primary assessment; Step 3, obtain a patient's medical history; Step 4, perform a secondary assessment; and Step 5, provide reassessment.
- The scene size-up is a general overview of the incident and its surroundings. On the basis of this information, you can make decisions about the safety of the scene, the type of incident, the mechanism of injury or illness, the number of patients, and the need for additional resources.
- During the primary assessment, determine and correct any life-threatening conditions. The steps of the primary assessment are: form a general impression of the patient, assess responsiveness, and perform a rapid exam to identify life threats that consists of checking and correcting problems with the patient's airway, breathing, and circulation. Finally, update responding EMS units.
- The purpose of obtaining a medical history is to gather a systematic account of the patient's past medical conditions, illnesses, and injuries to determine the signs and symptoms of the current condition. The SAMPLE history provides a framework to ask needed questions of the patient.
- The secondary assessment of the patient consists of a secondary assessment of the entire body used to assess non–life-threatening conditions. It is done only after completing the primary assessment and stabilizing any life-threatening conditions. This assessment helps you locate and begin management of the signs and symptoms of illness or injury. After completing the secondary assessment of the entire body, assess the patient's vital signs.
- It is essential that you reassess all patients carefully to evaluate them for any changes in their status. If the patient is stable, repeat the vital signs every 15 minutes. If the patient is unstable, repeat the vital signs every 5 minutes. If the patient's condition changes, repeat the primary assessment and identify any changes in the patient's condition.
- Provide a concise and accurate handoff report to EMS personnel.
- Patients can generally be divided into two main categories: medical and trauma. When examining medical patients, follow the patient assessment sequence:
  1. Size-up the scene.
  2. Perform a primary assessment.
  3. Obtain the patient's medical history using the SAMPLE format.
  4. Perform a secondary assessment. Examine the patient from head to toe and assess vital signs.
  5. Provide ongoing reassessment.
- When examining trauma patients, perform the secondary assessment before obtaining the patient's medical history.

▶ Vital Vocabulary

abdomen The body cavity between the thorax and the pelvis that contains the major organs of digestion and excretion.

arm Part of the upper extremity that extends from the shoulder to the elbow.

aspiration Breathing in foreign matter such as food, drink, or vomitus into the airway or lungs.

assessment-based care A system of patient evaluation in which the chief complaint of the patient and other signs and symptoms are gathered. The care given is based on this information rather than on a formal diagnosis.

auscultation Listening to sounds with a stethoscope.

AVPU scale A scale to measure a patient's level of consciousness. The letters stand for Alert, Verbal, Pain, and Unresponsive.

backboard A straight board used for splinting, extricating, and transporting patients with suspected spinal injuries.

bounding pulse A strong pulse (similar to the pulse that follows physical exertion such as running or lifting heavy objects).

brachial pulse Pulse located on the arm between the elbow and shoulder; used for checking the pulse in infants.

capillary refill The ability of the circulatory system to restore blood to the capillary blood vessels after it has been squeezed out by the examiner.

carotid artery The principal arteries of the neck; they supply blood to the face, head, and brain.

carotid pulse A pulse that can be felt on each side of the neck where the carotid artery is close to the skin.

chief complaint The patient's response to questions such as "What happened?" or "What's wrong?"

clavicle The collarbone.

cyanosis Blue discoloration of the skin resulting from poor oxygenation of the circulating blood.

diastolic pressure The measurement of pressure exerted against the walls of the arteries while the left ventricle of the heart is at rest.

Prep Kit *Continued*

exhalation Breathing out.

flail chest A condition that occurs when three or more ribs are each broken in two places and the chest wall lying between the fractures becomes a free-floating segment.

fractures Breaks in a bone.

hypertension High blood pressure.

hypotension Low blood pressure.

inhalation Breathing in.

leg The lower extremity; specifically, the lower portion, from the knee to the ankle.

lower extremity Consists of the thigh, leg, ankle, and foot.

palpation To examine by touch.

posterior tibial pulse Ankle pulse.

primary assessment The first actions taken to form an impression of the patient's condition; to determine the patient's responsiveness and introduce yourself to the patient; to check the patient's airway, breathing, and circulation; and to acknowledge the patient's chief complaint. The primary assessment is sometimes called the initial patient assessment.

pulse The wave of pressure that is created by the heart when it contracts as a result of forcing the blood out and into the major arteries.

pupils The circular openings in the middle of the eye.

radial pulse Pulse located on the inside of the wrist on the thumb side.

respiratory rate The speed at which a person is breathing (measured in breaths per minute).

SAMPLE history A patient's medical history. The letters stand for Signs and Symptoms, Allergies, Medications, Pertinent past medical history, Last oral intake, Events associated with or leading up to the illness or injury.

scene size-up A step within the patient assessment process that includes a visual survey, or an overview of the incident and its surroundings, and a quick assessment of the scene and the surroundings to provide information about scene safety and the mechanism of injury or nature of illness before you enter and begin patient care.

secondary assessment The step in the patient assessment sequence in which you carefully examine the patient from head to toe and measure vital signs.

sign A condition that you observe in a patient, such as bleeding or the temperature of a patient's skin.

symptom A condition the patient tells you, such as "I feel dizzy."

systolic pressure The measurement of blood pressure exerted against the walls of the arteries during contraction of the heart.

thready pulse A weak pulse.

trauma A wound or injury.

upper extremity Consists of the arm, forearm, wrist, and hand.

vital signs Measurements or critical parameters used to assess the patient's immediate health condition including pulse, capillary refill, skin condition, temperature, respirations, and blood pressure.

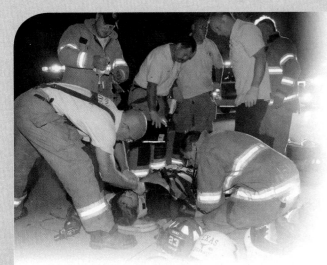

Assessment
in Action

You are dispatched to a convenience store for the report of a person who has fallen. On arrival, you find a 69-year-old man lying on the ground. He reports pain in the area of his left hip.

1. In what order should you perform the five steps of the patient assessment process on this patient?

   1. Secondary assessment
   2. Primary assessment
   3. History taking
   4. Scene size-up
   5. Reassessment

      A. 4, 2, 3, 1, 5
      B. 3, 1, 4, 2, 5
      C. 4, 2, 1, 3, 5
      D. 1, 3, 2, 5, 4

2. Which of the following steps should you perform first during the scene size-up?

   A. Take standard precautions.
   B. Ensure scene safety.
   C. Determine the need for additional resources and assistance.
   D. Determine the mechanism of injury/ nature of illness.

3. Place the following parts of the primary assessment in the order in which you should perform them.

   1. Assess the patient's airway.
   2. Assess the level of responsiveness.
   3. Assess the patient's circulation.
   4. Update the responding EMS units.
   5. Form a general impression of the patient.
   6. Assess the patient's breathing.

      A. 5, 2, 1, 6, 3, 4
      B. 6, 5, 3, 4, 1, 2
      C. 3, 2, 1, 5, 6, 4
      D. 2, 6, 3, 4, 5, 1

4. Which of the following measurements will give you the most information about this patient's condition?

   A. Taking blood pressure by palpation
   B. Taking blood pressure by auscultation

5. Your initial blood pressure reading on a patient who has been involved in a motor vehicle crash is 146/86 mm Hg. You reassess his blood pressure every 5 minutes and get the following readings: 142/82 mm Hg, 134/76 mm Hg, 126/68 mm Hg, and 106/54 mm Hg. What do these results tell you about this patient's condition?

   A. The patient's condition seems to be stable.
   B. The patient appears to be exhibiting signs of increasing shock.
   C. The patient is becoming more relaxed.
   D. The patient is probably not seriously injured.

6. How often do you need to monitor the vital signs of a patient in stable condition?

   A. Every 3 to 5 minutes
   B. Every 5 minutes
   C. Every 15 minutes
   D. Only when you see a change in the patient's condition

7. How often do you need to reassess a patient in unstable condition?

   A. Every 3 to 5 minutes
   B. Every 5 minutes
   C. Every 15 minutes
   D. Only when you see a change in the patient's condition

Assessment *in Action* Continued

8. Pale skin indicates which of the following conditions?

    A. Increased circulation to that part of the body

    B. Lack of oxygen

    C. A normal condition

    D. Decreased circulation to that part of the body

9. The SAMPLE mnemonic is part of which step in the patient assessment sequence?

    A. Primary assessment

    B. History taking

    C. Secondary assessment

    D. Reassessment

10. Why is it important to obtain a medical history on a patient who has sustained trauma?

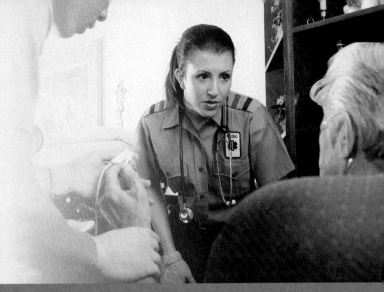

SECTION 4

Medical

Medical Emergencies

National EMS Education Standard Competencies

Medicine

Recognizes and manages life threats based on assessment findings of a patient with a medical emergency while awaiting additional emergency response.

Medical Overview

Assessment and management of a
> Medical complaint (pp 203–204)

Neurology

Anatomy, presentations, and management of
> Decreased level of responsiveness (p 204)
> Seizure (pp 204–206)
> Stroke (pp 210–211)

Abdominal and Gastrointestinal Disorders

Anatomy, presentations, and management of shock associated with abdominal emergencies
> Gastrointestinal bleeding (pp 214–215)

Endocrine Disorders

Awareness that
> Diabetic emergencies cause altered mental status (pp 213–214)

Cardiovascular

Anatomy, signs, symptoms, and management of
> Chest pain (p 207)
> Cardiac arrest (pp 207–209)

Respiratory

Anatomy, signs, symptoms, and management of respiratory emergencies including those that affect the
> Upper airway (Chapter 7, *Airway Management*)
> Lower airway (pp 209–210)

Genitourinary/Renal

> Blood pressure assessment in hemodialysis patients (p 215)

Knowledge Objectives

1. Describe the general approach to a medical patient. (p 203)
2. Explain the causes, signs, symptoms, and treatment of a patient with altered mental status. (p 204)
3. Explain the causes, signs, symptoms, and treatment of a patient with seizures. (pp 204–206)
4. Describe how to place an unconscious patient in the recovery position. (p 205)
5. Explain the causes of angina pectoris. (p 207)
6. Describe the signs, symptoms, and initial treatment of a patient with angina pectoris. (p 207)
7. Describe how to assist a patient with administering his or her nitroglycerin pills or spray. (p 207)
8. Explain the major causes of a heart attack. (p 207)
9. Describe the signs, symptoms, and initial treatment of a patient with a heart attack. (pp 207–209)
10. Explain the cause of congestive heart failure. (p 209)
11. Describe the signs, symptoms, and initial treatment of a patient with congestive heart failure. (pp 209–210)
12. Explain the causes of dyspnea. (p 210)
13. Describe the signs, symptoms, and initial treatment of a patient with dyspnea. (p 210)
14. Explain the causes of asthma. (p 210)
15. Describe the signs, symptoms, and initial treatment of a patient experiencing an asthma attack. (p 210)
16. Explain the major cause of stroke. (p 211)
17. Describe the signs, symptoms, and initial treatment of a patient with a stroke. (p 211)
18. Explain the use of the Cincinnati Prehospital Stroke Scale as a stroke assessment tool. (p 211)
19. Explain the causes of diabetes. (p 213)
20. Describe the signs and symptoms of hypoglycemia. (p 213)
21. Describe the initial treatment of a patient with hypoglycemia. (p 213)
22. Describe the signs and symptoms of a patient in a diabetic coma. (p 214)
23. Describe the initial treatment of a patient in a diabetic coma. (p 214)
24. Describe the causes, signs, and symptoms of an abdominal condition. (pp 214–215)
25. Describe the initial treatment of a patient with abdominal pain. (p 215)
26. Explain how to measure blood pressure in a dialysis patient. (p 215)
27. Discuss potential complications for dialysis patients. (p 215)

Skills Objectives

1. Demonstrate a patient assessment on a medical patient. (pp 203–204)
2. Demonstrate placing an unconscious patient in the recovery position. (p 205)

3. Demonstrate how to protect a patient who is seizing from sustaining further harm. (p 206)
4. Demonstrate how to assist a patient with administering his or her nitroglycerin pills or spray. (p 207)
5. Demonstrate how to support a patient experiencing a heart attack. (p 208)
6. Demonstrate care of a patient with congestive heart failure. (pp 209–210)
7. Demonstrate the steps to treat a patient with dyspnea. (p 210)

8. Demonstrate the use of the Cincinnati Prehospital Stroke Scale as a stroke assessment tool. (p 211)
9. Demonstrate treatment of a patient with hypoglycemia. (p 213)
10. Demonstrate treatment of a patient in a diabetic coma. (p 214)
11. Demonstrate treatment of a patient with abdominal pain. (p 215)
12. Demonstrate how to measure blood pressure in a dialysis patient. (p 215)

■ Introduction

This chapter on medical conditions has two parts. In the first part, you will learn about general medical complaints, including altered mental status and seizures. General medical complaints may result from a wide variety of medical conditions. You will learn the signs, symptoms, and common treatment steps for patients with these general medical complaints. The second part addresses some specific medical conditions you will encounter, including angina pectoris, heart attack, congestive heart failure, dyspnea, asthma, stroke, hypoglycemia, diabetic coma, and abdominal pain. You will learn the signs, symptoms, and treatment of patients with these specific medical conditions.

Treating patients with medical conditions can be some of the most challenging work you perform as an emergency medical responder (EMR). By carefully studying these conditions, you will be prepared to provide reassuring and sometimes life-saving care to patients who are experiencing medical emergencies.

▶ Patient Assessment in Medical Emergencies

Your approach to a patient who has a general medical complaint should follow the systematic approach outlined in the patient assessment sequence in Chapter 9, *Patient Assessment* **Figure 10-1**. Review your dispatch information to help you decide on possibilities for the

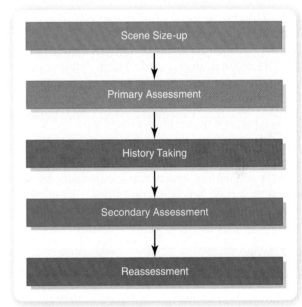

Figure 10-1 Patient assessment sequence.
© Jones & Bartlett Learning. Courtesy of MIEMSS.

patient's condition. Carefully assess the scene to determine safety issues for you and your patient. As you perform the primary assessment, first try to form an impression of the patient's condition. Then determine the patient's responsiveness, introduce yourself, check the patient's airway, breathing, and circulation (ABCs), and acknowledge the patient's chief complaint.

YOU ▶ are the Provider   CASE 1

Your alert tones go off at 0517 hours. You are dispatched to a residence about 4 miles (6 km) from your location for the report of a sick person. While you are responding, your dispatcher informs you that the patient is a 71-year-old woman. Her husband reports that his wife is having trouble speaking and she cannot move her right side.

1. What are your priorities for assessing this patient?
2. What tool do you have to help you with this assessment?
3. Why is it important for this patient to be transported without delay?

Usually, it is best to obtain a medical history on a patient experiencing a medical condition before you perform the secondary patient assessment. The medical history should be complete and include all factors that may relate to the patient's current illness.

The SAMPLE history format will help you secure the information you need:

S   Signs and symptoms
A   Allergies
M   Medications
P   Pertinent past medical history
L   Last oral intake
E   Events leading up to the illness or injury

Although the secondary assessment focuses on the areas related to the patient's current illness, the patient may not always be aware of all the aspects of his or her condition. It is better to perform a complete physical examination and find all the conditions than to perform a partial examination and miss an underlying condition. Obtain the patient's vital signs. Be sure to monitor your patient through ongoing reassessment if the arrival of additional emergency medical services (EMS) personnel is delayed.

As you perform the patient assessment, remember to reassure the patient. Any call for emergency medical care is a frightening experience for the patient. Stress aggravates many medical conditions. Reducing the patient's stress will go a long way toward making the patient more comfortable.

General Medical Conditions

General medical conditions may have different causes, but they result in similar signs and symptoms. By becoming skilled at recognizing the signs and symptoms of various general medical conditions and learning about general treatment guidelines, you will be able to provide immediate care for your patients even if you cannot determine the exact cause of the conditions. This initial treatment can stabilize the patient and allow other EMS and hospital personnel to diagnose and further treat the condition.

▶ Altered Mental Status

Altered mental status is a sudden or gradual decrease in the patient's level of responsiveness. This change may range from a decrease in the level of understanding to unresponsiveness. Any patient who is unresponsive has experienced a severe change in mental status.

When you are assessing altered mental status, remember the AVPU scale:

A   **Awake and alert.** An alert patient will answer simple questions accurately and appropriately.
V   **Responsive to Verbal stimuli.** A patient who is responsive to verbal stimuli will react to loud voices.

P   **Responsive to Pain.** A patient who is responsive to a painful stimulus will react to the pain by moving or crying out.
U   **Unresponsive.** An unresponsive patient will not respond to either verbal or painful stimuli.

When assessing the patient's mental status, consider two factors: the patient's initial level of consciousness and any change in that level of consciousness. A patient who is initially alert but later responds only to verbal stimuli has experienced a decrease in his or her level of consciousness.

Many different conditions may cause an altered level of consciousness, including:

- Head injury
- Shock
- Decreased level of oxygen to the brain
- Stroke
- Slow heart rate
- High fever
- Infection
- Poisoning, including drugs and alcohol
- Low level of blood glucose (diabetic emergencies)
- Insulin reaction
- Psychiatric condition

Some of the specific conditions that cause altered mental status are explained in the second part of this chapter. Even if you cannot determine what is causing the patient's altered level of consciousness, you can help by treating the symptoms of the condition.

In summary, complete the patient assessment sequence to ensure that the scene is safe and that you have properly assessed the patient's medical condition. Initial treatment consists of maintaining the patient's ABCs and normal body temperature and keeping the patient from additional harm. If the patient is unconscious and has not sustained trauma, place the patient in the recovery position or use an airway adjunct to help maintain an open airway. Be prepared to provide suctioning if there is a chance that the patient may vomit or not be able to handle secretions accumulating in the airway.

▶ Seizures

Seizures are caused by sudden episodes of uncontrolled electrical impulses in the brain. Instead of discharging electrical impulses in a controlled manner, the brain cells keep firing impulses. Seizures that produce shaking movements and involve the entire body are called **generalized seizures** (formerly called grand mal seizures). These seizures usually last 1 to 2 minutes, although prolonged seizures may continue for more than 2 minutes. Patients are usually unconscious during generalized seizures and do not remember them afterwards. Although seizures are rarely life threatening, they are a serious medical emergency and may be the sign of a life-threatening condition. After a seizure, you may need to assist the patient in maintaining an open airway. The patient may have a loss of bowel or bladder control, soiling his or her clothing.

One cause of generalized seizures is a sudden high fever. These seizures are called febrile seizures. Febrile seizures most commonly occur in infants and young children. Febrile seizures are discussed in Chapter 17, *Pediatric Emergencies*.

Some seizures result in only a brief lapse of consciousness. These seizures are called **absence seizures** (formerly called petit mal seizures). Patients experiencing absence seizures may blink their eyes, stare vacantly, or jerk one part of their body. Because these seizures are of brief duration and severity, the family or bystanders of the patient usually do not call EMS. A physician should examine patients exhibiting signs and symptoms of an absence seizure.

Many times you will find that you are not able to determine the cause of the patient's seizure. The patient's family may be able to tell you whether a physician has diagnosed the patient as having a seizure disorder. After a seizure, the patient may be sleepy, confused, upset, hostile, or out of touch with reality for up to an hour. You must monitor the patient's ABCs and arrange for *transport* to an appropriate medical facility.

the patient only if he or she is in a dangerous location, such as in a busy street or close to something hard, hot, or sharp.

During a seizure, the patient generally does not breathe and may turn blue. You cannot do anything about the patient's airway during the seizure, but once the seizure has stopped, it is essential that you ensure an open airway. Usually the best method to accomplish this is the head tilt–chin lift maneuver. Observe the seizure activity and report your observations and assessment findings to other EMS providers. This information may be important in determining the cause of the seizure.

After you have opened the airway, place the patient in the recovery position to help keep the airway open and to allow any secretions (saliva or blood from a bitten tongue) to drain out   Figure 10-2 . Patients who have experienced a seizure may have excess oral secretions.

Most patients start to breathe soon after the seizure ends. If the patient does not resume breathing after a seizure or if the seizure is prolonged, begin mouth-to-mask or mouth-to-mouth breathing (see Chapter 7, *Airway Management*). Supplemental oxygen should be administered as soon as it is available.

Words of Wisdom

There are many different types of seizures, and many factors that can cause them, including:

- Epilepsy
- Trauma
- Head injury
- Stroke
- Shock
- Decreased level of oxygen to the brain
- High fever
- Infection
- Poisoning
- Overdose of drugs or alcohol
- Brain tumor or infection
- Diabetic emergencies (low blood glucose)
- Complication of pregnancy
- Unknown causes

Treatment

Treatment for a seizure patient is as follows:

- Stay calm. You cannot stop a seizure once it has started.
- Do not restrain the patient.
- Time the duration of the seizure.
- Protect the patient from contact with hard, sharp, or hot objects.
- Loosen ties or anything else around the neck that may obstruct breathing.
- Do not force anything between the patient's teeth.
- Do not be concerned if the patient stops breathing temporarily during the seizure.
- After the seizure, turn the patient on his or her side and make sure breathing is not obstructed.
- If the patient does not begin breathing after a seizure, begin rescue breathing.

Usually, the seizure will be over by the time you arrive at the scene. If it has not ended, focus your treatment on protecting the patient from injury. Do not restrain the patient's movements. If you attempt to restrain the patient, you may cause further injury. If a patient experiences a seizure while on a hard surface, control the patient's arms by grasping them at the wrists. Allow the patient's arms to move but prevent the elbows from hitting the hard surface. To prevent the patient's head from hitting a hard surface, quickly slide the toes of your shoes under the patient's head. Move

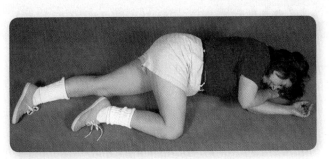

Figure 10-2 Recovery position for an unconscious patient.
© Jones & Bartlett Learning. Courtesy of MIEMSS.

Following a seizure, the patient will experience a state of confusion that may last for 30 to 45 minutes. The patient may also become anxious, hostile, or belligerent. Continue to monitor the patient to be sure he or she is breathing adequately. At this point, the patient needs privacy. Because the person is probably embarrassed about what happened or where it happened (perhaps in a public place such as a restaurant or shopping mall), move the patient to a more comfortable, private place if other EMS personnel have not arrived. Do not leave the patient, even if the patient insists that he or she is now awake and alert. Encourage any patient who experiences a seizure to go to a medical facility for examination and treatment.

Safety

Do not attempt to put anything in the mouth of a patient who is actively seizing. Remember, a person having a seizure cannot swallow his or her tongue.

The best treatment you can provide for a patient experiencing a seizure is to protect him or her from self-injury. After the seizure, ensure that the airway is open, the patient is breathing adequately, and the mouth is clear of secretions and blood.

Treatment

Although you may be inclined to quickly categorize patients as "medical patients" or as "trauma patients," many of the patients you encounter may have both a medical condition and a traumatic injury. For example, the altered level of consciousness experienced by a diabetic patient with severe hypoglycemia may contribute to a motor vehicle crash. As you study this chapter, try to imagine how you can use your knowledge to treat patients with a single condition or a variety of conditions. Remember to carefully assess each patient and treat the conditions that you identify.

■ Specific Medical Conditions

In the first part of this chapter, you learned how to assess general medical complaints and treat patients based on their signs and symptoms. This is the foundation for assessing and treating patients who present with medical conditions. You will find it helpful, however, to be knowledgeable about some of the more specific medical conditions you may encounter as an EMR. These include heart conditions, dyspnea, asthma, stroke, diabetic conditions, and abdominal pain.

Sometimes the patient or the patient's family will tell you that the patient has a certain medical condition. At other times, your careful assessment of the patient will reveal information that leads you to suspect a particular condition, allowing you to take specific steps to help the patient. The added knowledge you gain from the second part of this chapter will help you assess, treat, and communicate more effectively with patients who have medical conditions.

Words of Wisdom

Remember, many medical conditions can cause both altered mental status and seizures.

▶ Heart Conditions

The heart must receive a constant supply of oxygen or it will die. The heart receives its oxygen through a complex system of coronary (heart) arteries. As long as these arteries continue to supply the heart with an adequate amount of oxygen, the heart can continue to function properly.

As the body ages, however, the coronary arteries may narrow as a result of a disease process called **atherosclerosis**. Atherosclerosis causes layers of fat to coat the inner walls of the arteries. Progressive atherosclerosis can cause angina pectoris, heart attack, and even **cardiac arrest**.

YOU ▶ are the Provider   CASE 2

You are returning from a call and as you slow down for a traffic light ahead, you notice a small crowd of people on the sidewalk. When they see you, several people excitedly wave you down. You quickly pull your vehicle to the side and exit your vehicle. A patient is lying on the sidewalk. One of the bystanders tells you that the man was walking down the street and suddenly paused and then slumped to the ground. While you approach the patient, his legs and arms begin to vigorously contract in a seizure that seems to involve his whole body.

1. What can you do to prevent this patient from hurting himself during a seizure?
2. What actions should you take to provide care for this patient immediately after the seizure stops?
3. What additional care does this patient need during the first few hours after the seizure stops?

Angina Pectoris

As atherosclerosis progresses in the coronary arteries, it can reduce the blood (oxygen) supply to the heart enough to cause pain or pressure in the chest. This pain is known as **angina pectoris** or simply angina. The heart needs more oxygen than the narrowed coronary arteries can deliver.

When a patient has chest pain, first ask the person to describe the pain. Patients often describe angina as pressure or heavy discomfort. The patient may say something like, "It feels like an elephant is sitting on my chest." Angina attacks are usually brought on by exertion, emotion, or eating. The patient may feel crushing pain in the chest. The pain may radiate to either or both arms, the neck, jaw, or any combination of these sites. The patient is often short of breath and sweating, extremely frightened, and has a sense of doom. The patient may experience nausea and vomiting.

Ask whether the patient is already being treated for a diagnosed heart condition. If the answer is "yes," ask if the patient has a pill or spray to take for angina pain. A patient who has experienced previous episodes of angina usually has medication that he or she can place or spray under the tongue to relieve the pain. The most common medication of this type is **nitroglycerin**, and the patient may have already taken a dose by the time you arrive at the scene **Figure 10-3**.

If the patient has nitroglycerin but has not taken it during the past 5 minutes, help place one of the tiny pills under the patient's tongue or help the patient administer the aerosol spray. Follow your local protocols regarding the administration of nitroglycerin. Nitroglycerin usually relieves angina pain within 5 minutes. If the pain has not diminished after 5 minutes, help the patient take a second dose. If the pain still has not lessened 5 minutes after the second dose, assume the patient is having a heart attack. Before you assist with the administration of nitroglycerin, you need to receive training and have permission from your medical director.

Heart Attack

A heart attack (myocardial infarction) results when one or more of the coronary arteries is completely blocked. The two primary causes of coronary artery blockage are severe atherosclerosis and a blood clot from somewhere else in the circulatory system that breaks free and lodges in the artery. If one of the coronary arteries becomes blocked, the part of the heart muscle served by that artery is deprived of oxygen and dies **Figure 10-4**.

Blockage of a coronary artery causes the patient to experience immediate and severe pain. The pain of angina pectoris and a heart attack may be similar at first. Most heart attack patients describe the pain as crushing. The pain may radiate from the chest to the left arm, or to the jaw, or to the back **Figure 10-5**. Heart conditions do not cause all chest pain. Pneumonia and muscle strains to the chest wall can also cause chest pain. It is better for the patient to treat the pain as if it is a heart attack than to undertreat the symptoms. The patient is usually short of breath, weak, sweating, nauseated, and may vomit. Nitroglycerin pills or spray will not relieve the pain of a heart attack. The pain will persist, unlike the pain of angina, which rarely lasts more than 5 minutes. Giving one adult aspirin (325 mg) or 2 to 4 low-dose aspirins (81 mg each) may help to reduce the chance of death from a heart attack. Instruct the patient to chew the aspirin and then swallow it. Be sure the patient is not allergic to aspirin and has not had any recent internal bleeding such as a stomach ulcer.

If the area of heart muscle supplied by the blocked artery is either critical or large, the heart may stop completely. Complete cessation of heartbeat is called cardiac arrest. Cardiopulmonary resuscitation is your first emergency treatment for cardiac arrest (see Chapter 8, *Professional Rescuer CPR*, and Chapter 9,

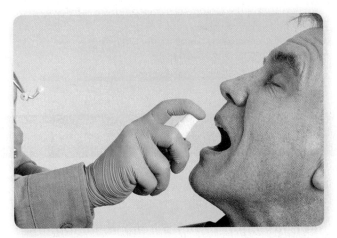

Figure 10-3 Nitroglycerin pills, ointment, patch, and spray relieve chest pain.
© Jones & Bartlett Learning.

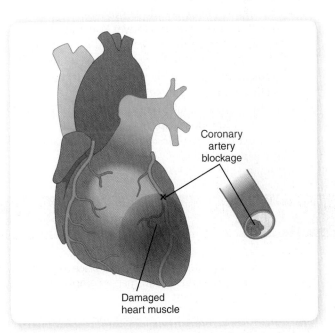

Coronary artery blockage

Damaged heart muscle

Figure 10-4 A blocked cardiac artery results in a heart attack.
© Jones & Bartlett Learning.

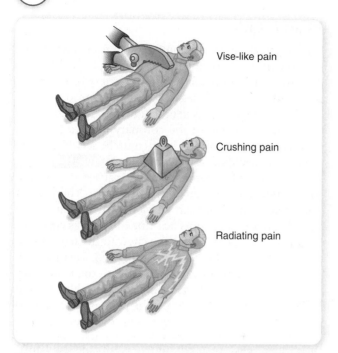

Vise-like pain

Crushing pain

Radiating pain

Figure 10-5 Descriptions of pain caused by heart attack.
© Jones & Bartlett Learning.

Patient Assessment). Most patients do not experience immediate cardiac arrest with a heart attack. To support the patient and reduce the probability of cardiac arrest, you can take the following actions:

- Summon additional help.
- Talk to the patient to relieve his or her anxiety.
- Touch the patient to establish a bond. Hold the person's hand.
- Reassure the patient that you are there to help. The person is afraid that death is close, and fear can create tension and make the pain worse.
- Move the patient as little as possible and do not allow the person to move! You and other bystanders must move the patient if necessary.
- Place the patient in the position he or she finds most comfortable. This is usually a semi-reclining or sitting position.
- Help the patient take one adult aspirin (325 mg) or 2 to 4 low-dose aspirins (81 mg each). Instruct the patient to chew and then swallow the aspirin tablets.

- If oxygen is available and you are trained to use it, administer it to the patient. Supplemental oxygen increases the amount of oxygen the blood can carry. The increase in oxygen reduces pain and anxiety. It also eases the minds of the patient's family and friends to see that you are doing something to relieve the patient's physical distress.
- Be prepared to administer cardiopulmonary resuscitation, if necessary.
- If an automated external defibrillator is available, have it brought to the patient and make sure it is ready for use if needed.

Because you do not have extensive equipment available to help a patient experiencing a heart attack, your primary role is to provide emotional support and arrange for *prompt transport* to an appropriate medical facility. Because the patient's emotional state can affect his or her physical condition, emotional support is valuable. It can help prevent cardiac arrest.

Words of Wisdom

Recent research has shown that the administration of one adult aspirin (325 mg) or 2 to 4 low-dose aspirins (81 mg each) may help to reduce the chance of death from a heart attack by reducing the size of the blood clot in the heart. The American Heart Association recommends that patients experiencing chest pain take aspirin as soon as possible. The patient should chew and then swallow the aspirin tablets. Check to be sure your patient is not allergic to aspirin and has not had any recent internal bleeding such as a stomach ulcer. Check with your supervisor or medical director to see if your department recommends aspirin administration in patients with chest pain.

Signs and Symptoms

The signs and symptoms of cardiac arrest are as follows:

- Unconsciousness
- Absence of respirations or only gasping
- Absence of a carotid pulse

YOU ▶ are the Provider   CASE 3

You are at a local diner where you have just placed your order for dinner when dispatch informs you that there is an incident just around the corner. A 58-year-old woman is complaining of not feeling right, but she cannot give any specific reason other than an odd sensation in her chest.

1. You ask if she has pain in her chest and she says no. Does that mean she is not having a heart attack?
2. The woman is nervous and repeatedly asks if she is going to die. What should you do?
3. Should you administer oxygen if you are trained to use it?

Treatment

Not everyone having a heart attack has severe chest pain. Older women and people with diabetes are more likely to have silent heart attacks. People experiencing silent heart attacks may report vague feelings of discomfort and not feel the classic chest pain associated with heart attacks. Do not discount vague complaints in these patients. The only way to rule out a heart attack is to have a thorough examination by a physician.

Treatment

Within the last 20 years, the use of clot-buster drugs and nonsurgical treatments, such as percutaneous coronary intervention (PCI), has been an important advance in treating patients experiencing a heart attack. Clot-buster drugs or PCI can often open the blocked coronary vessels and prevent the need for costly and painful surgery.

A specially trained physician must administer these treatments within a few hours of the start of a heart attack to be effective. Your prompt response and attentive care of a patient experiencing a heart attack may be the first step in returning that patient to a comfortable, healthy, and productive life.

Congestive Heart Failure

Congestive heart failure (CHF) is not directly caused by narrow or blocked coronary arteries, but by failure of the heart to pump adequately. As explained in Chapter 6, *The Human Body*, and Chapter 8, *Professional Rescuer CPR*, the heart has two sides. The right side receives deoxygenated blood from the body and sends it to the lungs; the left side receives fresh oxygenated blood from the lungs and pumps it to the body. If one side of the heart becomes weak and cannot pump as well as the other side, the circulatory system becomes unbalanced, resulting in circulatory congestion. In CHF, the failure is in the heart muscle, but the congestion is in the blood vessels.   Figure 10-6 shows what happens if CHF occurs on the left side of the heart, which sends blood to the body. Because the left side cannot send blood to the body as efficiently as the right side can send blood to the lungs, more blood goes to the lungs than to the body. This results in congestion (overload) in the blood vessels of the lungs.

The major symptom of CHF is breathing difficulty, not chest pain. If you are assisting a patient who has respiratory difficulty but no airway obstruction or signs of injury, look for the signs and symptoms of CHF. As

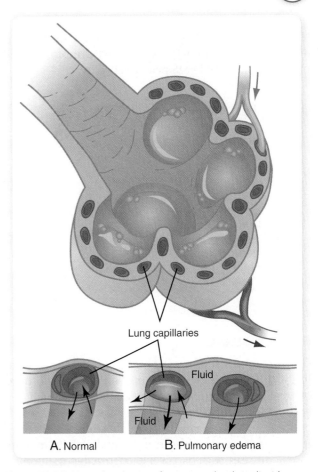

Figure 10-6 A. Normal exchange of oxygen and carbon dioxide between a capillary and an alveolus. **B.** Pulmonary edema: congestive heart failure causes fluid to leak from the capillary and build in the alveolus, impeding oxygen and carbon dioxide exchange.
© Jones & Bartlett Learning.

blood pressure builds in the vessels of the lungs, fluid is forced into the lung tissue, causing it to swell. The patient may make a gurgling sound when breathing and start spitting up a white or pink froth or foamy fluid. At this point, the patient is actually "drowning" in his or her own body fluids. The patient is very anxious but is usually in little or no pain (unless he or she is experiencing a heart attack coupled with CHF).

As soon as you determine that your patient is experiencing CHF, take these simple, life saving actions:

1. Place the patient in a sitting position, preferably on a bed or chair. Having the legs hang down over the edge of the bed or chair helps drain some of the fluid back into the lower parts of the body and may improve breathing.
2. Administer oxygen (if it is available and you are trained to give it) in large quantities and at a high flow rate.
3. Summon additional help.
4. Arrange for *prompt transport* to an appropriate medical facility.

The most important action you can perform is to place the patient in a sitting position with the legs down. This position helps relieve CHF symptoms until more highly trained EMS personnel arrive.

Signs and Symptoms

Signs and symptoms of congestive heart failure include the following:

- Shortness of breath
- Rapid, shallow breathing
- Moist or gurgling respirations
- Profuse sweating
- Enlarged neck veins
- Swollen ankles
- Anxiety

▶ Dyspnea

Dyspnea means shortness of breath or difficulty breathing. Although healthy people may experience shortness of breath during intense physical exertion or at high altitudes, this condition is not usually associated with serious heart or lung disease. Heart-related causes of dyspnea include angina pectoris, heart attack, and CHF. Pulmonary (lung) diseases such as **chronic obstructive pulmonary disease (COPD)**, emphysema, chronic **bronchitis**, pneumonia, and asthma can also cause dyspnea.

COPD and emphysema are caused by damage to the small air sacs (alveoli) in the lungs. This damage decreases the amount of working lung capacity, resulting in shortness of breath. Chronic bronchitis is caused by an inflammation of the airways in the lungs. Pneumonia is caused by an infection in the lungs. Asthma is caused by a clamping down or spasm of the smaller air passages.

As an EMR, you will not always be able to determine what is causing a patient to be short of breath. Do not spend too much time trying to determine the specific cause. Focus on treating the symptoms of dyspnea.

General treatment for patients with dyspnea consists of the following steps:

1. Check the patient's airway to be sure it is not obstructed.
2. Check the rate and depth of the patient's breathing. If the rate is less than 8 breaths per minute or more than 40 breaths per minute, be prepared to assist with mouth-to-mask or mouth-to-barrier device rescue breathing.
3. Place the patient in a comfortable position. A conscious patient is usually most comfortable when sitting.
4. Provide reassurance.

5. Loosen any tight clothing.
6. Administer oxygen if it is available and you are trained to do so.

Asthma

One common cause of dyspnea is **asthma**. Asthma is an acute spasm of the smaller air passages associated with excess mucus production and swelling of the lining of the respiratory passages. A type of allergic reaction can cause an asthma attack. Severe emotional stress, exercise, or a respiratory infection can also cause an asthma attack. Asthma is a common condition. According to the Centers for Disease Control and Prevention (CDC), more than 24 million people in the United States have asthma. It killed 3,630 people in the United States in 2013.

Patients experiencing an asthma attack have great difficulty exhaling through partially obstructed air passages. A patient experiencing an asthma attack is like a person trying to exhale though a narrow straw. You will hear a wheezing sound during exhalation. If there is a limited amount of air moving through the small air passages, wheezing may be absent. Fatigued patients may be so short of breath that they are unable to talk. Many patients with asthma will have taken medications before your arrival.

Treatment

Patients who are short of breath or receiving oxygen should have their breathing and pulse monitored at least every 5 minutes. Underlying illness or trauma may cause certain patients to stop breathing and require you to begin rescue breathing.

Patients can die during asthma attacks. It is important that you follow the steps just listed for treating dyspnea. In addition to these steps, you can instruct the patient to perform pursed-lip breathing. Ask the patient to purse his or her lips as if blowing up a balloon when exhaling. Tell the patient to blow out with force. Pursed-lip breathing relieves some of the internal lung pressures that cause the asthma attack. Treatment by paramedics or in the hospital includes medications that help to relax the constricted air passages. If advanced life support is not available, arrange for *prompt transport* to an appropriate medical facility.

▶ Stroke

Strokes are the fifth leading cause of death in the United States. Many more people suffer brain injury and disability as the result of strokes. According to the CDC, each year about 795,000 adults experience strokes, and approximately 130,000 of them die. Strokes are a leading cause of long-term disability. Most strokes (87%) are caused by a blood clot that lodges in an artery of the brain. The clot blocks the blood supply to a part of the brain. Without treatment, that part of the brain will be damaged or die. Think of a stroke as a "brain attack," similar to a heart attack. People with high blood pressure have an increased risk of having a stroke.

The signs and symptoms of a stroke vary depending on what portion of the brain is affected. They can be similar to the signs and symptoms of a head injury, hypoglycemia, or seizures. When you are caring for a stroke patient, the person may be alert, confused, or unresponsive. Responsive patients may not be aware that they have signs of a stroke. Some stroke patients are unable to speak; others are unable to move one side of their body. The patient may have a headache and may describe it as "the worst headache of my life." Some stroke patients experience seizures.

The Cincinnati Prehospital Stroke Scale is an easy-to-administer and accurate tool that you can use to determine whether a patient may have experienced a stroke. It requires no special equipment to administer. This test consists of three assessments: assessment of the facial muscles by having the patient smile, assessment of arm drift by having the patient hold his or her arms in front of him or her, and speech assessment by having the patient repeat a simple phrase. If the patient is not able to complete one or more of these tasks, suspect a stroke. **Table 10-1** describes the specific steps for administering the Cincinnati Prehospital Stroke Scale.

Your first priority is to maintain an open airway. Administer oxygen (if it is available and you are trained to use it) using a nasal cannula. If the patient is having a seizure, try to prevent further injury from occurring. Be prepared to administer rescue breathing if the patient stops breathing. Place an unresponsive patient in the recovery position to help maintain an open airway. This is especially important because some stroke patients are unable to swallow. Give emotional support by talking to and touching the patient. Be especially careful if you must move a patient because some patients may not be able to feel one side of their body.

Signs and Symptoms

The signs and symptoms of stroke include the following:

- Headache
- Numbness or paralysis on one side of the body
- Dizziness
- Confusion
- Drooling
- Inability to speak
- Difficulty seeing
- Unequal pupil size
- Unconsciousness
- Seizures
- Respiratory arrest
- Incontinence
- Unresponsiveness

Some stroke patients can be treated with special drugs to dissolve the blood clot in their brain. These clot-buster drugs must be administered in the hospital within the first few hours after the stroke. For this reason, it is important for you to determine the time the stroke began by questioning the patient, family, or bystanders. If the patient has signs or symptoms of a stroke, it is important for you to arrange for *prompt transport* of the patient to a medical facility that is equipped to treat stroke patients.

Table 10-1	The Cincinnati Prehospital Stroke Scale

The Cincinnati Prehospital Stroke Scale is a tool you can use to tell if there is a high probability that a patient has experienced a stroke. This scale requires you to quickly assess three things: Facial Droop, Arm Drift, and Abnormal Speech.

Facial Droop	**Have patient show teeth or smile.**
Normal	Both sides of the face move equally.
Abnormal	One side of the face does not move as well as the other side.

Arm Drift	**Patient closes eyes and holds both arms straight out for 10 seconds.**
Normal	Both arms move the same or both arms do not move.
Abnormal	One arm does not move or one arm drifts down compared with the other.

Abnormal Speech	**Have patient say, "You can't teach an old dog new tricks."**
Normal	Patient uses correct words with no slurring.
Abnormal	Patient slurs words, uses the wrong words, or is unable to speak.

Note: If any of these three signs is abnormal, the probability of a stroke is 72%.

© Jones & Bartlett Learning. Courtesy of MIEMSS.

Words of Wisdom

A stroke patient may be able to hear what you are saying even if he or she cannot speak or appears to be unconscious. Be careful not to say anything that would increase the patient's anxiety.

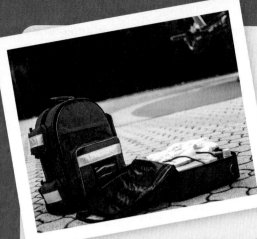

Voices *of* Experience

Some people end up attracting the same type of call throughout their shift or even series of shifts. That was me when I first started in EMS; I was almost guaranteed a seizure call.

Prior to my involvement with EMS, I had never witnessed a seizure. The terms *generalized seizure, status epilepticus,* and *postictal* were foreign.

> **❝ It was a little overwhelming to see someone writhing on the floor uncontrollably, and it took me a second to absorb what was happening. ❞**

We were dispatched to a community center for a male having a seizure. Seizures can have a variety of causes, but this patient was known to have epilepsy. When we arrived, people had cleared the area around him and he was still seizing. It was a little overwhelming to see someone writhing uncontrollably on the floor, and it took me a second to absorb what was happening. Then, the training kicked in. One of several concerns is the patient's airway, which is virtually impossible to assess while the patient is actively seizing. The patient's respiratory rate and tidal volume are compromised while he or she is in a seizure. The patient may vomit during and after the seizure, presenting the possibility of aspiration. We had suction ready along with a bag valve mask, high-flow oxygen, and an airway. The paramedic was prepared to start an IV line for both fluid and medication administration. Drugs like diazepam (Valium) are used to break or stop seriously prolonged seizure activity in a condition known as status epilepticus.

As the muscular activity subsided, the patient lay still. His breathing was shallow but present. We opened his airway, verified there were not any secretions, put a nonrebreathing mask on him, providing high-flow oxygen, and placed him on his side in the recovery position. He began to show purposeful movement and mumble a little. Seizure patients in their postictal phase (after the seizure, when the body is recovering) often are not able to communicate for some time, so it is our responsibility as EMRs to look out for what they may need. The paramedic started the IV line and we prepared to load the patient onto the gurney for our 35-minute transport to the nearest hospital.

Some patients will have a medical bracelet indicating their condition; some scenes will have family or friends available to give us a medical history. Other times, we have to wait until the patient is able to provide us with information, but obtaining a SAMPLE history helps us to provide the best care possible. It is also important to keep in mind that, while someone who has been prone to seizures might be a little more comfortable in communicating with us after a seizure, someone who has experienced one for the first time could be embarrassed or confused, complicating the information-gathering process. Either way, be patient and understanding. The worst part is over. Give the patient a gentle, comforting ride to the hospital.

Carl M. Prather, EMSI
Santa Fe Community College
Santa Fe, New Mexico

▶ Diabetes

Diabetes is caused by the body's inability to process and use glucose (sugar) that is carried by the bloodstream to the body's cells. Glucose is an essential nutrient. The body's cells need both oxygen and glucose to survive. The body produces a hormone (chemical) called insulin that enables glucose carried by the blood to move into individual cells, which use it as fuel.

If the body does not produce enough insulin, the cells become "starved" for glucose. This condition is called diabetes. Many people with diabetes must take supplemental insulin injections to bring their insulin levels up to normal. Oral medicine rather than insulin is sometimes used to treat mild diabetes.

Diabetes is a serious medical condition. Therefore, all patients with diabetes who are sick must be evaluated and treated in an appropriate medical facility. Two specific medical conditions can occur in patients in the course of managing their diabetes: hypoglycemia and diabetic coma. Consider both of these conditions as medical emergencies.

Hypoglycemia

Hypoglycemia, or low blood sugar, occurs if the body has enough insulin but not enough blood glucose. An older term for hypoglycemia is insulin shock. A person with diabetes may take insulin in the morning and then alter his or her usual routine by not eating or by exercising vigorously. In either case, the level of blood glucose drops and the patient experiences hypoglycemia.

The signs and symptoms of hypoglycemia (insulin shock) are similar to those of other types of shock. Suspect low blood sugar if your patient has a history of diabetes or is wearing medical emergency information, such as a medical alert necklace or bracelet.

Hypoglycemia is a serious medical emergency that can occur quickly, often within a few minutes. With very low levels of blood sugar, a person with diabetes may become unresponsive. If hypoglycemia is not diagnosed and corrected by the rapid administration of glucose in some form, the patient may die or experience permanent brain injury.

A person experiencing hypoglycemia may appear to be drunk or confused. This is an important fact for you to keep in mind. EMS personnel who misinterpreted hypoglycemia as intoxication have made mistakes. If you suspect that a patient is experiencing hypoglycemia, try to get answers to the following questions:

- Do you have diabetes?
- Did you take your insulin today?
- Have you eaten today?

If the patient has diabetes and has taken insulin that day, but has not yet eaten, suspect that the patient is going into hypoglycemia. If the patient is able to swallow, attempt to get the patient to eat or drink something sweet. For example, you could use a drink that has a high sugar concentration such as a cola or orange juice. Honey is another possibility. Do not give a diet beverage to these patients. Diet beverages do not contain the necessary sugar.

Signs and Symptoms

Signs and symptoms of hypoglycemia include the following:

- Pale, moist, cool skin
- Rapid, weak pulse
- Dizziness or headache
- Confusion or unconsciousness
- Sweating
- Hunger
- Rapid onset of symptoms (within minutes)

If the patient is unconscious, do not try to administer fluids by mouth because the patient may choke and aspirate the fluid into the lungs. Summon help immediately. Open the patient's airway, and assist breathing and circulation, if necessary. The patient must have glucose administered intravenously as soon as possible. A paramedic or a physician can do this.

Some EMRs carry glucose tablets or a tube of oral glucose gel. The preferred route for oral glucose administration is for the patient to swallow oral glucose tablets. If the patient is not able to safely swallow these, some people place a tablet or glucose gel inside the cheek. Some glucose will be absorbed through the inside of the patient's cheek **Figure 10-7**. Glucose can be administered orally to patients who are able to swallow. Even though the patient's body may absorb only a small amount of glucose, it may be enough to prolong consciousness until the patient receives further medical treatment.

Words of Wisdom

Progression into hypoglycemia is rapid and may be fatal; progression into diabetic coma usually takes several days.

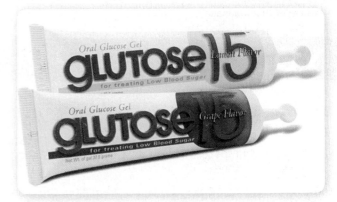

Figure 10-7 Instant glucose provides high concentrations of sugar.
Courtesy of Paddock Laboratories, Inc.

Diabetic Coma

Diabetic coma occurs when the body has too much blood glucose and not enough insulin. For example, a person with diabetes may fail to take insulin for several days, resulting in blood glucose levels that build to higher and higher levels, but there is no insulin to process it for use by the body's cells.

The patient may be unresponsive or unconscious. A patient experiencing a diabetic coma may appear to have the flu (influenza) or a severe cold. As with hypoglycemia, misdiagnosis is common. It is not always easy to tell the difference between hypoglycemia and diabetic coma **Table 10-2**.

If the patient is conscious and you cannot get definite answers to your questions to determine whether the patient is experiencing hypoglycemia or diabetic coma, you can do no harm by administering a liquid substance that contains sugar. In a patient who is experiencing low blood sugar, the sugar may improve the patient's condition. If the patient is experiencing a diabetic coma, the sugar will not raise blood glucose levels enough to do any further harm to the patient. In general, give conscious patients with diabetes sugar by mouth and arrange for *prompt transport* to an appropriate medical facility.

Treatment

During your initial examination of every patient, look for an emergency medical alert device (such as a necklace or bracelet) to find out whether the patient has a preexisting medical condition, such as diabetes.

If the patient with diabetes is unconscious, arrange for *prompt transport* to an appropriate medical facility. An ambulance must transport every patient with diabetes who is experiencing illness to an appropriate medical facility for further treatment and examination.

Signs and Symptoms

Signs and symptoms of diabetic coma include the following:

- History of diabetes
- Warm, dry skin
- Rapid pulse
- Deep, rapid breathing
- Fruity or acetone odor on the patient's breath
- Weakness, nausea, and vomiting
- Increased hunger, thirst, and urination
- Slow onset of symptoms (days)

Table 10-2	Comparing Hypoglycemia and Diabetic Coma
Hypoglycemia	**Diabetic Coma**
Pale, moist, cool skin	Warm, dry skin
Rapid, weak pulse	Rapid pulse
Normal breathing	Deep, rapid breathing
Dizziness or headache	—
Confusion or unresponsiveness	Confusion or unresponsiveness
Rapid onset of symptoms (minutes)	Slow onset of symptoms (days)

© Jones & Bartlett Learning. Courtesy of MIEMSS.

▶ Abdominal Pain

The abdomen is separated from the chest by the diaphragm. It is a crossroads for several body systems, including the circulatory, skeletal, nervous, digestive, and genitourinary systems. For example, the aorta carries blood from the heart through the abdomen to the lower parts of the body. Conversely, a large vein, the vena cava, carries blood back to the heart. The spine, with its large trunks of nerves, runs through this area. Parts of the rib cage surround the abdominal cavity. Most of the digestive system, including the stomach, small intestine, large intestine, liver, gallbladder, and pancreas, are in the abdomen. The kidneys and ureters are located in the abdominal area, as are parts of the male and female reproductive systems.

YOU are the Provider — CASE 4

You are dispatched to the Chippewa City Park for a report of a sick woman. After a 6-minute response, you arrive at the park and a concerned bystander directs you to a park bench. You find a 25- to 30-year-old woman slumped on the park bench. She is dressed in a jogging outfit. You introduce yourself and attempt to determine her primary complaint. The woman responds to verbal stimuli, but she seems confused when you ask her questions. You note that she is sweaty and has a weak pulse at the rate of 88 beats per minute.

1. What types of medical conditions or situations can cause confusion?
2. What steps can you take to determine the cause of the patient's confusion?
3. If you determine that this woman has diabetes, what steps can you take to improve her condition?

There are hollow and solid structures in the abdomen. Hollow structures, such as the small intestine, are really tubes through which contents pass. Solid structures, such as the pancreas and the liver, produce various substances used by the body. The structures in the abdomen are sometimes identified by quadrant, according to their location. As an EMR, you do not have to learn the names, types, and locations of all the abdominal structures, but it is helpful for you to have a basic understanding of the abdominal anatomy.

The abdomen occupies a large part of the body, and abdominal pain is a common complaint. Because of the number of body systems and organs located in the abdomen, even physicians may have a difficult time identifying the cause of abdominal pain. As an EMR, you need to be able to recognize that a patient has an abdominal condition. You do not have to determine the cause of the abdominal pain.

One condition you may encounter is called an **acute abdomen**. Irritation of the abdominal wall causes an acute abdomen. This irritation may be the result of infection or caused by the presence of blood in the abdominal cavity as the result of disease or trauma. A patient with an acute abdomen may have referred pain in other parts of the body such as the shoulder. The abdomen may feel as hard as a board. These patients may have nausea and vomiting, fever, and diarrhea as well as pain.

Some patients with abdominal pain will vomit blood because they are bleeding from the esophagus or the stomach. Bleeding from the lower part of the gastrointestinal tract may produce bloody stools that contain bright red blood, or the stools may be black and tarry. Treat these patients for shock. Arrange for *prompt transport* to an appropriate medical facility.

If a patient has abdominal pain, monitor vital signs, treat symptoms of shock, keep the patient comfortable, and arrange for *transport* to an appropriate medical facility. It is important for a physician to examine these patients.

One cause of an acute abdomen is an **abdominal aortic aneurysm (AAA)**. An abdominal aortic aneurysm occurs when one or more layers of the aorta become weak and separate from other layers of the aorta. Patients who have diabetes, high blood pressure, or atherosclerosis, as well as heavy smokers, are at high risk for developing an AAA. The weakening of the aorta causes a ballooning of the vessel, much like a weak spot on thin rubber tubing. If this weak spot or aneurysm ruptures, the patient will rapidly lose large quantities of blood into his or her abdomen. This massive internal blood loss will cause profound shock.

Patients with an AAA may report pain in the abdomen. Some patients describe this pain as a tearing sensation. They may have pain referred to the shoulder. If an AAA ruptures, the patient will experience severe pain and profound shock from the blood spilling into the abdomen.

Place any patient who experiences these signs and symptoms in a comfortable position. This is often a side-lying position with the legs drawn up. Treat the patient for shock. Handle these patients gently and arrange for *prompt transport* to an appropriate medical facility. The sooner these patients receive medical care, the better their chance of survival will be.

Signs and Symptoms

Signs and symptoms of an acute abdomen include the following:

- Nausea and vomiting
- Loss of appetite
- Pain in the abdomen
- Rigid abdomen
- Distention
- Shock

▶ Kidney Dialysis Patients

People with certain types of kidney disease are unable to filter waste products from their bloodstream. Many patients with chronic renal (kidney) failure must undergo a treatment called hemodialysis two or three times a week. During hemodialysis, the patient's blood passes through a machine that filters out the waste products and returns the cleansed blood to the patient. Most hemodialysis patients have a special device called a shunt implanted in their arm or leg. The shunt is a surgically created connection between an artery and a vein. The shunt is used to connect the patient to the hemodialysis machine. A shunt looks like a raised bump on the patient's arm or leg. If you have a patient who is on dialysis, find out if he or she has a shunt. If a shunt is in place, be sure to take the patient's blood pressure in the arm without the shunt to prevent damaging it.

Patients who are receiving dialysis treatment may experience medical emergencies related to the treatment. During or shortly after dialysis treatment, patients may experience a drop in blood pressure caused by the changes in their body from the treatment. This decrease in blood pressure can produce shock. Patients receiving dialysis treatment are also at risk for internal bleeding. Bleeding from stomach ulcers may result in the patient vomiting blood or having bloody stools. If the tubing that connects the patient's shunt to the dialysis machine separates, the patient can lose a significant amount of blood externally. Hemodialysis patients may also experience abnormal levels of electrolytes in their blood that can cause cardiac arrhythmias that sometimes result in cardiac arrest. For these conditions, treat the symptoms presented by the patient. Remember that the patient can most likely supply you with information about these situations. If not, question the patient's companions and caregivers because they are with the patient for many hours each week.

YOU ▸ are the Provider   SUMMARY

You are the Provider: CASE 1

1. What are your priorities for assessing this patient?

Obtaining information about the patient's condition before you arrive on the scene is always helpful. With this information, you can start thinking about what conditions might cause the signs and symptoms communicated to you. However, this information should not distract you from carefully completing the steps of the patient assessment sequence. For this situation, it is important for you to assess the scene for safety and then perform a primary assessment. Determine the patient's level of responsiveness, and then assess her airway, breathing, and circulation. Correct any problems, if necessary. For example, if the patient is having trouble handling her secretions, it may be necessary to place her lying on her side. Once you have completed the primary assessment, continue by obtaining the patient's medical history and performing a secondary assessment. After completing these steps, perform an ongoing reassessment every 5 minutes.

2. What tool do you have to help you with this assessment?

The Cincinnati Prehospital Stroke Scale is a valuable tool for assessing a person who has signs or symptoms of a stroke, or brain attack. If a patient shows signs of facial droop, arm drift, or abnormal speech, there is a 72% chance that he or she is experiencing a stroke. The results obtained from administering the Cincinnati Prehospital Stroke Scale also help the paramedics and physicians who will be treating the patient.

3. Why is it important for this patient to be transported without delay?

Some stroke patients can be treated with special drugs to dissolve the blood clot in their brain. These drugs must be administered within the first few hours from the time the stroke occurs. It is important that you try to determine when the patient's symptoms began and to arrange for prompt transport of this patient because she has signs and symptoms of a stroke. Your assessment and care help ensure this patient the best chance of a full recovery.

You are the Provider: CASE 2

1. What can you do to prevent this patient from hurting himself during a seizure?

Focus care for a patient experiencing a seizure on protecting the patient from further harm. Move any objects that the patient may strike or hit out of his way. Because this patient is seizing on a concrete sidewalk, try to prevent his head from violently striking the sidewalk. Slide your shoes under the back of the patient's head. This will provide a softer surface for the back of his head as he seizes. To prevent injury to his elbows as they strike the sidewalk, grasp each wrist with one of your hands and hold his wrists up in a position that prevents his elbows from forcefully striking the ground without restraining them. During the active phase of a seizure, it is not possible to control the patient's airway. Do not attempt to restrain the patient.

2. What actions should you take to provide care for this patient immediately after the seizure stops?

During a seizure, the patient generally does not breathe and may turn blue. As soon as the seizure stops, take steps to ensure that the patient has an open airway. The best way to accomplish this is to use the head tilt–chin lift maneuver. After you have opened the airway, make sure the patient starts to breathe. When you are sure the patient is breathing adequately, place the patient in the recovery position. This position will help to keep the airway open and to allow any secretions (saliva or blood from a bitten tongue) to drain from the patient.

3. What additional care does this patient need during the first few hours after the seizure stops?

After you have ensured that the airway is open and the patient is breathing adequately, the patient needs additional care. Remember that following a seizure, the patient will experience a state of confusion that may last 30 to 45 minutes. The patient may become anxious, hostile, or belligerent. Often this confusion will resolve with time and adequate respirations. Immediately after a seizure, the patient needs privacy. It may help to move the patient to a more comfortable private place until EMS personnel arrive. Arrange for transport to an appropriate medical facility. Usually you will not be able to determine the cause of a seizure. A physician needs to carefully evaluate the patient to determine the cause of the seizure. Once the physician determines the cause of the seizure, he or she can begin appropriate treatment. Remember that seizures can be caused by many different conditions, including stroke, epilepsy, head injury, shock, high fever, infection, poisoning, brain tumors, low blood sugar, and low levels of oxygen to the brain. Your role as an EMR is to ensure that the patient receives careful evaluation and further care at an appropriate health care facility.

You are the Provider: CASE 3

1. You ask if she has pain in her chest and she says no. Does that mean she is not having a heart attack?

Not every person having a heart attack has the classic symptom of chest pain. Older women and people with diabetes can have what is referred to as a silent heart attack with symptoms that tend to be vague. Like this woman, people experiencing a silent heart attack may report discomfort that does not seem like the classic crushing chest pain associated with most heart attacks. As an EMR, do not discount vague symptoms. Assure the woman that the best treatment is a thorough evaluation by an emergency department physician.

2. The woman is nervous and repeatedly asks if she is going to die. What should you do?

Patients with heart issues are often frightened and have a sense of doom. As always, as a trained EMR at the scene, you must remain calm. Your confidence will help reduce her stress. Reassure the woman that you are there to help. Establish a bond with the patient by talking with confidence, and hold her hand. Fear can create tension, resulting in additional pain or causing the condition to worsen. Your steps toward lowering her anxiety level may improve her condition. Make sure she is in a position of comfort and move her as little as possible.

3. Should you administer oxygen if you are trained to use it?

Yes, you should administer oxygen if allowed to do so. Supplemental oxygen boosts the amount of oxygen the blood can carry and can help reduce pain and anxiety. The simple action of administering oxygen can help ease the mind of family members by showing them that you are doing something to help their loved one. If providing oxygen, check the patient's breathing and pulse at least every 5 minutes.

You are the Provider: CASE 4

1. What types of medical conditions or situations can cause confusion?

There are many reasons a person may become confused. As an EMR, you will sometimes not be able to determine the cause of a patient's confusion. One way to approach a confused patient is to consider some of the conditions that might cause confusion. Confusion may be the result of trauma. Patients who have experienced an open or closed head injury, recently or in the past, may be confused. Shock from internal or external blood loss or other causes can result in confusion. A second category of conditions that may result in confusion is medical conditions. Some heart conditions can result in a slow heart rate and

in confusion. Heart attack and strokes can result in confusion. Patients with diabetes become confused because of low blood sugar. People who just had a seizure are confused. A third category that can result in confusion is improper levels of medications and drugs. The intentional or unintentional overdose of prescribed medications or unprescribed drugs or alcohol can result in confusion. Taking too small an amount of certain medications can have the same effect. A fourth category of conditions that can cause confusion is mental illness. Lack of proper medication or an overdose of certain medications can result in the patient being confused. Patients may have insufficient levels of oxygen for many reasons. Patients without sufficient oxygen will become confused. This list is a review of some conditions that can cause confusion. It is not a comprehensive list of all the possible causes of confusion. Rather, it gives you an idea of how you can systematically approach patients with this symptom.

2. What steps can you take to determine the cause of her confusion?

Always attempt to talk with the patient to gather as much information as possible. The SAMPLE history format provides a good framework to gather appropriate information. If the patient is not able to give you this information, consider other approaches. If there is a friend, relative, or caregiver with the patient, he or she can often assist you with gathering this information. Bystanders who have witnessed the scene before you arrive can sometimes help. Carefully look for any medical alert devices on the patient's neck, wrist, and ankle. Check to see if the patient has any identification with him or her. Often the patient will have information related to a medical condition that might result in an altered level of consciousness. If you are not able to determine the cause of the patient's confusion, treat any symptoms you find. Finally, make sure the next level of EMS personnel takes over the patient's care or the patient is transported to an appropriate medical facility.

3. If you determine that this woman has diabetes, what steps can you take to improve her condition?

If you suspect the patient has diabetes, try to ask her specific yes/no questions. Do you have diabetes? Have you taken your insulin today? When did you last have anything to eat? Even though she is confused, she may be able to answer these questions. Next, if she is able to swallow, try to give her some sugar to increase her blood sugar level. If you have some instant glucose tablets or gel, follow the instructions for administering this. If this is not available, try to find some orange juice or a carbonated drink that has sugar in it. These drinks can sometimes raise the blood sugar level enough to help the patient. If nothing is available to give the woman, remember that the EMS transport crew will be able to give her glucose either orally or through a vein. Make sure to turn over this patient to EMTs for additional care.

Prep Kit

▶ Ready for Review

- Your approach to a patient who has a general medical complaint should follow the systematic patient assessment sequence. Usually, it is best to collect a medical history on the patient experiencing a medical condition before you perform a physical examination. The SAMPLE history format will help you secure the information you need.

- General medical conditions may have different causes, but they result in similar signs and symptoms. By becoming skilled at recognizing the signs and symptoms of various general medical conditions and learning about general treatment guidelines, you will be able to provide immediate care for patients even if you cannot determine the exact cause of the condition.

- Altered mental status is a sudden or gradual decrease in the patient's level of responsiveness. When you are assessing altered mental status in a patient, remember the AVPU scale. Complete the patient assessment sequence to ensure scene safety and proper assessment. Initial treatment should consist of maintaining the patient's ABCs and normal body temperature and keeping the patient safe from incurring any additional harm. If the patient is unconscious and has not sustained trauma, place the patient in the recovery position or use an airway adjunct to help maintain an open airway.

- Seizures are caused by sudden episodes of uncontrolled electrical impulses in the brain. Usually, the seizure will be over by the time you arrive at the scene. If it has not ended, focus your treatment on protecting the patient from injury. Do not restrain the patient's movements. You cannot do anything about the patient's airway during the seizure, but once the seizure has stopped, it is essential that you ensure an open airway. After you have opened the airway, place the patient in the recovery position and arrange for transport to an appropriate medical facility.

- The second part of this chapter covers some specific medical conditions: angina pectoris, heart attack, congestive heart failure, dyspnea, asthma, stroke, hypoglycemia, diabetic coma, and abdominal pain. By learning the causes and knowing the signs and symptoms of these conditions, you may be able to provide specific care for the patient. Although a physician must diagnose and treat these conditions, you can greatly improve the patient's chances of survival by taking the simple actions described here until more highly trained EMS personnel arrive on the scene to assist you.

▶ Vital Vocabulary

abdominal aortic aneurysm (AAA) A condition in which the layers of the aorta in the abdomen weaken. This causes blood to leak between the layers of the artery, causing it to bulge and sometimes rupture.

absence seizures Seizures that are characterized by a brief lapse of attention. The patient may stare and not respond; formerly known as petit mal seizures.

acute abdomen The sudden onset of abdominal pain caused by disease or trauma that irritates the lining of the abdominal cavity and requires immediate medical or surgical treatment.

angina pectoris Chest pain with squeezing or tightness in the chest caused by an inadequate flow of blood to the heart muscle.

asthma A disease in which the airway becomes narrowed and inflamed, resulting in episodes of shortness of breath because of air being trapped in the small air sacs of the lungs.

atherosclerosis A disease characterized by thickening and destruction of the arterial walls and caused by fatty deposits within them; the arteries lose the ability to dilate and carry blood.

bronchitis Inflammation of the airways in the lungs.

cardiac arrest Sudden cessation of heart function.

chronic obstructive pulmonary disease (COPD) A slow process of destruction of the airways, alveoli, and pulmonary blood vessels caused by chronic bronchial obstruction (emphysema).

diabetes A disease in which the body is unable to use glucose normally because of a deficiency or total lack of insulin.

diabetic coma A state of unconsciousness that occurs when the body has too much glucose and not enough insulin.

dyspnea Shortness of breath or difficulty breathing.

generalized seizures Seizures characterized by contractions of all the body's muscle groups that may last for 1 to 2 minutes; formerly known as grand mal seizures.

hypoglycemia A condition of low blood sugar that occurs in a person with diabetes who has taken too much insulin or has not eaten enough food.

nitroglycerin A medication used to treat angina pectoris; increases blood flow and oxygen supply to the heart muscle and reduces or eliminates the pain of angina pectoris.

stroke A brain attack caused by a blood clot or a broken blood vessel in the brain. Strokes can result in trouble speaking, inability to move parts of the body, confusion, or unconsciousness.

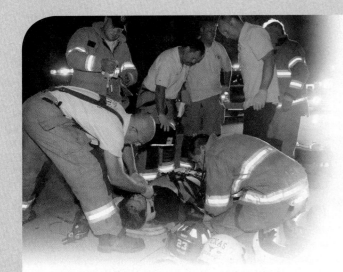

Assessment
in Action

You are sent to a local high school in the middle of a championship basketball game for a man experiencing chest pain. When you arrive at the scene, you find a 72-year-old man sweating, leaning forward, and breathing rapidly.

1. You begin to take a SAMPLE history. What does the *P* stand for?

   A. Pulse
   B. Patient
   C. Presumption
   D. Pertinent past medical history

2. Obtaining a medical history will give you all of the following information, EXCEPT:

   A. allergies.
   B. medications.
   C. signs and symptoms.
   D. name of the illness.

3. If the patient is not able to answer your questions, how should you obtain a medical history?

   A. Call the patient's physician.
   B. Ask the basketball coach if he knows the man.
   C. Ask the patient's son, who is standing nearby.
   D. Contact medical control.

4. Complete cessation of a heartbeat is called:

   A. cardiopulmonary resuscitation.
   B. angina.
   C. indigestion.
   D. cardiac arrest.

5. During your assessment of the man, you note that he has shortness of breath, moist or gurgling respirations, and enlarged neck veins. These are signs and symptoms of:

   A. asthma.
   B. diabetes.
   C. congestive heart failure.
   D. respiratory distress.

6. When you introduce yourself to the man, what are you looking for?

7. Why must the heart receive a constant supply of oxygen?

8. Which of the following is NOT a part of the Cincinnati Stroke Scale?

   A. Listening for abnormal speech
   B. Assessing arm drift
   C. Measuring the patient's blood pressure
   D. Looking for facial droop

9. Which of the following is NOT helpful for a person with diabetes who is suffering from low blood sugar?

   A. Instant glucose tablets
   B. Diet cola
   C. Orange juice
   D. Oral glucose gel

10. Which of the following is NOT a sign or symptom of an acute abdomen?

   A. Distention
   B. Nausea and vomiting
   C. Increased rate of respirations
   D. Pain in the abdomen

Poisoning and Substance Abuse

National EMS Education Standard Competencies

Medicine

Recognizes and manages life threats based on assessment findings of a patient with a medical emergency while awaiting additional emergency response.

Toxicology

Recognition and management of

> Carbon monoxide poisoning (pp 223–225)
> Nerve agent poisoning (p 228; p 230)
> How and when to contact a poison control center (pp 222–223; p 228)

Immunology

Recognition and management of shock and difficulty breathing related to

> Anaphylactic reactions (pp 225–227)

Pharmacology

Uses simple knowledge of the medications that the EMR may self-administer or administer to a peer in an emergency.

Medication Administration

Within the scope of practice of the EMR, how to

> Self-administer medication (p 223; pp 225–228; pp 231–233)
> Peer-administer medication (p 223; pp 225–228; pp 231–233)

Emergency Medications

Within the scope and practice of the EMR

> Names (p 223; pp 225–228; pp 231–233)
> Effects (p 223; pp 225–228; pp 231–233)
> Indications (p 223; pp 225–228; pp 231–233)
> Routes of administration (p 223; pp 225–228; pp 231–233)
> Dosages for the medication administered (p 223; pp 225–228; pp 231–233)

Knowledge Objectives

1. Define poison. (p 221)
2. Describe the signs and symptoms of ingested poisons. (p 222)
3. Explain how to treat a patient who has ingested a poison. (pp 222–223)
4. Describe the signs and symptoms of inhaled poisons. (p 224)
5. Explain how to treat a patient who has inhaled a poison. (p 225)
6. Describe the signs and symptoms of injected poisons. (p 226)
7. Explain how to treat a patient who has been injected with a poison. (pp 226–227)
8. Explain how to assist a patient with an auto-injector. (p 226)
9. Describe the signs and symptoms of absorbed poisons. (p 228)
10. Explain how to treat a patient who has absorbed a poison. (p 228)
11. Describe how to brush off a dry chemical from a patient and then flush with water. (p 228)
12. Describe how to use water to flush a patient who has come in contact with liquid poison. (p 228)
13. Describe the signs and symptom of exposure to a nerve agent. (p 228)
14. Describe the role of emergency medical responders (EMRs) in an incident involving exposure to a nerve agent. (p 228)
15. Explain how to administer a nerve agent auto-injector kit. (p 230)
16. Describe the signs and symptoms of a drug overdose caused by amphetamines, opioids, hallucinogens, and inhalants. (pp 231–232)
17. Explain the general treatment of a patient who has experienced a drug overdose. (p 223)
18. Explain how to administer intranasal naloxone for an opioid overdose. (pp 231–232)

Skills Objectives

1. Demonstrate treatment of a patient who has ingested a poison. (pp 222–223)
2. Demonstrate treatment of a patient who has inhaled a poison. (p 225)
3. Demonstrate treatment of a patient who has been injected with poison. (pp 226–227)
4. Demonstrate how to assist a patient with an auto-injector. (p 227)
5. Demonstrate treatment of a patient who has absorbed a poison. (p 228)
6. Demonstrate how to brush off a dry chemical from a patient and then flush with water. (p 228)
7. Demonstrate how to use water to flush a patient who has come in contact with liquid poison. (p 228)
8. Demonstrate administration of nerve agent auto-injector kits. (p 228)
9. Demonstrate treatment of a patient who has experienced a drug overdose. (p 233)
10. Demonstrate administration of intranasal naloxone for an opioid overdose. (pp 231–232)

Introduction

A **poison** is a substance that causes illness or death when eaten, drunk, inhaled, injected, or absorbed in relatively small quantities. This chapter covers the signs, symptoms, emergency care, and treatment of patients who have experienced accidental or intentional poisoning, bites or stings, or alcohol or substance abuse. You can save a patient's life by quickly recognizing and promptly treating a serious poisoning.

Patient Assessment for Poisoning

As an emergency medical responder (EMR), you need to be a good detective when caring for patients who have come in contact with poisons. Poisoning can be classified according to the way the poison enters the body.

Poisons can enter the body by four primary routes:

1. **Ingestion** occurs when a poison enters the body through the mouth and is absorbed by the digestive system.
2. **Inhalation** occurs when a poison enters the body through the mouth or nose and is absorbed by the mucous membranes lining the respiratory system.
3. **Injection** occurs when a poison enters the body through a small opening in the skin and spreads through the circulatory system. Injection can occur as a result of an insect sting, a snakebite, or the intentional use of a hypodermic needle to inject a poisonous substance into the body.
4. **Absorption** occurs when a poison enters the body through intact skin and spreads through the circulatory system.

Even though poisons can be introduced into the body by different routes, some of the effects of the poison on the body may be similar. In general, when you assess and treat patients who have been poisoned, begin with a thorough assessment that follows the patient assessment sequence Figure 11-1. If you suspect poisoning, obtain a thorough history from the patient or from bystanders. A good history of the incident will help guide you in your patient assessment.

Be alert for any visual clues that may indicate the patient has been in contact with a poison. These findings include traces of the substance on the patient's face and mouth (ingested poisons), traces of the substance on the skin (absorbed poisons), needle pricks or sting marks (injected poisons), and respiratory distress (inhaled poisons).

Much of the emergency care you provide will be based on the patient's signs and symptoms. A patient with a poisonous substance on the skin needs to have the substance removed, which may require special training or the assistance of a hazardous materials (HazMat) team. A patient who shows signs of respiratory distress needs to receive respiratory support. A patient who is exhibiting signs of digestive distress needs to receive support for that condition. Sometimes the patient's signs and symptoms will be less specific, and you will have to base your treatment on general signs and symptoms. The general signs and symptoms of poisoning are shown in Table 11-1.

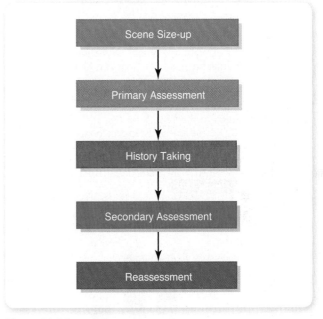

Figure 11-1 Patient assessment sequence.
© Jones & Bartlett Learning. Courtesy of MIEMSS.

Table 11-1	General Signs and Symptoms of Poisoning
History	History of ingesting, inhaling, injecting, or absorbing a poison
Respiratory	Difficulty breathing or decreased respirations
Digestive	Nausea and vomiting Abdominal pain Diarrhea
Central nervous system	Unconsciousness or altered mental status Dilation or constriction of the pupils Convulsions
Other	Excess salivation Sweating Cyanosis Empty containers at the scene

© Jones & Bartlett Learning. Courtesy of MIEMSS.

Safety

Conduct a scene size-up (overview) of the scene to determine whether it is safe for you to enter. Be alert for odors. Look for containers close to the patient. If you believe the scene is unsafe, stay a safe distance away and call for specialized assistance.

Ingested Poisons

An ingested poison is taken by mouth. More than 80% of all poisoning cases are caused by ingestion. Often, you will find chemical burns, odors, or stains around the patient's mouth. The person may also be experiencing nausea, vomiting, abdominal pain, or diarrhea. Later symptoms may include abnormal or decreased respirations, unconsciousness, or seizures.

Special Populations

The rate of deaths caused by drug poisoning varies widely across different age groups. In the past, the rate of deaths from accidental poisonings was higher in children between birth and age 12 years. The advent of child-resistant caps in the 1960s and other safety containers has significantly decreased poisoning deaths among children. According to the Centers for Disease Control and Prevention (CDC), the age-adjusted drug poisoning death rate has more than doubled between 2000 and 2013. Most of these deaths occur in adults and are the result of opioid overdose, such as hydrocodone, morphine, and oxycodone **Figure 11-2** .

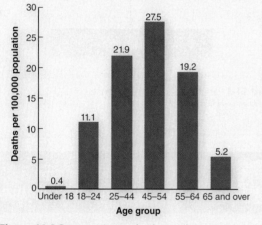

Figure 11-2 Drug poisoning death rates by age in the United States in 2013.
Data from CDC/NCHS, National Vital Statistics System 2013.

Signs and Symptoms

Signs and symptoms of ingested poisons include the following:

- Unusual breath odors
- Discoloration or burning around the mouth
- Nausea and vomiting
- Abdominal pain
- Diarrhea
- Any of the other signs and symptoms of poisoning listed in Table 11-1

▶ Treatment for Ingested Poisons

To treat a person who has ingested a poison, do the following:

- Identify the poison.
- Call the National Poison Center (1-800-222-1222) for instructions, and follow those instructions. If you are unable to contact the poison center, dilute the poison by giving large quantities of water, provided the patient is conscious and able to swallow.
- Arrange for *prompt transport* to a hospital.

When you encounter a patient who has ingested a poison, first attempt to identify the substance that has been ingested. Question the patient's family or bystanders and look for empty containers, such as empty pill bottles, that may indicate what the patient ate or drank. You should have the number of your local poison control center accessible in your EMR life

YOU are the Provider   CASE 1

Just as you are finishing your dinner at the station, you are dispatched to a residence in a middle-class neighborhood for a report of an unconscious patient experiencing an overdose. The dispatcher does not know the age of the patient.

1. If this patient is a young child, what types of overdose will you most likely encounter?
2. If this patient is a young adult, what types of overdose will you most likely encounter?
3. If this patient is an older adult, what types of overdose will you most likely encounter?

support kit. The poison control center can tell you if you should start any treatment before the patient is transported to the hospital.

Treatment

Place an unconscious patient in the recovery position to help keep the airway open and to facilitate the drainage of mucus and vomitus from the mouth and nose **Figure 11-3**.

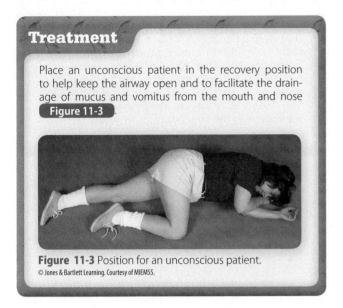

Figure 11-3 Position for an unconscious patient.
© Jones & Bartlett Learning. Courtesy of MIEMSS.

Special Populations

Laundry Detergent Pods and Children

Laundry detergent pods are a new category of cleaning product. Many people use them because they are premeasured, easy to handle, and do not spill. The coating on the pod dissolves in the wash, releasing the liquid detergent into the washing machine. These multicolored pods present a poisoning hazard for children, who may mistake them for candy and bite into them. Serious side effects can occur quickly and include difficulty breathing, severe vomiting, burns to the esophagus, and possible unconsciousness. In addition, the liquid detergent can cause burns to the skin and eyes.

If a child bites into a detergent pod, immediately remove it from the child's mouth. Wash the child's face and hands. Gently wipe out the child's mouth. Call Poison Control for assistance and arrange for transport to an appropriate medical facility.

Activated Charcoal

Administering activated charcoal is another method of treating ingested poisons **Figure 11-4**. Activated charcoal is a finely ground powder that is mixed with water to make it easier to swallow. It works by binding to the poison, thereby preventing the poison from being absorbed in the patient's digestive tract.

Activated charcoal may be used by some emergency medical services (EMS) systems to treat poisonings if the nearest medical facility is a long distance away. However, give activated charcoal only if you are trained in its use and have approval from your medical director or your poison control center. Do not give activated charcoal if

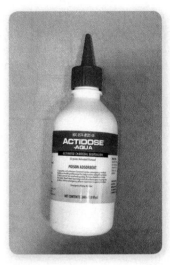

Figure 11-4 Activated charcoal.
© Chuck Stewart, MD.

the patient is unconscious or if he or she has ingested an **acid** (a chemical substance with a pH level of less than 7.0 that can cause severe burns) or a **base** (a chemical that has a pH level greater than 7.0, also known as an alkali or caustic). An example of a base is liquid drain cleaner. The usual dose of activated charcoal for an adult patient is 25 to 50 grams. The usual dose for a pediatric patient is 12.5 to 25 grams. Because the mixture looks like mud, you can serve the mixture in a covered cup and give the patient a straw. This step may make it easier for the patient to drink.

Treatment

Two general treatments for poisoning by ingestion are as follows:

1. Dilution using water
2. Activated charcoal

Follow the directions from your local poison control center or medical director.

Vomiting

Do not do anything to induce vomiting. In the past, syrup of ipecac was used to induce vomiting, but today, the American Association of Poison Control Centers does not endorse using ipecac in children or adults. It often can do more harm than good. Activated charcoal is considered more effective and safer than syrup of ipecac.

■ Inhaled Poisons

Poisoning by inhalation occurs if a **toxic** substance is breathed in and absorbed through the lungs. Some toxic substances such as carbon monoxide are poisonous but are not irritating to the respiratory tract. **Carbon monoxide** is an odorless, colorless, tasteless gas that cannot be detected by your normal senses. Other toxic gases such as chlorine gas and ammonia are irritating to the respiratory tract and will cause coughing and severe respiratory distress. These gases can be classified as irritants.

Signs and Symptoms

Signs and symptoms of inhaled poisons include the following:

- Respiratory distress
- Dizziness
- Cough
- Headache
- Hoarseness
- Confusion
- Chest pain
- Any other signs and symptoms of poisoning listed in Table 11-1

► Carbon Monoxide

One of the most common causes of carbon monoxide poisoning is an improperly vented heating appliance, such as a space heater, grill, or generator. Carbon monoxide is also present in smoke. People caught in building fires often experience carbon monoxide poisoning. When a person inhales even a relatively small quantity of carbon monoxide gas, severe poisoning can result because carbon monoxide combines with red blood cells about 200 times more readily than oxygen does. Therefore, a small quantity of carbon monoxide can "monopolize" the red blood cells and prevent them from transporting oxygen to all parts of the body.

The signs and symptoms of carbon monoxide poisoning include headache, nausea, disorientation, and unconsciousness. Low levels of carbon monoxide poisoning often cause signs and symptoms that are very similar to the flu. If you find several patients together who are all reporting these symptoms (especially in winter), suspect carbon monoxide poisoning and remove everyone from the structure or vehicle.

Safety

Residential carbon monoxide detectors have been installed in many homes. These detectors are designed to sound an alarm before the residents of the house show signs and symptoms of carbon monoxide poisoning. Once the residential carbon monoxide detector is activated, specially trained and equipped personnel must be summoned to investigate the source of the carbon monoxide and to verify that everyone is out of the building. Many newer detectors are combination alarms, which will activate in the presence of either smoke or carbon monoxide.

Signs and Symptoms

Signs and symptoms of carbon monoxide poisoning include the following:

- Headache
- Nausea
- Disorientation
- Unconsciousness
- Multiple people with flulike symptoms in the same location

► Irritants

Many gases irritate the respiratory tract. Two of the more frequently encountered gases are:

1. **Ammonia.** Inhalation of ammonia usually occurs in agricultural settings where it is used as a fertilizer Figure 11-5 . Ammonia is also a chemical that is used to manufacture amphetamine. It has a strong, irritating odor that is highly toxic. Inhaling large amounts of ammonia gas deadens the sense of smell and severely irritates the lungs and upper respiratory tract, causing violent coughing. Ammonia can also severely burn the skin. Anyone who enters an environment containing ammonia must wear a proper

YOU are the Provider CASE 2

On a rainy night, you are dispatched to a residence for a report of a sick man. As you are responding, your dispatcher informs you that the caller now reports the patient is unconscious. As you arrive on the scene and enter the house, you discover a 26-year-old man who is lying on the couch in the living room. He is not responsive to verbal stimuli, and as you check his pulse, you determine that he is breathing at a rate of about 6 breaths per minute. Your partner checks the empty pill bottles on the coffee table and tells you the drugs are pain medication and sleeping pills.

1. What should be your first concern when approaching the patient?
2. Where should you look for clues in this situation?
3. As you begin to care for the patient, his friend tells your partner that the patient's wife left him about 5 days ago and the patient called his friend this morning sounding depressed. Does this comment have any significance?

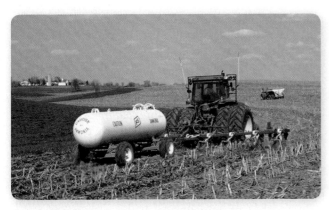

Figure 11-5 Fertilizer trucks on farms often carry ammonia.
Courtesy of Lynn Betts/NRCS.

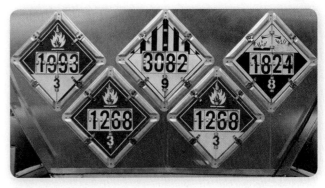

Figure 11-7 Placards used to identify the presence of hazardous materials.
© Mark Winfrey/Shutterstock.

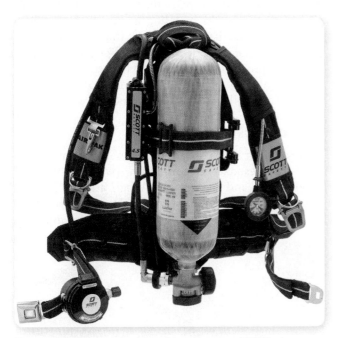

Figure 11-6 Self-contained breathing apparatus (SCBA).
Courtesy of Scott Health & Safety.

encapsulating suit with a **self-contained breathing apparatus (SCBA)** Figure 11-6 . This apparatus contains a mask, regulator, and air supply and delivers air to rescuers when they enter contaminated areas.

2. **Chlorine.** Chlorine gas is commonly found in large quantities around swimming pools and water treatment plants. The odor of chlorine is familiar to anyone who has used chlorine bleach or been in a swimming pool or hot tub. Chlorine gas can severely irritate the lungs and the upper respiratory tract, causing violent coughing. Chlorine gas can also cause skin burns. Anyone who enters an environment containing chlorine gas must wear a proper encapsulating suit with a SCBA.

The presence of hazardous materials that are toxic (poisonous) and those in which there is danger of fire or explosion should be indicated by the appropriate HazMat warning placard Figure 11-7 . Refer to

Chapter 21, *Incident Management*, for more information about HazMat.

▶ Treatment for Inhaled Poisons

The first step to take in treating a patient who has inhaled any poisonous gas is to remove him or her from the source of the gas. If the patient is not breathing, begin mouth-to-mask breathing. If the patient is breathing, administer large quantities of oxygen (if available and if you are trained to do so). Promptly transport any patient who has inhaled a poisonous gas to an appropriate medical facility for further examination because the patient may have a delayed reaction to the poison.

In some situations, your first response is to evacuate people. If you are called to the scene of a large poisonous gas leak (or other HazMat leak), you may have to evacuate large numbers of people to prevent further injuries. Once this has been done, begin to evaluate and treat the evacuees as necessary.

Safety

Do not venture into areas where poisonous gases may be present. Call an agency (such as the fire department) that is equipped with SCBA and other appropriate personal protective equipment. Be especially aware of the hidden dangers found in tanks, confined spaces, farm silos, sewers, and other below-ground structures. Every year, rescuers lose their lives by venturing into a silo, sewer, or pit to save a person who may already be dead. Often these calls are initially reported as a "sick person" or a person who has experienced a "heart attack." Confined space rescue is discussed further in Chapter 20, *Vehicle Extrication and Special Rescue*.

▪ Injected Poisons

The two major causes of poisoning by injection are (1) animal bites and stings and (2) toxic injection. This section covers animal bites and stings; toxic injection will be discussed later, as part of substance abuse. If a person has received a large amount of poison (for example, multiple bee stings) or if a person is especially sensitive to the poison (has an anaphylactic reaction), he or she may collapse and become unconscious.

Signs and Symptoms

Signs and symptoms of injected poisons from bites and stings include the following:

- Obvious injury site (bite or sting marks)
- Tenderness
- Swelling
- Red streaks radiating from the injection site
- Weakness
- Dizziness
- Localized pain
- Itching
- Any other signs and symptoms of poisoning listed in Table 11-1

▶ Treatment for Insect Bites and Stings

When a person has been bitten or stung by an insect, encourage the patient to keep calm and still. This step will help slow the spread of the poison throughout the patient's body. Wash the site with soap and water. Remove the stinger using gauze wiped over the area or by scraping a fingernail over the area. Never squeeze the stinger or use tweezers. Apply ice to reduce swelling, if available. Avoid scratching the sting as this may increase swelling, itching, and the risk of infection.

Some people experience an extreme allergic reaction to stings and bites and may go into anaphylactic shock (see Chapter 14, *Bleeding, Shock, and Soft-Tissue Injuries*). The signs and symptoms of **anaphylactic shock** include itching; **hives** (patches of swelling, redness, and intense itching on the skin); swelling; wheezing and severe respiratory distress; generalized weakness; unconsciousness; rapid, weak pulse; and rapid, shallow breathing. The patient's blood pressure drops, and the patient may develop hypovolemic shock and go into cardiac arrest.

Your first step should be to maintain the patient's airway, breathing, and circulation. Administer oxygen if available and if you are trained to do so. Treating the patient for shock may help in some cases. Remove the allergen if possible. Monitor the patient's vital signs. If the patient's condition progresses to the point of respiratory or cardiac arrest, begin mouth-to-mask breathing or cardiopulmonary resuscitation (CPR).

If a patient appears to be going into anaphylactic shock, immediately arrange for *rapid transport* to a medical facility where the patient can receive treatment with specific medications. Paramedics, nurses, and physicians can give medications that may reverse the allergic reaction. Some patients who have severe allergies carry an epinephrine auto-injector so they can give themselves a shot of epinephrine. If the patient has a prescribed auto-injector, help the patient to use it. Support the patient's thigh and place the tip of the auto-injector against the outer thigh. Using a quick motion, push the auto-injector firmly against the thigh and hold it in place for several seconds **Figure 11-8**. You can administer epinephrine if you have been trained in its use and have permission from your local medical director. Be aware of and follow your local protocols.

▶ Snakebites

There are four kinds of venomous snakes in the United States: rattlesnake, cottonmouth (water moccasin), copperhead, and coral snake. When a snake bites, it injects its venom into a person's skin and muscle with its fangs. This toxic venom can cause local injury to

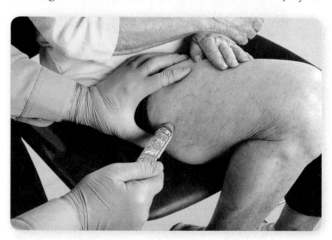

Figure 11-8 Depending on local protocols, EMRs may assist patients with the use of an auto-injector.
© Jones & Bartlett Learning.

YOU ▶ are the Provider   CASE 3

At 1337 hours, you are dispatched to a dairy farm about 7 miles (11 km) from your location for a report of an injured 32-year-old farm-worker.

1. What factors should you consider as you are responding?
2. As you arrive, the farmer's wife meets you and tells you that her husband spilled a concentrated pesticide on himself while he was filling the tanks on his tractor-mounted sprayer. He has washed himself off and is sitting under a shade tree away from the tractor. How does this information change your plan?
3. What are the first steps you should take to assess and treat this patient?

Treatment

The complete steps for administering epinephrine by auto-injector are as follows:

1. Remove the safety cap from the auto-injector. If possible, quickly clean the site with an alcohol pad, but do not delay administration of the drug. In extreme emergencies, it is possible to administer the auto-injector through the patient's clothing.
2. Place the tip of the auto-injector against the lateral part of the patient's thigh, halfway between the groin and the knee.
3. Push the injector firmly against the thigh until a click is heard. This sound indicates that the injector has activated and medication is being administered. Maintain steady pressure to prevent kickback from the spring in the syringe and to prevent the needle from being pushed out of the injection site too soon. Hold the injector in place for 10 seconds to administer all the medication.
4. Remove the injector from the patient's thigh and dispose of it in the proper container.
5. Rub the area for 10 seconds.
6. Reassess the patient's vital signs. If vital signs do not improve after 5 minutes, consider administering a second dose of the medication if available.

Signs and Symptoms

Signs and symptoms of anaphylactic shock include the following:

- Itching all over the body
- Hives, swelling
- Generalized weakness
- Unconsciousness
- Rapid, weak pulse
- Rapid, shallow breathing

Signs and Symptoms

Signs and symptoms of snakebites include the following:

- Immediate pain at the bite site
- Swelling and tenderness around the bite site
- Fainting (from the emotional shock of the bite)
- Sweating
- Nausea and vomiting
- Shock

The bite of the coral snake delivers a slightly different venom that may cause these additional conditions:

- Respiratory difficulties
- Slurred speech
- Paralysis
- **Coma** (state of unconsciousness from which the patient cannot be aroused)
- Seizures

▶ Treatment of Snakebites

The field treatment of a poisonous snakebite is basically the same as the treatment of shock (see Chapter 14, *Bleeding, Shock, and Soft-Tissue Injuries*). Keep the patient calm and still; have the patient lie down and try to relax. This step can slow the spread of venom. Gently wash the bite area with soap and water. If the bite occurred on the arm or leg, splint the affected extremity to decrease movement. Place the splinted extremity below the level of the patient's heart to decrease the absorption of the poison. Treat the patient carefully and arrange for *prompt transport* to the hospital or appropriate medical facility. The only effective treatment of venomous snakebites is the administration of **antivenin** in the hospital.

■ Absorbed Poisons

Poisoning by absorption occurs when a poisonous substance enters the body through the skin. Insecticides and industrial chemicals are two common poisons absorbed through the skin. Common household products can also result in poisoning by absorption. For example, because aspirin is included as an ingredient in many common ointments, excess amounts can be absorbed and result in poisoning, especially in young children. A person experiencing poisoning by absorption may have both localized and systemic signs and symptoms.

the skin and muscle and may even involve the entire extremity. Signs and symptoms may affect the entire body. A bite from a venomous snake is rarely fatal. The Centers for Disease Control and Prevention (CDC) estimate that 7,000 to 8,000 people per year receive venomous snakebites in the United States. Only about five people die from these bites each year. However, permanent injury can result if proper medical care is not obtained.

YOU are the Provider   CASE 4

You and a partner are out on a lunch break when dispatch calls on the radio. You are sent to a local park where a woman has called because she has been stung by a bee. She told the call center it felt like her throat was closing.

1. On arrival at the scene, what should you check first?
2. What are some of the signs and symptoms of anaphylactic shock?
3. What should you ask the woman about her past medical history?

Signs and Symptoms

Signs and symptoms of absorbed poisons include the following:

- Traces of powder or liquid on the skin
- Inflammation or redness of the skin
- Chemical burns
- Rash
- Burning
- Itching
- Nausea and vomiting
- Dizziness
- Shock
- Any other signs and symptoms of poisoning listed in Table 11-1

▶ Treatment for Absorbed Poisons

Your first step in treating a patient who has absorbed a poisonous substance through the skin is to ensure that the patient is no longer in contact with the toxic substance. Make sure that you do not come into contact with the poison. You may have to ask the patient to remove all clothing. Then brush off—do not wash—any dry chemical from the patient. Contact with water may activate the dry chemical and result in a burning or caustic reaction.

After removing all the dry chemical, wash the patient completely for at least 20 minutes. Use any water source that is available: an industrial shower, a home shower, a garden hose, or even a fire engine's booster hose. Do not forget to wash out the patient's eyes if they have been in contact with the poison. If additional EMS personnel are delayed, contact the poison control center or your medical director for additional treatment information.

If the patient is experiencing shock, have the patient lie down. If the patient is having difficulty breathing, administer oxygen if it is available and you are trained to use it.

Treatment

When in doubt in absorbed poison situations, have the patient remove all clothing so that he or she is no longer in contact with the toxic substance.

■ Nerve Agents

Nerve agents represent a special type of poison that attack the central nervous system. These agents can be absorbed through the skin, inhaled, or injected. Nerve agents are among the most deadly chemicals developed.

Small quantities of these chemicals can kill large numbers of people by causing cardiac arrest within minutes of exposure. Four of the most commonly mentioned nerve agents are sarin (GB), soman (GD), tabun (GA), and V agent (VX). Nerve agents were discovered by scientists who were in search of a superior pesticide; however, nerve agents are much stronger organophosphates than those found in insecticides. Nerve agents, like insecticides, block an essential enzyme in the nervous system. The symptoms listed in Table 11-2 can be remembered using the mnemonic SLUDGEM.

Additional symptoms include shortness of breath; slow heart rate; muscle weakness or paralysis; slurred speech; seizures; and loss of consciousness.

In the event you are called to the scene of an organophosphate or nerve agent poisoning, your primary responsibility is to keep yourself, other rescuers, and bystanders from becoming contaminated. A well-trained HazMat team in special protective equipment (SCBA and encapsulating suits) is needed to remove patients from the contaminated area and decontaminate them before they are turned over to you for treatment.

Treatment of exposed patients includes assessing and supporting the patient's airway, breathing, and circulation. A nerve agent antidote kit called the DuoDote Auto-Injector can be administered to exposed patients or to yourself if you have become exposed. Use the DuoDote kit only if you or the patient have signs and symptoms of organophosphate or nerve agent poisoning (SLUDGEM). You must have the approval of your medical director and have received proper training in its use. Organophosphate and nerve agents may require large quantities of medication.

The DuoDote kit contains one auto-injector syringe that contains two drugs, atropine and pralidoxime chloride. The instructions for using this kit are listed in Table 11-3.

Table 11-2	Symptoms of Exposure to an Organophosphate Insecticide or Nerve Agent
S	Salivation, sweating
L	Lacrimation (excessive tearing of the eyes)
U	Urination
D	Defecation, drooling, diarrhea
G	Gastrointestinal upset and cramps
E	Emesis (vomiting)
M	Muscle twitching, miosis (pinpoint pupils)

© Jones & Bartlett Learning. Courtesy of MIEMSS.

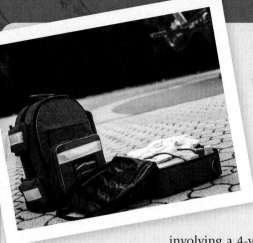

Voices *of* Experience

Early in my EMS career, I was assigned to an advanced life support unit in a rural setting. We received a call for an accidental ingestion involving a 4-year-old child. While en route, the dispatcher informed us that the child had ingested a large quantity of amitriptyline, a tricyclic antidepressant. We had recently been issued cellular phones for our EMS units and I had made a list of important numbers. One of those numbers was the Georgia Poison Center. I called them while en route to the call and was able to get some valuable information from the toxicologist.

On arrival, we found a lethargic child who responded to verbal stimulation. We began a rapid assessment and administered high-flow oxygen. An intravenous (IV) line was established and a normal blood glucose was obtained. We prepared the patient for rapid transport to our local critical access hospital because a pediatric hospital was over 45 miles (72 km) away and air transport was not readily accessible in those days.

While en route, the child became unresponsive. We secured the airway with an endotracheal tube and began to assist ventilations. I made contact with medical control to get orders for treatment recommended by the toxicologist, which was not part of our standing orders. The emergency department (ED) physician agreed and we administered an injection of sodium bicarbonate followed by a bicarbonate drip. Based on our report, the ED physician contacted a pediatric hospital and had a life flight helicopter start to the hospital.

The ED physician assessed the child on our arrival. The child's vital signs were stable and he was becoming more responsive. The child was sedated and prepared for air transport to the pediatric hospital. Thanks to some quick thinking and new technology, the child made a complete recovery.

> **Based on our report, the ED physician contacted a pediatric hospital and had a life flight helicopter start to the hospital.**

John A. Phillips III, RN, CEN, EMT-P
Director of Clinical Services
Rural Metro EMS
Atlanta, Georgia

Table 11-3	**Instructions for the Administration of a DuoDote Auto-Injector Kit***

1. Check the kit to be sure it contains the proper medication and that it has not expired.
2. Remove the gray protective cap.
3. Press the green end of the injector firmly against the lateral part of the patient's thigh.
4. Hold in place for 10 seconds to allow the medication to get into the muscle.
5. Dispose of the syringe in a medical sharps container.
6. Reassess the patient's vital signs and symptoms.

*Follow your local protocols.

© Jones & Bartlett Learning. Courtesy of MIEMSS.

■ Substance Abuse

Substance abuse is widespread in our society. According to the National Survey on Drug Use and Health, 8.1% of the US population (21.5 million people) have a substance use disorder; that is, they are dependent on alcohol or other drugs. Substance abuse results in an increased incidence of injuries and illness; therefore, many of your emergency calls will involve people who are under the influence of alcohol or other drugs. Even if the primary reason for the call is not substance abuse, it will still be a contributing factor in many calls.

▶ Alcohol

Alcohol is the most commonly abused drug in the United States today. Alcohol intoxication may be seen in people of any age, including children, teenagers, and older adults. According to the National Institute on Alcohol Abuse and Alcoholism, nearly 88,000 people die from alcohol-related deaths each year, which makes it the fourth leading cause of preventable death in the United States. In 2014, alcohol-impaired driving fatalities accounted for 32% of all driving fatalities. More than 10% of US children live with a parent with alcohol-related problems. More than one-half of all murders and more than one-third of all suicides are alcohol-related. Deaths as a result of alcohol abuse are two and one half times as numerous as deaths from motor vehicle crashes. In addition, people who have been drinking can be injured or suddenly develop a serious illness. As an EMR, many of the patients you encounter will be under the influence of alcohol.

When you have a patient who appears to be under the influence of alcohol, do not always assume that the symptoms (including the smell of alcohol on someone's breath) are caused by intoxication, because the symptoms of alcohol intoxication can be similar to those of other medical illnesses or severe injuries. If you are unsure about whether a patient who appears to be intoxicated has a serious injury or illness, be extra careful with your examination. Arrange for *prompt transport* to an appropriate medical facility, where a physician can make a complete assessment.

Alcohol is an addictive, depressant drug. A person who is physically dependent on alcohol and then is suddenly deprived of it may develop withdrawal symptoms, such as convulsions or seizures. The most severe withdrawal symptoms are called **delirium tremens (DTs)**. The signs and symptoms of DTs include shaking, restlessness, confusion, hallucinations, gastrointestinal distress, chest pain, and fever. These signs and symptoms usually appear 3 to 4 days after the person stops drinking. Arrange for *prompt transport* of a person suffering from DTs to an appropriate medical facility. DTs are a serious medical emergency and can be fatal.

Words of Wisdom

Public safety personnel are not immune to the seduction that draws people into addiction to alcohol and other drugs. If you are having a problem with alcohol or other drugs, seek help through your employee assistance program or through a self-help program such as Alcoholics Anonymous.

Treatment

Although a person may appear intoxicated, he or she actually may be experiencing any one of a number of serious illnesses or injuries. Insulin shock, diabetic coma, head injury, traumatic shock, and drug reactions may all display the same symptoms as alcohol intoxication.

▶ Drugs

In today's society, people of all ages abuse many different prescription and illegal street drugs. Drugs may be ingested, inhaled, injected, or absorbed into the body. As an EMR, you may not be able to identify the type of drug used, although this information will be helpful to medical providers. As you perform your scene size-up, look for clues that can indicate what type of drug was used and how it was administered. Today, the most commonly encountered drugs fall into four categories: amphetamines, opioids (painkillers), hallucinogens, and inhalants Figure 11-9 . The National Center for Health Statistics reported 47,055 deaths from drug poisoning in 2014. Of these, 82% were unintentional poisonings, 12% were suicides, and 6% were of undetermined causes. The drug poisoning rate was highest

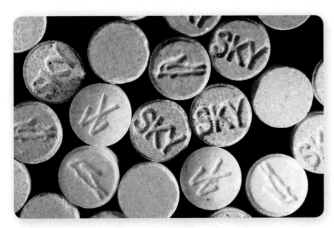

Figure 11-9 Types of drugs that are commonly abused.
Courtesy of DEA.

among adults aged 45 to 54 years. From 2000 to 2014, the age-adjusted poison death rate more than doubled from 6.2 deaths per 100,000 people to 14.7 deaths per 100,000 people.

In recent years, the abuse of prescription drugs has increased. Prescription drugs can have deadly effects when taken in large quantities and when mixed with other drugs. Many overdoses are the result of mixing alcohol with other drugs.

Amphetamines

Amphetamines are drugs that stimulate the **central nervous system (CNS)** (the brain and spinal cord). Drugs in this category are often called uppers, speed, ice, or crystal and include the drug **cocaine** (coke, crack, rock). People using these mind-altering substances show signs of restlessness, irritability, and talkativeness. Patients under the influence of these drugs may need to be kept from harming themselves and should be taken to a facility where they can be monitored until the effects of the drug wear off.

Synthetic stimulant-type drugs are called commonly called **bath salts** (synthetic cathinones). Bath salts should not be confused with products such as Epsom salt (magnesium sulfate). These drugs copy the effects of naturally occurring mind-altering drugs and can be strong and dangerous. Often labeled as "not for human consumption," these drugs can be swallowed, snorted, smoked, or injected. Bath salts can produce effects that include paranoia, panic attacks, inappropriate sexual behavior, hallucinations, and excited delirium.

Pain Relievers (Opioids) and Heroin

An **opioid** is a type of medication used to relieve pain by reducing the intensity of pain signals reaching the brain. Opioids also affect the areas of the brain that control emotion. This class of medications includes hydrocodone (Vicodin), oxycodone (OxyContin), morphine, and codeine. Opioids are named for the opium in poppy seeds, from which codeine and morphine are derived. When

used appropriately and as prescribed, opioids are a valuable part of medical care. However, if these medications are abused (that is, taken without a prescription or used in excess quantities), dependency or overdose can occur.

Heroin is an illegal street drug that is powerful and addictive. Heroin is made from morphine. According to the CDC, from 1999 to 2014, there have been more than 165,000 deaths attributed to drug poisoning caused by opioids (heroin or prescription painkillers).

An increasing number of drug overdoses are the result of taking a combination of drugs. One particularly deadly combination is heroin and fentanyl. Some drug dealers are using an illegal version of fentanyl, a drug used to induce anesthesia, to increase the potency of heroin that has been diluted. According to the Drug Enforcement Administration, fentanyl produced in illicit labs is up to 100 times more powerful than morphine and 30 to 50 times more powerful than heroin. This combination of drugs acts quickly and is deadly even in very small quantities.

Signs and Symptoms

Signs and symptoms of an opioid drug overdose include the following:

- Slow, difficult, shallow breathing, or no breathing
- Small or pinpoint pupils
- Weak pulse
- Low blood pressure
- Blue nails and lips
- Drowsiness
- Disorientation
- Delirium
- Coma

Treating a Patient With an Opioid Overdose. An overdose of opioid drugs can result in respiratory depression or arrest. A person who has overdosed on opioids may be breathing shallowly or not at all. If the person is not breathing, begin mouth-to-mask resuscitation. If cardiac arrest occurs, begin CPR immediately and arrange for prompt transportation to an appropriate medical facility.

Another treatment available for opioid overdose is naloxone (Narcan). Naloxone is a medication that can rapidly reverse the effects of opioid drugs on the central nervous system. In the past, naloxone was administered exclusively by injection or through an intravenous (IV) line and the use of this drug was limited to advanced life support (ALS) providers. Recently, however, naloxone has become available in a form that can be administered by spraying it into the patient's nostrils. This method of administration is called intranasal administration. **Figure 11-10** shows the administration of one type of naloxone by nasal spray.

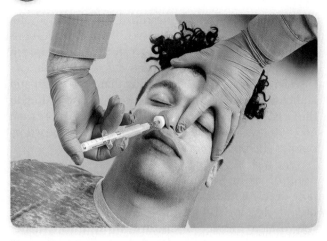

Figure 11-10 Depending on local protocols, some EMRs may administer naloxone intranasally to treat opioid overdose.
© Jones & Bartlett Learning.

Words of Wisdom

General Steps to Administer a Medication Intranasally

1. Obtain medical direction per local protocol.
2. Confirm correct medication and expiration date.
3. Attempt to determine whether the patient is allergic to any medications.
4. Prepare the medication and attach the atomizer. Never use a needle.
5. Place the atomizer in one nostril, pointing up and slightly outward (see Figure 11-10).
6. Administer a half dose (1 mL maximum) into each nostril.
7. Reassess the patient and document appropriately.

Naloxone is also available in the form of an auto-injector. In some communities, all law enforcement and EMS personnel have been trained in the use of this medication. As an EMR, you can give this medication only if you are trained in its use and have approval from your medical director.

Hallucinogens

Hallucinogens include PCP, LSD, peyote, mescaline, and some types of mushrooms. **Hallucinogens** are chemicals that cause people to see things that are not there. A patient who is hallucinating may become frightened and unable to distinguish between reality and fantasy. One hallucinogen, PCP, also blocks the body's pain receptors. People taking PCP may feel no pain and may seriously injure themselves or others. Large doses of PCP can produce convulsions, coma, heart and lung failure, or stroke. Your treatment for these patients is primarily supportive. Try to reduce auditory and visual stimulation. Avoid the use of bright lights and loud noises, including sirens.

Because some of the patients who have taken these drugs are prone to violent behavior, approach each emergency scene with caution. Maintain safety for yourself, other rescuers, bystanders, and the patient. Arrange for *transport* to an appropriate medical facility for treatment.

Abused Inhalants

Recently, the intentional inhalation of volatile chemicals (huffing) has increased, especially among teenagers who are seeking an alcohol-like high. Many of these substances can be bought in hardware stores and include gasoline, paint thinners, cleaning compounds, lacquers, and a wide variety of substances used as aerosol propellants. Users put the chemical in a plastic bag and inhale from the bag. The combination of a lack of oxygen and the effects of the poisonous substance can lead to unconsciousness and death. Some types of inhalants cause drowsiness or unresponsiveness, and others cause seizures. Some of the chemicals can overstimulate the heart and produce sudden cardiac death from ventricular fibrillation.

Treat these patients carefully. Try to keep them calm and still. Support the airway, breathing, and circulation. Give high-flow oxygen as soon as it is available and if you are trained to use it. Carefully monitor their vital signs and arrange for *prompt transport* to an appropriate medical facility.

Toxic Injection From Drugs

Drugs that are injected into the bloodstream can result in toxic injection. The patient's reaction depends on the quantity and type of drug injected. Because street drugs such as heroin and cocaine may be diluted (cut) with sugar or other substances that should not be injected into the bloodstream, the patient may be unaware of exactly what has been injected. After a toxic injection, the patient may report weakness, dizziness, fever, or chills. This type of emergency requires you to support the patient, treat the symptoms, and provide transport to an appropriate medical facility. You should also check the injection site for redness, swelling, and increased skin temperature. The presence of any of these signs may indicate an infection that requires medical care.

Safety

People who use IV drugs have a high incidence of blood-borne diseases such as hepatitis B and AIDS. Use standard precautions to reduce your chances of coming in contact with blood-borne pathogens.

▶ General Treatment for a Drug Overdose

Once you have determined that a patient is experiencing a drug overdose, your care should consist of the following:

- Provide basic life support (clear the airway and perform mouth-to-mask breathing or CPR, as necessary).
- Keep the patient from hurting himself or herself and others.
- Provide reassurance and emotional support.
- Arrange for prompt transport to a medical facility for treatment.

The effects of some drugs can be counteracted only by other drugs administered by a paramedic or a physician.

If a patient is acting out, speak to him or her in a calm, reassuring tone of voice and try to keep the patient from harming anyone. If a person reports seeing things that are not there, say, "I believe you are seeing those things; however, I do not see them myself." This statement lets the patient know that you understand his or her experience, but that in reality, the perceived object is not present.

Administer naloxone if you have been trained in its use and have the approval of your local medical director.

Patients who are experiencing adverse reactions from a drug overdose require specialized treatment. You and other EMS personnel should be aware of local facilities equipped to deal with such cases. Keep in mind that a person experiencing a drug overdose may also have other injuries or medical conditions that require medical treatment. Avoid classifying or judging the patient.

■ Intentional Poisoning

Intentional self-poisoning is attempted suicide and may involve ingested poisons (such as drugs) or inhaled poisons (such as carbon monoxide). Regardless of whether the poisoning was accidental or intentional, the medical treatment you provide is the same. A patient who has attempted suicide needs both medical and emotional support; however, the patient may not want your help and may be difficult to treat. Nevertheless, you and all other EMS personnel must make every effort to preserve life and offer reassurance to the patient.

Words of Wisdom

Excited Delirium

Excited delirium is a condition in which the patient shows a combination of agitation, anxiety, paranoia, violent and bizarre behavior, confusion, an inability to think or talk clearly, hallucinations, disorientation, insensitivity to pain, elevated body temperature, and superhuman strength. Excited delirium can result in sudden death, usually as the result of cardiac or respiratory arrest. Excited delirium is thought to involve multiple factors, including positional asphyxia, drug toxicity, and previous mental illness. It occurs most often in men with a history of serious mental illness and/or acute or chronic drug abuse—especially with cocaine, PCP, or methamphetamine. Alcohol withdrawal or head trauma may also be present. In some patients with excited delirium, a conducted electrical device may be used in an attempt to subdue the patient.

As part of the patient's health care team, your goal is to prevent the patient from going into respiratory and cardiac arrest. The use of physical restraints seems to worsen excited delirium in some patients, so try to minimize their use. ALS personnel can give medications to reduce the patient's anxiety, produce muscle relaxation, and sedate the patient. Spraying patients with a water mist or fanning their faces may help to reduce their body temperature. If the patient calms down enough for you to take vital signs, take them frequently. Arrange for prompt transportation of the patient to an appropriate medical facility.

YOU are the Provider   SUMMARY

You are the Provider: CASE 1

1. If this patient is a young child, what types of overdose will you most likely encounter?

Young children tend to put objects in their mouths. Medications without child-resistant safety caps that are left within the reach of unsupervised children may result in accidental overdoses. Young children are most at risk for ingesting cosmetics and personal care products, household cleaning supplies, pain medications, and foreign bodies that are within their reach.

2. If this patient is a young adult, what types of overdose will you most likely encounter?

Overdoses in young adults are frequently the result of attempted suicide or the result of an accidental overdose of alcohol or recreational drugs. Alcohol is the most widely abused drug in young adults. The majority of drug overdose deaths (more than six out of ten) involve opioid pain relievers. Since 1999, the rate of overdose deaths involving opioid or heroin has nearly quadrupled.

3. If this patient is an older adult, what types of overdose will you most likely encounter?

Many geriatric patients take a wide variety of medications for a multitude of ailments. Taking large numbers of medications, coupled with confusion, often leads to unintentional double dosing, synergistic reactions between medications, or overdoses of prescribed medications. There is also the risk that an older patient may unintentionally take a medication that is prescribed for his or her spouse. The most common patterns of overdose change with the age of the patient. Recognizing these patterns may help you to gain a better picture of a given incident.

You are the Provider: CASE 2

1. What should be your first concern when approaching the patient?

In every case, your safety is the first concern, so stop to make sure the scene is safe and that you will not be injured in approaching the patient. You should be concerned because you do not know what is wrong with this patient. Anytime a patient has taken medicine or drugs, he or she may have a variety of reactions to the drugs. Patients who are depressed sometimes try to end their lives with a gun. So you need to be sure there are no weapons around the patient. As with any patient interaction, take body substance isolation precautions.

Be alert for any needles that may have been used for drug administration. And continue to monitor the scene for safety.

2. Where should you look for clues in this situation?

As an EMR, you need to become a medical detective. Your partner has already told you that the empty bottles had contained pain medication and sleeping pills. Look around the patient for any other signs of drugs or medications. Check with family or friends to see whether they know how many pills had been in each bottle. Interviewing family members or friends about the patient may give you valuable information about the patient's condition and about any medications or drugs he or she may have been taking. As you gather this information, be sure that your partner is providing care to the patient.

3. As you begin to care for the patient, his friend tells your partner that the patient's wife left him about 5 days ago and the patient called his friend this morning sounding depressed. Does this comment have any significance?

The friend's comment is important because it may suggest that the potential poisoning was intentional, rather than accidental. From your perspective, the treatment should not change at all with this information; however, it is important that you share this information with the emergency department because it will be useful to them in terms of patient care. A patient who has intentionally ingested poison will need both medical and emotional assistance.

You are the Provider: CASE 3

1. What factors should you consider while you are responding?

While you are responding to the scene, review the dispatch information. Make sure you know how to get to the location of the call. See if you can arrange with the dispatcher to have someone meet you to take you to the patient. Remember that calls to rural locations may require you to travel off the road to get to patients. Be sure that adequate resources have been dispatched. Consider the hazards you may encounter at a farm, including heavy machinery, motorized equipment, electrical hazards, animals, tall structures, confined spaces, chemicals, and hazardous materials (HazMat) like pesticides, herbicides, and fertilizers.

2. As you arrive, the farmer's wife meets you and tells you that her husband has spilled a concentrated pesticide on himself while he was filling the tanks on his tractor-mounted sprayer. He has washed himself off and is sitting under a shade tree away from the tractor. How does this information change your plan?

This information changes your focus from dealing with one sick patient to dealing with an incident that involves materials that are hazardous to both the patient and to responders. First, ensure scene safety for all people working at this scene. Make sure that responders are not exposed to the pesticide, and remove the patient from the source of the pesticide. This type of call exceeds the limits of your training and requires additional resources. Inform the dispatcher that HazMats are involved and request a HazMat team to respond to your location.

3. What are the first steps you should take to assess and treat this patient?

The first step is to request a HazMat team. Determine how long it will take the team to arrive at your location. Because the farmer has washed off the pesticide and has removed himself from the source of the poison, it is probably safe for you to approach him to obtain a history of the incident and determine the actions he has taken. You can determine his level of consciousness and determine is if he is experiencing any signs of pesticide poisoning. If you have received training in HazMat and have protective gear, you may be able to provide additional care. One of the most important goals of a situation like this is to prevent other people from becoming contaminated. Contact your local poison control center for further information and assistance.

You are the Provider: CASE 4

1. On arrival at the scene, what should you check first?

The patient is concerned that her throat is closing, which suggests her airway could be at risk. Here, as in all cases, your first step (after scene safety) is to ensure the patient has a patent (open) airway. Place the patient on high-flow oxygen if available and if you are trained to do so. Ask the woman if she has an auto-injector, EpiPen, or other medication that she can take. If you have been trained to administer an EpiPen and have permission to use it, you can administer it.

2. What are some of the signs and symptoms of anaphylactic shock?

The signs and symptoms are itching; hives; swelling; rapid, shallow breathing; wheezing and respiratory distress; weakness; and a rapid, weak pulse. The patient's blood pressure will drop and he or she may develop hypovolemic shock and possible cardiac arrest.

3. What should you ask the woman about her past medical history?

Ask the patient if she knows if she is allergic to bee stings. Some people who have severe, life-threatening allergies carry an epinephrine auto-injector so they can give themselves an injection in those situations. If the woman has an auto-injector prescribed by a physician, you may help her use it. The injection is delivered through the clothes into the patient's outer thigh. Press the tip firmly against the woman's leg, press the injector into the woman's leg, and hold for several seconds. Rub the spot for a few moments after removing the injector. If the patient's condition does not improve, arrange for rapid transport to an appropriate medical facility.

Prep Kit

▶ Ready for Review

- This chapter discusses the signs, symptoms, and treatment of patients who have experienced accidental or intentional poisoning.
- The four primary routes by which poisons enter the body are (1) ingestion, (2) inhalation, (3) injection, and (4) absorption.
- An ingested poison is taken by mouth. Often, there are chemical burns, odors, or stains around the mouth. The person may also be experiencing nausea, vomiting, abdominal pain, or diarrhea.
- An inhaled poison is breathed in and absorbed through the lungs. Some toxic substances such as carbon monoxide are very poisonous but are not irritating to the respiratory tract. Other toxic gases such as chlorine gas and ammonia are very irritating and will cause coughing and severe respiratory distress.
- The two major causes of poisoning by injection are (1) animal bites and stings and (2) toxic injection.
- Poisoning by absorption occurs when a poisonous substance enters the body through the skin. A person experiencing absorption poisoning may have both localized and systemic signs and symptoms.
- Many nerve agents are the same types of chemicals as insecticides. Your primary role in incidents involving nerve agents is to keep yourself and others from becoming exposed.
- It is important to pay special attention to scene safety. Do not enter a hazardous environment without the proper training and equipment.
- Naloxone (Narcan) is a medication that can rapidly reverse the effects of opioid drugs on the central nervous system.

▶ Vital Vocabulary

acid A chemical substance with a pH level of less than 7.0 that can cause severe burns.

amphetamines Stimulants that produce a general mood elevation, improve task performance, suppress appetite, or prevent sleepiness.

anaphylactic shock Severe shock caused by an allergic reaction to food, medicine, or insect stings.

antivenin A serum that counteracts the effect of venom from an animal or insect.

base A chemical with a pH level of greater than 7.0. Bases are also called caustics or alkalis.

bath salts The common name for certain types of synthetic stimulant-type drugs.

carbon monoxide A colorless, odorless, tasteless, poisonous gas formed by incomplete combustion, such as in a fire.

central nervous system (CNS) The brain and spinal cord.

cocaine A powerful stimulant that induces an extreme state of euphoria. Legitimately, it is a potent local anesthetic. On the street, it is commonly known as coke. Crack cocaine, crack, or rock is a solid, smokable form of cocaine.

coma A state of unconsciousness from which the patient cannot be aroused.

delirium tremens (DTs) A severe, often fatal, complication of alcohol withdrawal that most commonly occurs 3 to 4 days after withdrawal (though it can occur as late as 10 days after withdrawal). It is characterized by restlessness, fever, sweating, confusion, disorientation, agitation, hallucinations, and convulsions.

hallucinogens Chemicals that cause a person to see visions or hear sounds that are not real.

hives An allergic skin disorder marked by patches of swelling, redness, and intense itching.

nerve agents Deadly toxic substances that attack the central nervous system.

opioids Medications that relieve pain, including prescription drugs such as morphine, oxycodone, and hydrocodone and illicit drugs such as heroin, which is produced from the morphine in poppy plants.

poison Any substance that may cause injury or death if relatively small amounts are ingested, inhaled, absorbed, applied to, or injected into the body.

self-contained breathing apparatus (SCBA) A complete unit for delivery of air to a rescuer who enters a contaminated area; contains a mask, regulator, and air supply.

toxic Poisonous.

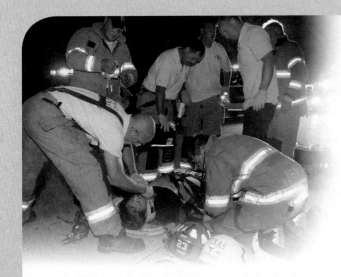

Assessment
in Action

Three days after a massive snowstorm, several parts of your response area are still without electricity. More than 30 inches (76 cm) of snow fell in the region. You and your partner are dispatched to a home in an area where the power has been out since the storm began. A family of four is complaining of flulike symptoms.

1. When you walk in the home, you notice a kerosene heater in the middle of the room. This appliance should be a clue to you that the family may be experiencing:

   A. heat exhaustion.
   B. carbon monoxide poisoning.
   C. the common cold.
   D. low body temperatures.

2. Which of the following is NOT a sign or symptom of carbon monoxide poisoning?

   A. Headache
   B. Vomiting
   C. Itching
   D. Disorientation

3. Carbon monoxide enters a person's body by what route?

   A. Ingestion
   B. Inhalation
   C. Absorption
   D. Injection

4. Carbon monoxide attaches to the red blood cells, affecting the transportation of:

   A. white blood cells.
   B. carbon dioxide.
   C. oxygen.
   D. glucose.

5. Which of the following drugs is NOT an opioid?

   A. Oxycodone
   B. Heroin
   C. Morphine
   D. Amphetamine

6. Opioid overdose can cause all of the following symptoms EXCEPT:

   A. pinpoint pupils.
   B. an increase in the rate of respiration.
   C. weak pulse.
   D. low blood pressure.

7. Which class of drugs includes the synthetic drugs commonly called bath salts?

   A. Amphetamines
   B. Opioids
   C. Inhalants
   D. Hallucinogens

8. A patient who is frightened and seeing things that are not there has most likely taken which type of drug?

   A. Amphetamine
   B. Opioid
   C. Inhalant
   D. Hallucinogen

9. If you find that a residential carbon monoxide detector is sounding an alarm, what should you do?

10. A patient who exhibits a weak pulse, shallow or absent breathing, delirium or coma, and blue lips is most likely suffering from which type of drug overdose?

Behavioral Emergencies

Opener photo: © Jones & Bartlett Learning. Courtesy of MIEMSS.

Introduction

Every emergency situation, whether it is an illness or an injury, has emotional and psychological effects on everyone involved—you, the patient, the patient's family and friends, and even bystanders. When you respond to the scene of a behavioral emergency, you will need to give psychological support as well as the necessary emergency medical care to your patient. This chapter explains the five major factors that cause behavioral emergencies: medical conditions, physical trauma conditions, psychiatric illnesses, mind-altering substances, and situational stresses.

The simple intervention techniques addressed in this chapter will help prepare you to care for patients and their families during the stressful experience of a medical emergency. Also, you will be better able to identify and understand the reactions to the grief that you observe.

Many patients experience high anxiety, denial, anger, remorse, and grief during a situational crisis. Three skills that are useful to you when communicating with patients in crisis are restatement, redirection, and empathy. This chapter provides information on how to deal with crowd control, domestic violence, violent patients, armed patients, suicide crises, sexual assault, posttraumatic stress disorder, and death and dying. Medical and legal considerations and the role of critical incident stress debriefings are also covered.

Patient Assessment in Behavioral Emergencies

When you are assessing a patient who appears to be experiencing a behavioral emergency, you should follow the steps of the patient assessment sequence. You should complete a scene size-up, being especially careful to ensure the scene is safe for you and for the patient. If the patient is oriented and responsive, you can complete your primary assessment by observing the patient's responsiveness, airway, breathing, and measuring the pulse to determine the rate and strength of the heartbeat. Use the SAMPLE mnemonic to aid you when obtaining the patient's past medical history. You may need to ask additional questions about the events leading up to the call for assistance. Do not neglect to ask about medical problems. Many of the calls you receive for situations that appear to be behavioral will have a medical cause or a medical component. It is important that you do not overlook this part of your examination.

The secondary assessment should rule out any obvious injuries and focus on signs of medical illnesses. Some patients experiencing a behavioral crisis may not be aware of injuries or illnesses that might contribute to their condition. Complete your secondary assessment by taking a set of vital signs. As you are performing your patient assessment, inform the patient what you are doing at each step of the way. Complete the last step of the patient assessment by reassessing the patient every 15 minutes for a stable patient and every 5 minutes for an unstable patient. Some patients will not let you assess them. In this case, try to help the patient understand that you are trying to help. However, in cases where you cannot complete the assessment, be sure to document your assessment findings and the reason for not completing all the steps. Figure 12-1 lists the steps of the patient assessment sequence.

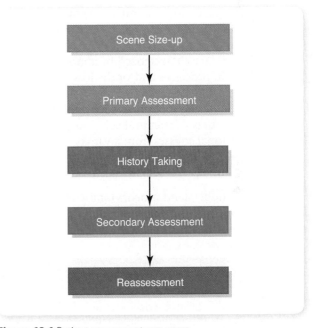

Figure 12-1 Patient assessment sequence.
© Jones & Bartlett Learning. Courtesy of MIEMSS.

YOU are the Provider CASE 1

In the middle of the night, you are dispatched for the report of a sick person at the bus stop at the corner of Pennsylvania Avenue and 6th Street. As you arrive on the scene, you find a middle-aged man pacing back and forth at the bus stop. He is shouting that he needs to get to Albuquerque tonight to stop his pain. He then asks you why you are there.

1. What types of conditions contribute to or cause a situational crisis?
2. What are the four phases of a situational crisis?
3. What are three communication tools you can use to help you communicate with this patient?

Behavioral Crises

As an emergency medical responder (EMR), you will encounter situations in which patients exhibit abnormal behavior. Sometimes this abnormal behavior is the primary reason that you have been called to the scene, and sometimes it is a secondary reaction to another situation such as an accident or illness. A behavioral emergency is a situation in which the patient exhibits abnormal behavior that is unacceptable or cannot be tolerated by the patient himself or herself or by family, friends, or the community. Some behavioral emergencies involve your patient, and others involve the patient's family or friends.

Five main factors contribute to behavioral changes. They are:

1. Medical conditions such as uncontrolled diabetes that cause low blood glucose, respiratory conditions that prevent the patient's brain from receiving enough oxygen, strokes, head injuries, high fevers, infections, and excessively low body temperature.
2. Physical trauma conditions such as head injuries and injuries that result in shock and an inadequate blood supply to the brain.
3. Psychiatric illnesses such as depression, panic disorders, or psychotic behavior (mental disturbance characterized by abnormal thought processes and/or the loss of contact with reality).
4. Mind-altering substances such as alcohol and a wide variety of chemical substances.
5. Situational stresses from a variety of emotional traumas such as death or serious injury to a loved one.

To better understand a behavioral crisis, you need to look at the phases a person experiences during a situational crisis.

What Is a Situational Crisis?

Simply put, a situational crisis is a state of emotional upset or turmoil. The crisis is caused by a sudden disruptive event such as a physical illness, a traumatic injury, or the death of a loved one. Every emergency creates some form of situational crisis for the patient and those people close to the patient. You will often encounter this type of crisis as an EMR. Some of the concepts covered here are similar to the concepts covered in Chapter 2, *Workforce Safety and Wellness*.

Most situational crises are sudden and unexpected (such as a motor vehicle crash), cannot be handled by the person's usual coping mechanisms, last only a short time, and can cause socially unacceptable, self-destructive, or dangerous behavior.

Phases of a Situational Crisis

There are four emotional phases to each situational crisis. Although a person may not experience every phase during a crisis, he or she will certainly experience one or more of the phases. If you understand what these phases are and why they occur, you can better understand how to help the people who are experiencing a behavioral crisis.

▶ High Anxiety or Emotional Shock

In the first phase of a situational crisis, a person exhibits high anxiety or emotional shock. High anxiety is characterized by rather obvious signs and symptoms: flushed (red) face, rapid breathing, rapid speech, increased activity, loud or screaming voice, and general agitation. Emotional shock is often the result of a sudden illness or accident or the sudden death of a loved one. Like most other types of shock, emotional shock is characterized by signs and symptoms including cool, clammy skin; a rapid, weak pulse; vomiting and nausea; and general inactivity and weakness.

> ### Words of Wisdom
>
> The emotional phases of a situational crisis are:
> - High anxiety or emotional shock
> - Denial
> - Anger
> - Remorse and grief

▶ Denial

The next phase of a situational crisis may be denial or a refusal to accept the fact that an event has occurred. For example, a child who has just suffered the loss of a parent may refuse to accept the death by telling everyone that the parent is sleeping or has gone away.

Allow the patient to express denial. Do not argue with the patient, but try to understand the emotional and psychological trauma that he or she is experiencing.

▶ Anger

Anger is a normal human response to emotional overload or frustration. Anger may follow denial or, in some cases, may occur instead of denial. For example, the spouse of a patient may, for no apparent reason, begin screaming at you, calling you incompetent, or using foul language or racial slurs. Although it may be difficult, you should remain calm and not respond angrily as well.

In crisis situations, it is often easier to vent angry feelings on an unknown person (the EMR) or an authority figure (a law enforcement officer) than on a friend or family member. Anger is perhaps the most difficult emotion to deal with objectively because the angry person seems to be directing his or her anger at you. Do not take the person's anger personally, but acknowledge that it is a reaction to stress.

Frustration and a sense of helplessness can often build to anger. If these emotions are not released, the anger may be expressed by aggressive physical behavior. For example, in a serious crash involving a school bus, you may have to demonstrate to bystanders that you and other rescue personnel are indeed removing children from the bus. If little activity is apparent to the bystanders, leading them to believe that nothing is being done, they may become angry, hostile, and even violent. In such situations, you must show confidence. Demonstrate that you are making progress. Always be professional and do not react to anger by becoming angry yourself. Remain calm and deliberate in your actions to prevent the escalation of violence. If necessary, a member of the emergency medical services (EMS) team may have to explain the situation—what is being done and why it appears to be taking so long. Acknowledge anger by saying something like, "What's the matter? Can you tell me what I can do to help?" Then allow the person to express his or her anger.

Treatment

Virtually every emergency call requires some degree of psychological intervention.

► Remorse or Grief

An acceptance of the situation may lead to remorse or grief Figure 12-2 . People may feel guilty or sorry about their behavior or actions during an incident. They may also express grief about the incident itself.

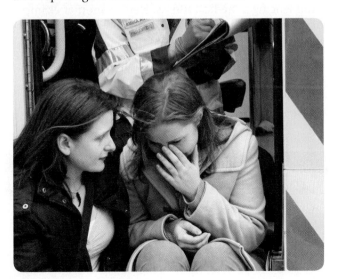

Figure 12-2 An acceptance of the situation may lead to grief.
© Jones & Bartlett Learning. Courtesy of MIEMSS.

■ Crisis Management

As an EMR, you should consider how you can best manage a patient's emotional concerns or crises. When you have a patient who is experiencing a behavioral or situational crisis, you need to approach the situation using the same general framework for patient assessment that applies to other types of patients.

In this section, you will learn about some additional skills that you can use for patients who are exhibiting behavioral crises or emotional stress.

► Role of the Emergency Medical Responder

Remember, as an EMR, your approach to a patient who may be exhibiting abnormal behavior is to follow the steps of your patient assessment sequence:

1. Perform a scene size-up.
2. Perform a primary assessment.
3. Obtain the patient's medical history (SAMPLE).
4. Perform a secondary assessment.
5. Provide ongoing reassessment.

After you complete the primary assessment, you may need to obtain the patient's medical history or perform a physical examination, depending on the needs of that individual patient. As you perform these steps, it is important that you remain calm and reassure the patient.

Your most important assessment skill may be your ability to communicate with the patient. Your communication skills will help you obtain needed information from the patient as you calm and reassure the patient.

► Communicating With the Patient

The first and most important step you can take in crisis management is to talk with the person. Talking lets the person know that someone cares. Introduce yourself to the patient, ask the patient his or her name, and ask what you can do to help. When you communicate with the patient, be honest, warm, caring, and understanding.

When you begin talking with the patient, your body language is as important as your words. Try to position yourself at eye level with the patient Figure 12-3 . If the person is lying down, kneel beside him or her. If the person is sitting, move down to his or her level. Do not stand above the person with your hands on your hips. This is a threatening position and communicates an uncaring attitude and indifference to the patient's problem Figure 12-4 .

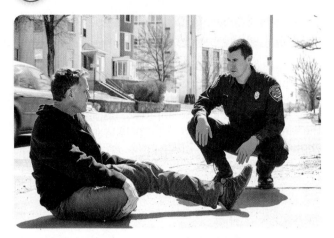

Figure 12-3 Crouch or seat yourself at the same level as the patient.
© Jones & Bartlett Learning.

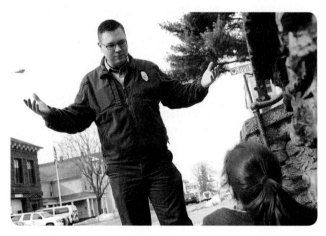

Figure 12-4 This body language communicates an uncaring attitude.
© Jones & Bartlett Learning.

When you establish eye contact with the person, you are assuring him or her that you are, indeed, interested in helping. Use a calm, steady voice when you talk to the person and provide honest reassurance. Avoid making false statements or giving false assurances. The patient does not want to be told that everything is all right when it obviously is not.

Try not to let negative personal feelings about the person or about the person's behavior interfere with your attempt to assist. Your function is to help the person cope with the events that caused the crisis. You should remain neutral and avoid taking sides in any situation or argument.

Sometimes a simple act, such as offering a tissue or a warm blanket, defuses the person's reaction to the immediate crisis. Simple acts of kindness can comfort and reassure the person that you are there to help. Some patients are comforted by your touch during an emergency. It provides a sense of presence, reassurance, and comfort to them. Other patients may find your touch offensive and may become upset or violent if you touch them without their permission. Be observant in determining when touch is appropriate.

Words of Wisdom

The following crisis intervention tips may help you at the scene of a behavioral emergency:

- Take your time.
- Remain calm.
- Reassure the patient.
- Use eye contact.
- Touch the patient, if appropriate.
- Talk in a calm, steady voice.
- Demonstrate confidence.
- Do not take the patient's comments personally.

Restatement

To show the person that you understand what he or she is saying, you can use a technique known as **restatement**. This means you rephrase a person's own words and thoughts and repeat them back to the person. Here is one example of restatement:

> *Patient:* I just don't think I can go on anymore. Nobody cares.
> *EMR:* You sound like you are very discouraged. Why do you feel you can't go on and that nobody cares?

These communication techniques can also be effective with patients who have sustained trauma or are experiencing a medical illness. Here is another example of restatement with an injured patient who is experiencing a crisis:

> *Patient with a broken arm:* I can't take any more of this pain!
> *EMR:* The pain may seem unbearable to you right now, but it will ease up when we finish applying this splint.

YOU are the Provider — CASE 2

It is 1600 hours when you are called to the local community center for the report of a 12-year-old girl who is having difficulty breathing. You arrive on scene and observe a young girl sitting on the ground, leaning against the wall. The girl is breathing rapidly. A counselor at the community center who is with the girl informs you that she became upset after being told her father was in a vehicle crash.

1. What actions should you take upon arriving on the scene?
2. What care can you give to this patient?

It is not usually helpful to say, "I know what you mean," or, "I know how you feel." You do not know exactly how the patient is feeling, even though you may have been through a similar experience. Be honest and give the patient hope, but do not give false hope.

Redirection

Sometimes, a patient may be embarrassed about being the center of attention or may be concerned about others involved in the situation. Redirection helps focus a patient's attention on the immediate situation or crisis. You should use redirection in an attempt to lessen the concerns the patient expressed and draw his or her attention back to the immediate situation. An example of redirection follows:

> *Patient involved in a motor vehicle crash:* Oh my God! Where are my children? What's wrong with my children?
>
> *EMR:* Your children are being taken care of by my partner; they are in good hands. Now, we must take care of you.

If the patient is in a public place such as on a sidewalk or in the lobby of a building, move the patient to a location that is quieter and more private, if the injury or illness permits.

Empathy

The ability to empathize involves the ability to sense someone else's emotions and to imagine what he or she might be thinking and feeling. Empathy helps you understand the emotional or psychological trauma the patient is experiencing. Ask yourself, "How would I feel if I was lying on the sidewalk with my clothes all torn and bloody and strangers were looking down at me?"

Empathy is one of the most helpful concepts you can use when caring for patients in crisis situations. To show empathy and to reassure the patient, you need to use a calm and caring approach.

Communication Skills

By using these various communication skills, you will be able to more effectively manage the patient's conditions. Practice these skills with another person until you are comfortable using them. Some principles you can use when assessing patients with a behavioral crisis are listed here:

1. Identify yourself and let the patient know you are there to help.
2. Inform the patient of what you are doing.
3. Ask questions in a calm, reassuring voice.
4. Allow the patient to tell you what happened. Do not be judgmental.
5. Show you are listening by using restatement and redirection.
6. Acknowledge the patient's feelings.
7. Assess the patient's mental status:
   - Appearance
   - Activity
   - Speech
   - Orientation to person, place, and time
   - Mood
   - Thought process
   - Memory

▶ Crowd Control

Performing simple crowd control may help reduce a patient's anxiety when there are too many people around. Encourage bystanders to leave. Sometimes too many emergency personnel have been dispatched

---

Special Populations

Communicating With Patients With Developmental Disabilities

Data from the Centers for Disease Control and Prevention indicate that 1 in 6 children have some type of developmental disability. Developmental disabilities range from learning disabilities and developmental delays to autism spectrum disorder. Some patients with developmental disabilities will present a challenge for you during an emergency. For example, patients with autism spectrum disorder might:

- Avoid eye contact and want to be alone.
- Not look at objects when another person points to them.
- Have trouble expressing their needs using typical words or motions.
- Appear to be unaware when people talk to them but respond to other sounds.
- Have trouble adapting when a routine changes.
- Prefer not to be held or cuddled.

Some of the behaviors listed above may make it difficult for you to determine the patient's illness or injury. These behaviors may make it harder to assess the patient and more difficult to provide needed treatment. If a family member or caregiver is present with the patient, he or she is often helpful. He or she can supply helpful information about the patient, help you determine the patient's problem, and he or she can often communicate more effectively with the patient. If no caregiver or relative is present, use the communication skills described in this chapter to help you. Remain calm, speak in a reassuring tone, and allow only one person to communicate with the patient.

to the scene. The presence of many uniformed personnel in a small apartment, for instance, is overwhelming or threatening to some people. Any emergency personnel who are not needed right away should leave the room or immediate area until the patient calms down.

During your initial overview of the emergency scene, look to see if there is a crowd that may become hostile. If you feel the potential exists, it is better to ask for assistance early on to deal with an unhappy crowd than it is to wait until the situation is unsafe for you and your patient.

▶ Domestic Violence

Domestic violence is common in today's society. It takes on different forms, including elder abuse, child abuse, and spousal and domestic partner abuse. As an EMR, you need to recognize the signs and symptoms of abuse and to understand the three phases in the cycle of abuse. Protecting yourself at the scene is also very important. When you respond to a situation involving domestic violence, you know how to maintain safety for yourself and for the patient and how to conduct an effective assessment and treatment in what could be a volatile situation. Finally, understand the requirements for reporting abuse in your state.

The signs of abuse include physical injuries, the emotional state of the patient, and the personality indicators of the abuser. Physical injuries from domestic violence include broken bones, cuts, head injuries, bruises, burns, and scars from old injuries. Internal injuries may also be caused by abuse. In some cases, injuries will be in varying stages of healing. The abused person's emotional scars and symptoms may include depression, suicide attempts, and abuse of alcohol or drugs. The patient may have feelings of anxiety, distress, and hopelessness. People who are abusers may be paranoid, overly sensitive, obsessive, or threatening. They often abuse alcohol or drugs and have access to weapons.

If you suspect abuse, your responsibility is to maintain safety for yourself and for the patient. Dealing with a violent person is covered later in this chapter. To defuse a tense situation, try to separate the patient from the person who may have been the abuser. This will create a safe place for the patient, give you a chance to gather needed information, and allow you to treat the patient's injuries. As you question the patient, express your concern. Ask the patient if she or he is all right. Avoid judging the patient. If the patient refuses to be transported, some agencies provide information about domestic abuse shelters. In some cases, the presence of law enforcement personnel will be helpful. Finally, learn the requirements for reporting cases of suspected abuse in your state.

Cycles of Abuse

Abuse has been described as a three-part cycle. In the tension-building phase, the abuser becomes angry and often blames the victim. If the victim has been in the relationship for some time, he or she may recognize the tension buildup and react by trying to calm the abuser. The victim may also try to minimize or deny the abuse. The tension phase is usually the longest part of the abuse cycle.

The second stage is the explosive, or acute battery, phase, when the abuser becomes enraged and loses control as well as the ability to think clearly. Most injuries to the victim occur during this stage. The third phase is the honeymoon or makeup phase. During this stage, the abuser may make all sorts of promises, which are seldom kept. This phase helps keep the abused person in the relationship with the abuser. As an EMR, you may enter a domestic scene anywhere in this cycle. Understanding this cycle will help you to anticipate the actions of both the abuser and the person being abused.

▶ Violent Patients

If you must treat an unarmed patient who is or may become violent, immediately attempt to establish verbal and eye contact with the patient. This begins the process of establishing rapport with the patient, which is important for communicating with a potentially violent person.

If family members or friends are present, ask them about the patient's history of violence. A patient with a history of violence is more likely to become violent again. Is the patient yelling or issuing verbal threats? Loud, obscene, or bizarre speech indicates emotional instability. Assess the patient's posture to determine

---

YOU are the Provider   CASE 3

It is 2430 hours on a rainy Friday night and your unit is called to the scene of a motor vehicle crash where a vehicle has rolled over and crashed into a ditch. The driver is out of the car, walking with an unsteady gait, and not talking clearly. The law enforcement officer says she thinks the driver may be drunk.

1. What actions should you take first with this patient?
2. What treatment do you need to give to this patient?

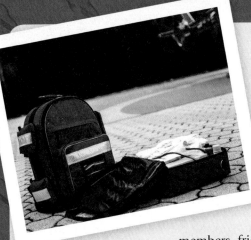

Voices *of* Experience

How many of us have experienced a personal behavioral situation when responding to an incident? We may also have family members, friends, or a coworker with some type of a personal situation we don't talk about. As responders, we should not forget that a patient in a behavioral emergency may be crying out for help or just need someone to talk to.

In the late 1990s, we responded to a call of a man cutting himself with glass. We were told to hold short until the Sheriff's Officer had secured the scene. The scene was declared safe within a few minutes. (Let's all remember that our safety comes first.) We arrived on scene and found a man in his late 20s stabbing himself in his upper legs with broken bottles.

> **Be willing to look beyond the situation at hand.**

After obtaining a brief history from family members, we found out that the patient was taking medications for mental illness and that he had had an argument with his father earlier that day. The family stated he had been off his medication for around a week.

We convinced the patient to stop hurting himself after a few minutes. He continued saying no one wanted him. He was transported to the local emergency department for treatment. During his stay in the emergency department, a nurse turned her back, and the patient left the emergency department and went to the woods across the street from the hospital. He was found there less than an hour later, stabbing himself with tree branches.

A second incident occurred about 3 months later, at the same residence. This time the patient had taken two broken beer bottles and had walked to the interstate near his home. He was found sitting on the guardrail with the necks of the bottles around his thumbs and resting at his neck veins. Several bystanders had stopped and were trying to convince him to remove them from his neck. This was making the situation worse.

After obtaining a history report, we found out that he and his father had been arguing again. After talking with him, I managed to convince him to be treated for small cuts to his neck. He kept saying no one liked him; we had to convince him to believe in himself. He was later removed from the family setting and hospitalized. After about 2 years of hospitalization he was released. We see him from time to time, and he is a changed person. His family lives in the area but will not see him. We have not had a call to his residence in several years.

Sometimes family members can contribute to a behavioral illness. When confronted with this type of situation, the responder has to remember that this could be his or her own family member. Be willing to look beyond the situation at hand. What caused this person to react this way? Remember, your safety comes first, then your crew's safety, and then the patient's safety.

Jimmy Talton
Fire Chief
Reece City Volunteer Fire Department
Attalla, Alabama

whether he or she is showing threatening behavior **Figure 12-5**. A person who is pacing, cannot sit still, or tries to protect his or her personal space is more likely to become violent. Patients who have been abusing alcohol or drugs are also at a high risk for developing violent behavior. Do not force the patient into a corner, and do not allow yourself to be cut off from a route of retreat.

In these situations, it is usually best to have only one person talk with the patient. Having more than one rescuer attempt conversation is often very threatening. The communicator should be the rescuer with whom the patient seems to have the best initial rapport.

If all other means of approach and intervention fail, it may be necessary for you to summon law enforcement personnel to control a violent patient.

▶ Violence Against EMRs

According to the National Institute for Occupational Safety and Health, the following factors increase the risk of violence in the workplace:

- Working alone or in small numbers
- Working late at night or early in the morning hours
- Working in high-crime areas
- Working in community settings

All of these factors describe your job as an EMR. You come in contact with all kinds of people at all hours of the day and night. You work in the community and may be called to high-crime areas. You should be alert when you respond to a call that has an increased chance for violence. These include crime scenes, incidents involving gangs, large gatherings of hostile or potentially hostile people, and domestic disputes (previously discussed). However, even though you are more likely than the average citizen to be involved in potentially violent situations, there are steps you can take to minimize the chance of injury to you and to your patients. Take steps to keep yourself and other rescuers safe at these scenes. Remember, always keep an escape route between you and the patient at scenes that may become dangerous.

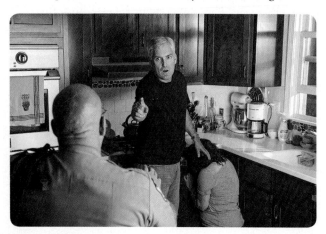

Figure 12-5 A patient's posture will indicate the potential for violent behavior.
© Jones & Bartlett Learning.

Prevention

Prevention is the best way to avoid violence. It is far better to avoid or prevent an incident of violence than to have actual violence erupt and then have to deal with it. You may have several different opportunities for preventing violence. Can you learn anything from the dispatch information you received about the incident? As you arrive at the scene, use your personal antenna to pick up any signs that you may be approaching a violent situation. (Review the section on scene safety in Chapter 2, *Workforce Safety and Wellness*.) Make sure you have an escape route in mind as you approach any suspicious scene.

Your ability to use good interpersonal communication skills will help prevent many situations from becoming violent. Empathy can often defuse tense situations. Practice the communication skills discussed in this chapter. If you think you need backup or law enforcement personnel, request it early. If you are unable to handle a situation by yourself, remember your escape route. Learn your local protocols for violent situations and take part in additional training for handling this type of situation.

Safety

If you have any doubts about your safety at a scene, wait at a safe distance and request for assistance from law enforcement officials.

▶ The Armed Patient

You may encounter a person who is armed with a gun, knife, or other weapon. It is not your role to handle this situation unless you are a law enforcement officer. Be alert for potentially threatening situations and summon assistance if you think the person is armed. Do not proceed into an area where there may be an armed person without assistance from law enforcement personnel. If you must wait for law enforcement personnel to arrive, stay with your vehicle in a safe location. If, despite caution, you are confronted by an armed person, immediately attempt to withdraw. Your best defense is to avoid confronting a person who is armed! Work with the law enforcement personnel in your area to learn what your role is in cases that might involve an armed person.

Safety

If you cannot withdraw from a dangerous scene:

- Stay calm.
- Do not turn your back on the patient.
- Do not make threatening moves.
- Try to talk with the person and explain that you are there to give emergency medical assistance.

Medical and Legal Considerations

To protect the rights of the patient and to protect yourself from any possible legal action, you must understand the laws of your state and community that relate to dealing with patients experiencing a behavioral emergency. If a patient agrees to be treated, there should be few legal issues. However, if a patient who appears to be disturbed refuses to accept treatment, it may be necessary to provide care against the patient's will. To do this, you must have a reasonable belief that the patient will harm himself, herself, or others. Usually, if patients are a threat to themselves or to others, it is possible to treat and transport them without their consent. As an EMR, you usually will not be responsible for transporting the patient, but you should know what the laws in your state permit you to do. This direction should come from your medical director and from legal counsel.

There may be times when it is necessary for you to apply reasonable force to keep a patient from injuring himself, herself, or others. If you are required to restrain a patient, you should consider the following factors: the patient's size and apparent strength, the sex of the patient, the type of abnormal behavior, the mental state of the patient, and the method of restraint. Whenever possible, you should avoid acts of physical force that may injure the patient. You may, however, use reasonable force to defend yourself against an attack by a behaviorally impaired patient.

To prevent legal issues if you must restrain a patient, seek assistance from law enforcement officials and from your medical director. It is also important to document the conditions present in cases where you must restrain or subdue a patient. To prevent accusations of sexual misconduct by behaviorally impaired patients, a caregiver of the same sex should take primary responsibility for the care of the patient, whenever possible.

Other Types of Emotional Crises

Four other types of emotional crises—attempted suicide, posttraumatic stress disorder, sexual assault, and death and dying—also require you to have good communication skills. Each of these situations is difficult for the patient and for the EMR.

Attempted Suicide

Each year, thousands of people, from teenagers to older adults, attempt suicide (self-inflicted death). People attempt suicide by ingesting poisons, jumping from heights or in front of motor vehicles or trains, cutting their wrists or neck, and shooting or hanging themselves. Not all suicide attempts result in death, and many patients who fail on their first attempt will try again to commit suicide. Most people who attempt suicide have a serious psychiatric illness, such as depression or alcohol or drug abuse. Many people attempt suicide while under the influence of alcohol or drugs. The underlying psychiatric disease is usually treatable, however, and with proper treatment the patient will no longer be suicidal. However, until that treatment is carried out, the patient must at all times be considered suicidal. All suicide attempts should be taken seriously. Do not be afraid to ask the patient questions about suicide such as: Do you feel depressed? Have you ever been prescribed medication for depression? Have you ever thought about suicide?

Management of an attempted suicide consists of the following steps:

1. Protect yourself and the patient from further harm.
2. Obtain a complete history of the incident.
3. Determine whether the patient still has a weapon or drugs on him or her.
4. Support the patient's airway, breathing, and circulation (ABCs), as needed.
5. Dress open wounds.
6. Treat the patient for spinal injuries, if indicated.
7. Do not judge the patient. Treat him or her for the injuries or conditions you discover.
8. Provide emotional support for the patient and family.

Talk with the patient as you are providing treatment. Remember, many suicide attempts are cries for help **Figure 12-6**. In addition to treating the patient, you should provide emotional support for the patient's family. Help the family understand that a suicide attempt usually indicates an underlying psychiatric illness and that it

---

YOU are the Provider   CASE 4

It has been a quiet Saturday night. Just after the bars close, you receive a report for an injured woman who has fallen. Your dispatcher reports she heard a man swearing loudly in the background while she was talking to the patient. As you and your partner approach the house, you are met by a 30-year-old man who appears to be agitated. He quickly tells you everything is all right and that there is no need for medical assistance. He tells you no one from this house called for assistance. As you glance in the front door you see a woman who has some abrasions on her face. She appears to be crying quietly. Her blouse appears torn.

1. What are your initial priorities in this case?
2. How should you proceed with treating the injured woman?

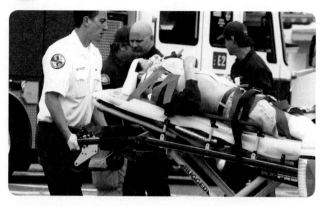

Figure 12-6 Many suicide attempts are cries for help.
© Michael Ledray/Shutterstock.

Special Populations

One of the main causes of suicide in older adults is terminal disease. A person who knows he or she is going to die from an incurable condition may choose to commit suicide to avoid the final disability and suffering associated with that disease. In these cases, the patient's family will be coping with the grief from the diagnosis of the terminal disease as well as the patient's suicide. This is a time when they need your comfort and understanding.

A second age group at high risk for attempted suicide is teenagers. For many teenagers, this is a difficult time of adjustment to growth and change. Stressors in this age group include school, interpersonal relationships, problems at home, and experimentation with drugs and alcohol. The rate of suicide among teenagers is high. Be especially alert for signs of depression and attempted suicide in teenage patients.

is not the fault of the family or friends. It is not your role as an EMR to pass judgment on a patient; it is your role to provide a caring attitude and good medical care.

Posttraumatic Stress Disorder

Posttraumatic stress disorder (PTSD) is a mental health or behavioral condition triggered by experiencing or witnessing a terrifying event. Although many people who experience traumatic events have difficulty coping and adjusting for a while, most get better with time and by taking care of themselves.

However, people experiencing PTSD get worse with time, and their anxiety often interferes with their normal day-to-day activities. General symptoms of posttraumatic stress disorder include severe anxiety, nightmares, flashbacks, and uncontrollable thoughts about the event. Symptoms may be broken into four different groups:

1. **Intrusive memories.** Includes unwanted distressing memories of the traumatic event, unsettling dreams, emotional distress when reminded of the event, or reliving the event.
2. **Avoidance.** People experiencing PTSD avoid places, activities, or people that remind them of the traumatic event.

3. **Negative feelings.** People with PTSD have negative changes in mood or thinking, such as the inability to experience positive emotions, experiencing negative feelings about themselves or others, a lack of interest in activities once enjoyed, difficulty maintaining close relationships, or feelings of hopelessness.
4. **Emotional reactions.** Being easily frightened, having difficulty sleeping, having trouble concentrating, engaging in self-destructive behavior, becoming irritable, or feeling overwhelmed with shame or grief.

Physicians are not sure why some people develop PTSD and others do not. It may be caused by a mixture of multiple factors, and certain risk factors may make some people more likely to develop PTSD. These risk factors include having a job that increases the risk of being exposed to traumatic events (such as military personnel or first responders), having a preexisting mental health condition, lacking a good support system or coping mechanisms, or having experienced a trauma earlier in life. Traumatic events that may lead to PTSD include physical attack, sexual assault, childhood neglect, military combat exposure, or being threatened with a weapon.

People experiencing PTSD may develop self-destructive behaviors including suicidal thoughts, eating disorders, or abuse of alcohol or drugs. They may also suffer from anxiety and depression or exhibit violent behaviors. Patients exhibiting any of these possible symptoms of PTSD need to receive appropriate medical care. PTSD is treated with a combination of psychotherapy and medications. It is important that these patients do not self-medicate and that they have a good support system to help them cope with their illness. As an EMR, you need to practice good communication skills when working with PTSD patients, always ensure your safety and the safety of your partner and your patient, and ensure your patient is transported to a facility where he or she can receive the necessary treatment.

Sexual Assault

Special consideration should be given to any person who has been sexually assaulted. These patients may be a man or a woman, old or young. Because sexual assault creates an emotional crisis, the psychological aspects of treatment are important. The patient may have a hard time coping with a rescuer who is the same sex as the person who committed the assault. You may have to delay all but the most essential treatment until a responder of the same sex as the patient arrives. Your first priority is the medical well-being of the patient, so treat any injuries the person may have (knife wounds, gunshot wounds, and so forth). However, because sexual assault is a crime, you should not remove any of the patient's clothing except to give medical care. Try to convince the patient not to bathe or use the toilet. Keep the scene and any evidence as undisturbed and intact as possible, and avoid aggressively questioning the patient as to what happened.

In addition to giving medical care, treat the patient with empathy. Maintain the patient's privacy by covering her or him with a sheet or blanket, and do not leave the patient alone. Contact your local law enforcement agency and the organization designated as the rape crisis center in your community.

Death and Dying

As an EMR, you will encounter death and dying from natural, accidental, and intentional causes. How well you can help the dying patient and the person's family or friends largely depends on your own feelings about death. The material presented here expands on the material introduced in Chapter 2, *Workforce Safety and Wellness*.

In some situations, there is nothing you can do and the patient dies. In other situations, the patient dies despite everyone's best efforts. In yet other situations, the patient's death is completely unexpected. In every case, you must do whatever you can to meet the patient's medical needs. Your attempts to save or give comfort to the patient help everyone (the patient, the family, and you) to cope emotionally with the patient's death.

Most people are afraid of dying. Witnessing the death of another person brings that fear to the forefront, if only for a brief time. You must work through your personal feelings about death so you can confront it in the field. Although you may be somewhat uncomfortable bringing up the subject, it helps to discuss it with others in the emergency care field. If you are uncomfortable talking with your peers, talk to a member of your hospital's emergency department staff.

Once you have done everything you can to medically treat a patient, consider the psychological needs of the patient and his or her family. Being there as an empathetic caregiver is helpful. Do not be afraid to touch. Putting an arm around a shoulder or holding the hand of the patient or a member of the family helps everyone, including you Figure 12-7 . Do not make false statements about the situation, but it is just as important not to destroy hope. Even if, in your judgment, the situation

is hopeless, try to give comfort by making such positive statements as, "We are here to help you, and we are doing everything we can. The ambulance is on its way, and you will be at the hospital as soon as possible."

As unfortunate as it may seem, coping with the deaths of others is a routine aspect of your job as an EMR. Therefore, you must constantly be on guard to prevent any callousness from entering into your interactions with patients and their families. For every call you respond to, always deliver compassionate medical care.

One specific type of death, sudden infant death syndrome (SIDS), is discussed in Chapter 17, *Pediatric Emergencies*.

▶ Critical Incident Stress Debriefing

Providing emergency care is stressful for you as well as for the patient. As an EMR, you will encounter patients experiencing high levels of stress and anxiety. In emergency situations, there may be times when you may not always be able to help patients. Some types of situations, such as rescue missions involving children or mass-casualty incidents, tend to produce more stress than others. You may need counseling to cope with these stressors.

If you let stress build up without releasing it in healthy ways, it can begin to have negative effects on you and your performance.

Signs and Symptoms

Signs and symptoms of extreme stress include:

- Depression
- Inability to sleep
- Weight changes
- Increased alcohol consumption or drug abuse
- Inability to get along with family and coworkers
- Lack of interest in food or sex

To help prevent excess stress and to relieve stress caused by critical incidents, some departments use a process called **critical incident stress debriefing (CISD)**. CISD brings rescuers and a trained professional together to talk about the rescuers' feelings. CISD may help rescuers understand the signs and symptoms of stress and receive reassurance from the group leader. It also allows people to obtain more help from trained professionals, if needed. Some public safety agencies have set up CISD teams to handle stressful events. These teams may be helpful to rescuers who have been through an overwhelming or stressful event. Other departments have trained professionals available to counsel members who have experienced a highly stressful event. Additional information about critical incident stress debriefing is presented in Chapter 2, *Workforce Safety and Wellness*. Check with your agency to see what types of counseling and CISD resources are available.

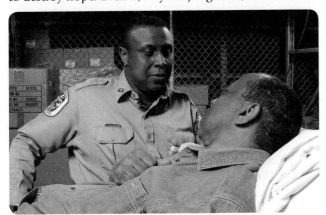

Figure 12-7 Do not be afraid to show empathy to patients and family members.
© Jones & Bartlett Learning.

YOU are the Provider   SUMMARY

You are the Provider: CASE 1

1. What types of conditions contribute to or cause a situational crisis?

As you begin your assessment of this situation, it is helpful to review the five types of conditions that can cause or contribute to a situational crisis:

- Medical conditions such as uncontrolled diabetes, low blood glucose, and conditions that prevent the patient's brain from receiving enough oxygen
- Physical trauma such as head injuries and shock
- Psychiatric illnesses such as depression, panic disorders, and psychotic behaviors
- Alcohol and drug abuse
- Situational stressors such as serious injury or death of a loved one

By evaluating the patient for each of these conditions, you can get a better idea of what might be causing the behavior you are observing.

2. What are the four phases of a situational crisis?

The four phases of a situational crisis are high anxiety or emotional shock, denial, anger, and remorse or grief. Even though not all patients go through these phases in this order, learning about the phases will often give you some idea of why a patient is acting in a certain way.

3. What are three communication tools you can use to help you communicate with this patient?

Your ability to communicate with the patient will help you determine the cause of his or her problem, and often you can begin to defuse the patient's anger. Three tools that are useful in this communication process are restatement, redirection, and empathy.

You are the Provider: CASE 2

1. What actions should you take upon arriving on the scene?

As you arrive on this scene it is important for you to avoid getting tunnel vision regarding what is happening. Complete all the steps of the patient assessment sequence. Be sure to consider all the possibilities regarding what may be happening. Shortness of breath is a scary event for anyone. As you approach this patient, be sure to introduce yourself, and let the patient know you are there to help her. Ask her what the problem is. She may respond that she is having an asthma attack or is upset about a stressful event. Perform a careful patient assessment, including a thorough SAMPLE history. Ask additional questions to follow up on any problems she identifies. Remember, you cannot determine if the problem is purely emotional until all medical causes have been ruled out, and that is something only a physician can do. There are many conditions that can cause difficulty breathing, including asthma, pneumonia, head injuries, diabetic coma, imbalance of medications, and emotional crises. Do not be led into the trap of believing the problem is purely emotional just because a patient is upset.

2. What care can you give to this patient?

The care that you give to this patient should be based on her signs and symptoms and on any problems that you identify from performing a patient assessment. Because shortness of breath produces anxiety, anything you can do to calm this patient will help relieve her anxiety. Treat any medical problems you identify. It is often reassuring to have a family member or close friend for support. Try to determine where her family members are and see if it is possible to reunite her with one of them. If her condition is caused by a behavioral crisis, she may become calmer as you talk with her. You should arrange for her to be transported to an appropriate medical facility for further treatment.

You are the Provider: CASE 3

1. What actions should you take first with this patient?

As you arrive on this scene, you should understand that the mechanism of injury in this case leads to the high possibility that this patient has suffered serious injuries. This is complicated by the fact that there appear to be barriers to clear communication with this patient. Whether you smell alcohol or not, it is important to conduct a complete patient assessment to determine all injuries and illness that this patient has sustained. Talk with the patient to ensure he knows you are there to help him. Help him to remember that he has experienced a vehicle crash. Take spinal precautions to prevent further injuries. Remember, if this patient is under the influence of alcohol or drugs, he is at high risk for trauma and injuries, and often a patient under the influence of alcohol will not realize that he is seriously injured.

2. What treatment do you need to give to this patient?

Your treatment should reflect the understanding that an incident such as this places the patient at high risk for serious trauma to any part of the body. Consider the possibility of head injuries, spinal injuries, chest and abdominal injuries, and extremity injuries. Take spinal precautions. Consider whether this patient may have a serious medical condition, such as diabetes or heart disease, that contributed to this situation. Because this patient may not be able to communicate his history to you, see if there is a friend or family member with him. Provide the best treatment you can, and arrange for transport to an appropriate medical facility as soon as possible. Remember, the odor of alcohol should serve as an indication for added caution and careful attention to assessment and treatment.

You are the Provider: CASE 4

1. **What are your initial priorities in this case?**

Your initial priorities in this case are to secure scene safety for yourself, for other rescuers, and for the patient. Unless you are a law enforcement officer trained to handle a situation such as this, you should not proceed into this residence. Back off to a safe location away from the house and call for immediate assistance from law enforcement personnel. It is their responsibility to

secure the scene for you and for the patient. Only after they have secured the scene may you approach the injured woman and begin to examine and treat her. Domestic disputes can be some of the most explosive situations you are called to deal with.

2. **How should you proceed with treating the injured woman?**

Once the scene has been secured by law enforcement personnel, you can approach the injured woman and begin to examine and treat her. In situations such as this, it is important to separate the woman from any people who may be threatening her. This gives her some feeling of safety. Realize that she may be afraid to talk about her experience for fear of punishment from her significant other. Try to be supportive; be a good listener. Remember, you must report cases of suspected domestic abuse to the proper authorities.

Perform a complete patient assessment in a calm manner. Treat any physical injuries you find. Ask her about any other abuse. Document the results of your examination and treatment. Arrange for transportation of the woman to an appropriate medical facility for further examination and treatment.

Prep Kit

▶ Ready for Review

- Only a small percentage of the patients you treat are severely mentally ill, but almost every patient you care for is experiencing some degree of a behavioral and emotional crisis. No matter what type of incident or crisis is taking place, your response must be to help the patient.
- Behavioral emergencies are situations in which a person exhibits abnormal, unacceptable behavior that cannot be tolerated by the patients themselves or by family, friends, or the community.
- The five major factors that contribute to behavioral crises: medical conditions, physical trauma conditions, psychiatric illnesses, mind-altering substances, and situational stresses.
- The four emotional phases to each crisis include high anxiety or emotional shock, denial, anger, and remorse or grief. Although a person may not experience every phase during a crisis, he or she will certainly experience one or more of the phases.
- Your role as an EMR consists of assessing the patient and providing physical and emotional care. Your most important assessment skill may be your ability to communicate with the patient.
- You must understand the laws of your state and community that relate to caring for patients experiencing a behavioral emergency. If a patient who is experiencing a behavioral emergency agrees to be treated, there should be few legal issues. However, if a patient who appears to be disturbed refuses to accept treatment, it may be necessary to provide care against the patient's will. To do this, you must have a reasonable belief that the patient would harm himself, herself, or others. Usually, if patients are a threat to themselves or to others, it is possible to treat and transport them without their consent.
- Even when you have thoroughly mastered the processes and tools for managing behavioral crises, it is important to remember that sometimes the best approach is to ask yourself, "How would I like to be treated if I were in this situation?"

▶ Vital Vocabulary

behavioral emergency A situation in which the patient exhibits abnormal behavior that is unacceptable or cannot be tolerated by the patient him- or herself or by family, friends, or the community.

critical incident stress debriefing (CISD) A system of psychological support designed to reduce stress on emergency personnel.

emotional shock A state of shock caused by a sudden illness, an accident, or the death of a loved one.

empathy The ability to share another person's feelings or ideas.

posttraumatic stress disorder (PTSD) A mental health or behavioral condition triggered by experiencing or witnessing a terrifying event.

psychotic behavior Mental disturbance characterized by abnormal thought processes and/or the loss of contact with reality.

redirection A means of focusing the patient's attention on the immediate situation or crisis.

restatement Rephrasing a patient's own statement to show that he or she is being heard and understood by the rescuer.

situational crisis A state of emotional upset or turmoil caused by a sudden and disruptive event.

suicide Self-inflicted death.

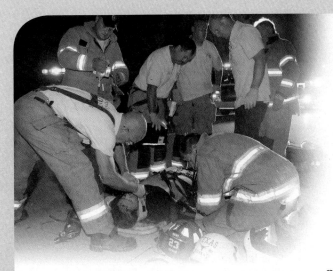

Assessment
in Action

You and your partner are dispatched to a single-family home for a report of a possible overdose. On arrival, a man claiming to be the patient's husband opens the door and begins yelling at you, stating he arrived home and found his wife unconscious on the floor of the bedroom with an empty bottle of diazepam (Valium). He thinks she took at least 40 pills. The husband is very agitated, flushed in the face, and obviously distraught. As your partner calms the man, you assess the woman and find her pulseless and not breathing. While you are performing CPR, the paramedics arrive and begin more advanced life support measures and provide transport to the hospital. The patient is pronounced dead on arrival at the hospital.

1. What emotional phase of a situational crisis is the husband exhibiting?

   A. High anxiety or emotional shock
   B. Denial
   C. Anger
   D. Remorse or grief

2. The signs and symptoms the husband is exhibiting are suggestive of:

   A. posttraumatic stress.
   B. high anxiety.
   C. hypovolemic shock.
   D. denial.

3. When performing your primary assessment of the woman, you should do all of the following EXCEPT:

   A. demonstrate confidence.
   B. provide emotional support for the family.
   C. allow personal feelings to influence your care.
   D. talk in a calm, steady voice.

4. What is the single most important personal history factor in an attempted suicide?

   A. Aggression
   B. Anxiety
   C. Excessive confidence
   D. Depression

5. All of the following skills are useful to you when communicating with patients in crisis EXCEPT:

   A. restatement.
   B. redirection.
   C. empathy.
   D. sympathy.

6. What is a behavioral emergency?

7. Describe the condition(s) under which you could take a behaviorally disturbed patient to a medical facility against his or her will.

8. Explain how redirection might be used to improve your communication in this situation.

9. List the general symptoms of posttraumatic stress disorder.

10. Describe the risk factors that make a person more likely to develop posttraumatic stress disorder.

Environmental Emergencies

National EMS Education Standard Competencies

Trauma

Uses simple knowledge to recognize and manage life threats based on assessment findings for an acutely injured patient while awaiting additional emergency medical response.

Environmental Emergencies

Recognition and management of:

> Submersion incidents (pp 261–262)
> Temperature-related illness (pp 256–259)

Knowledge Objectives

1. Describe the signs and symptoms of a patient experiencing heat cramps. (p 256)
2. Describe the treatment of a patient experiencing heat cramps. (p 256)
3. Describe the signs and symptoms of a patient experiencing heat exhaustion. (p 256)
4. Describe the treatment of a patient experiencing heat exhaustion. (p 256)
5. Describe the signs and symptoms of a patient experiencing heatstroke. (pp 256–257)
6. Describe the treatment of a patient experiencing heatstroke. (pp 256–257)
7. Describe the signs and symptoms of a patient experiencing frostbite. (pp 257–258)
8. Describe the treatment of a patient experiencing frostbite. (pp 257–258)
9. Describe the signs and symptoms of a patient experiencing hypothermia. (p 259)
10. Describe the treatment of a patient experiencing hypothermia. (p 259)
11. Discuss the relationship between hypothermia and cardiac arrest. (p 259)
12. Describe the signs and symptoms of a patient who sustained a submersion injury. (p 261)
13. Describe the treatment of a patient who sustained a submersion injury. (p 261)
14. Describe the signs and symptoms of a patient who has been struck by lightning. (p 262)
15. Describe the treatment of a patient who has been struck by lightning. (p 262)

Skills Objectives

1. Demonstrate patient assessment on a patient who has sustained an injury or illness from exposure to heat, exposure to cold, or submersion. (p 255)
2. Demonstrate cooling a patient who has experienced exposure to heat. (p 256)
3. Demonstrate treating a patient who has experienced exposure to cold. (pp 257–258)
4. Demonstrate treating a patient who has a submersion injury. (p 261)
5. Demonstrate treating a patient who has a lightning injury. (p 262)

Introduction

This chapter describes medical conditions that are caused by environmental conditions such as excessive heat, humidity, and cold and injuries and illnesses related to submersion in water. When a person is exposed to excessive heat, the body's mechanisms for controlling temperature can be overwhelmed, resulting in heat cramps, heat exhaustion, or heatstroke. Exposure to cold environments may result in conditions such as frostbite or hypothermia. You will learn about each of these conditions, including signs, symptoms, and common treatments. This chapter also discusses unintentional exposure to water leading to submersion injuries and drowning and the signs, symptoms, and treatment of these conditions. Special considerations for treating hypothermic patients in cardiac arrest are emphasized. Finally, this chapter outlines the injuries caused by lightning and emphasizes the importance of properly treating these patients.

Patient Assessment for Environmental Emergencies

Your approach to a patient who has signs and symptoms of an environmental emergency should follow the same patient assessment sequence described in Chapter 9, *Patient Assessment* Figure 13-1 . Review your dispatch information and evaluate it to help you consider the possible conditions or injuries the patient may be experiencing. Carefully assess the scene to determine safety issues for you and your patient. As you perform the primary assessment, first, try to form an impression of the patient's condition. Determine the patient's level of responsiveness as you introduce yourself. Then check the patient's airway, breathing, and circulation (ABCs), and acknowledge the patient's chief complaint.

Usually it is best to collect a medical history on the patient experiencing a medical problem before you

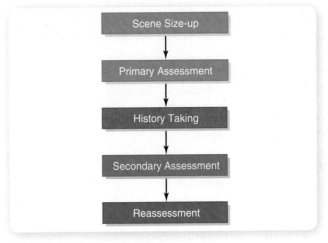

Figure 13-1 Patient assessment sequence.
© Jones & Bartlett Learning. Courtesy of MIEMSS.

perform a secondary assessment. The medical history should be complete and include all factors that may relate to the patient's current illness.

Use the SAMPLE mnemonic to help you secure the medical history information you need:

S Signs and symptoms
A Allergies
M Medications
P Pertinent past medical history
L Last oral intake
E Events associated with or leading up to the illness or injury

Although the secondary patient assessment should focus on the areas related to the patient's current illness, you should also recognize the patient may not always be aware of all the various aspects of his or her condition. It is better to perform a complete patient assessment and find all the problems than to perform a partial assessment and miss an underlying problem. Obtain the patient's vital signs and do not forget to monitor your patient through the use of ongoing reassessment if the arrival of additional emergency medical services (EMS) personnel is delayed.

YOU are the Provider   CASE 1

As you gather for the morning report at the beginning of your shift, you listen to your supervisor as she reviews the weather forecast for this July day. She reports the temperature is expected to reach 95° to 97°F (35° to 36°C), and the humidity is expected to be in excess of 80%. Just before ending her report, she encourages everyone to monitor his or her fluid intake to avoid dehydration. After the report you are dispatched to standby at an aid station for a local road race. Soon after you arrive, a 38-year-old female runner is assisted to the aid station by two runners. She is sweating and her clothes are completely wet. You check her pulse and discover it is weak and thready. She says she feels nauseous and was light-headed during the last part of the race.

1. As you evaluate the symptoms the patient relates to you and the signs she exhibits, what do you think is most likely wrong with this patient?
2. What steps should you take to treat this patient?

■ Exposure to Heat

As an emergency medical responder (EMR), you will encounter patients who have been exposed to excessive heat. Next, we will discuss the signs, symptoms, and treatment for patients experiencing heat cramps, heat exhaustion, and heatstroke to help you recognize and treat these patients.

▶ Heat Cramps

Heat cramps are painful involuntary muscle spasms. They often occur after vigorous exercise, especially in hot weather. They can also occur in factory or construction workers and even in well-conditioned athletes. The exact cause of heat cramps is not known, but it is thought to be partly related to the change in the electrolytes that occurs during exercise and partly as a result of the dehydration that accompanies exercise or working in a hot environment. A large amount of water loss occurs during vigorous physical activity. This loss of water may affect muscles that are stressed and cause them to go into spasm. Heat cramps occur most often in the leg or calf muscles. They may also occur in the abdominal muscles. When abdominal cramps occur, it may appear that the patient is having an acute abdominal problem.

The first step in treating heat cramps is to move the patient to a cool place. Have the patient lie down in a comfortable position to rest the affected muscles. Give the patient water to drink. A diluted balanced electrolyte solution, such as Gatorade, can also be given if it is available. Usually with rest and fluid the cramps will go away. If the cramps do not go away, or if the patient is young, old, or has a chronic medical condition, you should arrange to have the patient transported to an appropriate medical facility for a thorough evaluation and treatment.

▶ Heat Exhaustion

Heat exhaustion is a heat-related illness that occurs when a person is exposed to temperatures above 80°F (27°C), often in combination with high humidity. It may also occur as a result of vigorous exercise at lower temperatures. A person experiencing heat exhaustion sweats profusely and becomes light-headed, dizzy, and nauseated.

Certain risk factors may make some people more susceptible to heat-related illnesses. The very young, older adults (age 65 and older), and people who have preexisting medical conditions or who are taking certain medications are more likely to experience a heat-related illness. High air temperatures reduce the body's ability to cool itself by radiation. High humidity reduces the body's ability to lose heat through evaporation. Exercise results in greater production of sweat.

Signs and Symptoms

Signs and symptoms of heat exhaustion include the following:

- Dizziness, light-headedness
- Weak pulse
- Profuse sweating
- Nausea, vomiting

The patient's blood pressure may drop (causing a weak pulse), and the patient may frequently report feeling weak. Body temperature is usually normal. The signs and symptoms of heat exhaustion are similar to the early signs of shock, and its treatment is similar as well.

When you encounter a patient who is experiencing heat exhaustion, complete a scene size-up and a primary assessment. Patients experiencing heat exhaustion sweat heavily and are in mild shock from fluid loss. To treat heat exhaustion, move the patient to a cooler place (for example, from a baseball diamond to a shady spot under a tree) and treat him or her for shock. Unless the patient is unconscious, nauseous, or vomiting, give fluids by mouth to replace fluid loss through sweating. Drinking cool water is excellent treatment for patients experiencing heat exhaustion. Monitor the ABCs and arrange for transport to a medical facility.

▶ Heatstroke

Heatstroke occurs when the body is subjected to more heat than it can handle and the normal mechanisms for getting rid of the excessive heat, such as through sweating, are overwhelmed. The patient's body temperature rises until it reaches a level at which brain damage occurs. Without prompt and proper treatment, a patient with heatstroke will die.

The patient usually has flushed, dry skin that feels hot to the touch. Be alert for the fact that the patient's clothing may still be wet even though he or she has stopped perspiring. A person who is experiencing heatstroke may be semiconscious; however, as the body temperature rises, the patient will rapidly lose consciousness. These patients may have body temperatures in excess of 104°F (40°C).

Maintain the patient's ABCs. Move the patient from the heat and into a cool place as soon as possible **Figure 13-2**. Remove the patient's clothes, down to his or her underwear. Soak the patient with water. You can cool the patient with water from a garden hose, a shower in the home or factory, or a low-pressure hose from a fire truck. Ice packs can be placed on the groin and armpits. If the patient is conscious and not nauseated, give small amounts of cool water. Arrange for rapid transport to an appropriate medical facility for further treatment. **Table 13-1** compares the signs and symptoms of heat exhaustion with those of heatstroke.

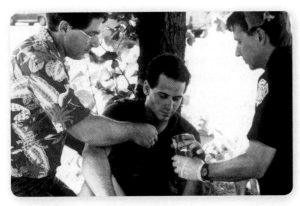

Figure 13-2 Move the patient from the heat as soon as possible.
© American Academy of Orthopaedic Surgeons.

Table 13-1	Comparing Heat Exhaustion and Heatstroke	
Heat Exhaustion	**Heatstroke**	
Normal body temperature	High body temperature	
Sweating	Dry skin (usually)	
Cool and clammy skin	Hot and red skin	
Dizziness and nausea	Semiconscious (or unconscious)	

© Jones & Bartlett Learning. Courtesy of MIEMSS.

Treatment

Heatstroke is an emergency that requires immediate action. The patient's body temperature must be lowered quickly!

Safety

Firefighters are at high risk for heat exhaustion and heatstroke when wearing heavy turnout gear because, in addition to working in hot environments, the turnout gear does not allow body heat to escape. Law enforcement personnel are also at high risk for heat-related conditions because of the heavy ballistic vests they wear for protection. It is important to keep hydrated and to take breaks when operating in hot environments.

■ Exposure to Cold

As an EMR, you will encounter patients who have been exposed to excessive cold. When you assess these patients, you should follow the steps of the patient assessment sequence discussed earlier. The signs and symptoms exhibited by the patient will guide you in your treatment. To help you recognize and treat these patients, the signs, symptoms, and treatment for frostbite and hypothermia are discussed next.

▶ Frostbite

Frostbite can result when parts of the body are exposed to a cold environment. It can occur outside on a winter day, in a walk-in food freezer, or in a cold-storage warehouse in the middle of the summer. It can also occur through exposure to super-cooled gases. Exposed body parts actually freeze. The body parts most susceptible to frostbite are the face, ears, fingers, and toes Figure 13-3 . Depending on the temperature and wind speed, frostbite can occur in a short period.

Increases in wind speed have the same effect as decreases in temperature. Imagine holding your hand outside an automobile traveling at 55 mph on a cold winter day. The combination of wind speed and low temperature produces a windchill factor Figure 13-4 . When the temperature is relatively mild, 35°F (2°C), an accompanying 20-mph wind will produce a windchill equivalent to an

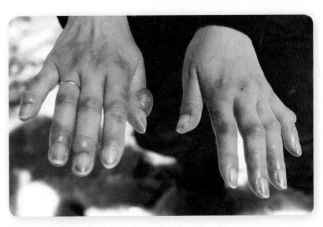

Figure 13-3 The fingers are one of the most common areas affected by frostbite.
Courtesy of Neil Malcom Winkelmann.

YOU are the Provider   CASE 2

It is now 1015 hours at the marathon when a runner is transported to the medical tent by the remote assistance team. The EMR handing off the patient to you indicates the runner is a 53-year-old man who collapsed at mile 18. He is responsive only to verbal stimuli and his skin is flushed, red, and hot to the touch. Treatment was not initiated in the field; the patient was immediately transported to the medical tent.

1. What signs would indicate this runner is experiencing heat exhaustion or heatstroke?
2. After completing the primary assessment, what is the most appropriate treatment for this runner?

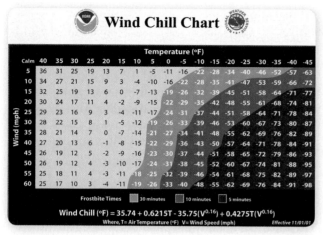

Figure 13-4 Windchill table.
Courtesy of the National Weather Service/NOAA.

actual temperature of 24°F (−4°C). If there is a combination of low temperature and high wind, protect yourself and your patient from the dangers of windchill.

People weakened by old age, medical conditions, exhaustion, or hunger are the most susceptible to frostbite. In superficial frostbite, sometimes called frostnip, the affected body part first becomes numb and then acquires a bright red color. Eventually the area loses its color and becomes pale. There may be a loss of feeling and sensation in the injured area. If the area is rewarmed, the patient may experience a tingling feeling.

Warming a frostbitten area or body part must be done quickly and carefully. Usually, putting the fingers, toes, or ears next to a warm body part is enough. For example, place frostbitten fingers in the armpits. Do not try to warm a frostbitten area by rubbing it with your hands or a blanket, and never rub snow or ice onto a suspected frostbitten area. Doing so will only make the problem worse. Treat the frostbitten patient for shock.

A patient with frostbite who has been outside for an extended period may have deep frostbite. In this situation, the patient's skin will be white and waxy, and it may be firm or frozen. Swelling and blisters may be present. If the skin has thawed, it may appear flushed with areas of purple and white color or it may be mottled and cyanotic. Follow the scene size-up, primary assessment, and secondary assessment sequence. Remove any jewelry the patient is wearing and cover the extremity with dry clothing or dry dressings. If possible, remove wet clothing and keep the patient warm to prevent hypothermia and further frostbite. Do not break blisters, rub the injured area, apply heat, or allow the patient to walk on an affected lower extremity. Patients with deep frostbite should receive prompt transport to a medical facility so they can be warmed under carefully controlled conditions. Remember, any patient with a frostbite injury may have been in the cold environment long enough to produce hypothermia.

Special Populations

Infants and small children have poorly developed heat-regulating mechanisms. They sometimes spike a fever with a minor infection. They are also susceptible to both heat and cold injuries. They are more susceptible to cold injuries because they cannot tell you when they are cold or take steps to change their environment. Also, their ability to generate and use up heat is limited.

Older adults are much more susceptible to heat and cold injuries. Many older adults have decreased sensation to heat and cold. Their bodies are not capable of generating heat as efficiently as younger adults. Some of the medications taken by many older adults reduce their ability to compensate for hot and cold conditions, and older adults generally tend to drink less fluids, which makes them more susceptible to dehydration. All of these factors make geriatric patients more susceptible to heat and cold injuries.

You should always be alert for the possibility of heat and cold injuries in infants, young children, and older adults.

Safety

Prevention is the only defense against frostbite. If you are going outside in freezing weather, dress warmly and make sure the vulnerable parts of your body are well covered and protected.

YOU ▶ are the Provider   CASE 3

On a cloudy cold day in November you and your partner are restocking the rig when you are dispatched to assist a man who has collapsed. After a 4-minute response, you arrive at the scene at his apartment building. As you enter the apartment, you and your partner notice the temperature in the room is very chilly. As you enter the bedroom, you discover an older man lying on the floor between his bed and the wall. Your initial assessment reveals an older man in light clothing who is experiencing violent shivers. He has a shallow and thready pulse and slow respirations. His skin temperature is cold to the touch. Although he seems a bit withdrawn, the man knows his name and the date and is aware of his surroundings. As you complete your patient assessment, the patient does not indicate any areas of tenderness or pain. You are not able to obtain a good medical history because the patient is confused and does not remember what happened to him.

1. What is your initial treatment for this patient?
2. What other conditions might be causing these symptoms?

▶ Hypothermia

When a person's body temperature falls to a subnormal range of below about 95°F (35°C), the condition is called **hypothermia** ("low temperature"). Hypothermia occurs when the body is not able to produce enough energy to keep the internal (core) body temperature at a satisfactory level.

Hypothermia does not only occur in the winter; it can occur in temperatures as high as 50°F (10°C). People who become cold because they do not have enough clothing or their clothing is wet are likely to experience hypothermia, especially if they are weakened by illness. Intoxicated patients and patients who have abused drugs are at an especially high risk for developing hypothermia. The initial signs of hypothermia include feelings of being cold, shivering, decreasing level of consciousness, and sleepiness. Shivering is the body's attempt to produce more heat. As the body temperature drops and hypothermia progresses, shivering stops. A patient who is so cold that he or she cannot shiver cools down even faster. Signs of increasing hypothermia include a lack of coordination, decreased level of consciousness, mental confusion, and slowed reactions. As the body's temperature goes below about 90°F (32°C), the patient will lose consciousness. Patients suffering from hypothermia may have weak or very slow pulse rates. Therefore, it is important to carefully monitor their pulse for at least 30 seconds to accurately determine the underlying heart rate. Without treatment and warming to reverse the downward trend in body temperature, the patient will eventually die **Table 13-2**.

If you suspect a patient is experiencing hypothermia, move the patient to a warm (or warmer) location. Remove wet clothing and place warm blankets over and under the patient to help retain body heat and begin the warming process. If the patient is conscious, give warm fluids to drink.

If you are outdoors and cannot easily take the patient inside a building, move the patient into a heated vehicle as soon as possible. If you cannot move the patient to a warmer environment, keep the patient dry and place as many blankets and insulating materials as possible around the patient. If transport is delayed or extended you may need to consider using your own body heat to warm the patient. Wrap blankets around yourself and the patient or get into a sleeping bag with the patient to use your body heat to start the warming process, even during transport. Handle the patient gently. Any patient experiencing hypothermia must be examined by a physician.

Cardiac Arrest and Hypothermia

If the patient's body temperature falls below 83°F (28°C), the heart may stop and you will need to begin cardiopulmonary resuscitation (CPR). As odd as it may seem, hypothermia may actually protect patients from death in some cases. Therefore, always start CPR and use an automated external defibrillator, if available, on hypothermic patients even if you believe they have been dead for several hours. Hypothermic patients should never be considered dead until they have been warmed in an appropriate medical facility.

Treatment

A special example of hypothermia protecting a patient from death is an apparent drowning in water colder than 70°F (21°C). Many children who fell in cold water and apparently drowned have been resuscitated successfully. Always start CPR on apparent drowning victims pulled from cold water.

Table 13-2	Characteristics of Systemic Hypothermia			
	Core Temperature			
	93° to 95°F (34° to 35°C)	89° to 92°F (32° to 33°C)	80° to 88°F (27° to 31°C)	< 80°F (< 27°C)
Signs and symptoms	Shivering, foot stamping	Loss of coordination, muscle stiffness	Coma	Apparent death
Cardiorespiratory response	Constricted blood vessels, rapid breathing	Slowing respirations, slow pulse	Weak pulse, dysrhythmias, very slow respirations	Cardiac arrest
Level of consciousness	Withdrawn	Confused, lethargic, sleepy	Unresponsive	Unresponsive

© Jones & Bartlett Learning. Courtesy of MIEMSS.

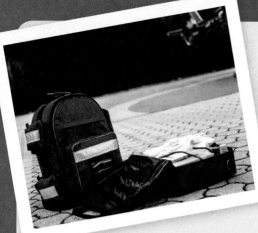

Voices *of* Experience

Don and Margaret had been happily married for 52 years and, as with any couple, they had had their ups and downs. Recently, things had gotten harder for Don. It seemed Margaret's dementia was getting worse. Sometimes she did not recognize Don, and sometimes she did not know where she was. But throughout it all, Don always provided for all of Margaret's needs.

It was a cold, wintery night when Don got up around 0300 hours to use the bathroom. As he was getting back into bed, he looked over and realized Margaret was not in bed. Had she been there when he got up? He couldn't remember. He called her name, but heard nothing in the house. As he entered the living room, he found the worst: the front door was open. Frantically he called 9-1-1 and reported his wife missing.

As emergency medical responders and law enforcement officers arrived, they began searching the area. Looking for footprints was difficult due to the rapidly falling snow. The National Weather Service was forecasting an additional 8 inches (20 cm) of snow, and a high of –20°F (–29°C). After approximately 8 minutes, a police officer called saying he had found her, but she was not moving. As we got over to Margaret, we found her unresponsive, but she was breathing and had a pulse. We rapidly moved her into the ambulance, turned up the heat as high as possible, and removed all of her wet clothing. Drying Margaret as much as we could, we applied hot packs to the appropriate areas and covered her with all the blankets we could find. As we were shutting the doors of the ambulance, I heard Don say, "You're all I know, Margaret. I love you and don't want to lose you." Hearing this brought tears to my eyes. I looked at Don and told him we would do everything we could to help his wife.

As we were en route to the local, rural hospital, I called in a report and advised the physician that the patient was cold, really cold. Once we arrived at the emergency room, we turned over care to the waiting staff. There was a lot frantic activity and I kept hearing, "Make sure the helicopter is coming." Just then we were dispatched to another call, so I could not follow up with the outcome of Margaret's care.

Almost a month later, my partner and I were sitting at our station watching television when there was a knock on the door. When I opened the door, I was met by Don and Margaret, along with a large plate of cookies. We invited our guests inside and Don immediately gave me a huge embrace and broke down in tears. He told us how the events surrounding that night unfolded. The doctors suspected that Margaret had become confused, had gone outside by herself, and had become disoriented. After a 2-week stay in the intensive care unit, Margaret was discharged and came home, with no lasting effects. Don is now working with a social worker to provide a safer home for Margaret.

As you study the material in this textbook, consider the following: while you may not know the patients whose life you will impact, someone deeply cares about that individual, and you need to provide the best care possible.

> **"** The National Weather Service was forecasting an additional 8 inches (20 cm) of snow, and a high of –20°F (–29°C). **"**

Brian J. Williams
EMS Chief
Pembina Ambulance Service
Pembina, North Dakota

Drowning and Submersion

Because EMRs are often the first trained people to arrive at the scene of a drowning, it is important for you to have some understanding of drowning and submersion injuries.

According to the Centers for Disease Control and Prevention, from 2005 to 2014, there was an average of 3,536 unintentional drownings annually, about 10 deaths per day. An additional 332 people died each year from drownings in boat-related incidents. An additional 12,000 people are hospitalized because of injuries resulting from submersion in water. Drowning is the second leading cause of injury and death among children 1 to 14 years. Fifty percent of the cases of infant drowning occur in the bathtub. In children ages 1 to 4 years, most drownings occur in swimming pools. For children ages 5 to 14 years, most of the drownings occur in rivers and lakes. Alcohol consumption and drug abuse are contributing factors in many cases of drowning involving teenagers and adults.

Drowning is defined as suffocation because of submersion in water or in other fluids. **Submersion injuries** are any injuries that result from being beneath the surface of water or another liquid.

Familiarize yourself with your emergency response area; consider the places a drowning could occur. Likely locations include streams, lakes, and swimming pools. Hot tubs, wading pools, public fountains, and storm drain ponds are also potential locations for drowning. Common hazards for drowning in infants and young children that are present in every household include bathtubs, toilets, and mop buckets. Remember, young children can drown in liquids as shallow as 6 inches (15 cm).

The process of drowning progresses through several stages. Usually, the initial stage is panic as the person realizes that something is wrong, such as a strong current that is overpowering. In other instances, the person becomes fatigued, injured, and cold; becomes entangled in seaweed or kelp; experiences a loss of orientation; or becomes ill.

The feeling of panic produces an inefficient breathing pattern. If a swimmer is not able to take in full breaths, the ability to float is lost, and exhaustion sets in as the person struggles to stay on the surface of the water. Small quantities of water reaching the larynx (voice box) cause a spasm of the larynx (**laryngospasm**), which makes it hard or impossible to breathe. If this cycle of panic is not corrected, respiratory and cardiac arrest can result. Signs and symptoms of a submersion injury include coughing, vomiting, difficulty breathing, respiratory arrest, and cardiac arrest. Some patients who have sustained submersion injuries may have broken bones or spinal injuries from hitting a hard surface. Hypothermia is an added risk when a patient is wet, especially if the water is cold or if the air temperature is low.

Follow the steps of the patient assessment sequence when examining and treating a patient who has sustained a submersion injury. Begin by assessing scene safety. If the patient is still in the water, do not exceed the limits of your training in an attempt to rescue the patient. Keep yourself safe and attempt rescue only if you can do so safely. Use the reach, throw, row, and go sequence outlined in Chapter 20, *Vehicle Extrication and Special Rescue*. Call for additional help if needed. If there is evidence of trauma and you need to move the patient, protect the spine from further injury as described in Chapter 20.

Perform a primary assessment. Correct any airway, breathing, and circulation (ABC) problems. You may need to carefully turn the patient on his or her side to allow water to drain out of the mouth. Begin CPR if indicated. If the patient is breathing adequately, administer high-flow oxygen as soon as it is available. As soon as the ABCs are stabilized, dry the patient because wet skin results in a significant loss of body heat. Then cover the patient with towels or blankets to help preserve body temperature. As soon as possible, perform a secondary assessment to check for other injuries. Obtain the patient's medical history from the patient if possible or from any family members present. Perform regular reassessments.

All patients who have sustained a submersion injury should be examined by a physician. These patients may appear to be uninjured immediately after submersion, but life-threatening respiratory problems can develop hours after the incident. You must arrange to have these

YOU are the Provider   CASE 4

On one of the first warm days of the summer, you and your family are enjoying a restful day at a small lake close to your home. As you are finishing a picnic lunch, you hear cries for help coming from the lakefront. A woman shouts that her 11-year-old son has fallen off a small ledge 2 feet (less than 1 m) above the water. As you begin to run toward the cries for help, you can see a boy fighting to keep his head above the surface of the water. As you approach the scene, another bystander reaches out and grabs one of the boy's arms and pulls him to shore.

1. If the boy were still in the water when you arrived at the lakefront what steps would you have taken to rescue him from the water?
2. What steps should you take to provide care for this boy?

patients transported to an appropriate medical facility for a complete examination by a physician.

▶ Cold Water Drowning

You should begin CPR on a drowning victim as long as the patient does not show definitive signs of death discussed in Chapter 4, *Medical, Legal, and Ethical Issues*. When a person is submerged in cold water, a protective mechanism called the *mammalian diving reflex* may be activated. This reflex slows the heart rate and metabolic rate and decreases the body's demand for oxygen. Because of the protection provided by the mammalian diving reflex, there have been cases in which a person has been in cold water for longer than 30 minutes and has been successfully resuscitated and recovered to a normal level of physical and mental functioning. Therefore, when you encounter a person who has been submerged in cold water even for an extended period, CPR should be started and continued until the person has been delivered to an appropriate medical facility. Resuscitating a cold water drowning patient often requires warming the patient in the hospital while continuing CPR.

Words of Wisdom

Do not put your life at risk by exceeding the limits of your training.

■ Other Environmental Emergencies

▶ Lightning Injuries

Lightning injuries are sometimes classified as environmental emergencies because they have an environmental cause. The electrical injury resulting from a lightning strike can cause cardiac irregularities or cardiac arrest. Treat patients who have been struck by lightning by supporting their ABCs. Oxygen administration, defibrillation, and CPR may be needed for some patients. Because there is a chance of cardiac problems occurring hours after the injury, it is important that patients who have been struck by lightning are transported to an appropriate medical facility for examination and treatment.

Lightning injuries also cause electrical burns. This type of burn is mainly internal and the extent of burn damage will not be visible right after the injury occurs. For this reason, it is also important to transport all patients who have been struck by lightning to an appropriate medical facility. Electrical burns are discussed in Chapter 14, *Bleeding, Shock, and Soft-Tissue Injuries*.

▶ Bites and Stings

Bites and stings are sometimes classified as environmental injuries. They are discussed in detail under the topic of poisoning in Chapter 11, *Poisoning and Substance Abuse*.

YOU ▶ are the Provider   SUMMARY

You are the Provider: CASE 1

1. **As you evaluate the patient's symptoms and the signs she exhibits, what do you think is most likely wrong with this patient?**

   The signs and symptoms of this patient seem to indicate that she may be experiencing heat exhaustion.

2. **What steps should you take to treat this patient?**

   The first step in treating this patient is to perform the patient assessment sequence to determine what problems the patient is experiencing. Ensure the scene is safe. Perform a primary assessment to determine the patient's level of responsiveness and assess the state of her airway, breathing, and circulation (ABCs). Obtain the patient's medical history and vital signs and complete the secondary assessment. The patient's signs and symptoms are consistent with heat exhaustion. Be alert for additional signs and symptoms that might indicate other conditions such as heart problems (eg, a heart attack or other medical conditions). Your treatment should include the following: remove or dry wet clothing. Try to get the patient in a place that has a comfortable temperature, and place the patient in a position of comfort (sitting or lying down). Slowly give water or other fluid with electrolytes if available. Finally, reassess the condition of the patient and arrange for transport to an appropriate medical facility.

You are the Provider: CASE 2

1. **What signs would indicate this runner is experiencing heat exhaustion or heatstroke?**

   This patient is showing signs and symptoms of a more serious heat illness, heatstroke. The patient has an altered level of consciousness, and his skin is red, hot, and flushed. Because he was running prior to the illness, his skin may still be moist.

2. After completing the primary assessment, what is the most appropriate treatment for this runner?

This patient needs immediate medical treatment. You should initiate rapid cooling by removing the patient's clothing down to his underwear and placing ice bags around the groin and in the armpits. Fanning the patient may help if the humidity and temperature are not too high. Run cool water over the patient if available. In the field it is very difficult to successfully cool a patient experiencing heatstroke. This patient needs continued assessment and immediate transport to a medical facility for more aggressive cooling.

You are the Provider: CASE 3

1. What is your initial treatment for this patient?

This patient needs to be warmed immediately to prevent further heat loss. After the primary assessment, the patient should be wrapped in blankets to help his body temperature return to a more normal level. Although he does not appear to have suffered any injuries, you cannot be sure given his current state of confusion. You should ask if anyone present is familiar with the medical history of the patient. Look for any medications that EMS might take to the hospital. When EMS arrives, the patient should be gently transported to the medical facility for more aggressive warming and monitoring. Handle the patient carefully to avoid causing cardiac dysrhythmias.

2. What other conditions might be causing these symptoms?

From the limited information available to you, it appears this patient is suffering from hypothermia. The actions described above are helpful in beginning to warm the patient to a more normal body temperature. It is important that this patient be transported to an appropriate medical facility for further testing to determine the underlying cause of his condition. This patient may have suffered a stroke, a cardiac dysrhythmia, a diabetic emergency, or a seizure. He may have forgotten to take his prescribed medication, or he may have taken an incorrect dosage. As an EMR, you do not have sufficient training or equipment to determine the underlying cause of his hypothermia, but you must take the initial steps to rewarm this patient and arrange for his prompt transport to an appropriate medical facility for further warming and treatment.

You are the Provider: CASE 4

1. If the boy had still been in the water when you arrived at the lakefront, what steps would you have taken to rescue him from the water?

When you are on the scene of any emergency as it is happening, remember to call for assistance as soon as possible. In this instance, you might have another family member, or bystander, call 9-1-1 as you rush to the scene. During water rescues, ensure your safety as well as the safety of the person in distress. Do not put your life in danger if there is little chance of saving a person. Also keep in mind your training and limitations. Follow the Reach, Throw, Row, and Go steps. Think first of reaching out to rescue the person. Extend your reach with any available object like a tree branch or ball bat. If you are not able to reach the person in distress, find a floatable object such as a ring buoy or improvise with any floatable object such as an almost empty jug or a picnic cooler. If this is not possible, see if any type of small boat is available. Only as a final resort, should you ever consider entering the water to rescue another person. In this case, an extended arm was enough to rescue this boy from the water.

2. What steps should you take to provide care for this boy?

As soon as the patient has been removed from the water, begin to assess his airway, breathing, and circulation (ABCs). If he has water in his mouth or throat, turn his head to the side to drain any retained water from his mouth. Support his ABCs as necessary. Since it is early summer, the water in the lake is probably cold. Therefore, it is especially important to remove all his wet clothing as soon as possible and cover him with any available dry clothing, tablecloths, or blankets that are available. Examine the patient for any injuries and treat as necessary. Obtain a medical history from the patient or his mother. Confirm EMS has been called and is responding to your location. Explain to the boy's mother that he may need to be transported to an appropriate medical facility for warming and for further treatment because of the possibility of delayed symptoms from his submersion into the cold water. Do not forget to always explain what you are doing to patients and their family members and to provide them with reassurance.

Prep Kit

▶ Ready for Review

- Your approach to a patient who has experienced an environmental emergency should follow the patient assessment sequence.
- Heat cramps are caused by electrolyte imbalance and dehydration. They usually involve muscles in the calf, leg, or abdomen. Usually the cramps disappear with rest and the administration of water.
- A person experiencing heat exhaustion sweats profusely and becomes light-headed, dizzy, and nauseated. Certain risk factors may make some people more susceptible to heat-related illnesses.
- Heatstroke results when a person has been in a hot environment for a long period, overwhelming the body's sweating mechanism. The patient's body temperature rises until it reaches a level at which brain damage occurs.
- The body parts most susceptible to frostbite are the face, ears, fingers, and toes. Warming the frostbitten part must be done quickly and carefully.
- Hypothermia occurs when a person's body is not able to produce enough heat to keep the internal (core) body temperature at a satisfactory level.
- The initial signs of hypothermia include feeling cold, shivering, decreasing level of consciousness, and sleepiness. Signs of increasing hypothermia include a lack of coordination, mental confusion, and slowed reactions.
- Hypothermic patients should never be considered dead until they have been warmed in an appropriate medical facility.
- Drowning can occur in a variety of settings around a home and outdoors. Signs and symptoms of a submersion injury include coughing, vomiting, difficulty breathing, respiratory arrest, cardiac arrest, and trauma.
- Lightning injuries are caused by a powerful jolt of electrical current that passes through part of the body. They may cause irregular heart rhythms or cardiac arrest. They also cause an electrical type of burn that damages tissue within the body.

▶ Vital Vocabulary

drowning Suffocation because of submersion in water or other fluids.

frostbite Partial or complete freezing of the skin and deeper tissues caused by exposure to the cold.

heat cramps Painful muscle spasms that usually occur after vigorous exercise in hot weather and are generally relieved by rest and drinking water.

heat exhaustion A form of shock that occurs from significant fluid loss and too many electrolytes through very heavy sweating after exposure to heat.

heatstroke A condition of rapidly rising internal body temperature that occurs when the body's mechanisms for the release of heat are overwhelmed. Untreated heatstroke can result in death.

hypothermia A condition in which the internal (or core) body temperature falls below 95°F (35°C) after prolonged exposure to cool or freezing temperatures.

laryngospasm A spasm of the muscles of the larynx or vocal cords resulting in an inability to breathe.

submersion injury An injury resulting from being beneath the surface of water or another liquid.

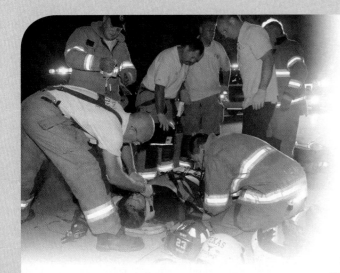

Assessment
in Action

You are dispatched to a residence for the report of a possible drowning. As you are responding, your dispatcher reports the patient is a 37-year-old man who has been removed from the backyard swimming pool. The dispatcher reports the police were called to this residence earlier in the evening for the report of a noisy party. When you arrive at the scene, you find your patient lying on the pool deck. He is pale and unresponsive.

1. Which of the following contributing factors should you consider as you examine and treat this patient?

   A. Possible injuries
   B. Possible alcohol or drug use
   C. The patient's age and size
   D. Possible injuries and possible alcohol or drug use

2. What added step in clearing the airway is sometimes needed in drowning situations?

   A. Rinse out the patient's mouth.
   B. Place a towel under the patient's shoulders.
   C. Roll the patient onto one side to allow water to drain out of the mouth.
   D. Place a towel under the patient's head.

3. In submersion injuries, small quantities of water reaching the voice box cause a(n) _____, which makes it hard or impossible to breathe.

   A. oropharynx block
   B. laryngospasm
   C. nasopharynx spasm
   D. tracheal spasm

4. Which of the following persons is at the highest risk for hypothermia?

   A. A person wearing cotton shorts and a T-shirt on a dry, windless 70°F (21°C) day
   B. A person sitting in the warm sun in a bathing suit
   C. A person wearing cotton jeans and a T-shirt on a rainy, windy 60°F (16°C) day
   D. A person running in a marathon with an outside temperature of 67°F (19°C)

5. What environmental condition is of concern in a situation that involves drowning?

   A. Heatstroke
   B. Heat exhaustion
   C. Hyperthermia
   D. Hypothermia

6. The mammalian diving reflex is activated when:

   A. the person has been under the water for a long time.
   B. the person is young.
   C. the water is cold.
   D. the water is warmer than the body temperature.

Assessment *in Action* Continued

7. Which of the following is NOT a sign of deep frostbite?

    A. Skin remains soft.
    B. Skin is white and waxy.
    C. Blisters may be present.
    D. Swelling may be present.

8. What are the typical stages in the drowning process?

9. Why should a person who has been submerged in cold water and is pulseless, not breathing, and cold *not* be pronounced dead at the scene?

10. Discuss the different signs and symptoms for early and late hypothermia.

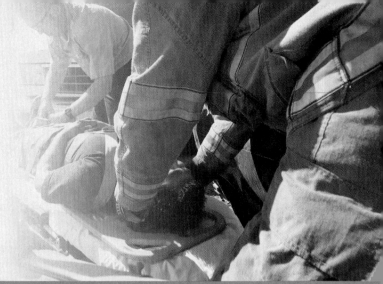

SECTION 5

Trauma

Bleeding, Shock, and Soft-Tissue Injuries

Skills Objectives

■ Introduction

This chapter presents the skills you need to recognize and care for patients who are experiencing shock, are bleeding, or have soft-tissue injuries. Because most soft-tissue injuries result in bleeding, maintaining good standard precautions is important when you are caring for patients with these types of injuries. The chapter describes four types of soft-tissue wounds: abrasions, lacerations, punctures, and avulsions. Techniques for controlling external bleeding are discussed, and you will learn the various techniques for dressing and bandaging wounds.

Damage to internal soft tissues and organs can cause life-threatening conditions. Internal bleeding causes blood loss in the circulatory system and results in shock. **Shock** is a state of collapse of the cardiovascular system that results in inadequate delivery of blood to the organs. More trauma patients die from shock than from any other condition. Your ability to recognize the signs and symptoms of shock and to take simple measures to aid shock patients will give them the best chance for survival. This chapter explains the causes and types of shock using an analogy of a pump, pipes, and fluid. You will learn how the failure of any part of the system can cause shock.

Burns are another type of soft-tissue injury. Burns may be caused by heat, chemicals, or electricity. They may damage any part of the body and are especially harmful if they occur inside the respiratory tract. This chapter examines the extent, depth, and cause of burns.

As you study this chapter, keep in mind the importance of maintaining standard precautions to prevent the spread of disease-carrying organisms.

Patient Assessment for Bleeding, Shock, and Soft-Tissue Injuries

It is important to follow the steps of the patient assessment sequence described in Chapter 9, *Patient Assessment*, when caring for patients who are bleeding, are in shock, or have soft-tissue injuries. Your scene size-up needs to include all the steps you learned previously to ensure safety for you and your patient. When performing the primary assessment, you may need to temporarily halt the assessment if the patient is losing a significant amount of blood. However, once you have managed this problem, you should immediately return to completing the assessment sequence, performing all the remaining steps to ensure no problems or injuries are overlooked.

During your secondary assessment, be alert for any signs and symptoms of shock from internal or external blood loss. When obtaining a SAMPLE history, ask the patient whether he or she is using a blood thinner, which may interfere with blood clotting. When performing a reassessment, watch the patient for signs and symptoms of shock such as pale skin, increasing pulse rate, or decreasing blood pressure.

For trauma patients, you will usually perform the secondary assessment before you obtain the SAMPLE history. Review the patient assessment sequence shown in Figure 14-1 .

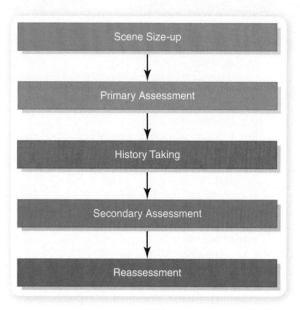

Figure 14-1 Patient assessment sequence. For trauma patients, you may perform the secondary assessment before obtaining a SAMPLE history.
© Jones & Bartlett Learning.

Safety

Most soft-tissue injuries involve some degree of bleeding. Always maintain standard precautions when you approach a patient with a potential soft-tissue injury.

Standard Precautions and Soft-Tissue Injuries

The concept of standard precautions assumes all body fluids are potentially infectious. Therefore, take appropriate measures to prevent contact with the patient's body fluids. Wear gloves to prevent contact with the patient's blood when caring for patients who have soft-tissue injuries. At times, you may also need to wear a surgical mask and eye protection if there is danger of blood splatter from a massive wound or if the patient is coughing or vomiting bloody material.

Parts and Function of the Circulatory System

The three parts of the circulatory system are the pump (heart), the pipes (arteries, veins, and capillaries), and the fluid (blood cells and other blood components). Figure 14-2 presents a schematic illustration of the circulatory system.

YOU are the Provider   CASE 1

On a crisp autumn day, you are dispatched for a report of an injured carpenter at the site of a new house under construction. As you are responding, the dispatcher informs you that your patient is a 38-year-old man who has cut his leg with a circular saw. He is "actively bleeding" from the wound.

1. What safety considerations should you keep in mind as you approach this situation?
2. What equipment and supplies do you want to take with you?
3. What are your treatment goals for this incident?

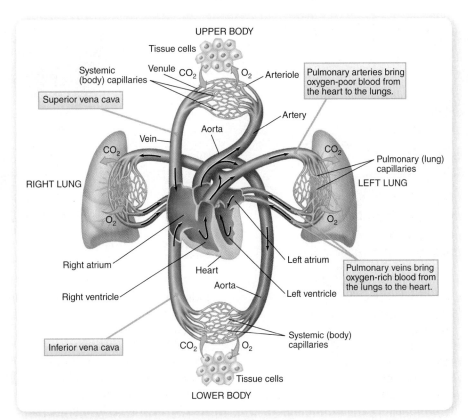

Figure 14-2 The circulatory system includes the heart, arteries, veins, and capillaries. At the center of the system is the heart, which pumps the blood.
© Jones & Bartlett Learning.

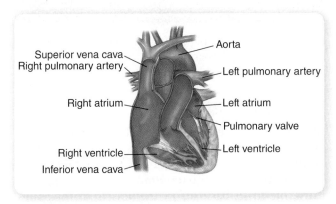

Figure 14-3 The heart functions as the pump of the human circulatory system.
© Jones & Bartlett Learning.

▶ The Pump

The heart functions as the human circulatory system's pump. The heart consists of four separate chambers: the two upper chambers on the top of the heart are called the left and right **atria** (a single chamber is called an atrium), and the two lower chambers on the bottom of the heart are called the left and right **ventricles**. The ventricles are the larger chambers and do most of the actual pumping. The atria are somewhat less muscular and serve as reservoirs for blood flowing into the heart from the body and the lungs **Figure 14-3** .

▶ The Pipes

The human body has three main types of blood vessels: arteries, capillaries, and veins. The arteries (big-flow, heavy-duty, high-pressure pipes) carry blood away from the heart. The capillaries (distribution pipes), the smallest of the blood vessels, form a network that distributes blood to all parts of the body. The smallest capillaries are so narrow that blood cells have to flow through them single file. The veins return the blood from the capillaries to the heart, where it is pumped to the lungs. There, the blood gives off carbon dioxide and absorbs oxygen **Figure 14-4** .

▶ The Fluid

Fluid in the circulatory system consists of blood cells and other blood components, each with a specific function. The liquid part of the blood is known as plasma. Plasma serves as the transporting medium for the solid parts of the blood, which are the red blood cells, white blood cells, and platelets. Red blood cells carry oxygen and carbon dioxide **Figure 14-5** . White blood cells have a "search and destroy" function. They consume bacteria and viruses to combat infections in the body. Platelets interact with each other and with other substances in the blood to form clots that help stop bleeding.

▶ Pulse

A pulse is the pressure wave generated by the pumping action of the heart. With each heartbeat, there is a surge

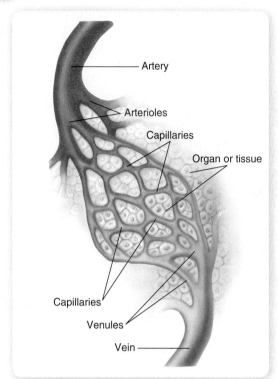

Figure 14-4 Blood enters an organ or tissue through the arteries and leaves through the veins.
© Jones & Bartlett Learning.

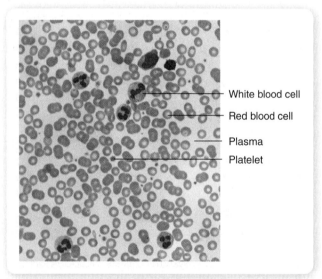

Figure 14-5 The components of blood.
© Donna Beer Stolz, PhD, Center for Biologic Imaging, University of Pittsburgh Medical School.

of blood from the left ventricle as it contracts and pushes blood out into the main arteries of the body. When you are counting the number of pulsations per minute, what you are actually counting is each heartbeat per minute. In other words, the pulse rate reflects the heart rate.

Usually you can feel a patient's radial and carotid pulses. In a conscious patient, you can easily find the radial (wrist) pulse at the base of the thumb. If the patient is unconscious, experiencing shock, or both, it may be impossible for you to feel a radial pulse. Therefore, it is vital that you know how to locate the carotid (neck)

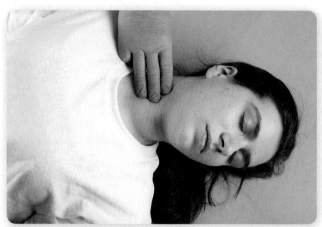

Figure 14-6 Taking the carotid pulse.
© Jones & Bartlett Learning.

pulse. If the patient appears to be in shock or is unconscious, attempt to locate the carotid pulse first. To locate the carotid pulse, place two fingers lightly on the larynx and slide the fingers off to one side until you feel a slight notch on the neck. You should be able to feel the carotid pulse at this location ▸ Figure 14-6 ◂. Practice locating the carotid pulse of another person in a dark room. You should be able to locate the pulse within 3 seconds of touching the person's larynx.

▣ Shock

Shock is failure of the circulatory system. Circulatory failure has many possible causes, but the three primary causes are discussed here.

▶ Pump Failure

Cardiogenic shock occurs if the heart cannot pump enough blood to supply the needs of the body. Pump failure can result if the heart has been weakened by a heart attack. Inadequate pumping of the heart can cause blood to back up in the vessels of the lungs, resulting in a condition known as **congestive heart failure (CHF)**.

▶ Pipe Failure

Pipe failure is caused by the expansion (dilation) of the capillaries to as much as three or four times their normal size. This causes blood to pool in the capillaries, instead of circulating throughout the system. When blood pools in the capillaries, the rest of the body, including the heart and other vital organs, is deprived of blood. Blood pressure falls and shock results. **Blood pressure** is the pressure of the circulating blood against the walls of the arteries.

In shock caused by sudden expansion of the capillaries, blood pressure may drop so rapidly in your patient that you are unable to feel either a radial or a carotid pulse.

Special Populations

In an infant, check the brachial (upper arm) pulse instead of the carotid pulse.

The least serious type of shock caused by pipe failure is fainting. Fainting, a form of **psychogenic shock**, is the body's response to a major psychological or emotional stress. As the nervous system reacts, the capillaries suddenly expand to three or four times their normal size. Blood then pools in the dilated vessels, resulting in reduced blood supply to the brain. Fainting is a short-term condition that corrects itself once the patient is placed in a horizontal position.

Anaphylactic shock is caused by an extreme allergic reaction to a foreign substance, such as venom from bee stings (see Chapter 11, *Poisoning and Substance Abuse*), penicillin, or certain foods. Shock may develop very quickly following exposure. The patient may suddenly start to sneeze or itch, a rash or hives may appear, the face and tongue may swell very quickly, and a blue color may appear around the mouth. The patient appears flushed (red) and breathing may quickly become difficult, with wheezing sounds coming from the chest. Blood pressure drops rapidly as the blood pools in the expanded capillaries. The pulse may be so weak that you cannot feel it. Pipe failure has occurred and death will result if prompt action to counteract the toxin is not taken.

Spinal shock may occur in patients who have sustained a spinal cord injury. The injury to the spinal cord allows the capillaries to expand, and blood pools below the level of the injury. The brain, heart, lungs, and other vital organs are deprived of blood, resulting in shock.

Words of Wisdom

Three types of shock caused by capillary expansion are as follows:

1. Shock induced by fainting
2. Anaphylactic shock
3. Spinal shock

▶ Fluid Loss

The third general type of shock is caused by fluid loss. Fluid loss caused by excessive bleeding (**hemorrhage**) is the most common cause of shock. Blood escapes from the normally closed circulatory system through an internal or external wound, and the system's total fluid level (blood volume) drops until the pump cannot operate efficiently. To compensate for fluid loss, the heart begins to pump faster to maintain pressure in the pipes. However, as the fluid continues to drain out, the pump eventually stops pumping altogether, resulting in cardiac arrest.

External bleeding is not difficult to detect because you can see blood escaping from the circulatory system to the outside of the patient's body. With internal bleeding, blood escapes from the system, but usually the bleeding cannot be seen. However, you may see signs of internal blood loss, such as bruising, swelling, and rigidity in the affected area. If the patient is conscious, he or she may report severe pain in the immediate area. Even though the escaped blood remains inside the body, it cannot reenter the circulatory system and it is not available to be pumped by the heart. Whether the bleeding is external or internal, if it remains unchecked, the result will be shock, eventual pump failure, and death.

An average adult has about 12 pints (6 L) of blood circulating in the system. The loss of a single pint of blood will not produce shock in a healthy adult. In fact, 1 pint (0.5 L) per donor is the amount that blood banks collect. However, the loss of 2 or more pints (1 L or more) of blood can produce shock. This amount of blood loss can result from such injuries as a fractured femur. **Figure 14-7** shows the amount of blood loss that can result from various injuries.

▶ Signs and Symptoms of Shock

Shock deprives the body of sufficient blood to function normally. As shock progresses, the body alters some of its functions in an attempt to maintain sufficient blood supply to its vital parts. A patient who is in shock may exhibit some or all of the signs and symptoms shown in the box below. Initially, the patient's breathing may

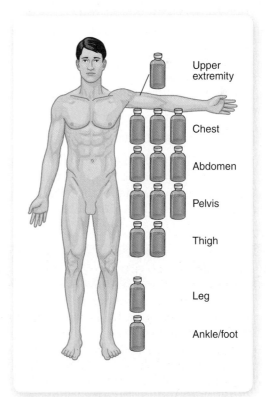

Figure 14-7 Potential blood loss from injuries in various parts of the body. Each bottle equals 1 pint (473 mL).
© Jones & Bartlett Learning.

be rapid and deep, but as shock progresses in severity, breathing becomes rapid and shallow.

Changes in mental status may be the first signs of shock; therefore, monitoring the overall mental status of a patient can help you detect shock. Any change in mental status may be significant. In severe cases of shock, the patient loses consciousness. If a trauma patient who has been quiet suddenly becomes agitated, restless, and vocal, you should suspect shock. If a trauma patient who has been loud, vocal, and aggressive becomes quiet, you should also suspect shock and begin treatment. If the patient has dark skin, you may not be able to use skin color changes to help you detect shock. Therefore, be especially alert for other signs of shock. The capillary refill test and the condition of the skin (cool and clammy) will help you recognize shock in patients who have dark skin.

Signs and Symptoms

Signs and symptoms of shock include:

- Confusion, agitation, restlessness, or anxiety
- Cold, clammy, sweaty, pale skin
- Rapid, shallow breathing
- Rapid, weak pulse
- Increased capillary refill time
- Nausea or vomiting
- Weakness or fainting
- Thirst

▶ General Treatment for Shock

As an emergency medical responder (EMR), you can combat shock from any cause and keep it from getting worse by taking several simple but important steps. Remember that the protocols for use of these skills may vary. Always follow the protocols approved by your medical director.

Position the Patient Correctly

If the patient has no head injury, extreme discomfort, or difficulty breathing, place the patient flat on his or her back (supine) on a horizontal surface. Place a blanket under the patient, if available. Elevate the patient's legs according to local protocol. If the patient has a head injury, spine injury, or lower extremity injury, position the patient flat on his or her back. If the patient is having chest pain or difficulty breathing (which is likely to occur in cases of heart attack and emphysema) and no spinal injury is suspected, place the patient in a sitting or semireclining position.

Treatment

Follow these steps for the general treatment of shock:

1. Position the patient correctly.
2. Maintain the patient's ABCs.
3. Treat the cause of shock, if possible.
4. Maintain the patient's body temperature by placing blankets under and over the patient.
5. Ensure the patient does not eat or drink anything.
6. Assist with other treatments (such as administering oxygen, if available).
7. Arrange for immediate and prompt transport to an appropriate medical facility.

Treatment

Do not allow a patient in shock to stand!

Maintain the Patient's ABCs

Check the patient's airway, breathing, and circulation (ABCs) at least every 5 minutes. If necessary, open the airway, perform rescue breathing, or begin cardiopulmonary resuscitation (CPR).

Treat the Cause of Shock, if Possible

Most patients who are in shock must be treated in the hospital, with care provided by specially trained physicians. However, you are able to treat one common cause of shock—external bleeding. By controlling external bleeding with direct pressure, elevation, tourniquet, or **pressure points**, you can treat this cause of shock temporarily until the patient can be transported to an appropriate medical facility for more advanced treatment.

YOU ▶ are the Provider   CASE 2

At 1515 hours you are dispatched to a residential neighborhood for a report of a gunshot wound. As you are responding, your dispatcher reports the police are on the scene, and they report it appears to be an accidental discharge. As you arrive on the scene, a sheriff's deputy takes you to the basement where you find a 43-year-old man sitting in a chair. He is holding his hand on his right thigh. There is blood seeping around his hand and some blood on the floor. A police officer has taken possession of the gun. There are no other weapons in sight. You cut off his trousers from around the gunshot wound. There is a small wound in the middle of his thigh that is moderately bleeding. You cannot locate an exit wound.

1. What are your initial steps in treating this patient?
2. How serious is an injury like this?

Maintain the Patient's Body Temperature

Attempt to keep the patient comfortably warm. A patient with cold, clammy skin should be covered. It is as important to place blankets under the patient to keep body heat from escaping into the ground as it is to cover the patient with blankets.

Do Not Allow the Patient to Eat or Drink

Even though a patient in shock is often very thirsty, do not give liquids by mouth. There are two reasons for this rule:

1. A patient in shock may be nauseated and eating or drinking may cause vomiting.
2. A patient in shock may need emergency surgery. Patients should not have anything in their stomachs before surgery.

If you are working in an area where ambulance response time is more than 20 minutes, you may give patients a clean cloth or gauze pad that has been soaked in water to suck on. This relieves dryness of the mouth but does not quench thirst. No matter how thirsty patients are, do not permit them to drink anything.

> **Treatment**
>
> In the summer or in hot environments, it is not necessary to cover every shock patient with blankets. You are trying to maintain body heat, not produce more.

Assist With Other Treatments

When an advanced life support (ALS) unit arrives at the scene, be ready to assist them with further treatment. Patients may be given oxygen or IV solutions. If you are trained in the administration of oxygen and have it available, provide it to shock patients. Oxygen benefits shock patients by ensuring that the reduced number of red blood cells are as oxygen saturated as they can be.

Advanced emergency medical technicians (AEMTs) or paramedics can administer **intravenous (IV) fluids**. Adding fluid to the body combats the loss of blood volume. Although rare, some emergency medical services (EMS) personnel sometimes use **pneumatic anti-shock garments (PASGs)** in the field to treat pelvic fractures; however, PASGs are no longer favored for shock treatment. PASGs are placed around the patient's legs and abdomen and inflated with air. As the PASG inflates, it exerts pressure around the legs and abdomen. Although, as an EMR, you will not use these devices yourself, you should know their purpose and function. It is also important to understand that PASGs must not be removed in the field. Removing PASGs must be done in a hospital and under the direct supervision of a physician.

Arrange for Transport

As soon as you determine that you have a patient who is in shock, make sure an ambulance has been dispatched. When the ambulance arrives, give EMS personnel a concise handoff report, emphasizing the signs and symptoms of shock that you noted. The EMS personnel will then ensure the patient is quickly prepared for *prompt transport* to an appropriate medical facility that can handle a patient with this type of condition. Usually, the most appropriate treatment for a patient in shock that is the result of injury or bleeding is surgical repair, and the sooner the patient gets to the hospital, the better the chance of his or her survival.

> **Words of Wisdom**
>
> A quiet patient is often a patient who is in shock. Other times, when you have a patient who suddenly becomes agitated, shock may be developing. Watch all patients carefully for signs of shock!

▶ Treatment for Shock Caused by Pump Failure

Patients experiencing pump failure may be confused, restless, anxious, or unconscious. Their pulse is usually rapid and weak, and their skin is cold and clammy, sweaty, and pale. Their respirations are often rapid and shallow. Pump failure is a serious condition. Your proper treatment and *prompt transport* by ambulance to an appropriate medical facility will give these patients their best chance for survival.

▶ Treatment for Shock Caused by Pipe Failure

Patients who have fainted, who are experiencing anaphylactic shock, or who have sustained a severe spinal cord injury will have pipe failure. Their capillaries may increase three or four times the normal size, causing signs and symptoms of shock.

Treatment for Anaphylactic Shock

The initial treatment for anaphylactic shock is similar to the treatment for any other type of shock. Anaphylactic shock is an extreme emergency, and the patient must be transported as soon as possible. Paramedics, nurses, and physicians can administer medications that may reverse the allergic reaction. Some patients who have severe allergies may carry an epinephrine auto-injector. If the patient has a prescribed auto-injector, you can administer the epinephrine if you have been trained in its use and have permission from your local medical director. Be aware of and follow your local protocols. Support the patient's thigh and place the tip of the auto-injector lightly against the outer thigh. Using a quick motion, push the auto-injector firmly against the thigh and hold it in place for several seconds. This will inject the medication. The detailed steps for administering epinephrine by auto-injector are outlined in Chapter 11, *Poisoning and Substance Abuse.*

▶ Treatment for Shock Caused by Fluid Loss

Shock may be caused by internal blood loss (blood that escapes from damaged blood vessels and stays inside the body) or by external blood loss (blood that escapes from the body). Excessive bleeding is the most common cause of shock.

Signs and Symptoms

Signs and symptoms of internal bleeding include the following:

- Coughing or vomiting of blood
- Abdominal tenderness, rigidity, bruising, or distention
- Rectal bleeding
- Vaginal bleeding in women
- Classic signs of shock

Shock Caused by Internal Blood Loss

Patients can die quickly and quietly from internal bleeding following abdominal injuries that rupture the spleen, liver, or large blood vessels. You must be alert to detect the earliest signs and symptoms of internal bleeding and to begin treatment for shock. If you are treating several injured patients, those with internal bleeding should be transported first to the medical facility because immediate surgery may be needed. (Chapter 19, *Transport Operations*, discusses how to decide which patients should receive care first.)

Bleeding from stomach ulcers, ruptured blood vessels, or tumors can cause internal bleeding and shock. This bleeding can be spontaneous, massive, and rapid, often leading to the loss of large quantities of blood by vomiting or bloody diarrhea.

It is important to recognize the signs and symptoms of internal bleeding and take prompt corrective action. In addition to the classic signs of shock (confusion, rapid pulse, cold and clammy skin, and rapid breathing), patients with internal bleeding may show additional signs and symptoms as depicted in the Signs and Symptoms box on this page.

Treatment

You cannot stop internal bleeding. You can only treat its symptoms and arrange for the patient to be promptly transported to an appropriate medical facility.

■ Bleeding

Blood loss can occur through external bleeding, which is visible, or through internal bleeding, which can be hard to detect. It ranges from minor cuts to massive blood loss that can kill a person in a few minutes. As an EMR, it is important for you to be able to recognize the signs and symptoms of external bleeding and internal bleeding. It is also important for you to know what steps to take to control bleeding and what care you can administer for patients who are experiencing internal blood loss and shock.

Words of Wisdom

Patients who regularly consume large quantities of alcohol are at high risk for internal bleeding. Heavy alcohol consumption damages the liver and reduces the production of clotting factors and platelets. Because platelets are needed for blood coagulation and clotting, these patients can experience life-threatening internal bleeding from relatively minor injuries. According to the Centers for Disease Control and Prevention (CDC), in 2013, 36,427 deaths were reported from liver failure. Remember that patients with liver disease are at a high risk for bleeding because liver disease interferes with blood clotting.

Alcohol also irritates the digestive system, which makes patients with alcoholism more likely to experience life-threatening bleeding from the esophagus or stomach.

▶ Controlling External Blood Loss

This section describes how to control external blood loss using direct pressure, elevation, tourniquets, and pressure points. Follow your local protocols for bleeding control. Some protocols may not permit the use of all these methods. They are all included because each technique may be beneficial to patients under certain circumstances.

There are three types of external blood loss: capillary, venous, and arterial **Figure 14-8**. The most common type of external blood loss is **capillary bleeding**. In capillary bleeding, the blood oozes out (such as from a cut finger). You can control capillary bleeding simply by applying direct pressure to the site.

The next most common type of bleeding is **venous bleeding**. This type of bleeding has a steady flow. Bleeding from a large vein may be profuse and life threatening. To control venous bleeding, apply direct pressure to the site for at least 5 minutes.

The most serious type of bleeding is **arterial bleeding**. Arterial blood spurts or surges from the laceration or wound with each heartbeat. Blood pressure in arteries is higher than in capillaries or veins, and unchecked arterial bleeding can result in death from loss of blood in a short time. To control arterial bleeding, exert and

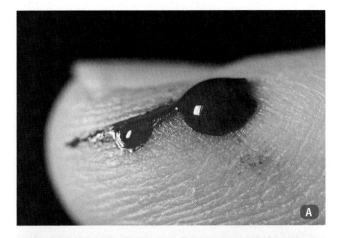

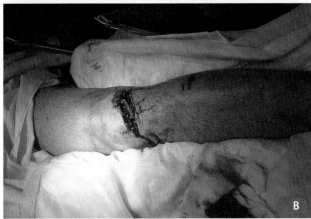

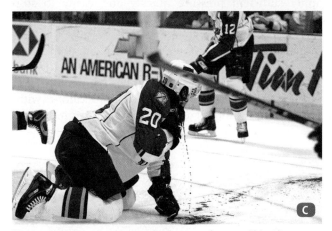

Figure 14-8 Recognizing the three types of external bleeding. **A.** Capillary **B.** Venous **C.** Arterial.

A: Sasha Radosavljevic/iStock/Getty; B: © E. M. Singletary, MD. Used with permission; C: © Brian Slichta/ AP Photo.

maintain direct pressure on the site, sufficient to stop the flow of blood, until EMS arrives. If available and permitted under your local protocol, apply a tourniquet between the heart and the site of the arterial bleeding.

Because many injured patients actually die from shock caused by blood loss, it is vitally important that you control external bleeding quickly.

Treatment

Follow these steps to treat shock caused by pump failure:

1. Keep the patient lying down unless the patient is able to breathe easier in a sitting position.
2. Maintain the patient's ABCs. Be prepared to perform CPR, if necessary.
3. Maintain the patient's normal body temperature.
4. Ensure the patient does not eat or drink anything.
5. Keep the patient quiet and do any necessary moving for him or her.
6. Provide reassurance.
7. Arrange for *prompt transport* by ambulance to an appropriate medical facility.
8. Provide high-flow oxygen as soon as it is available.

Follow these steps to treat shock caused by pipe failure:

Fainting

1. Examine the patient to ensure there is no injury.
2. Keep the patient lying down and elevate the legs if indicated by local protocol.
3. Maintain the ABCs.
4. Maintain the patient's normal body temperature.
5. Provide reassurance.

Anaphylactic Shock

1. Keep the patient lying down and elevate the legs if indicated by local protocol.
2. If the patient has an epinephrine auto-injector, help the patient use it if indicated by local protocol.
3. Maintain the patient's ABCs. Anaphylactic shock may cause airway swelling. In severe reactions, the patient may require mouth-to-mask breathing or full CPR.
4. Maintain the patient's normal body temperature.
5. Provide reassurance.
6. Arrange for *rapid transport* by ambulance to an appropriate medical facility.

Spinal Shock

1. Place the patient on his or her back. Because the spine may be injured, keep the patient's head and neck stabilized to protect the spinal cord (see Chapter 15, *Injuries to Muscles and Bones*).
2. Maintain the patient's ABCs.
3. Maintain the patient's normal body temperature.
4. Ensure the patient does not eat or drink anything.
5. Assist with other treatments. Help other medical providers place the patient on a backboard.

Follow these steps to treat shock caused by fluid loss:

Internal Blood Loss

1. Keep the patient lying down and elevate the legs if indicated by local protocol.
2. Maintain the patient's ABCs.
3. Maintain the patient's normal body temperature.
4. Ensure the patient does not eat or drink anything.
5. Provide reassurance.
6. Keep the patient quiet and do any necessary moving for him or her.
7. Provide high-flow oxygen as soon as it is available.
8. Monitor the patient's vital signs at least every 5 minutes.
9. Arrange for *prompt transport* by ambulance to an appropriate medical facility.

Treatment *Continued*

External Blood Loss

1. Control bleeding by applying direct pressure on the wound, elevating the injured part, and applying a tourniquet if one is available and permitted under your local protocols. Controlling bleeding using one of these methods is the most important step. Maintain standard precautions.
2. Ensure the patient is lying down and elevate the legs if indicated by local protocol.
3. Maintain the patient's ABCs.
4. Maintain the patient's normal body temperature.
5. Ensure the patient does not eat or drink anything.
6. Provide reassurance.
7. Provide high-flow oxygen as soon as it is available.
8. Arrange for *prompt transport* by ambulance to an appropriate medical facility.

Treatment

Three methods of controlling external bleeding are as follows:

1. Apply direct pressure.
2. Elevate the injured body part.
3. Apply a tourniquet if permitted and if available.

Direct Pressure

Most external bleeding can be controlled by applying direct pressure to the wound. Place a dry, sterile **dressing** directly on the wound and apply pressure to the wound with your gloved hand **Figure 14-9**. Wear the gloves from your EMR life support kit. If you do not have a sterile dressing or gauze bandage, use the cleanest cloth available. Wrap the dressing and wound snugly with a roller gauze bandage to maintain direct pressure on the

wound. Do not remove a dressing after you have applied it. If the dressing becomes blood soaked, place another dressing on top of the first and keep them both in place.

Elevation

If direct pressure does not stop external bleeding from an extremity, elevate the injured arm or leg as you maintain direct pressure. Elevation, in conjunction with direct pressure, will usually stop severe bleeding **Figure 14-10**.

Tourniquets

Use tourniquets in any situation where extremity bleeding cannot be easily and immediately controlled by direct pressure or elevation. High-velocity gunshot wounds and explosive devices can sever arteries in the arm or the leg. These types of injuries result in rapid and profound blood loss that lead to death within minutes. These devastating types of wounds occur in military combat situations and in noncombat situations where high-velocity weapons are used by civilians or law enforcement personnel.

Recent military experience in combat situations has resulted in some changes regarding the use of tourniquets. To reduce deaths from these types of wounds, the military has developed and adopted several modern versions of tourniquets that use simple laws of physics to apply sufficient pressure quickly and easily to stop life-threatening bleeding. These updated tourniquets can be applied in less than 1 minute. Because the tourniquets multiply the force you place on them, they require you to use only one hand to apply.

Recent medical research indicates that a tourniquet can be applied and left in place for up to 2 hours without causing additional damage to the injured limb. This

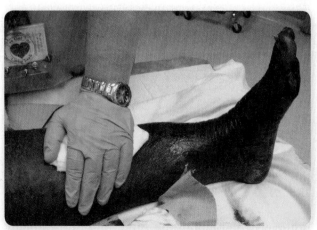

Figure 14-9 Applying direct pressure to a wound.
Courtesy of Rhonda Hunt.

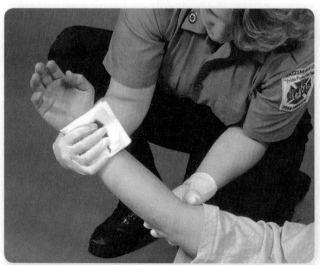

Figure 14-10 Elevate an extremity while maintaining direct pressure to control external bleeding.
© Jones & Bartlett Learning. Courtesy of MIEMSS.

means that the use of tourniquets seems to have great benefit to the patient without incurring a high risk of further damage to the limb.

Some EMS agencies teach their personnel the indications for the use of these tourniquets and how to apply them properly **Figure 14-11**. You should use tourniquets once you have completed proper instruction and have protocols in place that have been approved by your medical director.

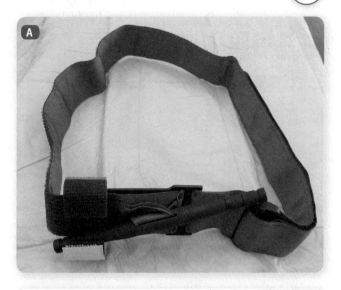

> ## Words of Wisdom
>
> Recent military research has resulted in the development of effective blood clotting or **hemostatic agents**. These are usually impregnated in gauze dressings or supplied as a powder. These agents can be packed into a wound and aid in the formation of a blood clot in a shorter period of time. The use of these clotting agents is usually not recommended for some wounds involving the head, neck, chest, or abdomen. They are useful for extremity wounds and for wounds in junctional areas, such as the groin, shoulder and armpit, or neck, where a tourniquet cannot be applied. Hemostatic agents are carried by some EMS agencies and are carried in special kits by some law enforcement agencies for rapid treatment of gunshot wounds. Use these clotting agents only if you have received special training and are permitted by your local protocols.

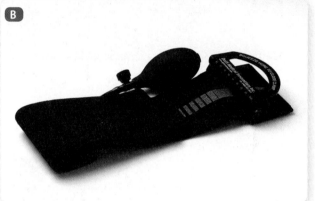

Follow the steps in **Skill Drill 14-1** to control bleeding with a tourniquet:

1. Apply direct pressure with a dry, sterile dressing **Step 1**.
2. Apply a pressure dressing **Step 2**.
3. Apply a tourniquet above the level of bleeding **Step 3**.

Pressure Points

Pressure points should be used for extremity wounds if direct pressure and elevation do not control the bleeding and only if you are not permitted to use a tourniquet (or if a tourniquet is not available). Pressure points can be difficult to use to control hemorrhage and are not always effective. However, using pressure points to attempt to control bleeding requires no special equipment and should be considered in cases where other options are unavailable.

For injuries too near to the body to allow for tourniquet application (for example, injuries that are too proximal or too close to the trunk to apply a tourniquet [junctional injuries]), direct pressure and use of pressure points may be effective. Tourniquets, however, can be improvised when commercially produced options are not available. Options for improvisation include belts and articles of clothing tied around the limb as proximal as possible to the zone of injury. If

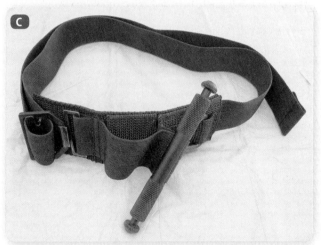

Figure 14-11 Different types of tourniquets used by EMS personnel. **A.** A CAT tourniquet. **B.** An EMT tourniquet. **C.** A SOF-T tourniquet.
A&C: Courtesy of Peter T. Pons, MD, FACEP; B: Courtesy of Delfi Medical Innovations, Inc.

you have a choice between using a pressure point or a tourniquet to control brisk bleeding in an extremity, use the tourniquet because it is more effective and will lessen the chance that the patient will die from serious hemorrhage.

Pressure points may theoretically be able to control bleeding by preventing blood from flowing into a

Skill Drill 14.1

Controlling Bleeding With a Tourniquet

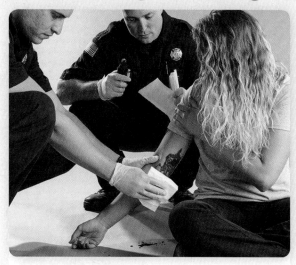

Step 1 Apply direct pressure with a sterile dressing.

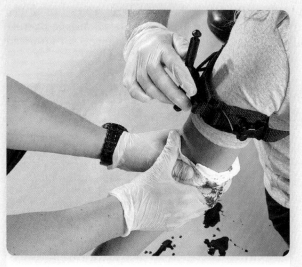

Step 2 Apply a pressure dressing.

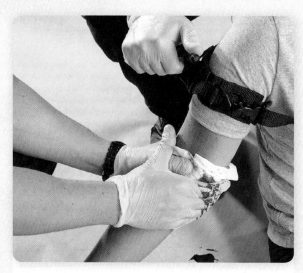

Step 3 If bleeding continues or recurs, apply a tourniquet above the level of bleeding.

© Jones & Bartlett Learning.

limb. This is accomplished by compressing a major artery against the bone at a specific location, a pressure point. Although there are several pressure points in the body, the **brachial artery pressure point** (in the upper arm) and the **femoral artery pressure point** (in the groin) are the most commonly described **Figure 14-12**.

Words of Wisdom

Pressure points should never be used as a tool to control hemorrhage in place of a tourniquet if one is available or if one can be improvised using readily available materials.

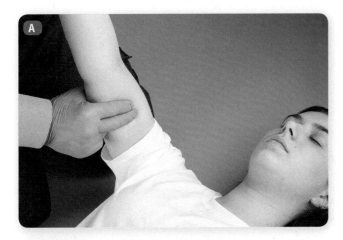

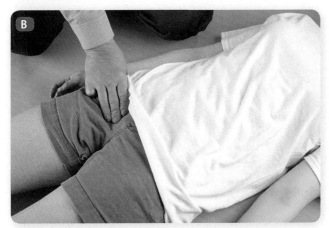

Figure 14-12 The location of the brachial **(A)** and femoral **(B)** pressure points.
A & B: © Jones & Bartlett Learning.

Safety

To prevent coming into contact with any blood that is present, wear gloves and other protective devices as necessary.

When you are applying pressure to the brachial artery, remember the words "slap, slide, and squeeze":

1. Position the patient's arm so the elbow is bent at a right angle (90°) and hold the upper arm away from the patient's body.
2. Gently "slap" the inside of the biceps with your fingers halfway between the shoulder and the elbow to push the biceps out of the way.
3. "Slide" your fingers up to push the biceps away.
4. "Squeeze" (press) your hand down on the humerus (upper arm bone). You should be able to feel the pulse as you press down.

Treatment

Do not hesitate to lean into the pressure point.

If the patient is sitting down, squeeze the arm by placing your fingers halfway between the shoulder and the elbow and your thumb on the opposite side of the patient's arm. If done properly, this technique (in combination with direct wound pressure and elevation) will quickly stop any bleeding below the point of pressure application.

The femoral artery pressure point is more difficult to locate and squeeze. Follow these steps to apply pressure to the femoral artery:

1. Position the patient on his or her back and kneel next to the patient's hips, facing the patient's head. You should be on the side of the patient opposite the extremity that is bleeding.
2. Find the pelvis and place the little finger of your hand closest to the injured leg along the anterior crest on the injured side.
3. Rotate your hand down firmly into the groin area between the genitals and the pelvic bone. This action compresses the femoral artery and usually stops the bleeding, when combined with elevation and direct pressure over the bleeding site.
4. If the bleeding does not slow immediately, reposition your hand and try again.

To effectively apply brachial and femoral pressure points, you must regularly practice each step of these skills.

▶ Standard Precautions and Bleeding Control

Certain communicable diseases such as hepatitis or HIV can be spread by contact with blood from an infected person. This risk is greatly increased when the infected blood comes into contact with a cut or an open sore on your skin. Although your risk of contracting hepatitis or HIV through intact skin is small, you should minimize this risk as much as possible by wearing nitrile or latex gloves whenever you might come in contact with a patient's blood or body fluids Figure 14-13 . Carry your gloves on top of your

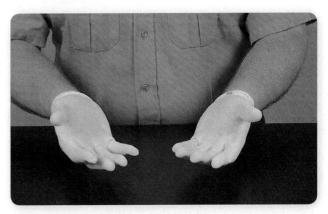

Figure 14-13 Wear gloves to minimize your risk of infection.
© Jones & Bartlett Learning. Courtesy of MIEMSS.

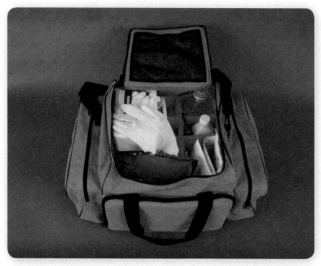

Figure 14-14 Keep your gloves on top in your EMR life support kit or in a pouch on your belt.
© Jones & Bartlett Learning.

EMR life support kit or in a pouch on your belt for quick access **Figure 14-14**. If you do get blood on your hands, wash it off as soon as possible with soap and water. If you are in the field and cannot wash your hands, use a waterless hand-cleaning solution that contains an effective germ-killing agent.

Wounds

A wound is an injury caused by any physical means that leads to damage of a body part. Wounds are classified as closed or open. In a **closed wound**, the skin remains intact; in an **open wound**, the skin is disrupted.

▶ Closed Wounds

The only closed wound is the **bruise** (contusion). A bruise is an injury of the soft tissue beneath the skin. Because small blood vessels are broken, the injured area becomes discolored and swells. The severity of these closed soft-tissue injuries varies greatly. A simple bruise heals quickly.

In contrast, bruising and swelling following an injury may also be a sign of an underlying fracture. Whenever you encounter a significant amount of swelling or bruising, suspect the possibility of an underlying fracture.

▶ Open Wounds

An open wound is one that results in a break in the skin. There are several types of open wounds, including abrasions, puncture wounds, lacerations, avulsions, and amputations. Each type is described below.

Abrasion

Commonly called a scrape, **road rash**, or rug burn, an **abrasion** occurs when the skin is rubbed across a rough surface **Figure 14-15**.

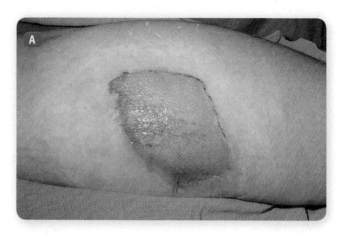

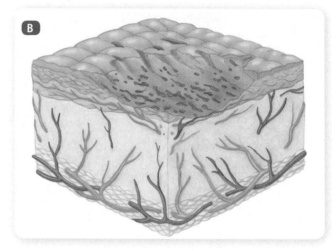

Figure 14-15 Abrasions involve variable depth of the skin; they are often called scrapes or road rashes.
A: © American Academy of Orthopaedic Surgeons; B: © Jones & Bartlett Learning.

Puncture

Puncture wounds are caused by a sharp object that penetrates the skin **Figure 14-16**. These wounds may cause a significant deep injury that is not immediately recognized. Puncture wounds do not bleed freely. If the object that caused the puncture wound remains sticking out of the skin, it is called an **impaled object**.

A **gunshot wound** is a special type of puncture wound. The amount of damage done by a gunshot depends on the type of gun used and the distance between the gun and the victim. A gunshot entry wound may appear as an insignificant hole but the bullet can cause massive damage to internal organs. Some gunshot wounds are smaller than a dime, and some are large enough to destroy significant amounts of tissue. Gunshot wounds usually have both an **entrance wound** and an **exit wound**. The entrance wound is usually smaller than the exit wound. Most deaths from gunshot wounds result from internal blood loss caused by damage to internal organs and major blood vessels as the bullet passes through the body. There is often more than one gunshot wound. It is important to conduct a thorough patient exam

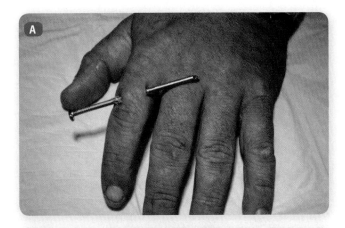

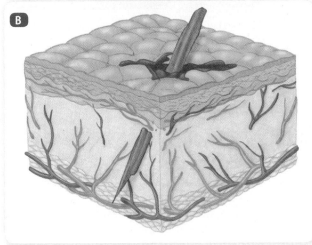

Figure 14-16 Puncture wounds may penetrate the skin to any depth.
A: © E. M. Singletary, MD. Used with permission; B: © Jones & Bartlett Learning.

▶ Principles of Wound Treatment

Very minor bruises need no treatment. Other closed wounds should be treated by applying ice and gentle compression and by elevating the injured body part. Because extensive bruising may indicate an underlying fracture, **splint** all major contusions. (Splinting involves using flexible or rigid support to prevent the movement of the injured body part; splinting is discussed more detail in Chapter 15, *Injuries to Muscles and Bones.*)

It is important to stop bleeding as quickly as possible using the cleanest dressing available. You can usually control bleeding by covering an open wound with a dry, clean, or sterile dressing and applying pressure to the dressing with your hand. If the first dressing does not

to ensure that you have discovered all of the entrance and exit wounds.

Laceration

The most common type of open wound is a **laceration** Figure 14-17 . Lacerations are commonly called cuts. Minor lacerations may require little care, but large lacerations can cause extensive bleeding and can even be life threatening.

Avulsions and Amputations

An **avulsion** is a tearing away of body tissue Figure 14-18 . The avulsed part may be totally severed from the body or it may be attached by a flap of skin. Avulsions may involve small or large amounts of tissue. If an entire body part is torn away, the wound is called a traumatic amputation Figure 14-19 . Any amputated body part should be located, placed in a clean plastic bag, kept cool, and taken with the patient to the hospital for possible reattachment (reimplantation). If the amputated part is small and a clean plastic bag is not available, use a surgical glove turned inside out. Use cold packs or ice water to keep the detached body parts cold. Do not allow ice to touch the body part directly.

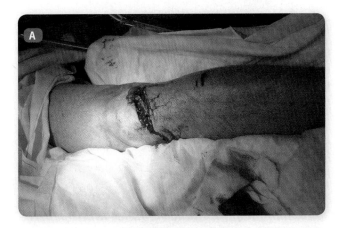

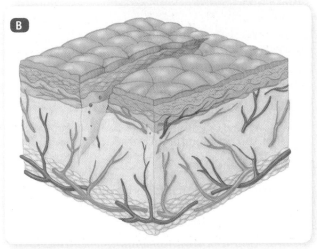

Figure 14-17 Lacerations are cuts produced by sharp objects.
A: © E. M. Singletary, MD. Used with permission; B: © Jones & Bartlett Learning.

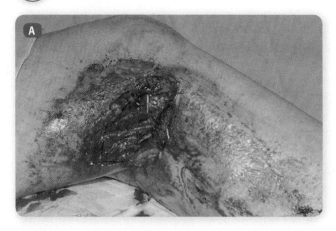

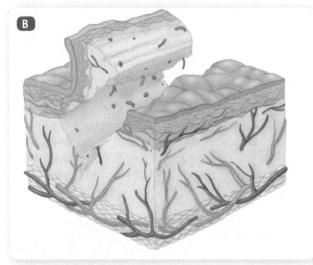

Figure 14-18 Avulsions raise flaps of tissue; significant bleeding is common.
A: © Jones & Bartlett Learning. Courtesy of MIEMSS; B: © Jones & Bartlett Learning.

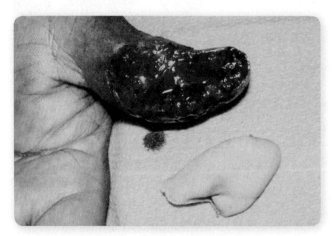

Figure 14-19 Amputated parts can often be reattached. Attempt to locate the body parts and transport them to the hospital with the patient.
© American Academy of Orthopaedic Surgeons.

control the bleeding, reinforce it with a second layer. Additional ways to control bleeding include elevating an extremity, applying a tourniquet, and using pressure points.

A dressing should cover the entire wound to prevent further contamination. Do not attempt to clean the

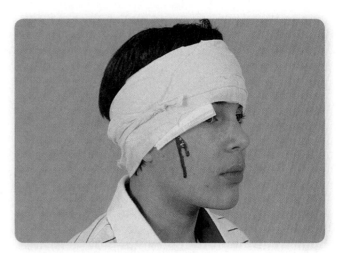

Figure 14-20 Head bandage.
© American Academy of Orthopaedic Surgeons.

contaminated wound in the field because cleaning will only cause more bleeding. A thorough cleaning will be done at the hospital. All dressings should be secured in place by a compression bandage.

Treatment

The major principles of open-wound treatment are to:
- Control bleeding.
- Prevent further contamination of the wound.
- **Immobilize** the injured part (reduce or prevent movement).
- Stabilize any impaled object.

Learning to dress and bandage wounds requires practice. As a trained EMR, you should be able to bandage all parts of the body quickly and competently **Figure 14-20**.

Treatment

Never remove an impaled object.

▶ Dressing and Bandaging Wounds

All wounds require bandaging; therefore, you should be familiar with the general principles of applying dressings and bandages to effectively cover and protect wounds.

Dressings and bandages are applied to achieve the following:

- Control bleeding
- Prevent further contamination
- Immobilize the injured area
- Prevent movement of impaled objects

Dressings

A dressing is an object placed directly on a wound to control bleeding and prevent further contamination. Once a dressing is in place, apply firm, direct manual pressure on it to stop any bleeding. It is important to stop severe bleeding as quickly as possible using the cleanest dressing available. If no dressing materials are available, you may have to apply direct pressure with your hand to a wound that is bleeding extensively; if this is the case, be sure to observe standard precautions and wear gloves.

Sterile dressings come packaged in many different sizes. The three most common sizes are gauze squares that measure 4 inches × 4 inches (10 cm × 10 cm) (commonly known as 4 × 4s), heavier pads that measure 5 inches × 9 inches (13 cm × 23 cm) (5 × 9s), and trauma dressings that are thick, sterile dressings that measure 10 inches × 30 inches (25 cm × 76 cm). Use a trauma dressing to cover a large wound on the abdomen, neck, thigh, or scalp—or as padding for splints Figure 14-21.

When you open a package containing a sterile dressing, touch only one corner of the dressing Figure 14-22. Place it on the wound without touching the side of the dressing that will be next to the wound. If bleeding continues after you have applied a compression dressing to the wound, put additional gauze pads over the original dressing. Do not remove the original dressing because the blood-clotting process will have already started and should not be disrupted. When you are satisfied that the wound is sufficiently dressed, you can proceed to bandaging the wound.

> ### Treatment
>
> If commercially prepared dressings are not available, use the cleanest cloth object available, such as a clean handkerchief, washcloth, disposable diaper, or article of clothing.

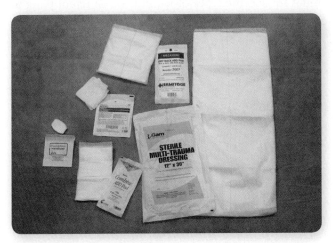

Figure 14-21 Common sizes of wound dressings are 10 inches × 30 inches (25 cm × 76 cm), 5 inches × 9 inches (13 cm × 23 cm), and 4 inches × 4 inches (10 cm × 10 cm).
© Jones & Bartlett Learning. Courtesy of MIEMSS.

Bandaging

A bandage is used to hold the dressing in place. Two types of bandages commonly used in the field are roller gauze and triangular bandages. The first type, conforming roller gauze, stretches slightly and is easy to wrap around the body part Figure 14-23. Triangular bandages are usually 36 inches (91 cm) across Figure 14-24. A triangular

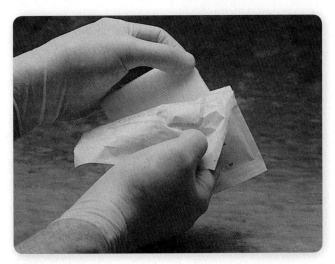

Figure 14-22 Open the package containing a sterile dressing carefully.
© Jones & Bartlett Learning.

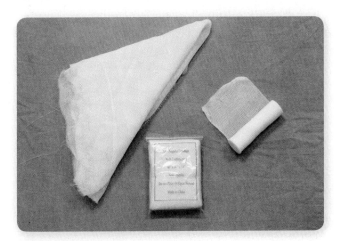

Figure 14-23 Roller gauze bandage.
© Jones & Bartlett Learning. Courtesy of MIEMSS.

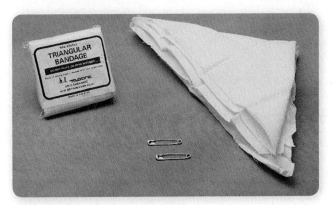

Figure 14-24 Triangular bandage.
© Jones & Bartlett Learning.

bandage can be folded and used as a wide **cravat** or it can be used without folding Figure 14-25. Roller gauze is easier to apply and stays in place better than a triangular bandage, but a triangular bandage is very useful for bandaging scalp lacerations and lacerations of the chest, abdomen, back, or thigh.

Follow certain principles if the bandage is to hold the dressing in place, control bleeding, and prevent further contamination. Before you apply a bandage, check to ensure the dressing covers the wound completely and extends beyond all sides of the wound Figure 14-26. Wrap the bandage just tightly enough to control bleeding. Do not apply it too tightly because it may cut off all circulation. It is important to regularly check circulation at a point farther away from the heart than the injury itself because swelling may make the bandage too tight. If this happens while the patient is under your care, remove the roller gauze or triangular bandage and reapply it, making sure that you do not disturb the dressing beneath.

Once you have completed applying the bandage, secure it so it cannot slip. Tape, tie, or tuck in any loose ends. Practice bandaging techniques for several types of wounds using both roller gauze and triangular bandages. Although the principles of bandaging are simple, some parts of the body are difficult to bandage. It is important to practice bandaging different parts of the body to ensure competency in emergency medical care situations.

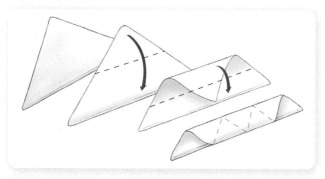

Figure 14-25 Folding a triangular bandage to make a cravat.
© Jones & Bartlett Learning.

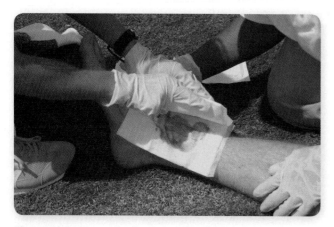

Figure 14-26 Ensure the dressing covers the wound completely.
© Jones & Bartlett Learning.

Treatment

Bandaging is a skill that requires practice. Apply bandages tight enough so they stay in place and apply sufficient pressure to stop the bleeding. However, do not apply bandages too tightly or they can occlude circulation to an extremity. Check bandages as part of your reassessment to ensure they are still applied correctly.

Standard Precaution Techniques for the EMR

Some infectious disease organisms, including the hepatitis and AIDS viruses, can be transmitted if blood from an infected person enters the bloodstream of a healthy person through a small cut or opening in the skin. Because you may have such a cut, it is important to wear gloves to avoid contact with patients' blood Figure 14-27. Wearing gloves also protects wounds from being contaminated by dirt or infectious organisms you may have on your hands. Nitrile or latex medical gloves can be stored on the top of your EMR life support kit or in a pouch on your belt, where they will be readily available. (See Chapter 2, *Workforce Safety and Wellness*, for more information on infectious diseases.)

Safety

Providing for your own safety and that of the patient is always a high priority when you are examining and treating open wounds.

Specific Wound Treatment

The preceding material discussed the general principles of wound treatment. The next section discusses treatment for specific types of wounds on different parts of the body.

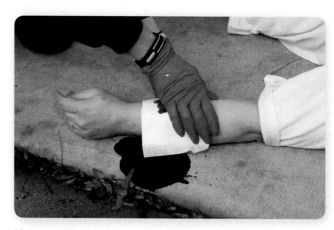

Figure 14-27 Always wear gloves when in contact with body fluids.
© Jones & Bartlett Learning. Courtesy of MIEMSS.

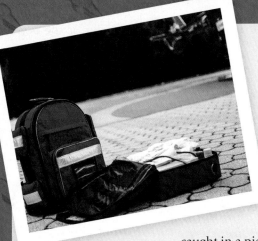

Voices *of* Experience

We were called to assist the ambulance at an accident at the local paper manufacturing facility. An adult male had his gloved hand caught in a piece of machinery and several of his fingers had been amputated. After we made contact with our patient, we simultaneously determined he had an open airway, was breathing adequately, and was bleeding from his hand. We were able to successfully stop the bleeding with direct pressure, all the while reassuring our patient.

We radioed ahead to the ambulance to let them know the status of our patient and that four of his fingers had been amputated at the knuckle level. The ambulance in turn requested a helicopter flight meet them at the hospital for rapid transit to a larger, Level One trauma center, which could perform intricate hand surgery.

I found all the fingers (sounds awful, but was not at all), wrapped them in gauze, put them in a plastic bag, and then placed the plastic bag into a container of cold ice water. The patient was transported to the hospital and on to the Level One trauma center.

About six months later, the patient made an unexpected visit to my place of business. He asked if I remembered him and I replied, "Of course!" He picked up his hand and waved at me, with all of his fingers intact and perfectly responding. He said, "I just wanted to say hi and say thank you."

He was back at work doing the same job, but being much more careful, and truly thankful for the quick action by the emergency medical responders.

> " **His gloved hand had gotten caught in a piece of machinery, and several of his fingers had been amputated.** "

Ellen A. Mathein, EMT, CPA
Nicolet Area Technical College
Tripoli, Wisconsin

Face and Scalp Wounds

The face and scalp have many blood vessels. Because of this generous blood supply, a relatively small laceration can result in significant bleeding. Although face and scalp lacerations may not be life threatening, they are always bloody and cause much anxiety for the patient.

You can control almost all facial or scalp bleeding by applying direct manual pressure. Direct pressure is effective because the bones of the skull are so close to the skin. Direct pressure compresses the blood vessels against the skull and stops the bleeding. If bleeding continues, do not remove the dressing. Instead, reinforce it with a second layer and continue to apply manual pressure. After the bleeding stops, wrap the head with a bandage Figure 14-28 .

For wounds inside the cheek, hold a gauze pad inside the cheek (in the mouth). If necessary, apply a pad outside the cheek. Always keep the airway open.

Severe scalp lacerations may be associated with skull fractures or even brain injury. If any brain tissue or bone fragments are visible, do not apply pressure to the wound. Instead, cover the wound loosely, being careful not to exert direct pressure on the brain or the bone fragments.

If the patient has a head injury, the neck and spine may also be injured. Move the head as little as possible and stabilize the neck. (Treatment of spinal injuries is discussed in Chapter 15, *Injuries to Muscles and Bones*.) In patients with a head injury, always evaluate the patient's level of consciousness. Carefully monitor the patient's airway and breathing and protect the spine.

Words of Wisdom

Remember, patients who have injuries or are bleeding will likely be worried. It is your job to reassure them that you are doing everything you can to treat them. Do not forget to show your patients and their families that you care!

Nosebleeds

Nosebleeds can result from injury, high blood pressure, or dry air. In some cases, there is no apparent cause. A nosebleed with no apparent cause is called a **spontaneous nosebleed**. In a patient with high blood pressure, increased pressure in the small blood vessels of the nose may cause one to rupture, resulting in bleeding. A patient with high blood pressure should be seen and treated by a physician.

Most nosebleeds can be controlled easily. Unless the patient is experiencing shock, have the patient sit down and tilt his or her head slightly forward. This position keeps the blood from dripping down the throat. Swallowing blood may cause coughing or vomiting and make the nosebleed worse.

Treatment

If you suspect that a patient may have high blood pressure, the patient must be evaluated by a physician.

After the patient is seated correctly, pinch both nostrils together for at least 5 minutes. The patient may wish to do this without assistance. This treatment usually controls nosebleeds Figure 14-29 . If the nosebleed persists or is very severe, arrange for transport to an appropriate medical facility. Instruct the patient to avoid blowing his or her nose because this will often cause additional bleeding.

Eye Injuries

All eye injuries are potentially serious and require medical evaluation. When an eye laceration is suspected, cover the entire eye with a dry gauze pad. Have the patient lie on his or her back and arrange for *transport* to an appropriate medical facility.

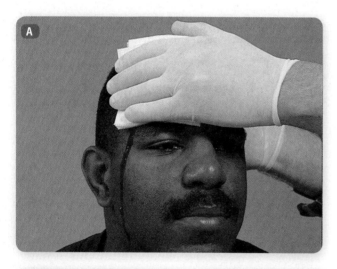

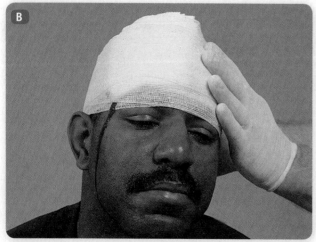

Figure 14-28 Bandaging a head wound. **A.** Apply direct pressure until bleeding stops. **B.** Wrap the head with a bandage.
A&B: © Jones & Bartlett Learning. Courtesy of MIEMSS.

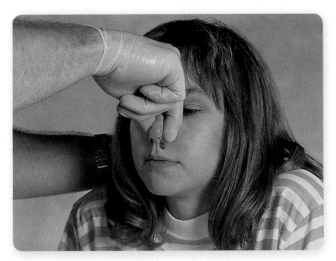

Figure 14-29 Pinch nostrils together to control a nosebleed.
© Jones & Bartlett Learning. Courtesy of MIEMSS.

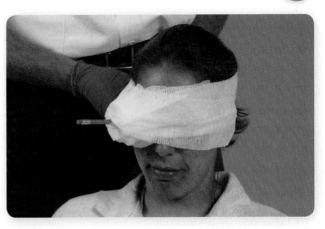

Figure 14-30 To bandage an eye impaled by an object, use a paper cup to cover the impaled object, then bandage both eyes to minimize eye movement.
© Jones & Bartlett Learning. Courtesy of MIEMSS.

If a small foreign object is lying on the surface of the patient's eye, you can use a saline solution, when available, to gently flush the object from the eye. Clean water can also be used, but it tends to irritate the injured eye. Flush from the nose side toward the outside to avoid flushing the object into the other eye. Even small foreign objects can leave a small scratch on the surface of the eye. It is always a good idea to transport the patient to an appropriate medical facility for further assessment and possible treatment.

Occasionally an object will be impaled in the eye. Immediately place the patient on his or her back and cover the injured eye with a dressing and a paper cup so the impaled object cannot move. Remember to bandage both eyes. This is an important step to help minimize eye movement because if the patient attempts to look at something with the uninjured eye, the injured eye moves in conjunction, further aggravating the injury **Figure 14-30** . Arrange for *transport* of the patient to the hospital.

Treatment

Whenever you must bandage both eyes, explain to the patient why you are doing so. Having both eyes covered may be distressing to the patient. Stay with the patient to provide reassurance.

Neck Wounds

The neck contains many important structures: the trachea, the esophagus, large arteries, veins, muscles, vertebrae, and the spinal cord. Because an injury to any of these structures may be life threatening, all neck injuries are considered serious.

Apply direct pressure to control bleeding neck wounds. Once bleeding is controlled, dress the neck **Figure 14-31** . In rare cases, you may have to exert finger pressure above and below the injury site to prevent further neck bleeding.

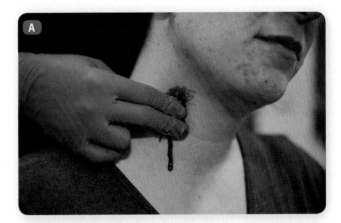

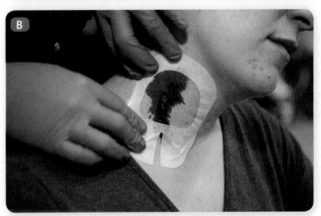

Figure 14-31 Dressing a neck wound. **A.** Apply direct pressure over the wound to control bleeding. **B.** Place the dressing over the wound.
A&B: © Jones & Bartlett Learning. Courtesy of MIEMSS.

Always keep in mind that major trauma to the neck may be associated with airway problems and with neck fracture or spinal cord injury. Therefore, maintain the patient's airway and stabilize the head and neck.

Chest and Back Wounds

The major organs affected by chest wounds and back wounds are the lungs, large blood vessels, and heart. Any wound involving these organs is a life-threatening injury. Place the patient with a chest injury in a comfortable position (usually sitting) (see Chapter 15, *Injuries to Muscles and Bones*).

If a lung is punctured, air can escape and the lung can collapse. The patient may cough up bright red blood. To help maintain air pressure in the lung, your first action should be to cover any open chest wound with an airtight material, thereby sealing the wound. This covering is called an **occlusive dressing**. Use a clear plastic cover from your medical supplies, aluminum foil, plastic wrap, gloves, or a special dressing that has been impregnated with petroleum jelly (Vaseline). Any material that will occlude (seal off) the wound is sufficient Figure 14-32 .

Administering oxygen is important early treatment for a patient with an injured lung. It should be given by EMS personnel when they arrive or by EMRs who are trained and have the equipment available.

Chest wounds may also damage the heart. Seal the wound in the manner described and monitor the patient's airway, breathing, and circulation. Treat the patient for shock and perform CPR, if necessary.

If the patient's breathing becomes more labored after you seal the chest wound, you may need to remove the seal briefly to allow excess air to escape and then reseal the wound.

Impaled Objects

If an object is impaled in the patient, apply a stabilizing dressing and arrange for the patient's *prompt transport* to an appropriate medical facility. Sometimes an impaled object is too long to permit the patient to be removed from the scene and transported to an appropriate medical facility. In these situations, it may be necessary to stabilize the impaled object and carefully cut it close to the patient's body. If you encounter a situation like this, stabilize the impaled object as well as you can and immediately request a specialized rescue team that has the tools and training to handle this type of incident.

If your patient has a knife or other object protruding from the abdomen, do not attempt to remove it. Instead, support the impaled object so it cannot move. Place a large roll of gauze or towels on either side of the object and secure the rolls with additional gauze wrapped around the patient's body. It is important to stabilize the object so it will not move while the patient is being transported to the hospital Figure 14-33 . Any movement of the object may cause further internal damage.

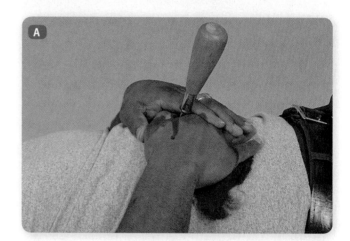

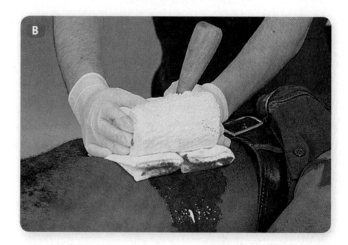

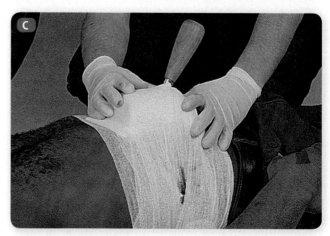

Figure 14-33 Bandaging an impaled object. **A.** Do not attempt to remove or move an impaled object. **B.** Stabilize the object in place with dressings. **C.** Place a bandage over the dressings.

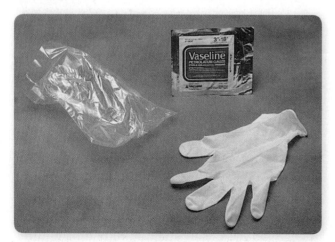

Figure 14-32 For occlusive dressings, use plastic wrap, petroleum jelly, or gloves.

Closed Abdominal Wounds

Closed abdominal wounds commonly occur as the result of a direct blow from a blunt object. Check for a closed abdominal wound whenever force has been applied to the abdomen. Look for bruises or other marks on the abdomen that indicate blunt injury.

Any time an injured patient is experiencing shock, you should remember that there may be internal abdominal injuries accompanied by bleeding. When there is internal bleeding, the abdomen may become swollen, rigid, or hard like a board. Treat patients with closed abdominal injuries and signs of shock by placing them on their backs (unless they are having difficulty breathing). Use blankets to help conserve their body heat and elevate the legs if indicated by local protocol.

If the patient is vomiting blood (ranging in color from bright red to dark brown), it may be an indication of bleeding from the esophagus or stomach. Monitor the patient's airway and vital signs carefully because shock may result. Give the patient nothing by mouth. Arrange for *prompt transport* to an appropriate medical facility.

Open Abdominal Wounds

Open abdominal wounds usually result from slashing with a knife or other sharp object and are always serious injuries.

If the intestines are protruding from the abdomen (an evisceration), place the patient on his or her back with the knees bent to relax the abdominal muscles. Cover the injured area with a sterile dressing **Figure 14-34** . Do not attempt to replace the intestines inside the abdomen.

You can make a bandage from a large trauma pad (10 inches × 30 inches [25 cm × 76 cm]) and several cravats to cover protruding abdominal intestines. Position the trauma pad to cover the whole area of the wound. Tie two or three wide cravats loosely over the trauma pad, just tightly enough to keep it firmly in place, but not tightly enough to push the intestines back into the abdomen.

EMTs and paramedics carry sterile **saline** (salt water) that can be poured on the dressing to keep the protruding organs moist so they do not dry out. Use only sterile saline.

Special Populations

Septic Shock

Septic shock is caused by a system-wide infection. It is a very serious condition that can result in rapid decrease of the patient's blood pressure. It is most common in older adults and people who have weakened immune systems. This recognition and treatment of this condition is discussed more fully in Chapter 18, *Geriatric Emergencies*.

Treatment

To treat an open abdominal wound, follow these steps:

1. Apply a sterile dressing to the wound.
2. Maintain the patient's body temperature.
3. Place the patient on his or her back with the knees bent.
4. Place the patient who is having difficulty breathing in a semireclining position.
5. Administer oxygen if it is available and you are trained to use it.

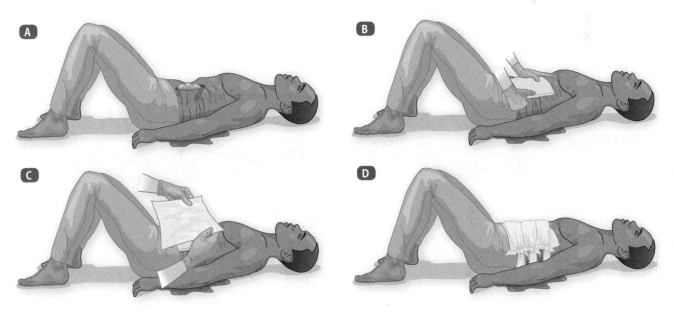

Figure 14-34 Bandaging an open abdominal wound. **A.** Place the patient on his or her back with the knees bent to relax the abdominal muscles. **B.** Cover the injured area with a sterile dressing. Do not attempt to replace the intestines inside the abdomen. **C.** Place a large trauma pad over the wound. **D.** Use several wide cravats to loosely cover the trauma pad. Place them just tight enough to hold the abdominal contents in place.

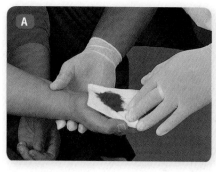
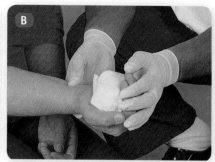
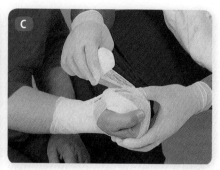

Figure 14-35 Bandaging a hand wound. **A.** Place a dressing over the wound. **B.** Place a gauze roll in the palm of the hand to apply pressure. **C.** Secure the dressing with a gauze roller bandage.

A, B & C: © Jones & Bartlett Learning.

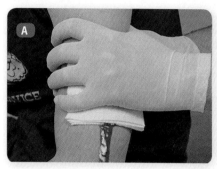
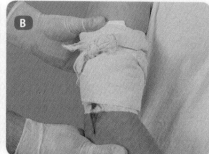
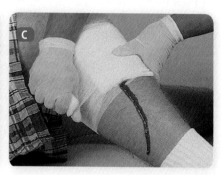

Figure 14-36 Bandaging an extremity wound. **A.** Place a dressing over the wound. **B.** Secure the dressing with a cravat. **C.** Secure the dressing with a roller bandage.

A, B & C: © Jones & Bartlett Learning.

Genital Wounds

Both male and female genitals have a rich blood supply. Injury to the genitals often results in severe bleeding. Apply direct pressure to any genital wound with a dry, sterile dressing. Direct pressure usually stops the bleeding. Although it may be embarrassing to examine the patient's genital area to determine the severity of the injury, you must do so if you suspect such injuries. The patient can experience a critical loss of blood if you do not find the injury and control the bleeding.

Extremity Wounds

To treat all open extremity wounds, apply a dry, sterile compression dressing and bandage it securely in place **Figure 14-35** and **Figure 14-36**. Elevate the injured part to help decrease bleeding and swelling. Splint all injured extremities prior to transport because there may be an underlying fracture.

Gunshot Wounds

Some gunshot wounds are easy to miss unless you perform a thorough patient examination **Figure 14-37**. Most deaths from gunshot wounds result from internal blood loss caused by damage to internal organs and major blood vessels. Because gunshot wounds are so serious, prompt and effective treatment is important. Gunshot wounds of the trunk and neck can cause spinal cord injuries. Because you cannot see the bullet's path

YOU are the Provider   CASE 3

It is almost midnight on Saturday when you are dispatched to the Friendly Bar & Lounge for a report of a stabbing. Your dispatcher quickly announces that the police have been notified. On the way to the scene, you cannot help but think about scene safety. After a 4-minute response, you arrive at the scene. A quick glance at the parking lot reveals at least four police cars on the scene. An officer approaches your vehicle as you are getting out and tells you the scene is secure. She leads you to an outdoor bench where your patient is sitting. You find a 30- to 35-year-old man, Alex, who is holding his abdomen with both hands. He appears to be in a lot of pain. As you begin to question him he tells you that he and Marco got into an argument and suddenly Marco pulled out a knife and stabbed him twice in the belly. Your patient exam reveals two small cuts on his stomach. Both cuts are seeping small amounts of blood. Your exam does not reveal additional injuries. Alex's pulse is 84 beats per minute, his blood pressure is 112/74 mm Hg, and his respirations are 22 breaths per minute. He is sweating. You are not surprised to detect a strong odor of alcohol on his breath.

1. What initial treatment can you give to this patient?
2. What additional care does this patient need?

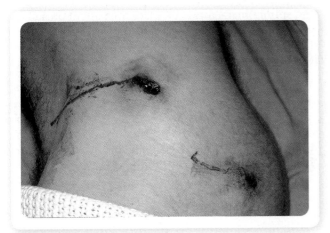

Figure 14-37 Bullet entry wound.
© Mediscan/Alamy.

through the body, you should treat these patients for spinal cord injuries.

To treat a patient with a gunshot wound, follow these steps:

1. Open the airway and establish adequate ventilation and circulation.
2. Control any external bleeding by covering wounds with sterile dressings and applying pressure with your hand or a bandage.
3. Examine the patient thoroughly to ensure you have discovered all entrance and exit wounds.
4. Treat for symptoms of shock by performing the following actions:
   - Maintain the patient's body temperature.
   - Place the patient on his or her back and elevate the legs if indicated by local protocol.
   - Place a patient who is having difficulty breathing in a semireclining position.
   - Administer oxygen, if available.
5. Arrange for *prompt transport* of the patient to an appropriate medical facility.
6. Perform CPR if the patient's heart stops as a result of loss of blood.

Bites

Bites from animals or humans may range from minor to severe. All bites carry a high risk of causing infection. Bites from an unvaccinated or wild animal may cause **rabies**. Minor bites can be washed with soap and water, if they are available. Major bite wounds should be treated by controlling the bleeding and applying a suitable dressing and bandage.

All patients who have been bitten by an animal or another person must be treated by a physician. In most states, EMS or hospital personnel are required to report animal bites to the local health department or a law enforcement agency. Check the laws in your local area to determine requirements.

Burns

The skin serves as a barrier that prevents foreign substances, such as bacteria, from entering the body. It also prevents the loss of body fluids. When the skin is damaged, such as by a burn, it can no longer perform these essential functions.

> ### Words of Wisdom
>
> Characteristics for burn classification include the following:
> - Depth
> - Extent (amount of the body injured by the burn)
> - Cause or type

▶ Burn Depth

There are three classifications of burns by depth: superficial (first-degree) burns, partial-thickness (second-degree) burns, and full-thickness (third-degree) burns. Although it is not always possible to determine the exact degree of a burn injury, it is important to understand this concept.

Superficial burns (first-degree burns) are characterized by reddened and painful skin. The injury is confined to the outermost layers of skin, and the patient experiences minor to moderate pain. An example of a superficial burn is sunburn, which usually heals in about a week, with or without treatment **Figure 14-38**.

Partial-thickness burns (second-degree burns) are somewhat deeper but do not damage the deepest layers of the skin **Figure 14-39**. Blistering is present, although blisters may not form for several hours in some cases. There may be some fluid loss and moderate to severe pain because the nerve endings are damaged. Partial-thickness burns require medical treatment. They usually heal within 2 to 3 weeks.

Full-thickness burns (third-degree burns) damage all layers of the skin. In some cases, the damage is deep

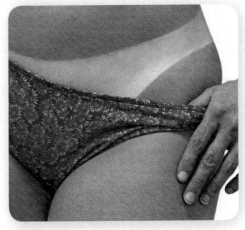

Figure 14-38 Superficial or first-degree burn.
© Amy Walters/Shutterstock.

enough to injure and destroy underlying muscles and other tissues Figure 14-40 . Pain is often absent because the nerve endings have been destroyed. Without the protection provided by the skin, patients with extensive full-thickness burns lose large quantities of body fluids and are susceptible to shock and infection.

If the patient has injuries in addition to the burn, treat the injuries before transporting the patient. For example, if a patient who has a partial-thickness burn of the arm has also fallen off a ladder and fractured both legs, splint the fractures and place the patient on a backboard, in addition to treating the burn injury.

▶ Extent of Burns

The **rule of nines** is a method used to determine what percentage of the body has been burned. Although this rule is most useful for EMTs and paramedics who report information to the hospital from the field, you should be able to roughly estimate the extent of a burn. Figure 14-41 shows how the rule of nines divides the body. In an adult, the head and arms each equal 9% of the total body surface. The front and back of the trunk and each leg are equal to 18% of the total body surface. For example, if one half of the back and the entire right arm of a patient are burned, the burn involves about 18% of the total body area. The rule of nines is slightly modified for young children, but the adult percentages serve as an adequate guide.

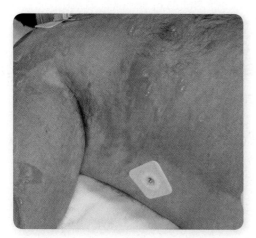

Figure 14-39 Partial-thickness or second-degree burn.
© E. M. Singletary, MD. Used with permission.

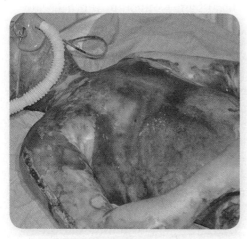

Figure 14-40 Full-thickness or third-degree burn.
© American Academy of Orthopaedic Surgeons.

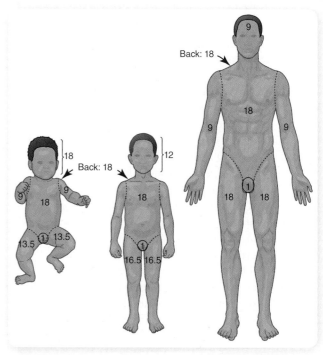

Figure 14-41 Use the rule of nines to determine the extent of burns.
© Jones & Bartlett Learning.

YOU are the Provider CASE 4

It is 2330 hours and you have been called to the local university for a report of a man who has burns as the result of a dormitory fire. You arrive at the scene to find a 20-year-old man with full-thickness burns to both forearms, from the wrist to the elbow. The patient indicates that while he was sleeping, his electric blanket caught fire. He attempted to put out the fire with his arms, which resulted in the severe burns on his arms. The fire department has extinguished the fire and removed the patient from the burned room.

1. What distinguishes a full-thickness burn from a partial-thickness burn?
2. Why is a person with full-thickness burns at an increased risk for shock?

▶ Cause or Type of Burns

Burns are an injury to body cells caused by excess exposure to heat (thermal burns), chemicals, or electricity. They may involve a small area of the body or involve the entire body. Burns can cause minor injuries affecting only the top layers of the skin or they can be deep, involving muscles, blood vessels, and nerves. Severe burns can involve damage to all the organs and systems of the body. This section discusses the three major causes of burns: heat, chemicals, and electricity. It discusses the impact the size and severity of the burn have on the patient, as well as the care and treatment you can provide to a burn patient.

Thermal Burns

Thermal burns are caused by heat. The first step in treating thermal burns is to cool the skin by putting out the fire. Superficial burns can be quite painful, but if there is clean, cold water available, you can place the burned area in cold water to help reduce the pain. You can also wet a clean towel with cold water and put it on superficial burns. After the burned area is cooled, cover it with a dry, sterile dressing or a large sterile cloth called a burn sheet (found in your EMR life support kit) **Figure 14-42**.

Treatment

Do not apply burn ointments, butter, grease, or cream to any burn!

Partial-thickness burns should be cooled if the burn area is still warm. Cooling helps reduce pain, stops the heat from further injuring the skin, and helps stop the swelling caused by partial-thickness burns.

If blisters are present, be very careful not to break the blisters. Intact skin, even if blistered, provides an excellent barrier against infection. If the blisters break, the danger of infection increases. Cover partial-thickness burns with a dry, sterile dressing or burn sheet.

Full-thickness burns, if still warm, should also be cooled with water to keep the heat from damaging more skin and tissue. Cut any clothing away from the burned area, but leave any clothing that is stuck to the burn. Cover full-thickness burns with a dry, sterile dressing or burn sheet **Figure 14-43**.

Patients with large superficial burns or any partial-thickness or full-thickness burns must be treated for shock and transported to a hospital.

Respiratory Burns

A burn to any part of the airway is a **respiratory burn**. If a patient has been burned around the head and face or while in a confined space (such as in a burning house), look for the signs and symptoms of respiratory burns listed in the Signs and Symptoms box.

Watch the patient carefully. Breathing problems that result from this type of burn can develop rapidly or slowly over several hours. Administer oxygen as soon as it is available and be prepared to perform CPR. If you suspect that a patient has sustained respiratory burns, arrange for *prompt transport* to a medical facility.

Signs and Symptoms

Signs and symptoms of a respiratory burn include the following:

- Burns around the face
- Singed nose hairs
- Soot in the mouth and nose
- Difficulty breathing
- Pain while breathing
- Unconsciousness as a result of a fire

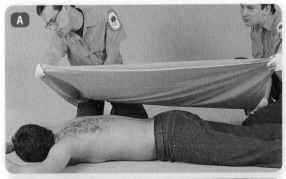

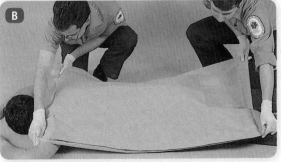

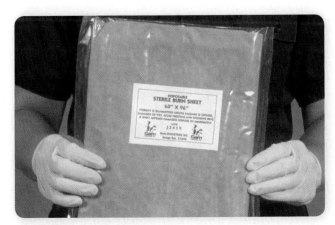

Figure 14-42 Sterile burn sheet.
© Jones & Bartlett Learning. Courtesy of MIEMSS.

Figure 14-43 Applying a sterile burn sheet.
A & B: © Jones & Bartlett Learning. Courtesy of MIEMSS.

Chemical Burns

Many strong substances can cause **chemical burns** to the skin, and chemicals are extremely dangerous to the eyes. These substances include strong acids such as battery acid or strong alkalis such as drain cleaners. Some chemicals are so strong or caustic that they can cause damage to the skin or eyes even if the exposure is very brief. The longer the chemical remains in contact with the skin, the more it damages the skin and underlying tissues, oftentimes resulting in superficial, partial-thickness, or full-thickness burns to the skin.

The initial treatment for chemical burns is to remove as much of the chemical as possible from the patient's skin. Brush away any dry chemical on the patient's clothes or skin, being careful not to get any on yourself. You may have to ask the patient to remove all clothing.

After you have removed as much of the dry chemical as possible, flush the contaminated skin with abundant quantities of water. Use water from a garden hose, a shower in the home or factory, or even the booster hose of a fire engine. It is essential that the chemical be washed off the skin quickly to avoid further injury. Flush the affected area of the body for at least 10 minutes, then cover the burned area with a dry, sterile dressing or a burn sheet and arrange for *prompt transport* to an appropriate medical facility.

Safety

Chemical burns are caused by hazardous materials. In situations like this, special protective equipment may be required. Follow your local protocols for these situations.

Chemical burns to the eyes cause extreme pain and severe injury. Gently flush the affected eye or eyes with water for at least 20 minutes Figure 14-44 . Hold the eye open to allow water to flow over its entire surface. Direct the water from the inner corner of the eye to the outward edge of the eye to avoid contaminating the unaffected eye. You may have to put the patient's face under a shower, garden hose, or faucet so the water flows across the patient's entire face. Continue flushing the eyes while the patient is being transported.

After flushing the eyes for 20 minutes, loosely cover the injured eye or eyes with gauze bandages and arrange for *prompt transport* to an appropriate medical facility. All chemical burns should be examined by a physician.

Electrical Burns

Electrical burns can cause severe injuries or even death, but they leave little evidence of injury on the outside of the body. These burns are caused by an electrical current that enters the body at one point (for example, the hand that touches the live electrical wire), travels through the body tissues and organs, and exits from the body at the point of ground contact Figure 14-45 .

Electricity causes major internal damage, rather than external damage. A strong electrical current can actually "cook" muscles, nerves, blood vessels, and internal organs, resulting in major damage. Patients who have been subjected to a strong electrical current can also experience irregularities of cardiac rhythm or even full cardiac arrest and death. Children often sustain electrical burns by chewing on an electrical cord or by pushing something into an outlet. Although the burn may not look serious at first, it is often quite severe because of underlying tissue injury.

Persons who have been hit or nearly hit by lightning frequently sustain electrical burns. Treat these

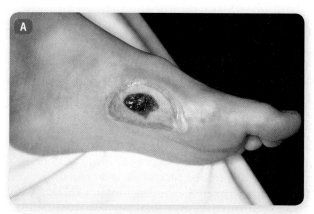
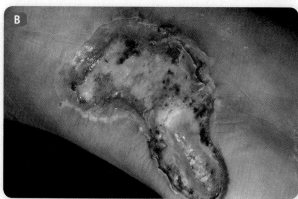

Figure 14-45 Electrical burns. **A.** An entrance wound is often small. **B.** An exit wound can be extensive and deep.
A&B: © Chuck Stewart, MD.

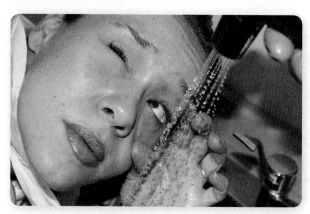

Figure 14-44 Flushing the eyes with water.
© American Academy of Orthopaedic Surgeons.

patients as you would electrical burn patients. Evaluate them carefully because they may also experience cardiac arrest. Arrange for *prompt transport* to an appropriate medical facility.

Before you touch or treat a person who has sustained an electrical burn, be certain the patient is not still in contact with the electrical power source that caused the burn. If the patient is still in contact with the power source, anyone who touches him or her may be electrocuted. If the patient is touching a live power source, your first act must be to unplug, disconnect, or turn off the power Figure 14-46 . If you cannot do this alone, call for assistance from the power company or from a qualified rescue squad or fire department.

If a power line falls on top of a motor vehicle, the people inside the vehicle must be told to stay inside until qualified personnel can remove the power line or turn the power off. After ensuring that the power has been disconnected, examine each electrical burn patient carefully, assess the ABCs, and treat the patient for visible, external burns. Cover these external burns with a dry, sterile dressing and arrange for *prompt transport* to an appropriate medical facility.

Monitor the airway, breathing, and circulation of electrical burn patients closely, and arrange to have these patients transported promptly to an appropriate medical facility for further treatment.

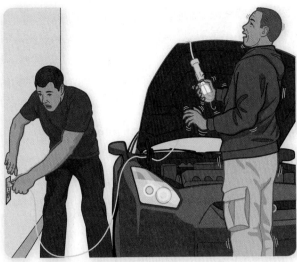

Figure 14-46 Do not touch the patient without unplugging, disconnecting, or turning off the power first.
© Jones & Bartlett Learning.

■ Multi-System Trauma

Multi-system trauma is an injury that affects more than one body system. The injuries in multi-system trauma can occur in one part of the body but involve different body systems. For example, an unrestrained patient who hits the steering wheel in a motor vehicle crash can sustain trauma to the chest. This trauma could result in injuries to both the heart (the circulatory system) and to the lungs (the respiratory system). Another patient in a vehicle crash might have injuries to different parts of body, for example, to the abdomen and to the head. Both of these patients have sustained multi-system trauma. As an EMR, you are not expected to diagnose a patient's injuries. However, it is important to remember that several body systems may be injured in situations that involve significant trauma. As you assess your patients, be alert for signs and symptoms of injury to each part of the body.

Safety

Avoid direct or indirect contact with live electrical wires. Direct contact occurs when you touch a live electrical wire. Indirect contact occurs when you touch a vehicle, a patient, a fence, a tree, or any other object that is in contact with a live electrical wire.

YOU ▶ are the Provider   SUMMARY

You are the Provider: CASE 1

1. What safety considerations should you keep in mind as you approach this situation?

Ensure the scene is safe for you, the patient, and bystanders. As you approach the scene, ensure there are no objects that can fall from above. Be certain that all power tools are turned off and unplugged. Be certain the saw blade and other sharp objects are out of the way. Maintain standard precautions to prevent the spread of bloodborne diseases. Remember to wear gloves to protect yourself from contact with blood. If there is a chance of blood splatter, consider the need for eye protection.

2. What equipment and supplies do you want to take with you?

For an incident such as this, there are three types of equipment you should take with you: equipment to maintain standard precautions, supplies for wound treatment, and equipment to treat the patient for shock. The equipment for standard precautions includes latex or nitrile gloves and eye protection for any possible blood splatter. Wound treatment equipment should include an adequate supply of dressings and bandages to treat the wound and supplies to immobilize the affected extremity. Equipment to treat for shock should include blankets to preserve body heat, a blood pressure cuff to assess blood pressure, and oxygen administration equipment if it is available and you have been trained in its use.

3. What are your treatment goals for this incident?

The goals for this incident include maintaining standard precautions, treating soft-tissue injuries by controlling external bleeding, preventing further contamination of the wound site, immobilizing the affected extremity, and treating the patient for shock.

You are the Provider: CASE 2

1. What are your initial steps in treating this patient?

Your initial treatment steps should include the following: ensure scene safety; look for any additional hidden weapons as you approach to examine the patient; take standard precautions to prevent contact with blood; control the external bleeding by placing a dressing over the wound, applying direct pressure, and then applying a pressure dressing; treat the patient for shock by placing him either in a supine position or a reclining position if he is having difficulty breathing and maintaining body temperature; take an initial set of vital signs; and ensure that an EMS transport unit is responding.

2. How serious is an injury like this?

A gunshot wound to the thigh is a serious injury. You cannot determine the pathway of the bullet or the parts of the leg that have been damaged. There is the possibility that the bullet may have traveled into the abdomen and caused additional damage. This type of injury often causes a significant amount of internal blood loss. There are no good ways for you to measure this blood loss. It is important for you to take repeat vital signs every 5 minutes to monitor the patient for signs of shock. The initial signs and symptoms of shock include: pale, cool, or clammy skin; increased heart rate and respiratory rate; and a sense of anxiety. It is also important to arrange for prompt transportation to an appropriate medical facility as soon as possible.

You are the Provider: CASE 3

1. What initial treatment can you give to this patient?

After you have completed your assessment of this patient, you need to put the pieces together to determine what type of injury you have found and then develop a treatment plan. This patient has two small wounds in his abdomen reportedly from a knife. There is no way for you to

determine how deep these wounds are, what organs have been damaged, or the amount of internal blood loss he has suffered. You need to understand that this type of wound can result in profound shock from internal blood loss; therefore your actions are to treat the patient for shock by placing him in a comfortable position—often for this type of injury, it will be lying supine with his legs drawn up or reclining—and maintaining his body temperature. Monitor his airway, breathing, and circulation. Monitor his vital signs every 5 minutes and be alert for the possibility that his vital signs may change rapidly. Apply a dressing to the abdominal wounds. Maintain standard precautions. Finally, ensure this patient is promptly transported to an appropriate medical facility that can provide evaluation and needed treatment.

2. What additional care does this patient need?

Advanced life support providers can provide additional treatment for shock by administering IV fluids. However, the care most needed by this patient can be provided only by a physician in a hospital setting. In the hospital, this patient will need to be taken into surgery to determine the extent of the damage to his abdominal organs and to stop the internal bleeding by surgically repairing the damaged organs. If not treated properly, this patient can develop life-threatening infections. Therefore, it is important for you to arrange for prompt transportation of this patient to an appropriate medical facility as soon as possible while continuing to monitor his vital signs and treating him for shock. If internal blood loss continues, his condition may deteriorate quickly.

You are the Provider: CASE 4

1. What distinguishes a full-thickness burn from a partial-thickness burn?

In partial-thickness burns, the burned area is very painful, the skin will be red, and blisters will form within a few hours. Full-thickness burns penetrate down through the dermis and epidermis, often into the underlying subcutaneous tissue, muscle, and bone. Full-thickness burns are usually blackened or charred. Pain in the burned area may be absent or diminished because of damage to the nerve endings. Many times it will not be possible to determine the thickness of burns immediately after they occur.

2. Why is a person with full-thickness burns at an increased risk for shock?

The integrity of the skin has been compromised in a full-thickness burn, allowing fluids to escape. The loss of body fluids can lead to hypovolemic shock. These patients can also develop severe infections if they do not receive proper and timely treatment.

Prep Kit

▶ Ready for Review

- This chapter covers the knowledge and skills you need to treat patients experiencing shock, bleeding, and soft-tissue injuries.
- Maintain standard precautions to prevent contact with the patient's body fluids.
- The three parts of the circulatory system are the pump (heart), the pipes (arteries, veins, and capillaries), and the fluid (blood cells and other blood components).
- Shock is a state of collapse of the cardiovascular system that results in inadequate delivery of blood to the organs. The three primary causes of shock are pump failure, pipe failure, and fluid loss. The general treatment for shock is positioning the patient correctly, maintaining the patient's ABCs, and treating the cause of shock, if possible.
- There are three types of external blood loss: capillary (blood oozes out), venous (bleeds at a steady flow), and arterial (blood spurts or surges). Most external bleeding can be controlled by applying direct pressure to the wound.
- A wound is an injury caused by any physical means that leads to damage of a body part. Wounds are classified as closed (skin remains intact) or open (skin is disrupted). Open wounds are classified as abrasions, punctures, lacerations, and avulsions or amputations.
- Control bleeding by covering an open wound with a dry, clean, or sterile dressing and apply pressure to the dressing with your hand. Additional ways to control bleeding include elevating an extremity, applying a tourniquet, and using pressure points.
- There are three classifications of burns by depth: superficial (first-degree) burns, partial-thickness (second-degree) burns, and full-thickness (third-degree) burns. Burns may be caused by heat, chemicals, or electricity.
- By learning to recognize and provide initial emergency treatment for patients experiencing shock, bleeding, and soft-tissue injuries, you will be able to provide physical and emotional assistance to these patients in their time of need. At times, your prompt recognition and treatment will make a real difference in the outcome.
- Injuries that affect more than one body system are called multi-system trauma. Multi-system trauma may be a result of an injury to one part of the body or it can be caused by injuries to different parts of the body.

▶ Vital Vocabulary

abrasion Loss or damage of skin as a result of a body part being rubbed or scraped across a rough or hard surface.

anaphylactic shock Shock caused by an extreme allergic reaction to certain foods, medications, or insect bites and stings.

arterial bleeding Serious bleeding from an artery in which blood frequently pulses or spurts from an open wound.

atria The two upper chambers of the heart.

avulsion An injury in which a piece of skin is torn completely loose or is left hanging as a flap.

blood pressure The pressure of the circulating blood against the walls of the arteries.

brachial artery pressure point Pressure point located in the arm between the elbow and the shoulder; also used in taking blood pressure and for checking the pulse in infants.

bruise Injury caused by a blunt object striking the body and crushing the tissue beneath the skin. Also called a contusion.

capillary bleeding Bleeding from the capillaries in which blood oozes from the open wound.

cardiogenic shock Shock resulting from inadequate functioning of the heart.

chemical burns Burns that occur when any toxic substance comes in contact with the skin. Most chemical burns are caused by strong acids or alkalis.

closed wound Injury in which soft-tissue damage occurs beneath the skin but there is no break in the surface of the skin.

congestive heart failure (CHF) Heart disease characterized by breathlessness, fluid retention in the lungs, and generalized swelling of the body.

cravat A triangular swathe of cloth used to hold a body part splinted against the body.

dressing Any of various materials placed directly on a wound to control bleeding and prevent further contamination.

electrical burns Burns caused by contact with high- or low-voltage electricity. Electrical burns have an entrance and an exit wound.

entrance wound Point where an object such as a bullet enters the body.

exit wound Point where an object such as a bullet passes out of the body.

femoral artery pressure point Pressure point located in the groin, in the middle of the bottom crease of the groin, between the groin and the upper thigh.

Prep Kit *Continued*

full-thickness burns Burns that extend through the skin and into the underlying tissues; the most serious class of burns.

gunshot wound A puncture wound caused by a bullet or shotgun pellets.

hemorrhage Excessive bleeding.

hemostatic agent A chemical compound that slows or stops bleeding by assisting with clot formation.

immobilize To reduce or prevent movement of a limb, usually by splinting.

impaled object An object such as a knife, splinter of wood, or glass that penetrates the skin and remains in the body.

intravenous (IV) fluids Fluids other than blood or blood products infused into the vascular system to maintain an adequate circulatory blood volume.

laceration An irregular cut or tear through the skin.

multi-system trauma An injury that affects more than one body system.

occlusive dressing An airtight dressing or bandage for a wound.

open wound Injury that breaks open the skin or mucous membrane.

partial-thickness burns Burns in which the outer layers of skin are burned; these burns are characterized by blister formation.

pneumatic antishock garments (PASGs) Trouser-like devices placed around a shock victim's legs and abdomen and inflated with air.

pressure points Points where a blood vessel lies near a bone; pressure can be applied to these points to help control bleeding.

psychogenic shock Commonly known as fainting; caused by a temporary reduction in blood supply to the brain.

puncture A wound resulting from a bullet, knife, ice pick, splinter, or any other pointed object.

rabies An acute viral infection of the central nervous system transmitted by the bite of an infected animal.

respiratory burn Burn to the respiratory system resulting from inhaling superheated air.

road rash An abrasion caused by sliding on pavement. Usually seen after motorcycle or bicycle accidents.

rule of nines Used to calculate the amount of body surface burned; the body is divided into sections, each of which constitutes approximately 9% or 18% of the total body surface area.

saline Salt water.

shock A state of collapse of the cardiovascular system; the state of inadequate delivery of blood to the organs of the body.

splint A means of immobilizing an injured part by using a rigid or soft support.

spontaneous nosebleed A nosebleed with no apparent cause.

superficial burns Burns in which only the superficial part of the skin has been injured; an example is a sunburn.

thermal burns Burn caused by heat; the most common type of burn.

venous bleeding External bleeding from a vein, characterized by steady flow; the bleeding may be profuse and life threatening.

ventricles The two lower chambers of the heart.

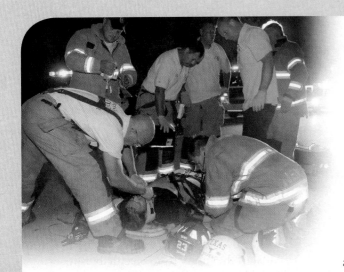

Assessment
in Action

You are dispatched to a lumber yard for a report of a log falling on a person. On arrival, you find a 21-year-old man lying in the supine position on the floor, holding his abdomen and reporting severe pain. He is also holding a blood-soaked T-shirt to his right forearm. Your primary assessment reveals a bruise approximately 3 inches (8 cm) in diameter to the right upper quadrant of the abdomen and a 1.5-inch (4-cm) flap of skin and fat that is loosely attached on his right arm, 2 inches (5 cm) below the elbow. Physical exam reveals a rigid abdomen. The patient has no pain in his head, neck, or spine. (Questions 1–6 relate to this scenario.)

1. What is your first concern as you arrive at the scene?

   A. The patient is bleeding profusely.
   B. How many patients are there?
   C. Do I have all the resources I need?
   D. Is the scene safe?

2. What is your primary concern about this patient?

   A. His back may be injured.
   B. He is bleeding into the abdomen and may go into shock.
   C. The cut on his arm may need a tourniquet.
   D. He is in a significant amount of pain.

3. What type of standard precaution is NOT needed when treating this patient?

   A. Gloves
   B. Eye protection
   C. Gown
   D. Face mask

4. What is the proper order to follow to control bleeding?

   1. Elevation
   2. Pressure points
   3. Direct pressure
   4. Tourniquet

      A. 3, 1, 4, 2
      B. 2, 3, 1, 4
      C. 3, 4, 2, 1
      D. 4, 1, 3, 2

5. What type of wound does this patient have on his arm?

   A. Avulsion
   B. Amputation
   C. Laceration
   D. Impaled object

6. If using a pressure point to assist in bleeding control for the forearm, which artery will you apply pressure to?

   A. Femoral
   B. Brachial
   C. Carotid
   D. Radial

7. Neck injuries may be life threatening because:

   A. they are close to the brain.
   B. they may result in injury to the parasympathetic nervous system.
   C. the neck contains many important structures.
   D. they result in shock.

8. Put the following steps for treating an impaled object in the proper order.

   1. Stabilize the object in place with dressings.
   2. Provide prompt transport to an appropriate medical facility.
   3. Do not attempt to remove the impaled object.
   4. Place a bandage over the dressings.

      A. 1, 4, 2, 3
      B. 3, 1, 4, 2
      C. 2, 3, 4, 1
      D. 3, 2, 1, 4

Assessment *in Action* Continued

9. Which of the following is NOT a recommended treatment for treating an open abdominal wound?

   A. Bandage the abdomen with a large trauma pad and several cravats.
   B. Place the patient on his or her back with his or her knees drawn up.
   C. Cover the intestines with a sterile dressing.
   D. Attempt to replace the intestines back in the abdomen.

10. Which of the following statements is NOT true about a patient who has come in contact with an electrical current?

   A. Electrical current often produces severe burns.
   B. Contact with an electrical current leaves little evidence of injury on the outside of the body.
   C. Electrical current may produce entrance and exit wounds.
   D. Most of the injury from electricity is to the skin.

Injuries to Muscles and Bones

National EMS Education Standard Competencies

Trauma

Uses simple knowledge to recognize and manage life threats based on assessment findings for an acutely injured patient while awaiting additional emergency medical response.

Orthopaedic Trauma

Recognition and management of:

› Open fractures (pp 307–325)
› Closed fractures (pp 307–325)
› Dislocations (p 308; pp 315–316; pp 319–320)
› Amputations (p 318)

Head, Facial, Neck, and Spine Trauma

Recognition and management of:

› Life threats (pp 327–334)
› Spine trauma (pp 330–334)

Knowledge Objectives

1. Discuss the anatomy and function of the musculoskeletal system. (pp 305–306)
2. Describe the mechanisms of injury for musculoskeletal injuries. (p 307)
3. Explain the characteristics of the following types of injuries:
   • Fractures (pp 307–308)
   • Dislocations (p 308)
   • Sprains and strains (p 308)
4. Explain the need for standard precautions when assessing or treating patients with musculoskeletal injuries. (p 308)
5. Explain how to assess a patient with a musculoskeletal injury. (p 309)
6. Explain how to check circulation, sensation, and movement in an injured extremity. (pp 309–312)
7. Describe how to splint the following injuries:
   • Shoulder girdle injury (p 315)
   • Shoulder dislocation (pp 315–316)
   • Elbow injury (p 316)
   • Forearm injury (pp 316–319)
   • Hand, wrist, or finger injury (pp 318–319)
   • Pelvic fracture (p 319)
   • Hip injury (pp 319–320)
   • Thigh injury (pp 321–323)
   • Knee injury (p 323)

   • Leg injury (pp 323–324)
   • Ankle or foot injury (pp 324–325)
8. List the signs and symptoms of open and closed head injuries. (p 328)
9. Describe the treatment of head injuries. (pp 328–329)
10. Describe the treatment of facial injuries. (pp 329–330)
11. Discuss the mechanism of spinal injuries. (pp 330–331)
12. List the signs and symptoms of spinal injury. (p 331)
13. Describe the treatment of spinal injury. (p 331)
14. Explain how to remove the mask on a sports helmet. (pp 332–333)
15. Explain how to remove a helmet. (pp 333–334)
16. Describe the signs, symptoms, and treatment of the following injuries:
    • Fractured ribs (p 335)
    • Flail chest (pp 335–336)
    • Penetrating chest wound (p 336)

Skills Objectives

1. Demonstrate use of standard precautions when assessing or treating patients with musculoskeletal injuries. (p 308)
2. Demonstrate assessment of a patient with a musculoskeletal injury. (p 309)
3. Demonstrate how to check circulation, sensation, and movement in an injured extremity. (pp 309–312)
4. Demonstrate how to splint the following injuries:
   • Shoulder girdle injury (p 315)
   • Shoulder dislocation (pp 315–316)
   • Elbow injury (p 316)
   • Forearm injury (pp 316–319)
   • Hand, wrist, or finger injury (pp 318–319)
   • Pelvic fracture (p 319)
   • Hip injury (pp 319–320)
   • Thigh injury (pp 321–323)
   • Knee injury (p 323)
   • Leg injury (pp 323–324)
   • Ankle or foot injury (pp 324–325)
5. Demonstrate the treatment of head injuries. (pp 328–329)
6. Demonstrate the treatment of facial injuries. (pp 329–330)
7. Demonstrate the treatment of spinal injury. (pp 330–331)
8. Demonstrate how to remove the mask on a sports helmet. (pp 332–333)
9. Demonstrate how to remove a helmet. (pp 333–334)
10. Demonstrate treatment of the following injuries:
    • Fractured ribs (p 335)
    • Flail chest (pp 335–336)
    • Penetrating chest wound (p 336)

Introduction

As an emergency medical responder (EMR), you will encounter many types of musculoskeletal injuries, including fractures, dislocations, sprains, strains, head injuries, spinal cord injuries, and chest injuries. You need to understand the basic anatomy and functioning of the musculoskeletal system and study the causes, or mechanisms, of injury. This will allow you to better understand the various injuries and know what care is needed.

Before you can treat musculoskeletal injuries, you must be able to recognize their signs and symptoms and to differentiate between open and closed injuries. Providing proper care at the scene can prevent additional injury or disability. This chapter describes how to manage injuries to the upper and lower extremities, the head, the spinal cord, and the chest. It also provides information on standard precautions and what steps you need to take to protect yourself when caring for a patient with musculoskeletal injuries.

Patient Assessment of Injuries to Muscles and Bones

When assessing a patient who has sustained an injury to the muscles and bones, you need to complete all five of the parts of the patient assessment sequence **Figure 15-1**. Begin with a thorough overview of the scene. This can often give you valuable information about the intensity and force of the incident. Do not get tunnel vision because the patient has an obvious injury. You need to complete all parts of the scene size-up to render the scene safe and to gain as much information as you can about the mechanism of injury. Be especially careful about following standard precautions to protect you and the patient from infectious diseases. When a patient has sustained a traumatic injury, there is a high chance that blood will be present.

Perform a complete primary assessment to determine whether the patient has any life-threatening

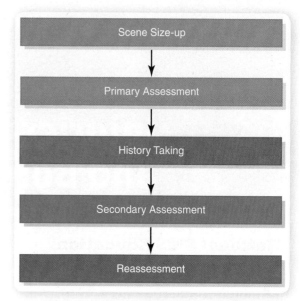

Figure 15-1 Patient assessment sequence.
© Jones & Bartlett Learning. Courtesy of MIEMSS.

conditions related to his or her airway, breathing, or circulation (including serious blood loss). Sometimes when a patient has an obvious soft-tissue injury or deformity of a limb, he or she may focus on that single injury and not be aware of additional conditions. These additional conditions may be more serious than the presenting problem (the chief complaint).

When performing a patient assessment on a trauma patient, it is often more efficient and helpful to perform the primary assessment and then immediately follow with the secondary assessment, holding off on obtaining the patient's medical history. Reordering the steps in this manner will give you a complete picture of all the physical findings about the patient. While you perform the secondary assessment, be thorough and systematic in examining all parts of the patient. However, do not get tunnel vision and assume that a trauma patient has no medical conditions. Heart conditions and low blood glucose levels in patients with diabetes can result in traumatic events. Be sure to perform a thorough SAMPLE medical history to determine whether the patient has any medical conditions that require attention. Finally, continue to reassess the patient every 15 minutes if the

YOU ▸ are the Provider　　　CASE 1

In the late afternoon on a clear, brisk autumn day, you are dispatched to a nearby park for the report of an injured person. Dispatch information reveals that your patient is a 14-year-old boy who has been injured while skateboarding. When you arrive at the scene, you find your patient lying on his side, complaining of severe pain in his left arm and elbow. He states that he was trying to skate along a ledge that was 2 inches (5 cm) high when he fell and landed on the parking lot. There appears to be significant deformity between his shoulder and elbow.

1. How should you conduct an assessment of this patient?
2. What type of injuries should you suspect with this patient?
3. Under what circumstances should you move this patient?

patient's condition is stable and every 5 minutes if the condition is unstable until other medical providers take over the care of the patient.

The Anatomy and Function of the Musculoskeletal System

The musculoskeletal system has two parts: the skeletal system, which provides support and form for the body, and the muscular system, which provides both support and movement.

▶ The Skeletal System

The skeletal system consists of 206 bones and is the supporting framework for the body. The four functions of the skeletal system are:

1. To support the body
2. To protect vital structures
3. To assist in body movement
4. To manufacture red blood cells

The skeletal system is divided into seven areas **Figure 15-2**:

1. Head, skull, and face
2. Spinal column
3. Shoulder girdle
4. Upper extremities
5. Rib cage (thorax)
6. Pelvis
7. Lower extremities

The bones of the head include the skull and the lower jawbone. The skull consists of many bones fused together to form a hollow sphere. It contains and protects the brain. The jawbone is a movable bone attached to the skull that completes the structure of the face.

The spine consists of a series of separate bones called vertebrae. The spinal vertebrae are stacked on top of each other. Muscles, tendons, disks, and ligaments hold them together. The spinal cord, a group of nerves that carry messages to and from the brain, passes through a hole in the center of each vertebra. In addition to protecting the spinal cord, the spine is the primary support structure for the entire body.

The spine has five sections **Figure 15-3**:

1. Cervical spine (neck)
2. Thoracic spine (upper back)
3. Lumbar spine (lower back)
4. Sacrum
5. Coccyx (tailbone)

The shoulder girdles form the third area of the skeletal system. Each shoulder girdle supports an arm and consists of the collarbone (clavicle) and the shoulder blade (scapula). The fourth area of the skeletal system, the upper extremities, consists of three major bones as

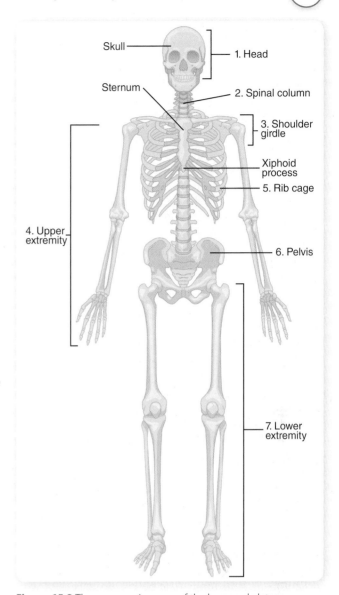

Figure 15-2 The seven major areas of the human skeleton.
© Jones & Bartlett Learning.

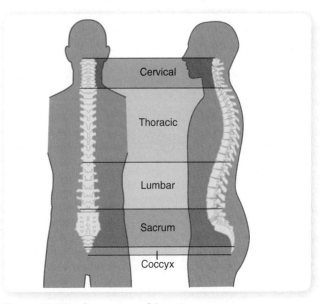

Figure 15-3 The five sections of the spine.
© Jones & Bartlett Learning.

well as the wrist and hand. The **arm** has one bone (the humerus), and the forearm has two bones (the radius and the ulna). The radius is located on the thumb side of the arm; the ulna is located on the side of the little finger. There are several bones in the wrist and hand. However, you do not need to learn their names at this time and you can consider them as one unit for the purposes of emergency treatment.

The fifth area of the skeletal system is the rib cage or chest (thorax). The 12 sets of ribs protect the heart, lungs, liver, and spleen. All of the ribs are attached to the spine **Figure 15-4**. The upper five rib sets connect directly to the sternum (breastbone). A bridge of cartilage connects the ends of the 6th through 10th rib sets to each other and to the sternum. The 11th and 12th rib sets are called floating ribs because they are not attached to the sternum. The sternum is located in the front of the chest. The pointed structure at the bottom of the sternum is called the xiphoid process.

The sixth area of the skeletal system is the pelvis, which links the body and the lower extremities. The pelvis also protects the reproductive organs and the other organs located in the lower abdominal cavity.

The lower extremities (the thigh and the leg) form the seventh area of the skeletal system. The **thighbone** (femur) is the longest and strongest bone in the entire body. The **leg** consists of two major bones, the tibia and fibula, as well as the ankle and foot. The kneecap (patella) is a small, relatively flat bone that protects the front of the knee **joint**. Like the wrist and hand, the ankle and foot contain a large number of smaller bones that can be considered as one unit.

A protective bony structure surrounds each of the body's essential organs. The skull protects the brain. The vertebrae protect the spinal cord. The ribs protect the heart and lungs. The pelvis protects the lower abdominal and reproductive organs. A vital but often overlooked function of the skeletal system is to produce red blood cells. Red blood cells are manufactured primarily within the spaces inside the bone called the marrow.

▶ The Muscular System

The muscles of the body provide both support and movement. Muscles are attached to bones by tendons and cause movement by alternately contracting (shortening) and relaxing (lengthening). Muscles are usually paired in opposition: As one member of the pair contracts, the other relaxes. This mechanical opposition moves bones and enables you to open and close your hand, turn your head, and bend and straighten your knee or other joints. To straighten the elbow, for example, the biceps muscle relaxes and an opposing muscle on the back of the arm contracts.

The musculoskeletal system gets its name from the coordination between the muscular system and the skeletal system to produce movement. Movement occurs at joints, where two bones come together. Ligaments hold the bones together. Ligaments are thick bands that arise from one bone, span the joint, and insert into the adjacent bone.

The body has three types of muscles: voluntary, involuntary, and cardiac. Voluntary, or skeletal, muscles are attached to bones and can be contracted and relaxed by a person at will. They are responsible for the movement of the body. Involuntary, or smooth, muscles are found on the inside of the digestive tract and other internal organs of the body. They are not under conscious control and perform their functions automatically. Cardiac muscle is found only in the heart **Figure 15-5**. Most musculoskeletal injuries involve skeletal muscles.

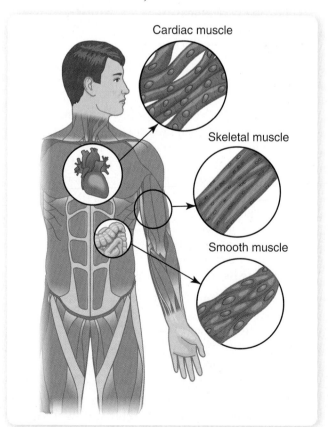

Figure 15-5 Three types of muscle in the human body.
© Jones & Bartlett Learning.

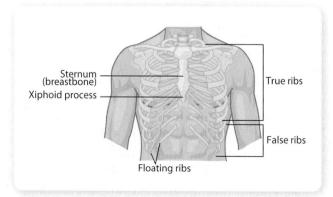

Figure 15-4 The rib cage.
© Jones & Bartlett Learning.

Mechanism of Injury

As an EMR, you must understand the **mechanism of injury (MOI)**, or how injuries occur. Three types of mechanisms of injury cause musculoskeletal injuries: direct force, indirect force, and twisting force **Figure 15-6**.

Examples of each mechanism and the type of injury it causes are as follows:

- **Direct force.** A car strikes a pedestrian on the leg. The pedestrian sustains a broken leg.
- **Indirect force.** A woman falls on her shoulder. The force of the fall transmits energy to the middle of the collarbone and the excess force breaks the bone.
- **Twisting force.** A football player is tackled as he is turning. As the leg twists, the knee sustains

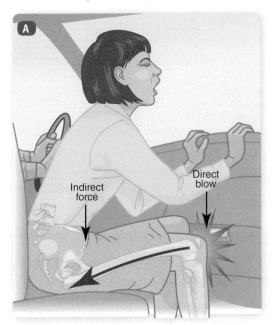

Indirect force

Direct blow

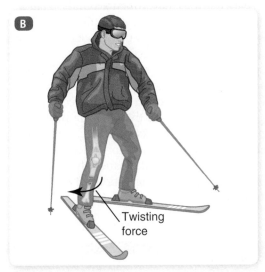

Twisting force

Figure 15-6 Three types of mechanisms of injury cause musculoskeletal injuries. **A.** Direct force and indirect force. **B.** Twisting force.

A&B: © Jones & Bartlett Learning.

a severe injury. Injuries can be caused by direct force at the site of impact or by indirect force at an impact site removed from the site of the injury.

As an EMR, you will see many different types of traumatic injuries. Some of these injuries will be the result of motor vehicle crashes involving one or more motor vehicles or a motor vehicle and a pedestrian; others will be the result of athletic activities, work-related accidents, falls, or violence. You will see injuries in people of all ages—from very young children to older people. Use the information provided by your dispatcher and gathered from your overview of the scene to identify the possible mechanisms of injury. You will gain additional information from examining and questioning the patient. By understanding the mechanism of injury (how the injury occurred), you will be better able to assess the patient and provide the needed treatment.

▶ A Word About Terminology

A patient's injuries can be described in different ways. You must rely on your senses of sight and touch to determine the type of injury the patient has experienced. You must also listen to the information that the patient gives you. However, keep in mind that, as an EMR, you do not have the training or tools to diagnose an injury as a physician can.

The next section defines fractures, dislocations, and sprains/strains. Although you are not expected to diagnose these injuries, the patient's signs and symptoms will lead you to suspect that a certain injury is most probable. Some instructors and medical directors may choose to identify musculoskeletal injuries strictly in terms of the signs and symptoms present, such as a painful, swollen, deformed extremity. Others may choose to use terms such as suspected or possible fracture, dislocation, or sprain. Regardless of the terminology used, the most important part of your job is to provide the best assessment and treatment for the patient.

Types of Injuries

It is often difficult to distinguish one type of musculoskeletal extremity injury from another. All three types are serious, and all extremity injuries must be identified so that appropriate medical treatment can be provided.

▶ Fractures

A fracture is a broken bone. A variety of mechanisms can cause a fracture, but a fracture most often occurs as a result of a significant force, unless the bone is weakened by a disease such as osteoporosis or cancer. Fractures are generally classified as closed or open **Figure 15-7**. In the more common **closed fracture**, the bone is broken but there is no break in the skin.

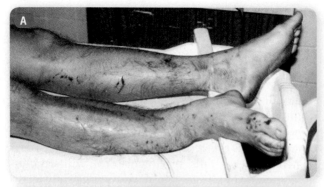

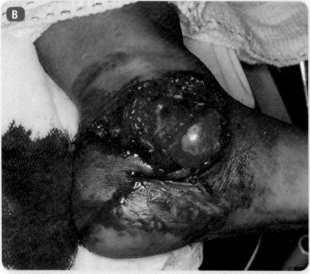

Figure 15-7 A. Closed fracture. **B.** Open fracture.
A&B: © Chuck Stewart, MD.

▶ Sprains and Strains

A **sprain** is a joint injury caused by excessive stretching of the supporting ligaments. Think of it as a partial dislocation. Strains are caused by stretching or tearing of a muscle.

In an **open fracture**, the bone is broken and the overlying skin is lacerated. The open wound can be caused by a penetrating object, such as a bullet, or by the fractured bone end itself protruding through the skin. Open fractures are likely contaminated by dirt and bacteria that may lead to infection. A patient with an open fracture requires more extensive care in the hospital to ensure that the associated wound is properly cleaned and the fracture properly treated to reduce the chance of developing a serious infection. Both open and closed fractures injure adjacent soft tissues, resulting in bleeding at the fracture site. Fractures can also injure nearby nerves and blood vessels, causing severe nerve injury and excessive internal or external bleeding.

▶ Dislocations

A **dislocation** is a disruption that tears the supporting ligaments of the joint. The bone ends that make up the joint separate completely from each other and can lock in one position. Any attempt to move a dislocated joint is very painful. Because many nerves and blood vessels lie near joints, a dislocation can damage these structures as well.

■ Standard Precautions and Musculoskeletal Injuries

While you examine and treat patients with musculoskeletal injuries, you need to practice standard precautions. These patients may have open wounds related to the musculoskeletal injury or to a separate, open soft-tissue injury. Assume that trauma patients have open wounds that pose a threat of infection. Always wear approved gloves. When you are responding to motor vehicle crashes or to other situations that may present a hazard from broken glass or other sharp objects, it is wise to wear heavy rescue gloves that provide protection from sharp objects. Some EMRs wear latex or nitrile gloves under the heavy rescue gloves for added protection from infectious body fluids. If the patient has active bleeding that may splatter, wear protection for your eyes, nose, and mouth as well.

Examination of Musculoskeletal Injuries

The three essential steps in examining a patient with a limb injury are as follows:

1. General assessment of the patient according to the patient assessment sequence
2. Examination of the injured part
3. Evaluation of the circulation, sensation, and movement in the injured limb

▶ General Patient Assessment

When caring for an injured patient, you must carry out all the steps in the patient assessment process before focusing your attention on any injured limb. Once you have checked and stabilized the patient's airway, breathing, and circulation (ABCs), you can then direct your attention to the injured limb identified during the physical examination.

Limb injuries are not life threatening unless there is excessive bleeding from an open wound. Therefore, it is essential that you first stabilize the patient's airway, breathing, and circulation (ABCs) before you focus on a limb injury, regardless of the pain or deformity that may be present at that injury site.

As you examine and treat patients with musculoskeletal injuries, remember that this is a frightening and painful experience for them. Explain what you are doing as you conduct your examination and stabilize the patient. Treat the patient with the same care and consideration that you would give to a close member of your own family.

▶ Examination of the Injured Limb

As an EMR, you should initially inspect the injured limb and compare it to the opposite, uninjured limb. To do this, gently and carefully cut away any clothing covering the wound, if necessary. (Never hesitate to cut a patient's clothing to uncover a suspected injury.)

> **Words of Wisdom**
>
> Listen to the patient. He or she is usually right about the location and type of injury.

When you examine the limb, you may find any one of the following:

- An open wound
- Deformity
- Swelling
- Bruising

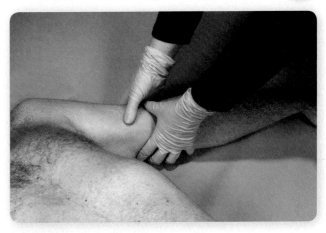

Figure 15-8 Examine the extremities.
© Jones & Bartlett Learning. Courtesy of MIEMSS.

After you uncover and look at the injured limb, gently feel it for any points of tenderness. Tenderness is the best indicator of an underlying fracture, dislocation, or sprain.

To detect limb injury, start at the top of each limb (where it connects to the body) and using both hands, squeeze the entire limb in a systematic, firm (yet gentle) manner, moving down the limb and away from the body Figure 15-8 . Make sure you examine the entire extremity.

As you carry out your hands-on examination, it is important to ask the patient where it hurts most; the location of greatest pain is probably the injury site. Also ask if the patient feels tingling or numbness in the extremity because this may indicate nerve damage or lack of circulation.

Careful inspection and a gentle hands-on examination will identify most musculoskeletal injuries. After you have made a careful visual and hands-on examination, and if the patient shows no sign of injury, ask the patient to move the limb carefully. If there is an injury, the patient will report pain and refuse to move the limb.

The signs or symptoms described earlier (deformity, swelling, bruising, tenderness, or pain with motion) indicate the presence of a limb injury. Only one sign is necessary to indicate an injury to the limb. Manage all limb injuries, regardless of type or severity, in the same way.

> **Treatment**
>
> If even the slightest motion causes the patient to report pain, NO further motion should be attempted.

▶ Evaluation of Circulation, Sensation, and Movement

Once you suspect limb injury, you must evaluate the circulation and sensation in that limb. Many important blood vessels and nerves lie close to the bones, especially around major joints. Therefore, any injury may have associated blood vessel or nerve damage. It is also essential to check circulation and sensation after any movement of the limb (such as for splinting). Moving the limb during splinting may cause a bone fragment to press against or even cut a blood vessel or nerve **Skill Drill 15-1** :

1. **Pulse.** Feel the pulse distal to the point of injury. If the patient has an upper extremity injury, check the radial (wrist) pulse **Step 1** . If the patient has a lower extremity injury, check the tibial (posterior ankle) pulse **Step 2** .

2. **Capillary refill.** Test the capillary refill in a finger or toe of any injured limb. Firm pressure on the tip of the nail causes the nail bed to turn white **Step 3** . Release the pressure and the normal pink color should return by the time it takes to say "capillary refill" **Step 4** . If the pink color does not return in this 2-second interval, it is considered to be delayed or absent and indicates a circulation condition in the limb. A cold environment will naturally delay capillary refill, so in that situation, do not use capillary refill to assess an injured limb. The absence of a pulse or capillary refill indicates that a limb is in immediate danger. Impaired circulation demands *prompt transportation* and prompt medical treatment at an appropriate medical facility.

Skill Drill 15-1

Checking Circulation, Sensation, and Movement in an Injured Extremity

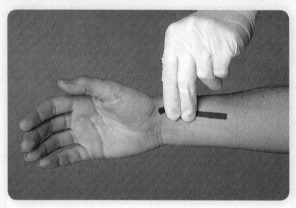

Step 1 Check for circulation. If upper extremity injury, check radial pulse.

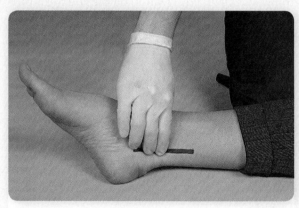

Step 2 If lower extremity injury, check posterior tibial pulse.

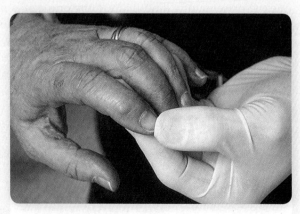

Step 3 Test capillary refill on finger/toe of injured limb.

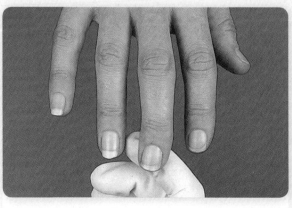

Step 4 Release pressure. Pink color should return.

Skill Drill 15-1 *Continued*

Checking Circulation, Sensation, and Movement in an Injured Extremity

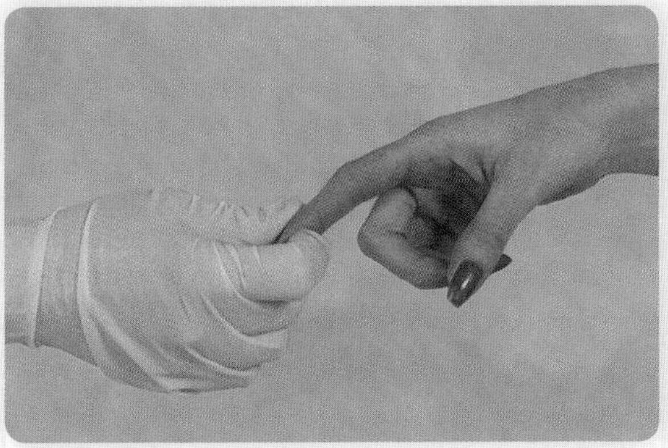

Step 5 Check for sensation at fingertips.

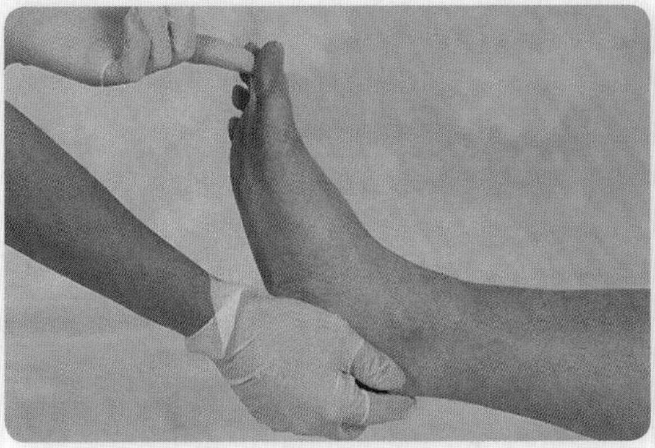

Step 6 Check for sensation at toes.

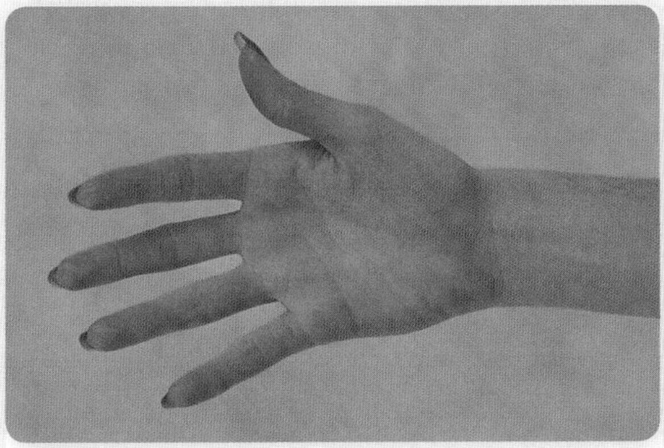

Step 7A Check for movement of the upper extremities by asking the patient to open (7A) and close (7B) the fist.

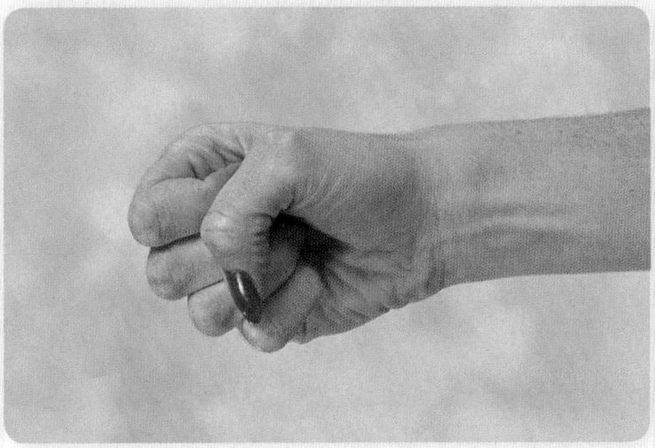

Step 7B

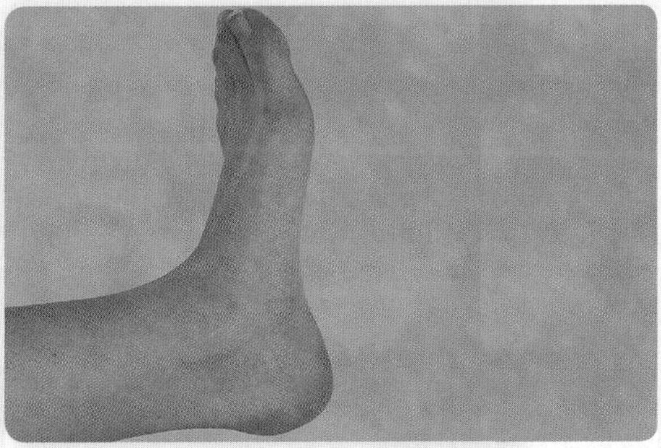

Step 8A Check for movement of the lower extremities by asking the patient to flex the ankle (or doriflex the ankle) (8A) and extend the ankle (or plantarflex the ankle) (8B).

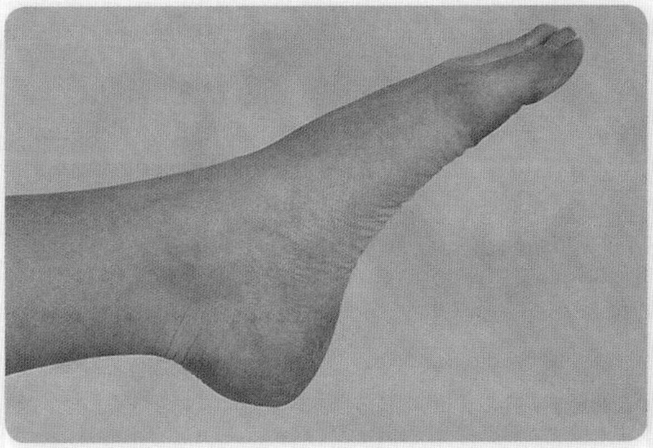

Step 8B

© Jones & Bartlett Learning. Courtesy of MIEMSS.

3. **Sensation.** The patient's ability to feel your light touch on the fingers or toes is a good indication that the nerve supply is intact. In the hand, check sensation by lightly touching the tips of the index and little fingers **Step 5** . In the foot, check the tip of the big toe and the top of the foot for sensation **Step 6** .

4. **Movement.** If the hand or foot is injured, do not have the patient perform this part of the test. When the injury is between the hand and the body or the foot and the body, have the patient open and close the fist **Step 7** or flex the foot of the injured limb **Step 8** . These simple movements indicate that the nerves to these muscles are working. Sometimes any attempt at motion will produce pain. In this situation, do not ask the patient to move the limb any further. Consider any open wound, deformity, swelling, or bruising of a limb evidence of a possible limb injury and treat it as such. Try to keep the extremity in a position of comfort for the patient.

Treatment

Examine the following factors for each injured limb:

- Pulse
- Capillary refill
- Sensation
- Movement

■ Treatment of Musculoskeletal Injuries

Regardless of their extent or severity, treat all limb injuries in the same way in the field. For all open extremity wounds, first cover the entire wound with a dry, sterile dressing, and then apply firm but gentle pressure to control bleeding, if necessary. The sterile compression dressing protects the wound and underlying tissues from further contamination. Apply a cold pack to painful, swollen, or deformed extremities. Then splint the injured limb.

▶ General Principles of Splinting

Splint all limb injuries before moving a patient, unless the environment prevents effective splinting or threatens the patient's life (or your life). Splinting prevents the movement of broken bone ends, a dislocated joint, or damaged soft tissues and thereby reduces pain. With less pain, the patient relaxes and the trip to the medical

facility is easier. Splinting also helps to control bleeding and decreases the risk of damage to the nearby nerves and vessels by sharp bone fragments. Splinting prevents closed fractures from becoming open fractures during movement or transportation.

All EMRs should know the following general principles of splinting:

1. In most situations, remove clothing from the injured limb to inspect the limb for open wounds, deformity, swelling, bruising, and capillary refill.
2. Note and record the pulse, capillary refill, sensation, and movement distal to the point of injury, both before and after splinting.
3. Cover all open wounds with a dry, sterile dressing before applying the splint.
4. Do not move the patient before splinting, unless there is an immediate danger to the patient or to you.
5. Immobilize the joint above and the joint below the injury site.
6. Pad all rigid splints.
7. When applying the splint, use your hands to support the injury site and minimize movement of the limb until splinting is completed.
8. Splint the limb without moving it unnecessarily.
9. When in doubt, splint.

▶ Materials Used for Splinting

Many different materials can be used as splints, if necessary. Even when standard splints are not available, you can bind an injured arm to a patient's chest and secure an injured leg to the other, uninjured lower extremity for temporary stability.

Rigid Splints

Rigid splints are made from firm material and are applied to the sides, front, or back of an injured extremity. Common types of rigid splints include padded board splints, molded plastic or aluminum splints, padded wire ladder splints, structured aluminum malleable (SAM) splints, and folded cardboard splints **Figure 15-9** . Padded wire ladder or SAM splints can be molded to the shape of the limb to splint it in the position found.

Treatment

Three basic types of splints are as follows:

1. Rigid
2. Soft
3. Traction

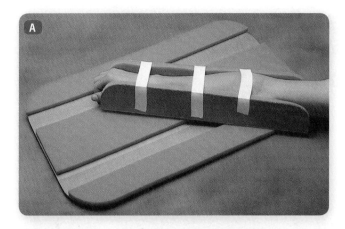

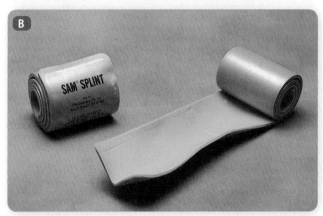

Figure 15-9 A. Rigid cardboard splints. **B.** SAM splints.
A&B: © American Academy of Orthopaedic Surgeons.

Soft Splints

Soft splints are flexible and easy to place around an injured limb 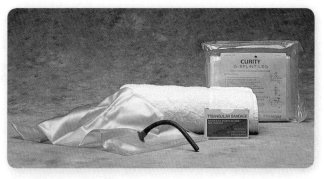 **Figure 15-10** . The most commonly used soft splints are **vacuum splints** and inflatable, clear plastic air splints. Vacuum splints become rigid when air is removed from the splint. Air splints become rigid when they are inflated with air.

Vacuum splints consist of an airtight covering that is shaped to fit around an arm or a leg. They are constructed with an inner layer of airtight fabric and an outer layer of the same fabric. Located between these two layers of fabric are small beads of a hard foam material surrounded by air. This makes the splint flexible and easy to mold to the contours of the patient's injured limb. When you remove air from inside the vacuum splint, it becomes more rigid and provides support for the injured limb. A vacuum pump to remove the air is included with the splint. Most vacuum splints have Velcro fasteners to make it easier to apply the splint.

Vacuum splints are not transparent so it is not possible to observe the limb once the splint is applied. Protect vacuum splints from damage from sharp objects. If they are punctured, the splint will become flexible and no longer be an effective splint. When using vacuum splints, you must monitor the pulse, movement, and sensation of the injured limb and the status of the vacuum splint itself. Changes in altitude and temperature can affect the

Figure 15-10 Soft splints.
© American Academy of Orthopaedic Surgeons.

rigidity of a vacuum splint. The steps for applying a vacuum splint are illustrated in **Skill Drill 15-2** .

1. Assess distal pulse and motor and sensory function.
2. Your partner supports and stabilizes the injured limb, applying traction if needed **Step 1** .
3. Gently place the injured limb onto the vacuum splint, and wrap the splint around the limb **Step 2** .
4. Draw the air out of the splint through the suction valve and then seal the valve. Once the valve is sealed, the vacuum splint becomes rigid, conforming to the shape of the deformed limb and stabilizing it **Step 3** .
5. Check distal circulation and nervous functions, and monitor them en route.

Air splints are constructed of a clear, flexible, plastic material. They are manufactured in a variety of sizes and shapes, with or without a zipper that runs the length of the splint **Figure 15-11** . Air splints are applied around the limb and then inflated by blowing into a specially constructed valve. Do not use a pump to inflate an air splint. The pressure from the air forms the air splint around the injured limb in a manner opposite from the way a vacuum splint works. Air splints are largely transparent, so it is possible to monitor the appearance of the injured limb after you apply one. Air splints provide support and are comfortable for the patient. Because they provide uniform pressure, you can use an air splint to apply pressure on a bleeding wound.

Protect air splints from sharp objects that could puncture them. When using air splints, monitor the pulse, motor function, and sensation of the injured limb. Also monitor the level of inflation of the air splint. Changes in altitude and temperature can affect the rigidity of an air splint.

Safety

NEVER use anything but the air from your mouth to inflate air splints!

Skill Drill 15-2

Applying a Vacuum Splint

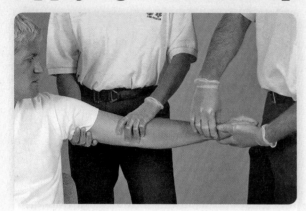

Step 1 Assess distal pulse and motor and sensory functions. Your partner stabilizes and supports the injury.

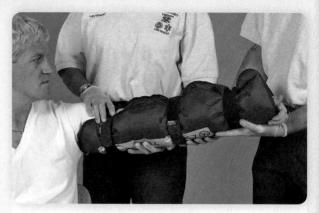

Step 2 Place the splint, and wrap it around the limb.

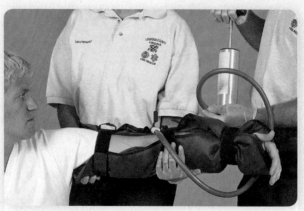

Step 3 Draw the air out of the splint through the suction valve and then seal the valve. Assess distal pulse and motor and sensory functions.

© Jones & Bartlett Learning. Courtesy of MIEMSS.

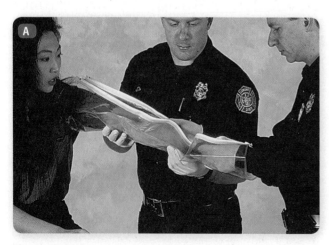

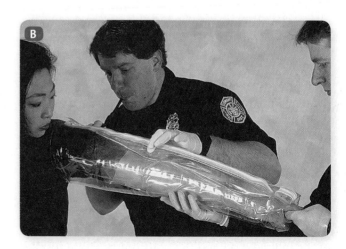

Figure 15-11 A. A zippered air splint. **B.** An unzippered air splint.
A&B: © Jones & Bartlett Learning. Courtesy of MIEMSS.

Traction Splints

A **traction splint** holds a lower extremity fracture in alignment by applying a constant, steady pull on the extremity. Properly applying a traction splint requires two well-trained emergency medical technicians (EMTs) working together; one person cannot do it alone. While most EMRs do not learn the skills necessary to apply this type of splint, you may be asked to assist trained medical personnel in the placement of a traction splint, and you should be familiar with the general techniques, as shown later in Skill Drill 15-6. There are several different types of traction splints. If you will be helping to apply a traction splint, you need instruction on the device used by your service.

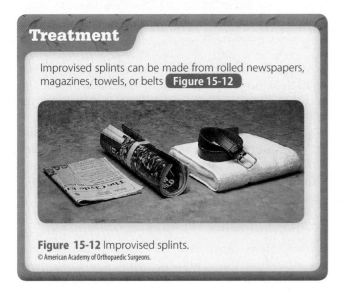

Treatment

Improvised splints can be made from rolled newspapers, magazines, towels, or belts **Figure 15-12**.

Figure 15-12 Improvised splints.
© American Academy of Orthopaedic Surgeons.

▶ Splinting Specific Injury Sites

A person with EMR training and with materials readily available can carry out the treatment techniques described here. Most splinting techniques are two-person operations. One person stabilizes and supports the injured limb while the other person applies the splint.

Shoulder Girdle Injuries

The easiest way to splint most shoulder injuries is to apply a **sling** made of a triangular bandage and to secure the sling (and arm) to the patient's body with swathes around the arm and chest. Apply the sling by tying a knot in the point of the triangular bandage, placing the elbow into the cup formed by the knot, and passing the two ends of the bandage up and around the patient's neck. Tie the sling so the wrist is slightly higher than the elbow **Figure 15-13**.

To keep the arm immobilized, fold another triangular bandage until you have a long swathe that is 3 to 4 inches (8 to 10 cm) wide **Figure 15-14**. Tie one or two swathes around the upper arm and chest of the patient. This easily applied splint adequately immobilizes fractures of the collarbone, most shoulder injuries, and fractures of the arm.

Shoulder Dislocation

The dislocated shoulder is the only shoulder girdle injury that is difficult to immobilize with a sling and swathe. In a shoulder dislocation, there is often a space between the upper arm and the chest wall. Fill this space with a pillow or a rolled blanket before applying a sling and swathe as for other shoulder injuries **Figure 15-15**.

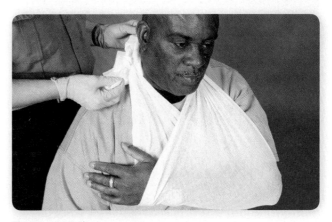

Figure 15-13 Sling.
© Jones & Bartlett Learning. Courtesy of MIEMSS.

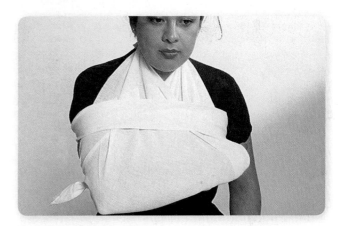

Figure 15-14 Sling and swathe.
© Jones & Bartlett Learning. Courtesy of MIEMSS.

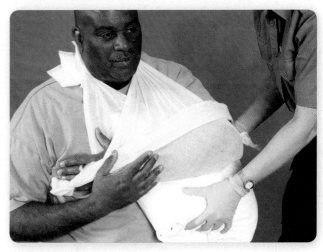

Figure 15-15 Splint the dislocated shoulder in a position of comfort by placing a pillow or towel between the arm and the chest before applying a sling and swathe.
© Jones & Bartlett Learning. Courtesy of MIEMSS.

Words of Wisdom

When triangular bandages are not available, loop a length of gauze (or even a belt) around the patient's wrist and suspend the limb from the neck **Figure 15-16**. Secure the arm gently, but firmly, to the chest wall with another length of gauze or belt. If you have not cut away the coat a patient is wearing, you can also pin a coat sleeve to the front of the patient's coat as a temporary splint **Figure 15-17**. This technique is less secure than a sling and swathe, but it may be of use in cold weather areas.

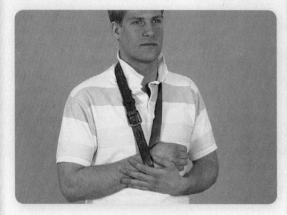

Figure 15-16 Improvised sling using a belt.
© American Academy of Orthopaedic Surgeons.

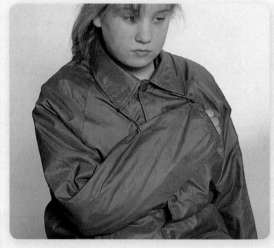

Figure 15-17 Improvised sling using safety pins.
© American Academy of Orthopaedic Surgeons.

Elbow Injuries

Do not move an injured elbow from the position in which you find it. You must splint the elbow as it lies because any movement can cause nerve or blood vessel damage. If the elbow is straight, splint it straight. If the elbow is bent at an unusual angle, splint it in that position.

After splinting the injured elbow of a patient who does not have a significant shoulder injury (and only if it does not cause pain), gently move the splinted injury to the patient's side for comfort and ease of transport.

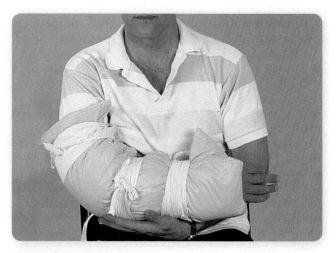

Figure 15-18 Pillow splint.
© American Academy of Orthopaedic Surgeons.

An effective splint for an injured elbow is a pillow splint. Wrap the elbow in a pillow, add additional padding to keep the elbow in the position found, and secure the pillow as shown in **Figure 15-18**.

The patient is usually transported in a sitting position with the splinted elbow resting on his or her lap. A padded wire ladder or SAM splint is also effective for splinting elbows that are found in severely deformed positions.

Forearm Injuries

Several splints can be used to stabilize the **forearm**: the air splint, the cardboard splint, the SAM splint **Skill Drill 15-3**, and even rolled newspapers and magazines. Be sure to pad all rigid splints adequately.

1. Support and stabilize the injured limb.
2. Form the SAM splint to the injured forearm **Step 1**.
3. Place the splint under the injured limb **Step 2**.
4. Secure the splint in place with gauze **Step 3**.
5. Recheck the pulse, capillary refill, and sensation of the injured forearm.

An air splint can be applied quickly, and it immobilizes the forearm quite well. Of the several types of air splints available, the one with a full-length zipper is easiest to use **Skill Drill 15-4**.

1. Apply gentle traction to the limb and support the site of injury. Have your partner place the open, deflated splint around the limb **Step 1**.
2. Zip up the splint and inflate it by mouth. Then test the pressure in the splint. With proper inflation, you should just be able to compress the walls of the splint together with a firm pinch between the thumb and index finger near the edge of the splint **Step 2**.
3. Check and record pulse and motor and sensory functions, and monitor them periodically until the patient reaches the hospital.

Skill Drill 15-3

Applying a SAM Splint

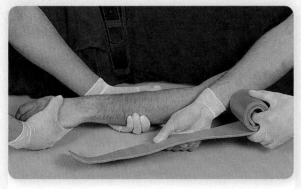

Step 1 Stabilize the injured limb. Form the SAM splint.

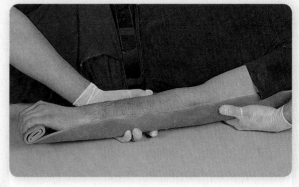

Step 2 Place the splint under the injured limb.

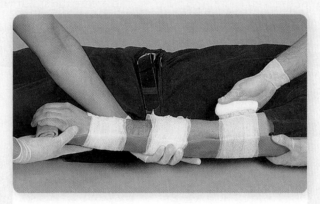

Step 3 Secure with gauze.

© Jones & Bartlett Learning. Courtesy of MIEMSS.

Skill Drill 15-4

Applying a Zippered Air Splint

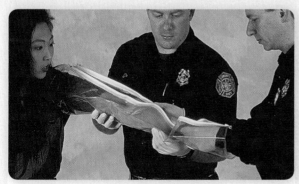

Step 1 Support the injured limb and apply gentle traction as your partner applies the open, deflated splint.

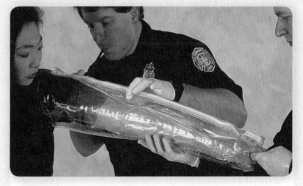

Step 2 Zip up the splint, inflate it by mouth, and test the pressure. Check and record distal pulse and motor and sensory functions.

© Jones & Bartlett Learning. Courtesy of MIEMSS.

The steps for applying an air splint without a zipper are illustrated in Skill Drill 15-5 .

1. Assess distal pulse and motor and sensory functions.
2. Your partner supports the patient's injured limb until splinting is complete.
3. Place your arm through the splint. Extend your hand beyond the splint, and grasp the hand or foot of the injured limb Step 1 .
4. Apply gentle traction to the hand or foot while sliding the splint onto the injured limb. The hand or foot of the injured limb should always be included in the splint Step 2 .
5. Your partner inflates the splint by mouth Step 3 .
6. Test the pressure in the splint. You must do this with either type of air splint.
7. Check and record pulse and motor and sensory functions, and monitor them en route.

Hand, Wrist, and Finger Injuries

As an EMR, you will see a variety of hand injuries, all of which can be potentially serious. The functions of the fingers and hand are so complex that any injury, if poorly or inadequately treated, may result in permanent deformity and disability. Treat even seemingly simple lacerations carefully. You can use a bulky hand dressing and a short splint to immobilize all injuries of the wrist, hand, and fingers. Send any amputated parts to the hospital with the patient by placing them in a sealed plastic bag. Cool the plastic bag by placing it in a cold water bath; never place the amputated part directly on ice.

To treat injuries of the hand, wrist, or fingers, first cover all wounds with a dry, sterile dressing. Then place the injured hand and wrist into the position of function Figure 15-19 . Place one or two soft roller dressings into the palm of the patient's hand. Apply a splint to hold the wrist, hand, and fingers in the position of function and secure the splint with a soft roller bandage.

Skill Drill 15-5

Applying an Unzipped Air Splint

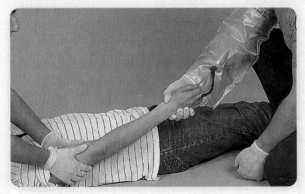

Step 1 Assess distal pulse and motor and sensory functions. Your partner supports the injured limb. Place your arm through the splint to grasp the patient's hand or foot.

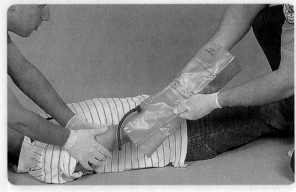

Step 2 Apply gentle traction while sliding the splint onto the injured limb.

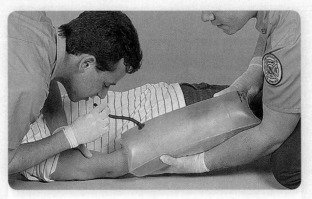

Step 3 Your partner inflates the splint by mouth. Assess distal pulse and motor and sensory functions.

Figure 15-19 Position of function for the hand and wrist.
© American Academy of Orthopaedic Surgeons.

Treatment

If you have to improvise a splint for a forearm injury, **Figure 15-20** shows how to apply a splint made of magazines and newspapers.

Figure 15-20 Applying an improvised splint using magazines. **A.** Immobilize the fracture above and below the fracture site. **B.** Place improvised splinting material around injured extremity. **C.** Secure in place with gauze, cravats, or other available material.
A, B, & C: © American Academy of Orthopaedic Surgeons.

Pelvic Fractures

Fractures of the pelvis often involve severe blood loss because the broken bones can easily lacerate the large blood vessels that run directly beside the pelvis. These vessels can release a large amount of blood into the pelvic area. Pelvic fractures commonly cause shock. Therefore, you must always treat the patient for shock.

The most definite sign of a pelvic fracture is tenderness when you use both your hands to firmly compress the patient's pelvis **Figure 15-21**. Immobilize fractures of the pelvis with a long backboard, as illustrated in **Figure 15-22**. EMTs may apply a pelvic compression binder or a pneumatic antishock garment to stabilize the fracture and treat shock.

Hip Injuries

Two types of hip injuries are common: dislocations and fractures. Both injuries may result from high-energy **trauma**. When a passenger in the front seat of a motor vehicle is not wearing a seat belt and the vehicle crashes, the person is thrown forward and crashes against the dashboard. The impact of the knee against the dashboard is transmitted up the shaft of the thighbone (femur), injuring the hip and often producing either a dislocation or a fracture, or both **Figure 15-23**.

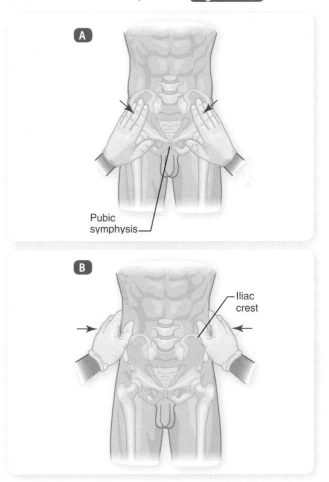

Pubic symphysis

Iliac crest

Figure 15-21 Examining the patient for pelvic fracture. **A.** Push down. **B.** Push in.
A&B: © Jones & Bartlett Learning.

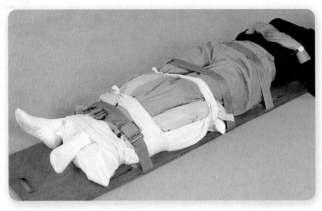

Figure 15-22 Immobilization of hip or pelvic injuries using a backboard.
© American Academy of Orthopaedic Surgeons.

Hip fractures actually occur at the upper end of the femur, rather than in the hip joint itself. High-energy trauma is not the only cause of hip fractures. They can occur in older adults, especially women, after only minimal trauma (such as falling down). These fractures in older adults occur because bone weakens and becomes more fragile with advancing age, a condition called **osteoporosis**. Patients with osteoporosis may sustain major fractures from minor falls.

A dislocated hip is extremely painful, especially when any movement is attempted. The joint is usually locked with the thigh flexed and rotated inward across the midline of the body. The knee joint is often flexed as well. Fractures of the hip region usually cause the injured limb to become shortened and externally (outwardly) rotated   Figure 15-24 .

Treat all hip injuries by immobilizing the hip in the position found. Use several pillows and/or rolled blankets, especially under the flexed knee. The patient should be placed on a backboard for transportation. The patient and the limb should be well stabilized to eliminate all motion in the hip region (see Figure 15-22).

Because fractures of the upper end of the femur are so common in older patients, any older person who has fallen and reports pain in the hip, thigh, or knee—even if there is no deformity—should be splinted and transported to the hospital for radiographic evaluation.

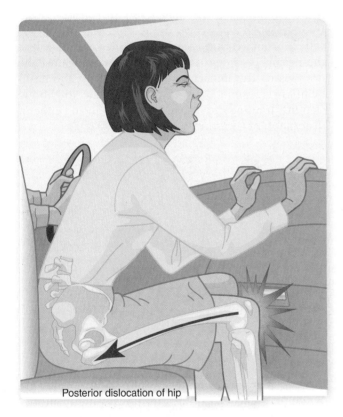

Posterior dislocation of hip

Figure 15-23 Posterior dislocation of the hip can occur as a result of the knee hitting the dashboard in a motor vehicle crash.
© Jones & Bartlett Learning.

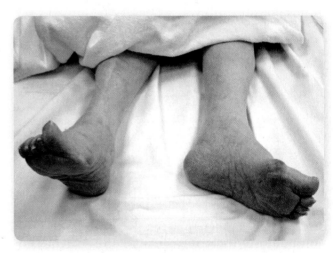

Figure 15-24 Signs of a hip fracture may include external rotation and shortening of the injured leg.
© E. M. Singletary, MD. Used with permission.

YOU are the Provider   CASE 2

On one of your days off from the station, you volunteer as an EMR at the local community college during events. Today you are working the softball tournament when one of the women slides safely into home plate with her right arm and hand outstretched. After making impact with the home plate, she immediately stands up, yelling in pain and cradling and protecting her right hand. Examination reveals considerable deformity on the palm side of the right hand. The patient reports significant pain in the hand and wrist and does not want to move the hand.

1. What type of examination should you perform on the patient's right arm?
2. Describe how you should splint this patient's injury.

Thigh Injuries

Trauma to the thigh can bruise the muscles or fracture the shaft of the femur. A fractured femur is very unstable and usually produces significant thigh deformity, with much bleeding and swelling.

The treatment of femoral fractures requires skill and proper equipment. As an EMR, you can treat for shock and help prevent further injury. Place the patient in as comfortable a position as possible, treat for shock, and call for additional personnel and equipment.

However, there are times, such as after a motor vehicle crash, when you may have to move the patient quickly before proper equipment and additional personnel arrive. Learn and practice emergency temporary splinting for lower extremity injuries. Secure both legs together with several swathes, cravats, or bandages to immobilize the two lower extremities as one unit. This technique allows you to remove the patient from a dangerous environment quickly.

A traction splint is the most effective way to splint a unilateral fractured femur. Traction splints are designed specifically for this purpose. Although you most likely do not have a traction splint in your EMR life support kit, you should learn this technique and know how it works in general, so that you can assist other EMS personnel, as needed.

Before applying a traction splint, trained EMTs align deformed fractures by applying manual longitudinal traction. Once manual traction is applied, it must be maintained until the traction splint is fully in place Figure 15-25 . Because many different types of traction splints are available, you should learn to use the one that your department uses. Most are applied using basically the same method. Skill Drill 15-6 illustrates the steps for applying a Hare traction splint.

Skill Drill 15-6

Applying a Traction Splint

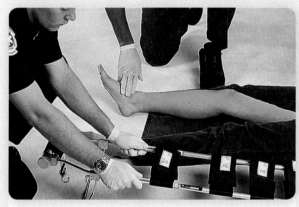

Step 1 Place the splint beside the uninjured limb, adjust the splint to the proper length, and prepare the straps.

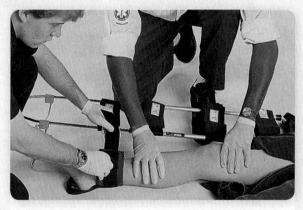

Step 2 Support the injured limb while your partner fastens the ankle hitch about the foot and ankle.

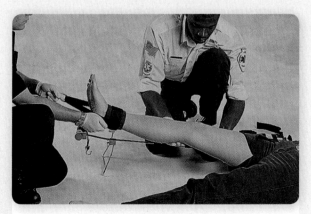

Step 3 Continue to support the limb while your partner applies gentle traction to the ankle hitch and foot.

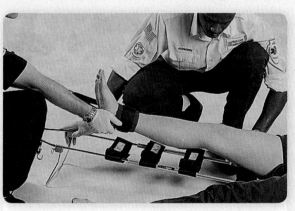

Step 4 Slide the splint into position under the injured limb.

© American Academy of Orthopaedic Surgeons.

Skill Drill 15-6 *Continued*

Applying a Traction Splint

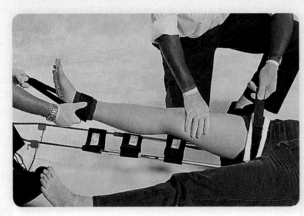

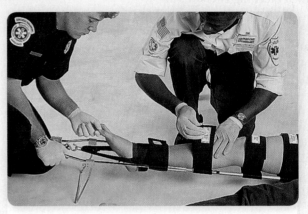

Step 5 Pad the groin and fasten the strap around the midthigh.

Step 6 Connect the loops of the ankle hitch to the end of the splint while your partner continues to maintain traction. Fasten the support straps to hold the limb securely in the splint.

© American Academy of Orthopaedic Surgeons.

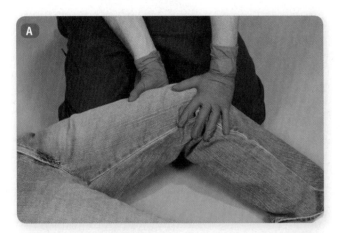

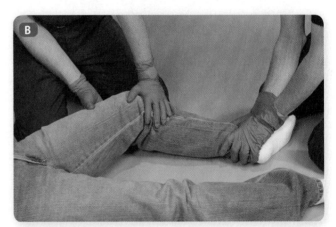

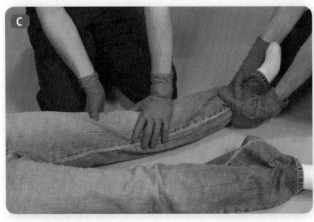

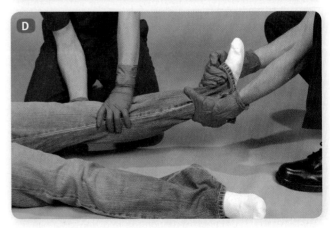

Figure 15-25 Straightening an injured leg for splinting. **A.** The first rescuer grasps the injured leg at the knee and applies traction in the long axis of the body. **B.** The second rescuer grasps the ankle. **C.** The second rescuer straightens the leg. **D.** The second rescuer maintains traction by leaning back.

A: © Jones & Bartlett Learning; B, C, & D: © Jones & Bartlett Learning. Courtesy of MIEMSS.

1. Place the splint beside the patient's uninjured leg and adjust it to the proper length. Open and adjust the four support straps. Position the support straps at the midthigh, above the knee, below the knee, and above the ankle **Step 1**.
2. The first rescuer supports and stabilizes the injured limb while the second rescuer fastens the ankle hitch about the patient's ankle and foot **Step 2**.
3. The first rescuer supports the leg at the site of the suspected injury while the second rescuer manually applies gentle traction to the ankle hitch and foot. Use only enough force to reposition the limb so it will fit into the splint **Step 3**. The first rescuer slides the splint into position under the patient's injured limb **Step 4**.
4. Pad the groin area and gently apply the strap around the midthigh **Step 5**.
5. The first rescuer connects the loops of the ankle hitch to the end of the splint while the second rescuer continues to maintain traction. Apply gentle traction to the connecting strap between the ankle hitch and the splint, just strongly enough to maintain limb alignment.
6. Once the proper traction is applied, fasten the support straps to hold the limb securely in the splint. Check all support straps to make sure they are secure **Step 6**.

To apply proper traction using this type of splint, it is essential that the foot end of the traction splint be elevated 6 to 8 inches (15 to 20 cm) off the ground. If the heel of the injured leg touches the ground, you will lose traction and have to reapply it. Most traction splints include a foot stand that elevates the limb. Check and recheck the pulse, capillary refill, and nerve function before and after a splint is applied **Figure 15-26**. If your department uses a different type of traction splint, you will need to be instructed in how to apply it properly.

Knee Injuries

Always immobilize an injured knee in the same position that you find it. If it is straight, use long, padded board splints or a long-leg air splint. If there is a significant deformity, place pillows, blankets, or clothing beneath the knee **Figure 15-27**, secure the splint materials to the leg with bandages, swathes, or cravats, and secure the injured leg to the uninjured leg. Then place the patient on a backboard.

Leg Injuries

Like fractures of the forearm, fractures of the leg can be splinted with air splints, cardboard splints, and even magazines and newspapers. **Skill Drill 15-7** shows how to apply an air splint to the leg. It takes two trained

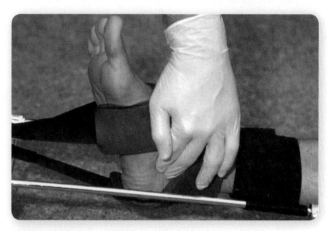

Figure 15-26 Checking the ankle pulse.
© Jones & Bartlett Learning. Courtesy of MIEMSS.

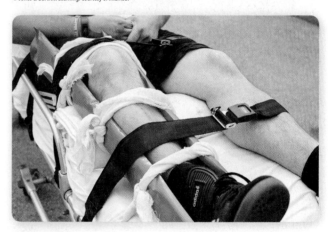

Figure 15-27 Immobilizing an injured knee.
© Jones & Bartlett Learning.

YOU are the Provider   CASE 3

It is a quiet Sunday morning. At 1043 hours you are dispatched to a local church for a report of a woman who has fallen in a religious education room. When you arrive at the scene, an usher takes you to your patient. The woman is lying on her back and has her left leg pulled up in an abnormal position. She complains of pain in her left hip area. In response to your questions, she tells you that she is 73 years old and that she takes medication for high blood pressure and diabetes and calcium supplements. She tells you that she got up from her chair, and when she tried to take a step, her left leg seemed to buckle. She thinks she heard a snap as she fell. Your assessment reveals moderate pain in her left hip area and an externally rotated and shortened left leg.

1. What type of injury do you believe is most likely based on her pain and on your patient assessment?
2. Because the patient did not experience significant trauma, what underlying factors may have contributed to this injury?
3. How should you immobilize this patient and prepare her for transport?

people to splint an injured leg. One person supports the leg with both hands (above and below the injury site), while the other person applies the splint.

1. The first rescuer supports the injured limb.
2. The second rescuer slides the splint under the limb **Step 1**.
3. The second rescuer places the splint around the limb **Step 2**.
4. The first rescuer slides his or her hands out of the splint while the second rescuer inflates the splint **Step 3**.
5. Either rescuer rechecks the pulse, capillary refill, and sensation of the injured leg.

Ankle and Foot Injuries

You can splint fractures of the ankle and foot with a pillow or an air splint. Place the pillow splint around the injured ankle and foot, and tie or pin it in place **Skill Drill 15-8**:

1. Place a pillow under the injured limb **Step 1**.
2. Mold the pillow around the foot and ankle.
3. Secure the pillow with cravats, swathes, or bandages **Step 2**.
4. Recheck the pulse, capillary refill, and sensation **Step 3**.

Skill Drill 15-7

Applying an Air Splint to the Leg

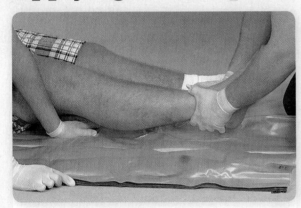

Step 1 Your partner supports the injured limb while you slide the splint under the limb.

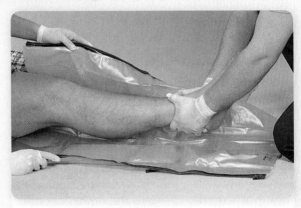

Step 2 Place the splint around the limb.

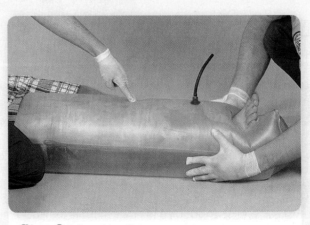

Step 3 Inflate the splint.

Skill Drill 15-8

Applying a Pillow Splint for Ankle or Foot Injury

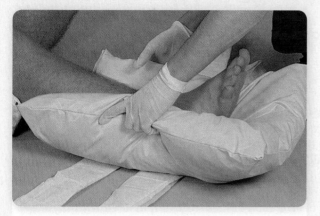

Step 1 Place a pillow under the injured limb.

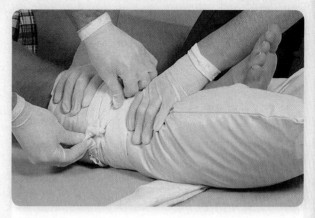

Step 2 Secure with cravats, swathes, or bandages.

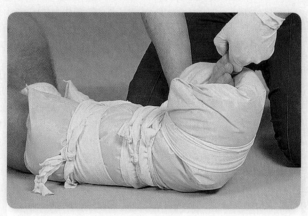

Step 3 Recheck the pulse, capillary refill, and sensation.

© Jones & Bartlett Learning. Courtesy of MIEMSS.

Safety

DO NOT elevate the injured leg when treating for shock.

► Additional Considerations

Remember that extremity injuries are not, in themselves, life threatening unless excessive bleeding is present. You may not always have the equipment or help you need to manage all types of extremity injuries. You may not even have time to splint an injury before additional EMS personnel arrive. There will be times, however, when you are the only trained person at the scene of an incident. To prepare for such situations, practice splinting until you can quickly and competently apply the principles in any situation. Because you may find patients in a variety of positions and locations, practice splinting both a sitting and a prone volunteer.

It takes two people to splint most limb injuries adequately: one person to stabilize and support the extremity and one person to apply the splint. Most of the principles and techniques of splinting covered in this chapter require that you work with another member of the EMS team. Learn how the team functions as a unit during stressful situations and be prepared to work with any member of the EMS team who arrives to assist you.

Voices *of* Experience

Early in my career, when faced with a patient who had a painful, bruised, or swollen injury, I would complete a full primary and secondary assessment. Upon completion of my assessment, and after realizing that the patient had only an isolated musculoskeletal injury, I would put my splinting and immobilizing knowledge and skills to use. Many times we would splint extremities with padded boards or padded metal splints, then tape or use cravats to secure the splint to the extremity to prevent continued movement and pain.

> **A fancy splint, especially if it required manipulating the injured extremity, was not necessary.**

Looking back, I believe many times we manipulated the injury more than necessary by applying the splint at the scene and then removing it at the emergency department. In many cases, we caused more movement and pain than if we had used simple splinting material or had the patient self-splint their injury. When delivering the patient to the hospital after completing a detailed splint, we would often get funny looks from the hospital staff as they were removing our splint. Over the years, I have realized that a fancy splint, especially if it required manipulating the injured extremity, was not necessary.

On one occasion, we moved a patient with a chief complaint of hip pain from her couch onto a scoop stretcher. We then secured her to a backboard, making sure we did not move her excessively. We then put her on the ambulance cot and transported her to the hospital, which was a 45-minute transport. Really!

With the experience I have now gained, I would do a three-person lift, placing her directly on the soft ambulance cot with blankets and pillows under her knees and her head raised for comfort. I would also call for an advanced life support intercept if the patient needed medications for pain. Not only can you immobilize the hip on the stretcher with pillows and straps, but you can avoid making your patient lie on a hard, flat backboard where bed sores can start forming within 20 minutes.

You've probably heard the phrase "Keep it simple." many times, and in EMS, this holds true most of the time. Use simple equipment that minimizes movement and pain and that can be applied and removed easily. Vacuum splints make splinting very easy. Don't forget to put a cold compress and a gauze or towel on the injury to decrease swelling. Keep it simple, and have a great career in EMS.

Mark Weber
EMS Director
Golden Heart Services
Heart of America Medical Center
Rugby, North Dakota

Treatment

Pad all rigid splints to provide the best stabilization and pain relief. Do not apply any splint too tightly. Recheck the pulse, capillary refill, and sensation after applying the splint to make sure that no damage has been done **Figure 15-28** .

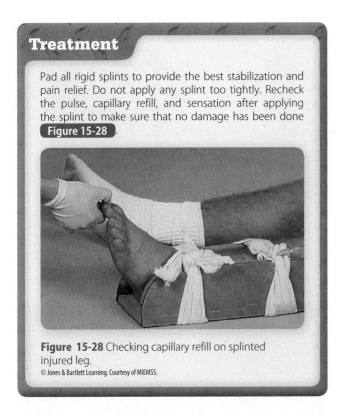

Figure 15-28 Checking capillary refill on splinted injured leg.
© Jones & Bartlett Learning. Courtesy of MIEMSS.

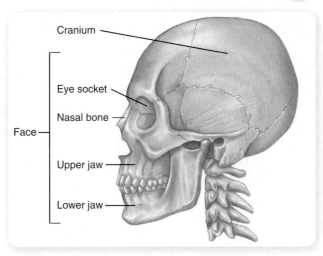

Figure 15-29 Cranium and face of the human skull.
© Jones & Bartlett Learning.

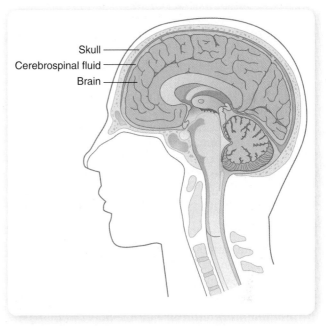

Figure 15-30 The brain.
© Jones & Bartlett Learning.

Injuries of the Head (Skull and Brain)

Severe head and spinal cord injuries can result from many different kinds of trauma. These injuries are common causes of death and can lead to irreversible **paralysis** and permanent brain damage. Improperly handling a patient after an incident can cause further injury or death. For example, well-intentioned citizens pulling a patient from a wrecked car or poor treatment from inadequately trained emergency personnel can cause spinal injuries. As an EMR, you must know what to do to provide prompt treatment and avoid errors that may make the injury worse.

The human skull has two primary parts **Figure 15-29** :

1. The cranium, a tough four-bone shell that protects the brain.
2. The facial bones, which give form to the face and furnish frontal protection for the brain.

▶ Mechanisms of Injury

Head injuries are common with certain types of trauma. Of patients involved in motor vehicle crashes, 70% sustain some degree of head injury. Imagine the cranium as a rigid bowl, containing the delicate brain **Figure 15-30** . Between the skull and brain, a fluid called **cerebrospinal fluid (CSF)** cushions the brain from direct blows. A direct force such as a hammer blow can injure the skull and the brain inside. Indirect forces can also cause injury, such as in a motor vehicle crash when the head strikes the windshield and causes the brain to bounce against the inside of the skull.

Spinal injury is often associated with head injury. The force of direct blows to the head is often transmitted to the spine, producing a fracture or dislocation. The injuries may damage the spinal cord or at least put it at risk for injury. Any time you suspect or identify an injury to the head or skull, suspect injury to the neck and spinal cord as well. Therefore, immobilize the cervical spine of all patients with head injuries to protect the spinal cord.

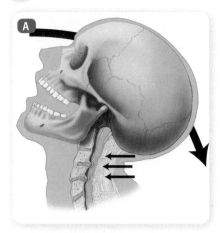
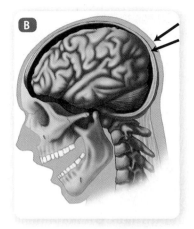
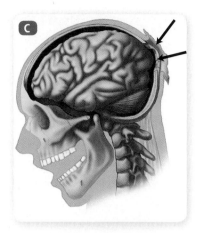

Figure 15-31 Open and closed head injuries. **A.** A head injury may occur in conjunction with a cervical spine injury. **B.** A closed head injury. **C.** An open head injury.

A, B, & C: © Jones & Bartlett Learning.

▶ Types of Head Injuries

Injuries of the head are classified as open or closed Figure 15-31 . In a **closed head injury**, bleeding and swelling within the skull may increase pressure on the brain, leading to irreversible brain damage and death if it is not relieved. An open injury of the head usually bleeds profusely. Severe open head injuries are serious but not always fatal.

Examine the nose, eyes, and the wound itself to see if any blood or CSF is seeping out. The CSF is clear, watery, and straw-colored. In severe cases of open head injury, brain tissue or bone may be visible.

▶ Signs and Symptoms of Head Injuries

A patient who sustained a head injury may exhibit some or all of the signs and symptoms shown in the following Signs and Symptoms box. A serious head injury may also produce raccoon eyes and Battle sign. Raccoon eyes look like the black eyes that develop after a fistfight. Battle sign appears as a bruise behind one or both ears Figure 15-32 .

Signs and Symptoms

Signs and symptoms of head injuries include the following:

- Confusion
- Unusual behavior
- Unconsciousness
- Nausea or vomiting
- Blood from an ear
- Decreasing consciousness
- Unequal pupils
- Paralysis
- **Seizures** (sudden episodes of uncontrolled electrical activity in the brain)
- External head trauma: bleeding, bumps, and contusions

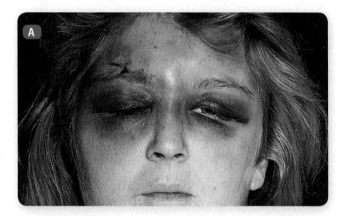
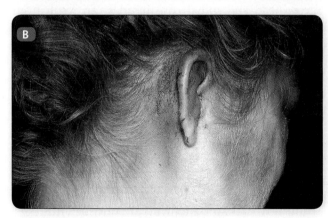

Figure 15-32 Signs of head injury. **A.** Raccoon eyes. **B.** Battle sign.

A&B: © American Academy of Orthopaedic Surgeons.

▶ Treatment of Head Injuries

When any one sign or symptom of head injury is present, proceed as follows:

1. Immobilize the head in a neutral position. Stabilize the patient's neck and prevent movement of the head. If returning the head to neutral is met with resistance, leave it in the position found.

2. Maintain an open airway. Use the jaw-thrust maneuver to open the airway (see Chapter 7, *Airway Management*). Be prepared to suction if the patient vomits. Avoid movement of the head and neck.

3. Support the patient's breathing. Be sure that the patient is breathing adequately on his or her own. If not, institute mouth-to-mask or mouth-to-barrier ventilation. Administer oxygen as soon as it is available if you are trained to use it. Oxygen helps minimize swelling of the brain.

4. Monitor circulation. Be prepared to support circulation by performing full cardiopulmonary resuscitation (CPR) if the patient's heart stops.

5. Check to see if CSF or blood is seeping from a wound or from the nose or ears **Figure 15-33**. CSF is clear, watery, and straw colored. Do not try to stop leakage of CSF from a wound or any other opening because leakage from inside the skull relieves internal pressure.

6. Control bleeding from all head wounds with dry, sterile dressings. Use enough direct pressure to control the bleeding without disturbing the underlying tissue.

7. Examine and treat other serious injuries.

8. Arrange for *prompt transport* to an appropriate medical facility.

Safety

If a patient has a head injury, assume that an associated neck or spinal cord injury is also present. Do nothing that would cause undue movement of the head and spine. Always immobilize the entire spine before moving the patient.

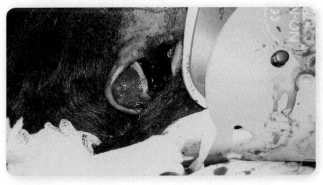

Figure 15-33 Blood or cerebrospinal fluid draining from the ear indicates head injury.
© E. M. Singletary, MD. Used with permission.

Words of Wisdom

A **concussion** is a type of closed brain injury. Concussions can occur without visible signs of trauma. The signs and symptoms of a concussion can be subtle and may not be immediately apparent. Some symptoms of concussions may be immediate or they may appear hours or days after the injury. The most common symptoms of a concussion are headache, loss of memory, and confusion. Other signs and symptoms of concussion include:

- Temporary loss of consciousness
- Headache or feeling of pressure in the head
- Confusion or seeming to be dazed
- Not remembering the traumatic event
- Dizziness or seeing stars
- Nausea and vomiting

Any time you see that a patient has suffered a traumatic event and exhibits these signs and symptoms, assess the patient and then prepare him or her for transport to an appropriate medical facility for evaluation by a physician.

Injuries of the Face

Facial injuries commonly result from the following types of incidents:

- Motor vehicle crashes in which the patient's face hits the steering wheel or windshield
- Assaults
- Falls

Airway obstruction is the primary danger in severe facial injuries. Severe damage to the face and facial bones can cause bleeding and the collapse of the facial bones, leading to airway conditions. If the patient has facial injuries, also suspect a spinal injury. Although facial injuries may bleed considerably, they are rarely life threatening unless the airway is obstructed.

▶ Treatment of Facial Injuries

When facial injuries are present, proceed as follows to care for the patient:

1. Immobilize the head in a neutral position. Stabilize it to prevent further movement of the neck.

2. Maintain an open airway. Use the jaw-thrust maneuver to open the airway. Clear any blood or vomitus from the patient's mouth with your gloved fingers.

3. Support breathing. Be prepared to ventilate the patient, if necessary.

4. Monitor circulation.

5. Control bleeding by covering any wound with a dry, sterile dressing and applying

direct pressure. Be sure to check for wounds inside the mouth. Try to prevent the patient from swallowing blood because this can cause vomiting. Have suction ready for use.

6. Look for and stabilize other serious injuries.
7. Arrange for *prompt transport* to an appropriate medical facility.

If these measures do not keep the airway clear or if you are unable to control severe facial bleeding, log roll the patient onto his or her side, keeping the head and spine stable and rolling the whole body as a unit. Turn the head and body at the same time. Do not allow the neck to twist **Figure 15-34** .

Bandage facial injuries as described in Chapter 14, *Bleeding, Shock, and Soft-Tissue Injuries*. If possible, leave the patient's eyes clear of bandages so he or she can see what is happening. Being able to see reduces the patient's tendency to panic.

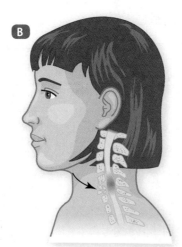

Figure 15-34 Keep the head and spine in alignment by using the log-roll technique.
© Jones & Bartlett Learning.

Safety

If a patient has head or spine injuries, use a log roll to move the patient onto his or her side. Do not place these patients in the recovery position. Provide support for the head and neck.

■ Injuries to the Spine

Spinal injuries can cause irreversible paralysis. As an EMR, you must know how to handle a patient properly and provide prompt treatment. Errors may make the injury worse.

▶ Mechanisms of Injury

If one or more vertebrae are injured, the spinal cord may also be injured. A displaced vertebra, swelling, or bleeding may put pressure on the spinal cord and damage it **Figure 15-35** . In severe cases, the cord may be severed. If all or part of the spinal cord is cut, nerve impulses (which are like signals in a telephone cable) cannot travel to and from the brain. Without the conduction of these nerve impulses, the patient is paralyzed below the point of injury. Injury to the spinal cord high in the neck paralyzes the diaphragm and results in death. Gunshot wounds to the chest or abdomen may produce spinal cord injury at that level. Falls, motor vehicle crashes, and stabbings are other common causes of spinal injuries. Suspect a spinal injury if the patient has sustained high-energy trauma.

Some common causes of spinal cord injuries are:

- Athletic collisions
- Diving injuries

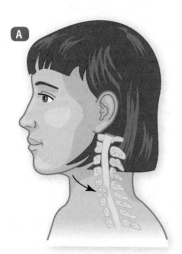
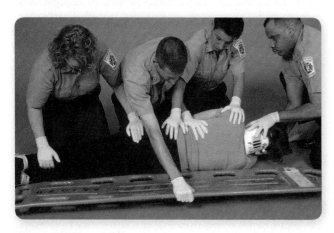
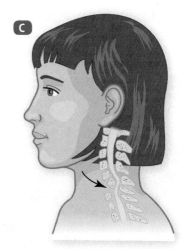

Figure 15-35 Types of spinal cord injuries. **A.** Pressure on the spinal cord from swelling or fracture. **B.** Bruising of the spinal cord by broken vertebrae. **C.** Injury by displacement and fractured vertebrae.
A, B, & C: © Jones & Bartlett Learning.

- Gunshot wounds and stabbings to the chest or neck
- Falls of greater than three times the patient's height
- Hangings
- Motorcycle crashes at speeds of over 20 mph
- Motor vehicle crashes with the following conditions:
  - Patient is ejected from vehicle
  - Patient is unrestrained
  - Speed is more than 40 mph
  - There is at least 12 inches (30 cm) of intrusion into the passenger compartment

Signs and Symptoms of Spinal Cord Injury

To determine whether a patient has sustained an injury to the spinal cord, talk to the patient and perform a careful examination to help determine the mechanism of injury. Gently conduct a hands-on examination, as described in Chapter 9, *Patient Assessment*, to detect paralysis or weakness. Ask the patient to describe any points of tenderness or pain. Do not move the patient during your examination, and ask the patient to keep still. The key signs and symptoms of a spinal injury are noted in the following Signs and Symptoms box. During your examination, be extremely careful and take your time. Position yourself so that the patient will not need to move his or her head to communicate with you. Do not move patients unless they are in a hazardous area.

Signs and Symptoms

Signs and symptoms of spinal injuries include:

- Laceration, bruise, or other sign of injury to the head, neck, or spine
- Tenderness over any point on the spine or neck
- Pain in the neck or spine or pain radiating to an extremity
- Extremity weakness, numbness, paralysis, or loss of movement
- Loss of sensation or movement or tingling or burning sensation in any part of the body below the neck
- Loss of bowel or bladder control

Treatment of Spinal Injuries

If any one sign or symptom of spinal injury is present, proceed as follows:

1. Place the head and neck in a neutral position. Avoid unnecessary movement of the head.
2. Stabilize the head and prevent movement of the neck.
3. Maintain an open airway. Use the jaw-thrust maneuver to open the airway to avoid movement of the head and neck. Clear any blood or vomitus from the mouth with your gloved fingers.
4. Support the patient's breathing. A spinal cord injury may paralyze some or all of the respiratory muscles, resulting in abnormal breathing patterns. In some cases, only the diaphragm may be working. Breathing using the diaphragm only is called **abdominal breathing**. The abdomen (not the lungs) swells and collapses with each breath. Help the patient breathe by administering oxygen (if available) and by keeping the airway open.
5. Monitor circulation.
6. Assess the pulse, movement, and sensation in all extremities.
7. Examine and treat other serious injuries.
8. Do not move the patient unless it is necessary to perform CPR or to remove him or her from a dangerous environment.
9. Assist in immobilizing the patient using a long or short backboard. (The steps for applying long and short backboards are covered in Chapter 3, *Lifting and Moving Patients*.)
10. Arrange for *prompt transport* to an appropriate medical facility.

Safety

If you suspect the presence of a spinal injury, it is essential to immobilize and protect the injury until hospital tests rule out a spinal cord injury. Do not move patients unless it is necessary to perform CPR or remove them from a dangerous environment.

Stabilizing the Cervical Spine

The cervical spine is initially stabilized manually, as shown in Skill Drill 15-9:

1. Stabilize the head and prevent movement of the neck. Place the head and neck in a neutral position Step 1.
2. In this position, the rescuer can maintain an open airway with the jaw-thrust maneuver Step 2. Do not manipulate or twist the head and neck. After you have manually stabilized the head and neck, you must maintain support until the entire spine is fully immobilized. Use a rigid collar and a long or short backboard to immobilize the cervical spine. Review the steps for applying a cervical collar and a short backboard device, which are covered in Chapter 3, *Lifting and Moving Patients*.

Skill Drill 15-9

Stabilizing the Cervical Spine and Maintaining an Open Airway

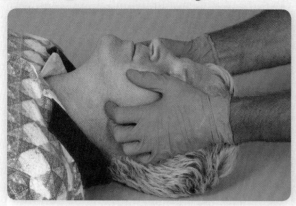

Step 1 Stabilize the head and neck in a neutral position.

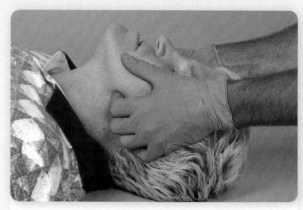

Step 2 Use the jaw-thrust maneuver to open the airway and avoid head or neck movement.

© Jones & Bartlett Learning. Courtesy of MIEMSS.

Words of Wisdom

Once you have applied spinal immobilization measures, maintain them until the care of the patient is turned over to more highly trained prehospital EMS personnel or hospital-based personnel. Spinal immobilization may be removed in the hospital after a physician evaluates the patient and often after radiographs or other diagnostic tests are conducted. Some EMS systems have adopted specific protocols that permit EMTs and paramedics to remove spinal immobilization in certain specific situations after they have completed a thorough patient assessment process that follows a specific protocol approved by their medical director.

The steps for evaluating a patient to determine if spinal immobilization can be removed are not taught in this course. Continue to apply spinal immobilization until you turn the care of the patient over to more highly trained EMS or hospital personnel, but be aware that they may employ a process that results in discontinuation of the immobilization procedures that you very appropriately initiated.

► Motorcycle and Sports Helmets

Many patients with neck injuries are motorcyclists or sports players who are wearing protective helmets. In almost all instances, it is not necessary to remove a helmet. Helmets are frequently snug and cradle the head; therefore, they can be secured directly to the spinal immobilization device.

Remove part or all of a helmet under only two circumstances:

1. When the face mask or visor interferes with adequate ventilation or with your ability to restore an adequate airway.
2. When the helmet is so loose that securing it to the spinal immobilization device will not provide adequate immobilization of the head.

When part of a motorcycle helmet interferes with ventilation, lift the visor away from the face. In the case of a football helmet, remove the face guard. Some newer football helmets have a tough plastic strap fixing the face guard to the mask. Trainers and coaches should have a special tool readily available that can remove the face guard. Also, loosen the chin strap to facilitate the jaw-thrust maneuver. In most instances, exposing the face and jaw allows you access to the airway to secure adequate ventilation. Most football face guards are fastened to the helmet by four plastic clips, which can be cut with a sharp knife or unscrewed with a screwdriver to remove the face guard, as shown in Skill Drill 15-10 :

1. Stabilize the patient's head and helmet in a neutral, in-line position Step 1 .
2. Then remove the mask in one of two ways:
   a. Unscrew the retaining clips for the face mask Step 2 .
   b. Use a trainer's tool designed for cutting retaining clips Step 3 .
3. Assess the patient's airway.

Skill Drill 15-10

Removing the Mask on a Sports Helmet

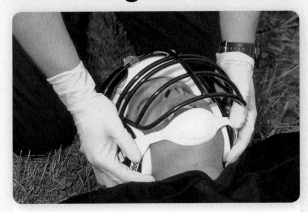

Step 1 Stabilize the patient's head and helmet in a neutral, in-line position. Then remove the mask in one of the following two ways.

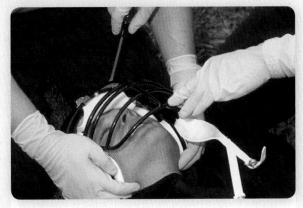

Step 2 Use a screwdriver to unscrew the retaining clips for the face mask or perform Step 3.

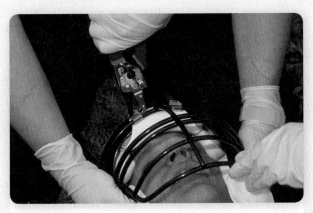

Step 3 Use a trainer's tool designed for cutting retaining clips.

The second indication for helmet removal is a loose helmet that will not ensure adequate immobilization of the head when secured to the spinal immobilization device. A loose helmet can be removed easily while the head and neck are being stabilized manually. The procedure for helmet removal in this circumstance is shown in **Skill Drill 15-11**. Note that this procedure requires two experienced people.

1. Kneel down at the patient's head and open the face shield so that you can assess the airway and breathing. Remove the eyeglasses if the patient is wearing them.
2. Stabilize the helmet by placing your hands on either side of it, ensuring that your fingers are on the patient's lower jaw to prevent movement of the head. Your partner can then loosen the strap **Step 1**.
3. After the strap is loosened, your partner should place one hand on the patient's lower jaw and the other behind the head at the occiput **Step 2**.
4. Once your partner's hands are in position, gently slip the helmet off about halfway and then stop **Step 3**.
5. Have your partner slide his or her hand from the occiput to the back of the head to prevent the head from snapping back once the helmet is removed **Step 4**.
6. With your partner's hand in place, remove the helmet and stabilize the cervical spine. Apply a cervical collar and then secure the patient to a long backboard **Step 5**. Note: With large helmets or small patients, you may need to pad under the shoulders.

Skill Drill 15-11

Removing a Helmet

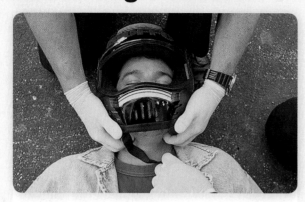

Step 1 Kneel down at the patient's head and open the face shield to assess the airway and breathing. Stabilize the helmet by placing your hands on either side of it, ensuring that your fingers are on the patient's lower jaw to prevent movement of the head. Your partner can then loosen the strap.

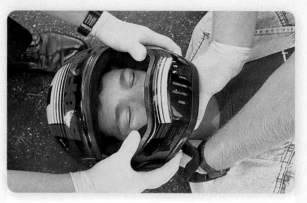

Step 2 Your partner should place one hand on the patient's lower jaw and the other behind the head at the occiput.

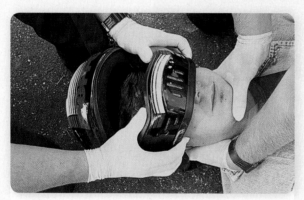

Step 3 Gently slip the helmet off about halfway and then stop.

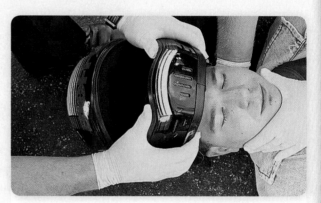

Step 4 Your partner slides his or her hand from the occiput to the back of the head to prevent the head from snapping back once the helmet is removed.

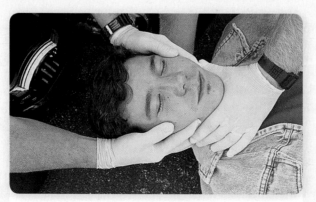

Step 5 With your partner's hand in place, remove the helmet and stabilize the cervical spine. Apply a cervical collar and then secure the patient to a long backboard.

Injuries of the Chest

The chest cavity contains the lungs, the heart, and several major blood vessels. The cavity is surrounded and protected by the chest wall, which is made up of the ribs, cartilage, and associated chest muscles. The most common chest injuries are fractures of the ribs, flail chest, and penetrating wounds.

▶ Fractures of the Ribs

Injury may produce fracture of one or more ribs. Even a simple fracture of one rib produces pain at the site of the fracture and difficulty breathing **Figure 15-36**. Multiple rib fractures result in significant breathing difficulty. The pain may be so intense that the patient cannot breathe deeply enough to take in adequate amounts of oxygen. Rib fractures may be associated with injury to the underlying organs.

To determine whether a rib is bruised or broken, apply some pressure to another part of the rib. Pain in the injured area indicates a bruise, crack, or fracture. If the injury is to the side of the chest, place one hand on the front of the chest and the other on the back and

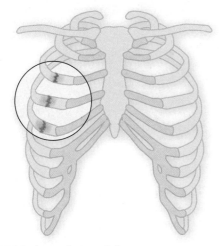

Figure 15-36 Broken or fractured ribs.
© Jones & Bartlett Learning.

gently squeeze. To check an injury to the front or back of the rib cage, put your hands on either side of the chest and gently squeeze. If there is no pain, the rib is probably not broken. In patients with rib fractures, be alert for signs and symptoms of internal injury, particularly shock.

Treatment of Rib Fractures

Try to reassure and make a patient with rib fractures more comfortable by placing a pillow against the injured ribs to splint them. Prevent excessive movement of the patient as you prepare for transport to an appropriate medical facility. Administer oxygen if it is available and you are trained to use it.

▶ Flail Chest

If three or more ribs are broken in at least two places, the injured portion of the chest wall does not move at the same time as the rest of the chest. The injured part bulges outward when the patient exhales and moves inward when the patient inhales. This condition is called a **flail chest** **Figure 15-37**. A flail chest decreases the amount of oxygen and carbon dioxide exchanged in the lungs, and it causes breathing problems that will progressively worsen.

You can identify a flail chest by examining the chest wall and observing chest movements during breathing. If the injured portion of the chest moves inward as the rest of the chest moves outward (and vice versa), the patient has a flail chest **Figure 15-38**.

Treatment of Flail Chest

If the patient is having difficulty breathing, do not attempt to restrict the movement of the chest while the patient is inhaling. It may be helpful to support the patient's breathing with positive pressure ventilation. This can be done by using a bag valve mask and supplemental oxygen. Monitor and support the patient's ABCs and arrange for *prompt transport* to an appropriate medical facility.

YOU ▶ are the Provider   CASE 4

At 0727 hours you are dispatched to a residence in a part of town where most houses were built about 50 years ago. After a 5-minute response, you arrive at the scene. The first thing you notice is that there are three trucks parked on the street and in the driveway. They all display the logo of the J & D Roofing Company. Before you can get out of your vehicle, an excited roofer directs you to follow him to the side of the house. While you are walking to the side of the house, he tells you that Alex was on the roof and slipped on a wet spot on the tin roof. He fell about 25 feet (8 m) and landed on a small walkway on the side of the house. As you approach, you find Alex lying on the sidewalk. He says he is not sure why he fell. He seems to be alert and oriented. You examine him and note some bruises and scrapes on his back and one spot that is very painful when you touch the back of his neck. When you ask him to squeeze your hands, you note that his right hand is much weaker than his left hand. You examine his lower extremities, and you ask Alex to move his toes. You do not detect any movement in his feet or toes.

1. What signs and symptoms of injuries does this patient exhibit?
2. How would you treat this patient?

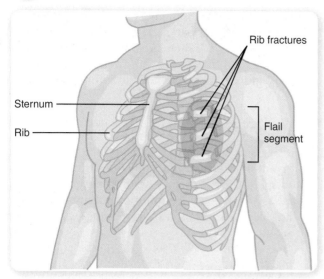

Figure 15-37 A flail chest occurs when three or more ribs are broken in at least two places.
© Jones & Bartlett Learning.

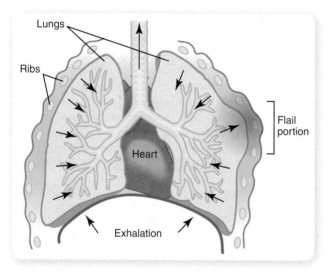

Figure 15-38 As the patient breathes, the flail portion of the chest moves in the opposite direction.
© Jones & Bartlett Learning.

▶ Penetrating Chest Wounds

If an object (usually a knife or bullet) penetrates the chest wall, air and blood escape into the space between the lungs and the chest wall **Figure 15-39** . The air and blood cause the lung to collapse. Lung collapse greatly reduces the amount of oxygen and carbon dioxide that is exchanged and can result in shock and death. Blood loss into the chest cavity can produce shock.

Treatment of Penetrating Chest Wounds

Quickly seal an open chest wound with a material that will prevent more air from entering the chest cavity. (Occlusive dressings are discussed in Chapter 14, *Bleeding, Shock, and Soft-Tissue Injuries,* and are shown in **Figure 15-40** .) You can use petroleum jelly-impregnated gauze, aluminum foil, plastic wrap, or a latex glove. In rare cases, sealing the wound may

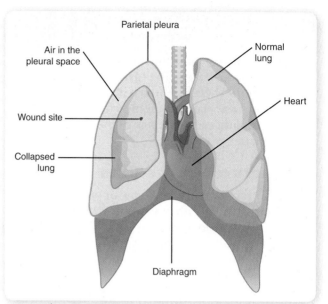

Figure 15-39 A penetrating chest wound may cause the patient's lung to collapse.
© Jones & Bartlett Learning.

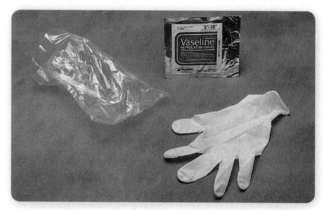

Figure 15-40 Occlusive dressings.
© Jones & Bartlett Learning. Courtesy of MIEMSS.

increase the patient's breathing difficulty. If it is harder for a patient to breathe after you seal the wound, uncover one corner of the occlusive dressing to see if the breathing improves. Administer oxygen if it is available and you are trained to use it. If a knife or other object is impaled in the chest, do not remove it. Seal the wound around the object with a dressing to prevent air from entering the chest. Stabilize the impaled object with bulky dressings.

Any chest injury that results in air leakage and bleeding requires prompt attention. For these reasons, patients with severe chest injuries require *rapid transport* to an appropriate medical facility.

A conscious patient with chest trauma may demand to be placed in a sitting position to ease breathing. Unless you must immobilize the spine or treat the patient for shock, help the patient assume whatever position eases his or her breathing. If oxygen is available, administer it. If the patient's respirations are excessively slow or absent, perform mouth-to-mask breathing. A bag valve mask may also be used by trained personnel. If the patient's heart stops, begin chest compressions, regardless of whether there are chest injuries.

YOU are the Provider

SUMMARY

You are the Provider: CASE 1

1. How should you conduct an assessment of this patient?

Use the patient assessment sequence to conduct a systematic and complete assessment of this patient. Start with a scene size-up to be sure that you and the patient are safe. Perform a primary assessment to evaluate and correct the patient's airway, breathing, and circulation. Acknowledge the painful injury to the patient's arm and then perform a secondary assessment by examining the patient from head to toe for additional injuries. As you examine the extremities, remember to check for circulation by checking pulses and capillary refill. Check for sensation and movement in each limb. Be especially aware of the potential for head and spinal injuries from the trauma of falling from the wall and landing on the hard surface of the parking lot. Look for open wounds. Perform a complete SAMPLE history to determine whether any medical conditions contributed to this fall. Finally, reassess the patient to ensure that he is stable.

2. What type of injuries should you suspect with this patient?

In any fall or trauma of this type, examine the patient for signs and symptoms of a head injury. This is especially important if the skateboarder was not wearing a helmet. Stabilize the head and neck as well as you can with the personnel and equipment available to prevent any further damage to the patient's spine. Examine the patient thoroughly for additional injuries to bones and joints besides the obvious injuries to his arm and elbow. Check for soft-tissue injuries. Do not forget to treat the patient for shock, especially because it is a cool autumn day.

3. Under what circumstances should you move this patient?

Do not move the patient unless a dangerous situation exists or you need to start lifesaving treatment. If the patient is in a place where there is uncontrolled traffic or other danger, you need to consider moving him. If you are unable to open the patient's airway, it may be necessary to move the patient to secure an open airway. However, if you can safely leave the patient in the location found, this is generally the best solution because you will need three or four people and a backboard to safely move this patient. Wait until you have adequate equipment and a sufficient number of trained personnel.

You are the Provider: CASE 2

1. What type of examination should you perform on the patient's right arm?

After completing a full primary assessment, expose the patient's right arm. Cut away any clothing that may interfere with a complete examination of the injured area. Confirm circulation in the arm, including checking for pulses and testing capillary refill in the fingers. Evaluate the patient for normal movement and sensation in the affected arm and compare the findings with the uninjured limb. Palpate the arm to determine the extent of the injury from the hand to the elbow.

2. Describe how you should splint this patient's injury.

Immobilize the lower part of the right arm using a rigid splint extending from the hand to the elbow. Pad the splint to fill any voids between the limb and the splint. Immobilize the hand in the position of function by placing one or two roller bandages in the hand. Secure the limb to the splint using roller gauze. Then secure the entire arm using a sling to minimize movement and a swathe to secure it to the body. Recheck circulation, sensation, and motion after the sling is in place.

You are the Provider: CASE 3

1. What type of injury do you believe is most likely based on her pain and on your patient assessment?

The full-body assessment revealed moderate pain in the left hip area. The patient's left leg is bent at an abnormal angle and her left leg appears to be shorter than her right leg. These signs and symptoms are consistent with a hip fracture.

2. Because the patient did not experience significant trauma, what underlying factors may have contributed to this injury?

Osteoporosis is a chronic health condition that affects older people, more commonly women. Osteoporosis results in a weakening of bone. In people with osteoporosis, fractures can occur with a low-force mechanism of injury. Based on the mechanism of injury and the fact that this woman takes calcium, it is likely that she has osteoporosis, which contributed to the hip fracture during the low-impact fall.

3. How should you immobilize this patient and prepare her for transport?

Using as much padding as possible, immobilize the hip in the position found. Then secure the patient to a long backboard with ample padding to provide support for the injured leg. In some situations, you may be responsible for immobilizing the fracture site and preparing her for transport. In other cases, your role will be to keep her as comfortable as possible, maintain her body temperature to prevent shock, monitor her vital signs, and reassure her until additional EMS personnel and equipment arrive. Sometimes your role is to help prevent unnecessary movement of the patient, which prevents further pain or injury.

You are the Provider: CASE 4

1. What signs and symptoms of injuries does this patient exhibit?

In a situation like this, use all the available information to make the best determination of the patient's injuries and to determine what treatment the patient needs. You can quickly get valuable information by evaluating the history of the incident. In this case, it appears that the roofer fell about 25 feet (8 m) from a roof onto a hard concrete sidewalk. A fall from this distance onto a hard surface has a high likelihood of producing a serious injury. A thorough patient examination will provide much information. This patient has abrasions and scrapes on his back indicating the possibility of internal injuries. He complains of pain on one part of his neck when you touch it. You note that one of his hands has a weaker grip than the other, which may

indicate an injury to his spinal cord. Most important, you determine that he is not able to move his feet. These are all important signs and symptoms of a possible spinal cord injury. When performing an assessment on a patient who has suffered trauma, do not get tunnel vision when you find one injury. Continue your assessment to be sure you have completed a thorough patient examination to identify all the injuries the patient may have suffered. Always carefully assess and monitor the patient's airway, breathing, and circulation. These indicators help you determine if there are additional injuries that might cause shortness of breath or shock.

2. How would you treat this patient?

Carefully assess and monitor the patient's airway, breathing, and circulation. These help you determine if there are internal injuries and the patient's overall condition. Because this patient has suffered a significant fall and is showing multiple signs and symptoms of a spinal injury, you need to stabilize the patient's neck and back to prevent movement that may cause additional injury. This patient will need to be moved using a spinal immobilization device such as a backboard. However, there does not appear to be a need to move the patient before the arrival of additional EMS personnel and equipment. As long as the patient's neck is stabilized, there is no need to move him. Cover him to treat him for shock. Update responding EMS units and provide encouragement to the patient and to his coworkers. Sometimes an important role of the first responder is to prevent unnecessary movement and further injury to the patient because of the unwise actions of untrained people.

Prep Kit

▶ Ready for Review

- Musculoskeletal injuries are caused by three types of mechanism of injury: direct force, indirect force, and twisting force.
- A fracture is a broken bone. Fractures can be closed (the bone is broken but there is no break in the skin) or open (the bone is broken and the overlying skin is lacerated).
- A dislocation is a disruption that tears the supporting ligaments of the joint.
- A sprain is a joint injury caused by excessive stretching of the supporting ligaments.
- The three steps in examining a patient with a limb injury include:
  - General assessment of the patient
  - Examination of the injured part
  - Evaluation of the circulation, sensation, and movement in the injured limb
- Regardless of their extent or severity, treat all limb injuries the same way in the field. For all open extremity wounds, first cover the entire wound with a dry, sterile dressing. Then apply firm but gentle pressure to control bleeding, if necessary. Then splint the injured limb.
- The three basic types of splints are rigid, soft, and traction.
- It takes two people to splint most limb injuries adequately: one to stabilize and support the extremity and one to apply the splint.
- Severe head and spinal cord injuries can result from many different kinds of trauma. These injuries are common causes of death and can lead to irreversible paralysis and permanent brain damage.
- Injuries of the head are classified as open or closed. In a closed head injury, bleeding and swelling within the skull may increase pressure on the brain, leading to irreversible brain damage. An open injury of the head usually bleeds profusely.
- When a sign or symptom of a head injury is present, immobilize the head and stabilize the patient's neck; maintain an open airway; support breathing; monitor circulation; check to see if cerebrospinal fluid or blood is seeping; control bleeding with dry, sterile dressings; treat other serious injuries; and arrange for prompt transport.
- Airway obstruction is the primary danger in severe facial injuries.
- When facial injuries are present, immobilize the head and stabilize the patient's neck; maintain an open airway; support breathing; monitor circulation; control bleeding with a dry, sterile dressing and apply direct pressure; treat other serious injuries; and arrange for prompt transport.
- When you suspect a spinal injury, do not move the patient during the examination. Further, do not allow the patient to move.
- When a sign or symptom of spinal injury is present, place the head and neck in a neutral position; stabilize the head and prevent movement of the neck; maintain an open airway; support breathing; monitor circulation; assess pulse, movement, and sensation; examine and treat other serious injuries; assist in immobilizing the patient using a long or short backboard; and arrange for prompt transport.
- The most common chest injuries are rib fractures, flail chest, and penetrating wounds.

▶ Vital Vocabulary

abdominal breathing Breathing using only the diaphragm.

arm The upper portion of the upper extremity; from the shoulder to the elbow.

cerebrospinal fluid (CSF) A clear, watery, straw-colored fluid that fills the space between the brain and spinal cord and their protective coverings.

closed fracture A fracture in which the overlying skin has not been damaged.

closed head injury Injury where there is bleeding and/or swelling within the skull.

concussion A closed head injury that alters the way the brain functions; symptoms of a concussion include headache, loss of memory, and confusion.

dislocation Disruption of a joint so that the bone ends are no longer in alignment.

flail chest A chest injury in which three or more ribs are broken in two or more places, resulting in the injured part of the chest moving in the opposite direction from the rest of the chest.

forearm The lower portion of the upper extremity; from the elbow to the wrist.

joint The point where two bones come in contact with each other.

leg The lower portion of the lower extremity; from the knee to the foot.

mechanism of injury (MOI) The means by which a traumatic injury occurs.

open fracture Any fracture in which the overlying skin has been damaged.

Prep Kit *Continued*

osteoporosis Abnormal brittleness of the bones in older people caused by loss of calcium; affected bones fracture easily.

paralysis Inability of a conscious person to move voluntarily.

rigid splint Splint made from firm materials such as wood, aluminum, or plastic.

seizure Sudden episode of uncontrolled electrical activity in the brain.

sling A bandage or material that helps to support the weight of an injured upper extremity.

soft splint A splint made from supple material that provides gentle support.

sprain A joint injury in which the joint is partially or temporarily dislocated and some of the supporting ligaments are either stretched or torn.

thighbone The upper portion of the lower extremity; from the hip joint to the knee.

traction splint A splint that holds a lower extremity fracture in alignment by applying a constant, steady pull on the extremity.

trauma A wound or injury, either physical or psychological.

vacuum splint A soft splint that becomes rigid when air is removed from the splint.

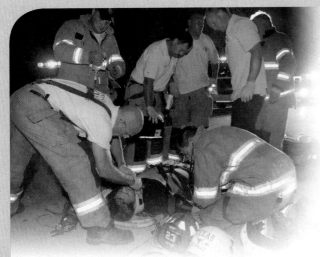

Assessment
in Action

You are dispatched to a single-family two-story home for a report of a fall from the roof. On arrival, you find a 32-year-old man who was stepping onto a ladder from the roof when the ladder moved away from the house, causing the patient to fall to the ground. The patient reports that he landed upright on both of his feet, probably because he was reaching for branches as he fell. The patient reports severe pain in the right lower leg and knee and is obviously frightened.

1. What kind of assessment should you perform on this patient?

   A. Examine only the areas that are painful.
   B. Examine only the upper extremities.
   C. Perform a full-body assessment.
   D. Complete a primary assessment only.

2. If a patient fell from the roof of a second story house and appeared to suffer from multiple injuries, which of the following would be the most appropriate way to move the patient?

   A. Perform a direct ground lift.
   B. Have the patient slide onto the stretcher.
   C. Log roll the patient onto a long backboard.
   D. Use a scoop stretcher.

3. If you identify pain and deformity of the lower leg, what type of splint should you apply?

   A. A sling
   B. A rigid splint
   C. A sling and swathe
   D. A traction splint

4. Do you need to immobilize this patient's neck?

   A. Yes
   B. No
   C. Only if he reports pain
   D. Only if there is pain and bruising

5. You discover swelling, deformity, and an open wound on the patient's lower leg. How should you treat this wound?

   A. Splint the leg.
   B. Leave the wound exposed because it is associated with a possible fracture.
   C. Cover the wound with a sterile dressing and then splint the leg.
   D. Stop the bleeding with direct pressure, cover the wound with a sterile dressing, and splint the leg.

Assessment *in Action* Continued

6. What is the general rule for splinting a fracture?

   A. Immobilize the fracture site.
   B. Immobilize the fracture site and the joint above it.
   C. Immobilize the fracture site and the joint below it.
   D. Immobilize the fracture site and the joints above and below it.

7. What is the general rule for splinting a joint?

   A. Immobilize the joint only.
   B. Immobilize the joint and the bone above it.
   C. Immobilize the joint and the bone below it.
   D. Immobilize the joint and the bones above and below it.

8. Why is it important to check and regularly recheck circulation, sensation, and movement in a patient with a limb injury?

9. Why is it important to consider the mechanism of injury when evaluating and treating patients who may have suffered a spinal injury?

10. Why do patients with severe penetrating chest injuries require rapid transport to an appropriate medical facility?

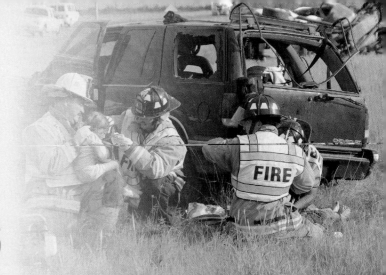

SECTION 6

Special Patient Populations

Childbirth

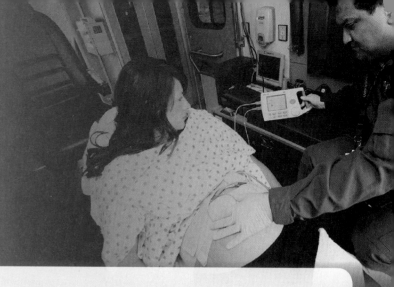

National EMS Education Standard Competencies

Special Patient Populations

Recognizes and manages life threats based on simple assessment findings for a patient with special needs while awaiting additional emergency response.

Obstetrics

Recognition and management of
> Normal delivery (pp 346–351)
> Vaginal bleeding in the pregnant patient (pp 353–354; p 356)

Neonatal Care

> Newborn care (p 352)
> Neonatal resuscitation (pp 352–353)

Medicine

Recognizes and manages life threats based on assessment findings of a patient with a medical emergency while awaiting additional emergency response.

Gynecology

Recognition and management of shock associated with
> Vaginal bleeding (pp 353–354; p 356)

Trauma

Uses simple knowledge to recognize and manage life threats based on assessment findings for an acutely injured patient while awaiting additional emergency medical response.

Special Considerations in Trauma

Recognition and management of trauma in
> Pregnant patient (p 356)
> Pediatric patient (Chapter 17, *Pediatric Emergencies*)
> Geriatric patient (Chapter 18, *Geriatric Emergencies*)

Knowledge Objectives

1. Describe the anatomy and function of the female reproductive system. (p 345)
2. Explain the three stages of the labor process. (p 346)
3. Discuss how to determine whether there is time to transport the woman to the hospital for delivery. (p 346)
4. Describe preparation for delivery of a newborn. (p 347)

5. Discuss the use of standard precautions in childbirth. (pp 347–349)
6. List the equipment emergency medical responders (EMRs) should have for an emergency childbirth situation. (p 349)
7. Explain how to assist with delivery of a newborn. (pp 349–351)
8. Discuss the delivery of the placenta. (p 351)
9. List the steps in resuscitating a newborn. (pp 352–353)
10. Describe the signs and symptoms and treatment for the following complications of childbirth:
    • Ectopic pregnancy and shock (pp 353–354)
    • Miscarriage and vaginal bleeding (p 354)
    • Premature birth (p 354)
    • Unbroken bag of waters (p 354)
    • Prolapse of the umbilical cord (p 354; p 356)
    • Breech birth (p 356)
    • Stillborn delivery (p 356)
    • Multiple births (p 356)
    • Excessive bleeding after delivery (p 356)
11. Explain how to care for a pregnant woman who has been in a motor vehicle crash. (p 356)

Skills Objectives

1. Describe preparation for delivery of a newborn. (p 347)
2. Demonstrate the use of standard precautions in childbirth. (pp 347–349)
3. Demonstrate how to assist with delivery of a newborn. (pp 349–351)
4. Demonstrate delivery of the placenta. (p 351)
5. Demonstrate resuscitation of a newborn. (pp 352–353)
6. Demonstrate treatment for the following complications of childbirth:
    • Ectopic pregnancy and shock (pp 353–354)
    • Miscarriage and vaginal bleeding (p 354)
    • Premature birth (p 354)
    • Unbroken bag of waters (p 354)
    • Prolapse of the umbilical cord (p 354; p 356)
    • Breech birth (p 356)
    • Stillborn delivery (p 356)
    • Multiple births (p 356)
    • Excessive bleeding after delivery (p 356)

■ Introduction

As an emergency medical responder (EMR), you must sometimes assist in the birth of a child. A planned childbirth is an exciting, dramatic, and stressful event in itself. An unplanned childbirth, where you are called to assist, can be even more dramatic and stressful. However, if you remember some easy steps, you can effectively assist in the birth process and offer comfort and support to both the mother and the newborn.

Childbirth is a normal and natural part of life. If you are concerned about your ability to handle such a situation, just remember that hundreds of thousands of deliveries occur in the world each day and result in healthy babies. In many countries, medical assistance at childbirth is the exception, not the rule.

You may not have the time or necessary assistance to transport the pregnant woman to the hospital. Therefore, you must be prepared to help your patient deliver the newborn wherever she is. In most cases, during the birth process, the newborn is literally being pushed out of the body; therefore, your part involves helping, guiding, and supporting the newborn as he or she is born. Following the birth, ensure that the newborn is breathing adequately and being kept warm.

Generally, pregnancy is not a surprise for the mother and she may be knowledgeable and well prepared for the birth process. However, there will be times when the timing of the childbirth catches everyone by surprise or a complication has developed, thus requiring a call to emergency medical services (EMS). In this chapter, you will learn about the three stages of the birth process. The two key indicators of an impending birth are the frequency of the **contractions** and the appearance of the newborn's head during a contraction, or **crowning**.

■ The Anatomy and Function of the Female Reproductive System

The major female reproductive organs are the ovaries, which produce eggs, and the **uterus (womb)**, which holds the fertilized egg as it develops during a pregnancy (the usual gestational period is 40 weeks). The egg released by the ovaries travels through the fallopian tube to the uterus. The external opening of the female reproductive system is called the **birth canal**, which includes the lower part of the uterus and the **vagina**. The developing newborn (**fetus**) is covered in an amniotic sac for support and floats in amniotic fluid. The **placenta**, or afterbirth, draws nutrients from the wall of the woman's uterus. These nutrients and oxygen are delivered to the fetus through the **umbilical cord**. **Figure 16-1** shows the anatomy of a pregnant woman.

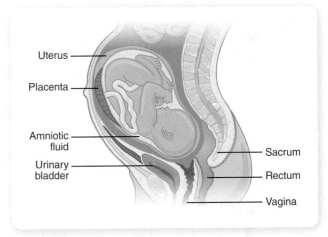

Figure 16-1 Anatomy of a pregnant woman.
© Jones & Bartlett Learning.

YOU are the Provider

CASE 1

Just as you are completing your dinner, you and your partner are dispatched to a nearby office building for the report of a 27-year-old woman in labor. As you are responding, your dispatcher reports that the woman's "water has broken" and that her contractions are 4 minutes apart. The nearest EMS transport unit is 9 minutes away.

1. What information do you need to know before determining whether there is time to transport this woman to the hospital or if you will need to assist her with the delivery?
2. What standard precautions do you need to take when assisting with the emergency delivery of a newborn?
3. What are the risks to a pregnant woman and fetus if they are involved in a motor vehicle crash?

Assessing the Birth Situation

Should you help deliver the newborn on the scene or arrange to transport the pregnant woman to the hospital? To make this decision, you need to understand that **labor** (the process of delivering a newborn) consists of three distinct stages.

▶ Stages of Labor

The first stage of labor is when the pregnant woman's body prepares for birth. This stage is characterized by the following conditions: initial contractions occur, the **bag of waters** breaks (rupture of the amniotic sac, which is the fluid in which the fetus floats), the **bloody show** (a plug of mucus often mixed with blood) occurs, but the newborn's head does not appear during the contractions. Check the woman's vaginal opening to determine whether the newborn is crowning. Report your findings to the responding ambulance crew so that they can make a decision on whether the woman is close to delivery or transport to the hospital is necessary.

The second stage involves the birth of the newborn. You will see the newborn's head crowning during contractions, at which time you must prepare to assist the woman with delivery Figure 16-2 . There is no time for transport now!

The third stage is the final stage. It involves delivery of the placenta (afterbirth). You must assist in stabilizing the condition of the mother and newborn and delivering the placenta.

▶ Is There Time to Reach the Hospital?

The following questions will help you to determine how close the pregnant woman is to delivery and whether there is time to transport her to the hospital or whether you need to prepare for a delivery.

1. **Is this the woman's first pregnancy?** The length of labor for a first-time mother is usually longer than for a woman who has had children. A woman who is experiencing her first labor will usually have more time to reach the hospital. It is also helpful to ask the woman the newborn's due date, although labor can start before this date.

2. **Has the woman experienced a bloody show?** As the newborn starts to descend toward the birth canal, the bloody show is expelled from the cervix and discharged from the vaginal opening. This occurs as the first stage of labor is about to begin.

3. **Has the bag of waters broken?** The bag of waters usually breaks toward the end of the first stage of labor and may give some idea of the progress of the birth process. In some women, the bag of waters may not break until the birth is actually occurring (discussed later in the chapter).

4. **How frequent are the contractions?** If the contractions are more than 5 minutes apart, you can usually transport the woman to the hospital. Contractions less than 2 minutes apart usually indicate that delivery will occur soon and you need to prepare for delivery. If the contractions are 3 to 4 minutes apart, take the other factors listed here into account to make your decision.

5. **Does the woman feel an urge to move her bowels?** When the newborn's head is in the birth canal, it presses against the rectum and the woman may feel the urge to move her bowels. Do not allow her to go to the toilet. This urge is an indication that she is close to delivery.

6. **Is the newborn's head crowning?** Crowning indicates that the newborn will be born in the next few minutes and you need to be ready.

7. **Is transportation available?** Find out whether the ambulance is responding and how far it is to the hospital. Will bad weather, a natural disaster, or rush hour traffic prevent prompt arrival of transportation?

▶ Timing Contraction Cycles

When you care for a patient in labor, time the contraction cycles from the beginning of one contraction to the beginning of the next Figure 16-3 . Do not time the interval between contractions. If contractions are less than 3 minutes apart, delivery is close.

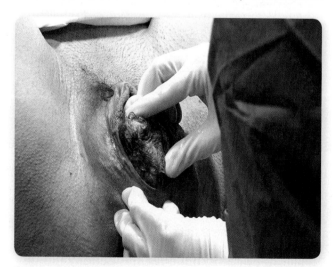

Figure 16-2 Crowning occurs when the newborn's head appears at the vaginal opening.
© University of Maryland Shock Trauma Center/MIEMSS.

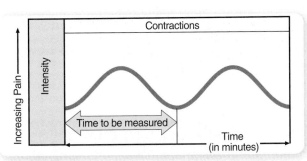

Figure 16-3 Time the contractions from the beginning of one to the beginning of the next.
© Jones & Bartlett Learning.

▶ Detecting Crowning

To determine whether the newborn's head is crowning, you must observe the vaginal opening during a contraction. If you see the head crowning during the contraction, prepare for delivery (see Figure 16-2). Do not risk transporting the woman to the hospital.

Words of Wisdom

Do not forget that pregnant women can experience trauma or medical emergencies too! It is important to perform a patient assessment to determine whether your patient has any additional medical conditions or has sustained a recent injury. It is easy to focus on the pregnancy and neglect other conditions.

▶ Preparing for Delivery

As you prepare to assist the patient in the delivery, keep these two things in mind:

1. Calm the woman. Delivery is a natural process.
2. Calm yourself. You are there to help.

Because you are not in a hospital, you will not be able to maintain sterile conditions. However, be as clean as possible. Wash your hands thoroughly. If you do not have a sterile delivery kit, use the gloves from your emergency medical responder (EMR) life support kit (or even clean kitchen gloves, if they are available). Place the patient on a firm surface that is padded with blankets, folded sheets, or towels. Elevate her hips 2 inches to 4 inches (5 cm to 10 cm) with pillows and blankets. Allow the patient to get in a comfortable position. This is often on her back with knees bent and feet flat on the surface beneath her.

Have plenty of clean towels ready to cover the newborn and to clean the mother after delivery has occurred. Childbirth involves blood and body fluids, so place towels or sheets on the floor around the delivery area to help soak up the fluids and to protect the mother and the newborn.

■ Standard Precautions and Childbirth

As the woman's contractions become more forceful, the newborn is gradually pushed down the birth canal. Because a woman in childbirth will expel both blood and body fluids, take standard precautions during the delivery. Try not to get any more blood or fluids on you than is absolutely necessary. Use sterile gloves during any delivery whenever possible. Sterile gloves protect not only the woman and newborn from infection but also protect you from any blood-borne diseases the woman might have Skill Drill 16-1 .

1. Carefully open the sterile glove package without touching the gloves Step 1 .
2. Pick up the first glove by grasping one edge Step 2 .
3. Pull on the first glove, being careful not to touch the outside of the glove Step 3 .
4. Grasp the second glove by sliding two fingers of your gloved hand into the rolled edge Step 4 .
5. Put on the second glove Step 5 .
6. Keep the gloves as sterile as possible Step 6 .

Because body fluids could splatter on your face during the delivery process, wear face and eye protection to keep possible splatter out of your eyes, nose, and mouth. Wearing a surgical gown can help keep fluids off your body. As an EMR, you will not have all the protective equipment that is available in a hospital. Do what you can to prevent unnecessary exposure

YOU are the Provider   CASE 2

Shortly after 0100 hours, you and your partner are dispatched to the home of a pregnant 32-year-old woman. When you arrive, you find her on the living room sofa. She is complaining of pain in her abdomen and says she is having contractions. She is sweating and generally uncomfortable.

1. What questions should you ask the patient about the contractions?
2. Why is it important to know whether this is her first pregnancy?
3. What stage of labor is she in?

Skill Drill 16-1

Putting on Sterile Gloves

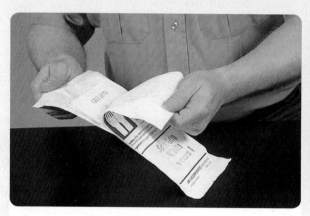

Step 1 Open sterile glove package.

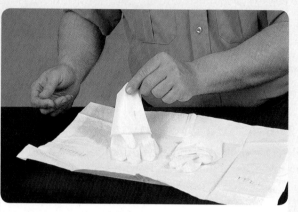

Step 2 Pick up first glove by grasping it as shown.

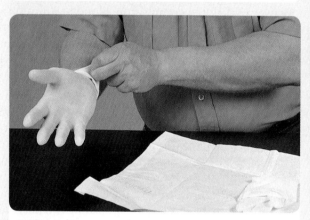

Step 3 Put on first glove.

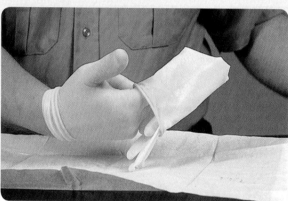

Step 4 Grasp second glove as shown.

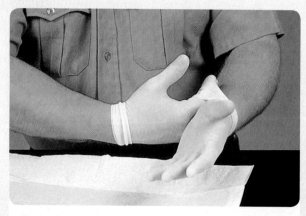

Step 5 Put on second glove.

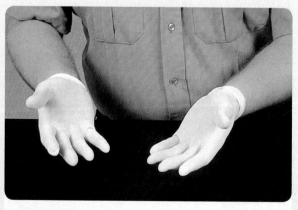

Step 6 Keep gloves as sterile as possible.

to body fluids and report all direct exposures of blood or fluids to the emergency physician or to your medical director.

Equipment

You should have a prepackaged obstetric (OB) delivery kit in your emergency care equipment Figure 16-4. The delivery kit includes the following materials:

- Sterile gloves
- Umbilical cord clamp
- Sterile drapes and towels
- Sanitary pads
- Gauze pads (4 inch × 4 inch [10 cm × 10 cm])
- Towel or blanket for the newborn
- Bulb syringe
- Plastic placenta bag

In addition, you will need the following:

- Sheets or towels for the mother
- Suction (if available)
- Oxygen (if available and if you are trained to use it)
- Newborn-sized face mask

If you do not have an OB delivery kit, look for appropriate substitute materials. You can find most of these items in your EMR life support kit or in most homes. Even if you do not have any equipment, remember that you can still assist in delivering a newborn with only common sense and gloved hands.

Assisting With Delivery

As you prepare to assist with delivery, remember that there are two lives to be considered in this situation: the life of the mother and the life of the newborn. Do not neglect to perform a patient assessment on the woman. Determine whether she has any medical conditions.

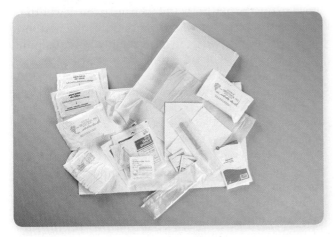

Figure 16-4 Commercial obstetric (OB) kit.
© Jones & Bartlett Learning.

Obtain a baseline set of vital signs and repeat them at least every 15 minutes. Throughout the delivery process, continue to monitor her airway, breathing, and circulation.

Remember, your primary purpose is to assist in the delivery of the newborn. The woman is going to feel pressure in the vaginal area, as if she has to move her bowels. This feeling is normal during the delivery process. Do not let her go to the bathroom and do not hold her legs together.

Be as clean as possible during the entire delivery process. Take standard precautions. Do not touch the vaginal area except during the delivery. If you have a partner, have him or her stay with you during the delivery.

The newborn's head should emerge slowly to prevent undue stress on the newborn and tearing of the vaginal tissues. As the head emerges, support the newborn's head and tell the woman to stop pushing. To help her stop pushing, tell her to take quick, short breaths (advise her to blow like she is blowing out a candle). Some EMS systems advise their personnel to use the palm of the hand to provide slight counterpressure over the newborn's head to slow down the birth process. Be sure to check with your medical director and follow your local protocols for the appropriate treatment in this situation.

Do not attempt to pull the newborn during the delivery. In a normal birth, the newborn will turn to the side by himself or herself after the head emerges, and the rest of the body will be delivered spontaneously Figure 16-5. Usually, the upper shoulder will deliver first. Continue to support the newborn's head and be ready to grasp the newborn in a clean towel. Remember, the newborn will be wet and slippery. As the torso and the legs are delivered, support the newborn with both hands. Grasp the newborn's feet as they are delivered. Keep the newborn's head at about the level of the woman's vagina. If the amniotic sac has not broken as the newborn's head starts to deliver, tear it with your fingers and push it away from the newborn's head and mouth. As the head emerges, check to make sure the umbilical cord is not wrapped around the newborn's neck. If the cord is wrapped around the neck, attempt to slip the cord over the newborn's head. If you cannot slip the cord over the head, attempt to reduce the pressure on the cord. Never pull on the umbilical cord; it is extremely fragile. In a normal delivery, there is no need for you to cut the umbilical cord.

▶ Caring for the Newborn

As soon as you are holding the newborn in a clean towel, lay him or her down between the mother's legs and immediately clear blood and mucus from the newborn's mouth and nose using a gauze pad or the

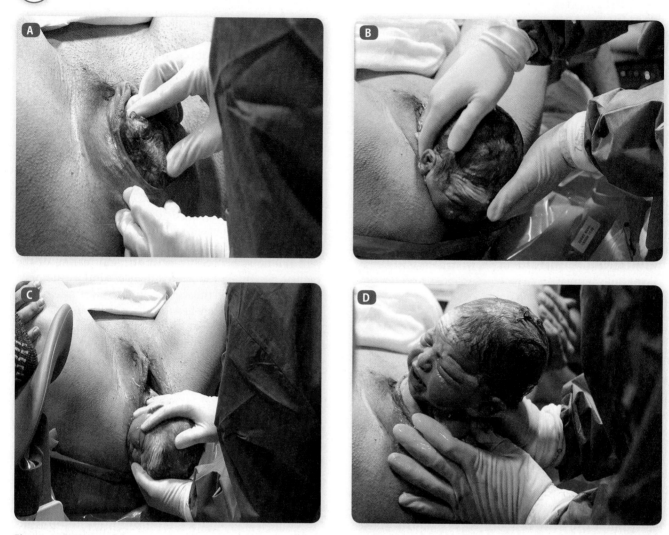

Figure 16-5 Phases of the second stage of labor. **A.** The head begins to deliver. **B.** Delivery of the head. **C.** Delivery of the upper shoulder. **D.** Delivery of the lower shoulder.

© University of Maryland Shock Trauma Center/MIEMSS.

cleanest object available. Many newborns will begin to breathe or cry without further assistance. If the baby does not begin to breathe spontaneously within a few seconds, **suction** the newborn's mouth and nose. Use a bulb syringe from the delivery kit if one is available **Figure 16-6** . Suction the mouth first and then the nostrils. Be careful not to reach all the way to the back of the newborn's mouth. Discard the fluid into a towel, and repeat the procedure two to three times until the mouth and nostrils are clear. If a bulb syringe is not available, wipe the newborn's mouth and nose with a gauze pad. Drying and suctioning the newborn usually provides enough stimulation to induce breathing.

Place the newborn on the mother's abdomen if the mother and the newborn are breathing adequately. This step allows skin-to-skin contact and will help keep the newborn warm. Wipe blood and mucus from the newborn's mouth and nose with sterile gauze or with the cleanest object available. If the newborn is still not breathing, suction the newborn's mouth and nose again.

Rub the newborn's back or flick the soles of the newborn's feet to stimulate breathing **Figure 16-7** . Use the towel to dry the newborn and then wrap the newborn in a blanket to keep him or her warm. Place the newborn on his or her side with the head slightly lower than the trunk. This step will aid in the drainage of secretions from the airway.

When the umbilical cord stops pulsating, clamp it with an umbilical cord clamp or tie it with gauze between the mother and the newborn. Remember, there is no need for you to cut the umbilical cord in a normal delivery. However, if you have sterile equipment and are trained to use it, you can cut the cord with sterile supplies. Keep the newborn warm and wait until more highly trained EMS personnel arrive. They will have the proper equipment to clamp and cut the umbilical cord in an approved manner.

Note the time of the delivery so it can be properly reported on the newborn's birth certificate. In the rare event of multiple births, prepare for the second delivery.

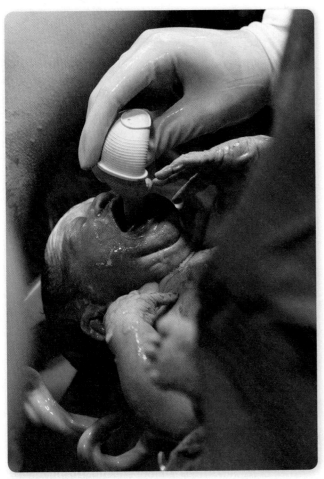

Figure 16-6 Suction the mouth and nose to clear the airway of mucus and amniotic fluid. Use a bulb syringe in a newborn's mouth first, then use the bulb syringe to suction the newborn's nose.
© University of Maryland Shock Trauma Center/MIEMSS.

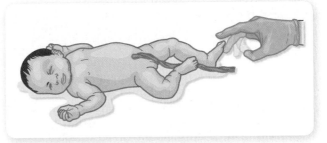

Figure 16-7 Gently flick your fingers against the soles of the feet to stimulate breathing in the newborn.
© Jones & Bartlett Learning.

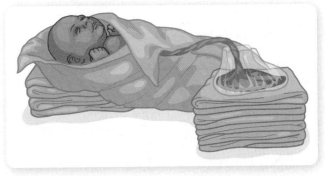

Figure 16-8 If sterile supplies are unavailable and you cannot cut the umbilical cord, keep the placenta, still attached at the cord, at the same level as the newborn during transport to the hospital.
© Jones & Bartlett Learning.

▶ Delivery of the Placenta

The placenta will deliver on its own, usually within 30 minutes after delivery. Never pull on the umbilical cord to help deliver the placenta.

The safest and best method for the mother and the newborn is to leave the umbilical cord uncut and attached to the placenta and the newborn—at least until the transporting EMS unit arrives. After the placenta is delivered, wrap it in a towel or newspaper with three-quarters of the umbilical cord, place it in a plastic bag, and transport it to the hospital with the mother and newborn so it can be examined by a physician. Try to keep the placenta at the same level as the newborn to help prevent any blood from the newborn flowing back out into the placenta. This step is especially important if you are unable to tie the umbilical cord Figure 16-8. The mother can be transported to the hospital before the placenta is delivered, if necessary.

Bleeding usually stops after the placenta is delivered. If bleeding does not stop, you can massage the uterus to help stop the bleeding. To massage the uterus, place one hand with fingers fully extended just above the mother's pubic bone. Use your other hand to press down into the abdomen and, using a circular motion, gently massage the uterus until it becomes firm. This process should take 3 to 5 minutes. As the uterus firms up, it should feel about the size of a softball or large grapefruit.

YOU are the Provider   CASE 3

You are dispatched to an apartment for a pregnant woman who is in labor. As you arrive on the scene, you find a 17-year-old who is 9 months pregnant. The teenager says she feels like she needs to move her bowels. As you examine the patient, you can see the top of the newborn's head.

1. What should be your first action?
2. What can you do to stimulate breathing in a newborn?

■ Aftercare of the Mother and Newborn

Continue to observe the mother and newborn carefully and keep them both warm. Cover the newborn's head and body to prevent the loss of body heat. About every 3 to 5 minutes, recheck the uterus for firmness. Also recheck the vagina for any excessive bleeding. In a normal delivery, the mother will have about 10 fluid ounces to 16 fluid ounces, or 1 cup to 2 cups (300 mL to 500 mL) of blood loss. Continue to massage the uterus using a circular motion if it is not firm or if bleeding continues. Allowing the newborn to nurse at the mother's breast causes a hormone to be released that helps to contract the uterus and reduce bleeding after childbirth.

Clean the mother with clean, moist towels or cloths. Cover the vaginal opening with a clean sanitary pad or large dressing, but do not pack any materials in the vagina. Replace the used towels or sheets with clean ones, if possible. If the mother is thirsty, you can give her small amounts of water to drink.

Special Populations

The newborn should begin to cry right after birth. You should observe the following vital signs in a healthy, conscious newborn:

- A respiratory rate of greater than 40 breaths per minute
- A pulse rate of greater than 100 beats per minute (Check the brachial pulse located at the inside of the infant's upper arm. Even for experienced health care providers, it is hard to accurately measure rapid heart rates.)

■ Resuscitating the Newborn

If the newborn does not cry and breathe on his or her own within the first minute after birth, proceed with the steps listed in Skill Drill 16-2.

1. Tilt the newborn's head down and to the side to encourage drainage of mucus **Step 1**. Use a gauze pad to clear secretions from the newborn's mouth and nose.
2. Suction the mouth and nose with a bulb syringe (if available). Other ways to stimulate breathing include gently flicking your fingers against the soles of the newborn's feet and/or rubbing the newborn's back. Do not handle the newborn roughly. A newborn responds best to simple, gentle techniques, but if the newborn is still not breathing, proceed to the next step **Step 2**.
3. Begin mouth-to-mouth-and-nose or mouth-to-mask breathing by gently puffing twice into the newborn's mouth and nose with only enough force to cause the newborn's chest to rise **Step 3**. If the newborn begins to cry and breathe on his or her own, support and assist respirations and recheck the airway to be sure it remains clear (see Chapter 7, *Airway Management*).
4. If the newborn is still not breathing, continue mouth-to-mouth-and-nose or mouth-to-mask breathing and check for a brachial pulse **Step 4**.
5. If you cannot feel a brachial pulse or if the heart rate is less than 60 beats per minute, begin closed-chest cardiac compressions.

Skill Drill 16-2

Resuscitating a Newborn

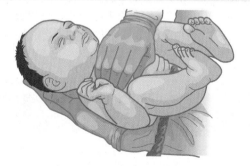

Step 1 Tilt the newborn so the head is down and to the side to clear the airway.

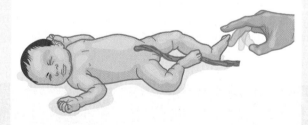

Step 2 Gently flick your fingers on the soles of the newborn's feet.

Skill Drill 16-2 *Continued*

Resuscitating a Newborn

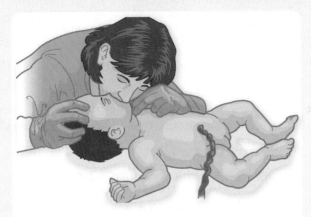

Step 3 Begin rescue breathing.

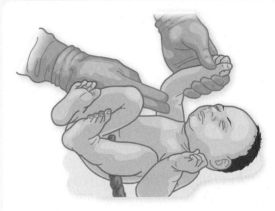

Step 4 Check for a brachial pulse.

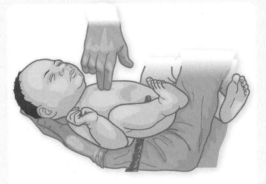

Step 5 Begin chest compressions using the two middle fingers.

© Jones & Bartlett Learning.

Use your two middle fingers to depress the newborn's chest **Step 5** (see Chapter 8, *Professional Rescuer CPR*).

6. Continue cardiopulmonary resuscitation (CPR) until the newborn begins breathing adequately and has a strong pulse of over 60 beats per minute or until the newborn is pronounced dead by a physician. Provide rapid transport to the hospital. Do not give up!

Throughout this process, try to dry the newborn and wrap the newborn in a blanket to keep him or her warm.

Special Populations

Newborns must be kept warm. Dry the newborn and keep the body and head covered to prevent loss of body heat and hypothermia.

■ Complications of Pregnancy and Childbirth

Although most pregnancies and births are normal, be aware of possible complications that can occur any time between early in the pregnancy until after the delivery. These complications include ectopic pregnancy and shock, miscarriage and vaginal bleeding, premature birth, unbroken bag of waters, prolapse of the umbilical cord, breech birth, stillborn delivery, multiple births, and excessive bleeding after delivery.

▶ Ectopic Pregnancy and Shock

Any woman of childbearing age who presents with severe abdominal pain or signs and symptoms of shock (pale skin, dizziness, rapid pulse, decreased blood pressure, fainting) needs to be evaluated by a physician to determine whether she has experienced a ruptured ectopic pregnancy. An ectopic pregnancy occurs when a fertilized egg becomes implanted in the fallopian tube rather than in the uterus. As the embryo starts to grow, it expands and causes the fallopian tube to rupture. This rupture causes sudden abdominal pain, internal bleeding, and shock. You will not be able to determine that an ectopic pregnancy has occurred, but you must be able to recognize this life-threatening condition if you encounter a woman of childbearing age who reports the sudden development of severe abdominal pain and has signs and symptoms of shock. As an EMR, your treatment begins with a complete patient assessment. Be sure to measure the patient's vital signs. Treat the woman for shock and arrange for *prompt transport* to an appropriate medical facility.

▶ Miscarriage and Vaginal Bleeding

A miscarriage (spontaneous abortion) is the delivery of an incomplete or underdeveloped fetus. A fetus before 20 weeks of pregnancy cannot survive outside the womb. If a miscarriage occurs, save the fetus and all the tissues that pass from the vagina. Control the woman's bleeding by placing a sanitary pad or other large dressing at the vaginal opening. Also treat her for shock. Arrange for *prompt transport* to a hospital so that a physician can examine her and the fetal tissues and control any additional bleeding.

Vaginal bleeding in a pregnant woman is often the first sign of a miscarriage. It can also indicate a variety of other complications with the pregnancy. Anytime a pregnant woman experiences vaginal bleeding, perform a patient assessment, obtain a good medical history, and obtain a set of vital signs to determine whether she is experiencing shock. A pregnant woman who experiences vaginal bleeding should be examined by a physician. Arrange for *transport* to an appropriate medical facility for further treatment.

A woman who miscarries will be upset about the loss of the newborn and will need your emotional support as well as emergency medical care. Be sensitive to the needs and concerns of the woman and other members of the family.

Words of Wisdom

When you conduct a patient assessment on a pregnant woman, be sure to check her blood pressure. Recall from Chapter 6, *The Human Body*, that the normal systolic blood pressure for adults is 90 mm Hg to 140 mm Hg. High blood pressure in pregnant women can be a sign of a serious condition (preeclampsia) that leads to seizures and can be life threatening to the woman and fetus. If you obtain a high blood pressure reading in a pregnant woman in labor, arrange for prompt transportation to an appropriate medical facility. Also, be sure to communicate this information to other emergency medical providers.

▶ Premature Birth

Any newborn weighing less than 5 pounds (2 kg) or delivered before 36 weeks of pregnancy is called premature. A premature newborn is smaller, thinner, and usually has redder skin than a full-term newborn.

You must keep premature newborns warm because loss of body heat occurs rapidly. Wrap the newborn in a clean towel or sheet and cover the head. Wrapping a premature newborn in an additional length of aluminum foil can also help maintain body temperature. Arrange for *prompt transport* to a medical facility.

▶ Unbroken Bag of Waters

In rare instances, the bag of amniotic fluid that surrounds the newborn does not break. If the newborn is surrounded by the bag of waters, carefully break the bag and push it away from the nose and mouth so the newborn can breathe. Be careful not to injure the newborn in the process. Then suction the newborn's mouth, followed by the nose, to help the newborn begin to breathe.

▶ Prolapse of the Umbilical Cord

On rare occasions, the umbilical cord appears from the vaginal opening before the fetus is delivered. This condition is called a prolapsed umbilical cord. The cord may be compressed between the newborn and the woman's pelvis during contractions, cutting off the newborn's blood supply. This condition is a serious emergency that requires immediate transport to a hospital.

YOU are the Provider   CASE 4

At 0317 hours, you are dispatched to 927 Fallow Run for a report of a sick woman. You know the address is in a suburban part of town, but you wish you had more information about this call. As you arrive at the scene, you are met at the front door by an excited man wearing a robe over his nightclothes. He leads you to the bedroom and tells you that his wife woke him up just before he called 9-1-1 and reported severe pain in her abdomen. As you obtain a medical history from the 31-year-old patient, you learn that she has no medical conditions, no allergies, and takes no medications except for a vitamin pill. The last time she saw her physician was 3 months ago for strep throat.

1. What additional information do you need from this patient?
2. What type of care does this patient need?

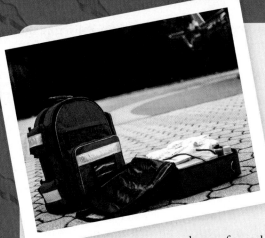

Voices *of* Experience

It was the morning of the 2004 Super Bowl; I was ending a 24-hour shift at the fire station and was looking forward to going home for a day of rest, relaxation, and football. We were finishing up the station duties when the dispatcher came on the radio and dispatched us for a 23-year-old woman who was reporting abdominal pain. As the address came across the radio, I could not help but think that it seemed oddly familiar. It took me a moment to process it; the address was mine. I was hit with a whirlwind of emotions and thought, "Is this really happening?" My wife and I had just found out that she was pregnant the previous week.

As we responded, I began running through the possible causes of her abdominal pain. There are a number of things that it could have been, but one thing was coming out on the top of my list: an ectopic pregnancy. We arrived to find my wife experiencing severe abdominal pain at 9/10 on a 0 to 10 scale. We placed her on oxygen, started an intravenous line (IV), loaded her into the ambulance, and began the drive to the hospital. We were fortunate that day. After having a battery of tests, we found out the baby was fine; the reason for her pain was a kidney stone.

> **There are a number of things that it could have been, but one thing was coming out on the top of my list: an ectopic pregnancy.**

The next 8 months went by and she and the baby were doing well, until the 38th week. Suddenly, she began experiencing the signs and symptoms of preeclampsia; she started having some unusual swelling in her hands and lower legs and said she just was not feeling quite right. Her obstetrician ordered bed rest. Two weeks later, my wife woke me up in the middle of the night; her water had broken. Because it was her first pregnancy we knew we did not have to rush to the hospital. We contacted our physician and patiently waited and timed her contractions. Suddenly, she started complaining of a headache and began having tremors in her arms.

I called 9-1-1, and within a few moments paramedics arrived. I explained that she had been diagnosed with preeclampsia 2 weeks earlier. They took her blood pressure and it was 190/110 mm Hg. We again loaded her into the ambulance for the drive to the hospital. I had never been so scared, but I knew I needed to be calm so that she did not become alarmed and risk making her situation worse. The last thing a patient with preeclampsia needs is extra stress. We were lucky for a second time when she delivered a healthy 6 pound 5 ounce (3 kg) baby boy.

As we progress through our training and then into our careers, we should always keep something in mind: you just never know who is going to benefit from the knowledge you gain and the lives that you will touch.

Richard Main, BS, NREMT-P
Lead EMT Instructor
National Center for Technical Instruction
Las Vegas, Nevada

Place the patient on her back and prop her hips and legs higher than the rest of her body with pillows, blankets, or articles of clothing. Keep the umbilical cord covered and moist, and do not try to push it back into the vagina. Administer oxygen to the patient if it is available and you are trained to use it. Arrange for *rapid transport* to the hospital.

Some EMS systems recommend placing the woman in a kneeling position (knee-chest position) to take the pressure off the umbilical cord. Check with your medical director regarding local procedures.

▶ Breech Birth

In a breech birth, the newborn's buttocks come down the birth canal first, rather than the head. This abnormal delivery can result in injury to the newborn and the woman.

If, instead of the normal crowning, you see a **breech presentation**, make every attempt to arrange for *prompt transport* to a medical facility. A breech birth slows the labor, so there will be more time for transport to the emergency department. If you are stranded and cannot transport the patient to the emergency department, you will have to assist with the breech birth.

Support the newborn's buttocks and legs as they are delivered; the head usually follows on its own. If the head does not deliver within 3 minutes, arrange for *prompt transport* to a hospital. Insert a gloved hand into the vagina and use your fingers to keep the newborn's airway open by forming a pocket over the newborn's nose and mouth.

In very rare cases, the arm or the leg is the first part of the newborn to appear in the birth canal. This circumstance, called limb presentation, is an extreme emergency that cannot be handled in the field. You must arrange for *rapid transport* to the hospital by ambulance.

Safety

When a newborn is in the breech position, do not attempt to pull the newborn out of the vagina!

▶ Stillborn Delivery

Start and continue resuscitation on all newborns who are not breathing. However, sometimes a newborn dies in the uterus long before labor. The fetus will generally have an unpleasant odor and will not exhibit any signs of life. A lifeless fetus is referred to as a stillborn. In a situation like this, carefully wrap the stillborn newborn in a blanket and turn your attention to the mother to provide physical care and emotional support.

▶ Multiple Births

In the event of multiple births (such as twins), another set of labor contractions will begin shortly after the delivery of the first newborn. A pregnant woman generally knows of a multiple birth in advance. However, there are times when a multiple birth has not been previously diagnosed. Do not worry—just get ready to repeat the procedures you completed for delivering the first newborn.

▶ Excessive Bleeding After Delivery

In addition to the early bloody show that precedes birth, about 1 cup or 2 cups (300 mL to 500 mL) of blood loss occurs during normal childbirth. If the mother is bleeding severely, place one or more clean sanitary pads at the opening of the vagina, treat her for shock, and arrange for *rapid transport* to the hospital by ambulance.

Remember to encourage the newborn to nurse at the mother's breast because nursing contracts the uterus and can often help stop the bleeding. Massage the uterus with your hand, as described earlier in this chapter.

If the area between the mother's vagina and **anus** is torn and bleeding, treat it as you would an open wound. Apply direct pressure using sanitary pads or gauze dressings.

Safety

Pregnant women showing signs and symptoms of shock should be transported while lying on the left side to prevent putting pressure on the major abdominal organs and vein, the inferior vena cava.

■ Vehicle Collisions and Pregnant Women

A pregnant woman who is involved in a motor vehicle crash or who has sustained other trauma should be examined by a physician. The forces involved in even a minor crash may be great enough to injure the woman or the unborn child, even though the fetus is usually well protected in the uterus.

Promptly assess and transport a pregnant woman who has been involved in a motor vehicle crash to the hospital. If the woman exhibits signs or symptoms of shock, monitor the airway, breathing, and circulation. Arrange for administration of high-flow oxygen if available and if you are trained to use it. Have the woman lie on her left side rather than on her back. This position will relieve pressure on the uterus and the abdominal organs and will allow blood to return through the major veins in the abdomen.

In rare circumstances, a crash can be severe enough to kill the pregnant woman but not the fetus. Provide CPR to the woman while transporting her to the closest medical facility.

Words of Wisdom

As part of your patient assessment, check to see whether the patient was wearing a seat belt. Pregnant women are at lower risk for injury to the fetus and to themselves if they wear a seat belt.

YOU are the Provider SUMMARY

You are the Provider: CASE 1

1. What information do you need to know before determining whether there is time to transport this woman to the hospital or if you will need to assist her with the delivery?

Consider the following seven factors to help you determine whether there is time to get the pregnant woman to the hospital before the newborn is born:

- Is this the woman's first pregnancy?
- Has the woman experienced a bloody show?
- Has the bag of waters broken?
- How frequent are the contractions?
- Does the woman feel an urge to move her bowels?
- Is the infant's head crowning?
- Is transportation available?

2. What standard precautions do you need to take when assisting with the emergency delivery of a newborn?

During normal childbirth, a woman expels blood and body fluids. It is important to prevent yourself from coming into contact with blood and body fluids as much as possible. Use sterile gloves to protect you and to protect the woman. Protect your face and eyes from splatter by putting on face and eye protection if it is available, as well as a surgical gown if it is available. Be sure to thoroughly wash your hands or shower as soon as possible after you have completed the call.

3. What are the risks to a pregnant woman and fetus if they are involved in a motor vehicle crash?

Whenever a pregnant woman is involved in a motor vehicle crash, remember that there are two lives at risk: the life of the woman and the life of the unborn child. Any pregnant woman involved in a crash should be examined by a physician. Even a minor crash may injure the woman or fetus. Injuries may not be obvious right after the crash. As an emergency medical responder (EMR), you do not have the training or equipment to assess the seriousness of injuries to a pregnant woman and fetus. Treat the pregnant woman with special care and monitor her carefully for signs and symptoms of injuries and shock. Transport her to an appropriate medical facility as soon as possible.

You are the Provider: CASE 2

1. What questions should you ask the patient about the contractions?

Ask the patient how long she has been having contractions and how frequently she is having contractions. The answers to these key questions will determine your next course of action. If the contractions are more than 5 minutes apart, you should be able to transport the woman to a nearby hospital. However, if the contractions are less than 2 minutes apart, she could be close to delivery. It is important for you to measure the contractions because many people either do not know how to measure the time between contractions or they do not accurately measure them in their excited state.

2. Why is it important to know whether this is her first pregnancy?

The time from the beginning of labor until the time of delivery is usually longer with the first child than with subsequent deliveries. Knowing whether the patient has had other children, along with the time between contractions, can help you make an informed decision about whether to transport or to prepare for an on-scene delivery.

3. What stage of labor is she in?

The woman is in the first stage of labor, in which her body is preparing for the birth. There are three stages of labor, beginning with the preparation of the woman's body for birth, which includes the breaking of the bag of waters, the bloody show, and contractions. The second stage is the actual birth, and the third stage is the delivery of the placenta.

You are the Provider: CASE 3

1. What should be your first action?

Prepare for the immediate birth of the newborn and prepare the area where the delivery is going to take place. If your medical gear includes a sterile delivery kit, use it. If not, use your EMR skills and improvise. Cover the area with clean towels and sheets. Use whatever personal protective equipment you may have because you will be exposed to blood and body fluids during the delivery.

YOU are the Provider   **SUMMARY** *Continued*

2. What can you do to stimulate breathing in a newborn?

If the newborn is not breathing, suction the mouth and nose. You can also try rubbing the newborn's back or flicking the soles of the feet to stimulate breathing. If these techniques do not work, give two small mouth-to-mouth-and-nose rescue breaths. Dry the newborn as soon as possible and keep the newborn warm.

You are the Provider: CASE 4

1. What additional information do you need from this patient?

You need to determine what the patient had to eat last evening and ask her how she felt last evening. Ask the date of her last menstrual period to determine if there is any chance she is pregnant. Obtain a set of vital signs to see if she is in shock. Ask the patient if she has ever had pain like this before. Determine the severity of her pain using a 0 to 10 scale (10 being unspeakable pain).

2. What type of care does this patient need?

Sudden onset of severe abdominal pain in a young, healthy woman often indicates a serious condition. Low blood pressure may indicate that she is in shock, but a normal blood pressure does not rule out a serious condition in its early stages. If the patient reports her menstrual period is late, suspect that she might be suffering from a ruptured ectopic pregnancy, which is a medical emergency. The only way to determine the cause of her pain is to arrange for her to be transported to an appropriate medical facility for evaluation by a physician.

Prep Kit

▶ Ready for Review

- Childbirth is usually a happy event. As an emergency medical responder (EMR), your role is to assist in the delivery and offer comfort and support to the mother and newborn. In most cases, deliveries result in healthy babies.
- To estimate how soon a delivery will occur, assess the time between contractions and whether the newborn's head appears during a contraction (crowning). By using these two key indicators, you can determine whether to transport the woman to a medical facility or whether the birth will occur outside the hospital.
- Normal labor consists of three distinct stages:
  - Stage one is characterized by the following conditions: initial contractions occur; the bag of waters breaks; the bloody show occurs, but the newborn's head does not appear.
  - Stage two involves the actual birth. You will see the newborn's head crowning during contractions, at which time you must prepare to assist the woman with delivery.
  - Stage three involves delivery of the placenta. You must assist in stabilizing the condition of the mother and newborn and delivering the placenta.
- Take standard precautions when assisting with delivery of a newborn.
- After the delivery, you have two patients to care for—the mother and the newborn.
- If the infant does not breathe on his or her own within the first minute after birth, proceed with the steps to resuscitate.
- Although most pregnancies and births are uneventful, be aware of possible complications, including ectopic pregnancy and shock, vaginal bleeding and miscarriage, premature birth, unbroken bag of waters, prolapse of the umbilical cord, breech birth, stillborn delivery, multiple births, and excessive bleeding after delivery.
- Promptly assess and arrange transport for a pregnant woman who has been involved in a motor vehicle crash to the hospital.

▶ Vital Vocabulary

anus The distal or terminal ending of the gastrointestinal tract.

bag of waters The amniotic sac and fluid that surround the fetus before birth.

birth canal The vagina and the lower part of the uterus.

bloody show The plug of mucus that is discharged from the vagina when labor begins.

breech presentation A delivery in which the newborn's buttocks appear in the birth canal first, rather than the head.

contractions Muscular movements of the uterus that push the newborn out of the birth canal.

crowning Appearance of the newborn's head during a contraction as he or she is pushed outward through the birth canal.

ectopic pregnancy A pregnancy that occurs outside the uterus, usually in a fallopian tube; usually terminates with the rupture of the fallopian tube.

fetus A developing newborn in the uterus or womb.

labor The process of delivering a newborn.

miscarriage Delivery of an incomplete or underdeveloped fetus before it is mature enough to survive outside the womb (about 20 weeks of pregnancy); also called spontaneous abortion.

placenta Life-support system of the fetus; also called the afterbirth.

premature newborn A newborn delivered before 36 weeks of gestation or who weighs less than 5 pounds (2 kg) at birth.

prolapsed umbilical cord A condition in which the umbilical cord appears before the newborn does; the newborn's head may compress the cord and cut off all circulation.

suction To aspirate (suck out) fluid by mechanical means.

umbilical cord Ropelike attachment between the pregnant woman and fetus; nourishment and waste products pass to and from the fetus and the woman through this cord.

uterus (womb) Muscular organ that holds and nourishes the developing fetus.

vagina The opening through which the newborn emerges.

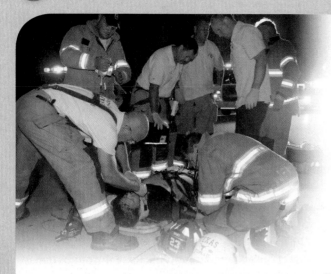

Assessment
in Action

You and your partner are on standby at a high school football game when a man runs up to you screaming that his wife is "having a baby." The man tells you that his wife suddenly started having contractions and the next thing he knew, her water broke. He tells you his wife is 9 months pregnant with their first child and she is waiting in their vehicle. You grab your medical bag and head to the patient's vehicle.

1. Which of the following steps is NOT indicated in this case?

   A. Gain information about the patient's pregnancy and medical history.
   B. Put on gloves and prepare for birth.
   C. Contact dispatch to request an EMS crew and a transport unit.
   D. Massage the patient's abdomen to speed up the delivery process.

2. The patient is sitting in the back seat of the vehicle and is clearly in distress. She says her contractions are 2 minutes apart. What should you do?

   A. Conduct a full patient assessment, including a secondary assessment.
   B. Prepare to deliver the newborn.
   C. Prepare for transport to the hospital.
   D. Move the patient into a position of comfort.

3. Moments later, you see that the newborn's head is visible at the vaginal opening. What is this called?

   A. Breech
   B. Prolapse
   C. Neonatal
   D. Crowning

4. Because the head of the newborn is visible and you are in the field, what is the next most appropriate step?

   A. Wait for emergency medical providers with a higher level of training.
   B. Have a supply of clean towels ready.
   C. Tell the woman to breathe slowly and push.
   D. Tell the woman to stop pushing.

5. As soon as the head of the newborn is delivered, what should you do?

   A. Look, listen, and feel for breathing.
   B. Pull on the newborn's shoulders to get the rest of the body out.
   C. Check the newborn's neck to be sure the umbilical cord is not wrapped around it.
   D. Clamp the umbilical cord.

6. If the bag of waters has not broken once the newborn's head has delivered, what should you do?

   A. Tear the bag with your fingers and push it away from the newborn's face.
   B. Place your hand on the newborn's head to keep it from moving.
   C. Be prepared to suction the newborn's mouth and nose with a bulb syringe.
   D. Arrange for immediate transport.

7. Which of the following steps is NOT indicated if you have just delivered a healthy newborn?

   A. Begin chest compressions.
   B. Suction the airway if the newborn is having difficulty breathing.
   C. Thoroughly dry the newborn.
   D. Place the newborn on the mother's abdomen to allow skin-to-skin contact.

8. The newborn starts breathing and appears healthy. After wrapping the newborn in towels and placing the newborn on the mother's abdomen, what is your next step?

9. When should the umbilical cord be cut?

10. Why is a ruptured ectopic pregnancy a life-threatening emergency?

CHAPTER 17

Pediatric Emergencies

National EMS Education Standard Competencies

Special Patient Populations

Recognizes and manages life threats based on simple assessment findings for a patient with special needs while awaiting additional emergency response.

Pediatrics

Age-related assessment findings and age-related assessment and treatment modifications for pediatric-specific major diseases and/or emergencies

> Upper airway obstruction (pp 369–371)
> Lower airway reactive disease (p 373)
> Respiratory distress/failure/arrest (pp 371–372)
> Shock (p 379)
> Seizures (p 375)
> Sudden infant death syndrome (p 378)

Patients With Special Challenges

> Recognizing and reporting abuse and neglect (pp 380–381)

Medicine

Recognizes and manages life threats based on assessment findings of a patient with a medical emergency while awaiting additional emergency response.

Respiratory

Anatomy, signs, symptoms, and management of respiratory emergencies including those that affect the

> Upper airway (pp 366–372; pp 373–374)
> Lower airway (p 373)

Trauma

Uses simple knowledge to recognize and manage life threats based on assessment findings for an acutely injured patient while awaiting additional emergency medical response.

Special Considerations in Trauma

Recognition and management of trauma in

> Pregnant patient (Chapter 16, *Childbirth*)
> Pediatric patient (pp 378–379)
> Geriatric patient (Chapter 18, *Geriatric Emergencies*)

Anatomy and Physiology

Uses simple knowledge of the anatomy and function of the upper airway, heart, vessels, blood, lungs, skin, muscles, and bones as the foundation of emergency care.

Knowledge Objectives

1. Describe the differences between a child's and an adult's anatomy. (pp 363–364)
2. Discuss the examination process for a child. (pp 364–366)
3. Describe how to implement the pediatric assessment triangle. (pp 364–365)
4. Discuss the normal rates of respiration and pulse for a child. (p 366)
5. Discuss the symptoms and effects of high body temperature in a child. (p 366)
6. Explain the differences between performing the following skills on a child and on an adult:
   - Opening the airway (p 367)
   - Basic life support (p 367)
   - Suctioning (pp 367–368)
   - Inserting an oral airway (p 368)
7. Describe how to treat a child and an infant with:
   - A mild (partial) airway obstruction (p 369)
   - A severe (complete) airway obstruction (pp 369–372)
   - A swallowed object (p 371)
   - Respiratory distress (p 371)
   - Respiratory failure (pp 371–372)
   - Circulatory failure (p 372)
8. Describe how to treat the following illnesses and medical emergencies:
   - Altered mental status (pp 372–373)
   - Asthma (p 373)
   - Croup (pp 373–374)
   - Epiglottitis (p 374)
   - Drowning (pp 374–375)
   - Heat illnesses (p 375)
   - High fever (p 375)
   - Seizures (p 375)
   - Vomiting and diarrhea (p 377)
   - Abdominal pain (p 377)
   - Poisoning (pp 377–378)
   - Sudden infant death syndrome (p 378)
9. Describe the patterns of pediatric injury. (pp 378–379)
10. Describe the signs and symptoms of shock in pediatric patients. (p 379)
11. Discuss the effects of child restraint laws and car seat use on pediatric trauma. (pp 379–380)
12. Explain the steps you should take to care for a child who has signs of child abuse or sexual assault. (p 380)
13. Describe the need for emergency medical responder critical incident stress debriefing. (pp 380–381)

Skills Objectives

1. Demonstrate the examination process for a child. (pp 364–366)
2. Demonstrate implementation of the pediatric assessment triangle. (pp 364–365)
3. Demonstrate how to determine the respiration and pulse rates for a child. (p 366)
4. Demonstrate performance of the following skills on a child:
   - Opening the airway (p 367)
   - Basic life support (p 367)
   - Suctioning (pp 367–368)
   - Inserting an oral airway (p 368)
5. Demonstrate how to treat a child and an infant with:
   - A mild (partial) airway obstruction (p 369)
   - A severe (complete) airway obstruction (pp 369–372)
   - A swallowed object (p 371)
   - Respiratory distress (p 371)
   - Respiratory failure (pp 371–372)
   - Circulatory failure (p 372)
6. Demonstrate how to treat the following illnesses and medical emergencies:
   - Altered mental status (pp 372–373)
   - Asthma (p 373)
   - Croup (pp 373–374)
   - Epiglottitis (p 374)
   - Drowning (pp 374–375)
   - Heat illnesses (p 375)
   - High fever (p 375)
   - Seizures (p 375)
   - Vomiting and diarrhea (p 377)
   - Abdominal pain (p 377)
   - Poisoning (pp 377–378)
   - Sudden infant death syndrome (p 378)

■ Introduction

Sudden illnesses and medical emergencies are common in children and infants. This chapter covers the special knowledge and skills you will need to assess and treat children and infants. This chapter also covers the differences between the anatomy of an adult and a child and highlights the special considerations for examining pediatric patients. It describes how the pediatric assessment triangle gives you a first impression of the severity of the child's illness or injury.

Respiratory care for children is extremely important. This chapter reviews the following respiratory skills: opening the airway, basic life support, suctioning, and relieving airway obstructions. It explains the signs of respiratory distress, respiratory failure, and circulatory failure in children and infants.

It is important that you learn some basic information and treatment for the following conditions: altered mental status, asthma, croup, epiglottitis, drowning, heat illnesses, high fever, seizures, vomiting and diarrhea, abdominal pain, poisoning, and sudden infant death syndrome. Because trauma is the leading cause of death in children, this chapter covers patterns of injury and the signs of traumatic shock in children. Finally, it is important for you to be able to recognize some of the signs and symptoms of child abuse and sexual abuse of children so you can take the appropriate steps to get help from the proper authorities.

■ General Considerations

Managing a pediatric emergency can be one of the most stressful situations you face as an emergency medical responder (EMR). The child is frightened, anxious, and usually unable to communicate the problem to you clearly. The parents are anxious and frightened. In an atmosphere where everyone involved is tense, you must remain calm and behave in a controlled and professional manner.

Emergency medical services (EMS) personnel often have mixed feelings when treating a child. In some situations, the child reminds them of someone they know. Even the most experienced personnel respond emotionally to a seriously ill or injured child. Unless you are prepared, your anxiety and fear may interfere with your ability to deliver proper care.

▶ The Parents

The child's parents or caregivers can be either allies or a potential problem. You must respond to them as much as to the child, although in a different way. Talk to both the parents and the child as much as possible. Parents are understandably concerned about their child's condition, especially if they do not clearly understand the situation or if they think the situation is more serious than it is. For example, imagine a parent's reaction to a bleeding laceration on his or her child's forehead. You know that scalp wounds can bleed profusely, but you also know that you can easily control such bleeding with direct pressure. However, many parents are not aware of this fact and may become emotionally distressed by the large amount of blood. Other parents can be extremely helpful. They know the child well and can tell you how the child's behavior is different from his or her usual behavior.

Children get many of their behavioral cues from their parents; therefore, if you calm the parents, talk with them, and ask for their assistance in calming the child, it is likely that the child will become less agitated. It is a good idea to allow a parent to hold the child if the illness or injury permits. If the injury is such that the parent cannot hold the child on his or her lap, let the parent hold the child's hand or keep the parents where the child can see them.

Quickly try to develop a rapport with the child. Tell the child your first name, find out what the child's name is, and use the child's name as you explain what you are doing. Do not stand over the child. Squat, kneel, or sit down to place yourself at the level of the child and establish eye contact. Ask the child simple questions about the pain and ask the child to help you by pointing to (or touching) the painful area.

Be honest with the child. For example, if you must move an arm or leg to apply a splint, tell the child what you are going to do and explain that the movement may hurt. In talking to the child, you can also request his or her help, asking the child to help you by being calm, lying still, or holding a bandage. The level of understanding and cooperation you can receive from an ill or injured child is often remarkable and may surprise you. Some emergency service agencies provide the child with a trauma teddy bear to hold while being examined **Figure 17-1**.

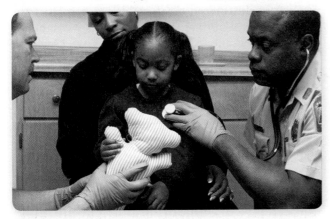

Figure 17-1 The trauma teddy bear helps keep a child calm while being examined.
© Jones & Bartlett Learning. Courtesy of MIEMSS.

Pediatric Anatomy and Function

Children and adults have the same body systems that perform the same functions. However, there are certain differences, particularly in the airway, that you need to understand. A child's airway is smaller in relation to the rest of the body. Therefore, secretions or swelling from illnesses or trauma can more easily block the child's airway. Because a child's tongue is relatively larger than the tongue of an adult, a child's tongue can more easily block the airway if the child becomes unresponsive **Figure 17-2**. Because a child's upper airway anatomy is more flexible than that of an adult, you must remember to avoid hyperextending (overextending) the neck of an infant or child when attempting to open the airway. Position the head in a neutral or slight sniffing position, but do not hyperextend the neck. Hyperextension of

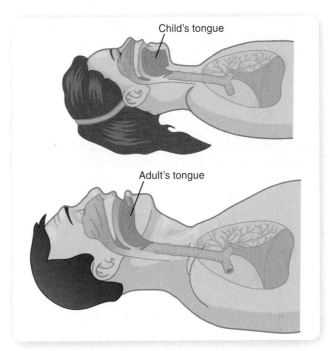

Figure 17-2 The anatomy of a child's airway differs from that of an adult. The tongue is proportionally larger and can more easily block the airway. Also, the back of a child's head is larger, so head positioning requires more care.
© Jones & Bartlett Learning.

YOU are the Provider — CASE 1

At 1037, you are dispatched to a residence that provides day care for five children. Upon your arrival, you are led to a small room where one of the caregivers is holding a 26-month-old boy in her arms. She tells you that the toddler was more fussy than usual when his mother dropped him off at the center at 0730 hours. He has remained fussy, with periods of crying. She thinks he may have a fever and has noted that his breathing is noisy.

1. What factors do you need to consider as you evaluate the first side of the pediatric triangle?
2. What factors do you need to consider as you evaluate the second side of the pediatric triangle?
3. What factors do you need to consider as you evaluate the third side of the pediatric triangle?

a child's neck can occlude the airway. For at least the first 6 months of their lives, infants can breathe only through their noses. If mucus blocks an infant's nose, the infant cannot breathe through the mouth. Therefore, it is important to clear the nose of an infant to enable breathing.

When the demands on a child's respiratory system change, the child is able to quickly compensate by increasing his or her breathing rate and breathing efforts. However, these compensatory mechanisms will function for only a short period of time, because the child will become exhausted. When this happens, the child may begin to show signs of severe respiratory distress and rapidly progress into respiratory failure if left untreated. Therefore, it is important for you to perform a thorough patient assessment and monitor the child's vital signs at least every 5 minutes when caring for seriously ill or injured pediatric patients.

Infants and children also have limited abilities to compensate for changes in temperature when compared with adults. Children have a greater surface area relative to the mass of their body. This means that they lose relatively more heat than adults do. Therefore, you need to keep the body temperature of children as close to normal as possible and warm them if they become chilled.

■ Examining a Child

It is important for you to perform a thorough and systematic assessment of a child to determine the extent of his or her illness or injury. The examination of a child should consist of the same five steps used in the patient assessment sequence that you learned for adult patients. First, perform a scene size-up to ensure that the scene is safe for you and for the patient. Then complete a primary assessment to form a general impression of the patient; to determine the patient's level of responsiveness; and to assess the status of the airway, breathing, and circulation (ABCs). Next, complete a secondary assessment by examining the child from head to toe. Obtain a medical history. Finally, perform reassessments as needed.

▶ The Pediatric Assessment Triangle

It is important for you to be able to quickly determine when a child is seriously ill or injured. The **pediatric assessment triangle (PAT)** was developed to help you quickly form a general impression of a pediatric patient's condition as part of your primary assessment. It does not change the steps of the patient assessment sequence you already learned.

The PAT is a valuable tool that allows you to quickly form a general impression of the child using only your

senses of sight and hearing. It provides you with an accurate initial picture of the functioning of the child's airway, breathing, circulation, and level of responsiveness. It will help you begin to identify whether the child is experiencing a serious condition. It will help you assess a child from a distance and determine what steps to take first. The three components of the PAT are: (1) the child's overall appearance, (2) the work of breathing, and (3) circulation to the skin **Figure 17-3** . Each of these three components is discussed in this section.

Appearance

The first element of the PAT is appearance. Does the child appear to be ill or injured? The child's general appearance is important when you are trying to determine the severity of the child's illness or injury. The general appearance is an indicator of how well the heart and lungs are working. Appearance is also a good indication of how well the central nervous system is working. As you assess a child, compare his or her appearance and actions with what you would expect from a healthy child of the same age.

Look at the child to see whether he or she has good muscle tone. Is the child crying or able to speak? Infants and young children normally cry in response to fear or pain; a child who is not crying may have a decreased level of consciousness, an upper airway infection, or swelling in the airway. If the child is crying, does the cry sound like a normal, healthy cry or is it a subdued whimper? Does the child have a blank, unfocused stare or does he or she look at others? Carefully evaluate a child who is unresponsive, lackluster, and appears ill, because lack of activity and interest can signal serious illness or injury. Is the child able to interact in a manner that is age appropriate? If the child is conscious, it is better to start your assessment from across the room than to disturb the child by removing him or her from the caregiver's arms. A child with good eye contact, good muscle tone, and good color would seem to be normal.

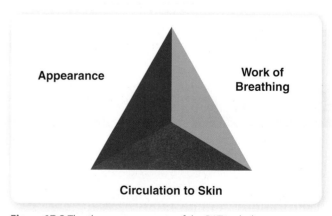

Figure 17-3 The three components of the PAT include appearance, work of breathing, and circulation to the skin.

Source: Used with permission of the American Academy of Pediatrics, Pediatric Education for Prehospital Professionals, © American Academy of Pediatrics, 2000.

A child who makes poor eye contact and is pale and listless should be of concern to you. As you evaluate the initial appearance of a child, keep in mind that the child's appearance can change quickly. Therefore, you need to reassess the child's appearance regularly. **Table 17-1** lists the characteristics of appearance you should look for in a pediatric patient.

Work of Breathing

The second element of the PAT is the work of breathing. In children, assessing the work of breathing is a more accurate indicator of a child's condition than merely determining the rate of respirations. You can determine the child's work of breathing by measuring four factors: (1) abnormal breath sounds, (2) abnormal positioning, (3) retractions of the neck or chest, and (4) flaring of the nostrils. Abnormal breath sounds include noisy breathing, snoring, crowing, grunting, or wheezing. Abnormal positioning includes leaning forward while supporting themselves with their arms and a refusal to lie down. Retractions can occur above the collarbone or between the ribs. Flaring of the nostrils occurs during inspiration. Assess these four factors to determine the work of breathing **Table 17-2**. You can perform this assessment from across the room without touching the child.

Circulation to the Skin

The third element of the PAT is circulation to the skin. The three characteristics for determining circulation to the skin are paleness, mottling, and cyanosis. Check the child's skin for paleness or pallor. White or pale skin indicates an inadequate blood flow to the skin. The second characteristic of circulation to the skin is **mottling**, a patchy skin discoloration that is caused by too little or too much circulation to the skin. The third characteristic used in assessing the skin is cyanosis. Cyanosis is a blue discoloration of the skin caused by low levels of oxygen in the blood **Table 17-3**. You can establish the status of the circulation to the skin without touching the child.

Based on the findings of the PAT, you should now be able to form a general impression of a pediatric patient and determine the severity of the child's illness or injury. Use the PAT with the other parts of the patient assessment sequence that you learned in Chapter 9, *Patient Assessment*. This helpful tool allows you to quickly obtain valuable information without touching and agitating the child, and it helps set the priorities for further assessment and treatment.

Table 17-1 Characteristics of Appearance

Characteristic	Healthy Reaction	Unhealthy Reaction
Movement	Moving vigorously	Limp, listless, flaccid
Interaction	Reaches for a toy Reacts to a person or sound	Uninterested in playing or toys
Reassurance	Reassured by caregivers	Crying or agitated Unrelieved by gentle reassurance
Eye movement	Eyes follow movement of a person or toy	Glassy-eyed stare
Speech	Age-appropriate speech	Garbled or confused speech
Cry	Strong cry	Weak or high-pitched cry

© Jones & Bartlett Learning.

Table 17-2 Characteristics of Work of Breathing

Characteristic	Features to Look For
Abnormal breath sounds	Noisy breathing, snoring, crowing, grunting, or wheezing
Abnormal positioning	Leaning forward while using the arms for support
Retractions	Retractions above the collarbone or between the ribs
Flaring	Flaring of the nostrils

© Jones & Bartlett Learning.

Table 17-3 Characteristics of Circulation to the Skin

Characteristic	Features to Look For
Pallor	White or pale skin or mucous membranes
Mottling	Patchy skin discoloration caused by too much or too little blood flow to the skin
Cyanosis	Blue discoloration of the skin and mucous membranes

© Jones & Bartlett Learning.

▶ Respirations

To calculate the respiratory rate of a child, count respirations for 30 seconds and multiply by two. Counting for less than 30 seconds can cause inaccurate results because children often have irregular breathing patterns.

As you examine children, look to see how much work they are doing to breathe. This work of breathing will help to determine whether they are in respiratory distress. Look for abnormal breath sounds such as noisy breathing, snoring, crowing, grunting, or wheezing. Look to determine whether they are holding themselves in an abnormal position. Are they supporting themselves with their arms while leaning forward (known as the tripod position) or do they refuse to lie down? Check for retractions of the neck or chest. Look for flaring of the nostrils. These signs and symptoms of breathing difficulty are the same as the ones you use to assess breathing difficulty as part of the PAT.

The presence of any of these signs indicates that the child is having some difficulty breathing and may be experiencing respiratory distress. Respiratory distress is discussed in the section on respiratory care.

Special Populations

From birth to about 6 months of age, children are "nose breathers." They have not yet learned to breathe through their mouths.

▶ Pulse Rate

The normal pulse rate of a child is faster than an adult's normal rate. For a child younger than 1 year, palpate a brachial pulse, which is located halfway between the shoulder and the elbow on the inside of the upper arm or directly over the heart Figure 17-4 . Table 17-4 describes the usual, normal vital signs for children at various ages.

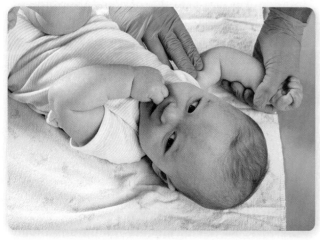

Figure 17-4 The best place to take the pulse in an infant is over the brachial artery or directly over the heart.
© Jones & Bartlett Learning.

▶ High Body Temperature

Flushed, red skin, sweating, and restlessness often accompany high temperatures in children. You can often feel a high temperature just by touching the child's chest and head. A child's heart rate increases with each degree of temperature rise.

■ Respiratory Care

Neither adults nor children can tolerate a lack of oxygen for more than a few minutes before permanent brain damage occurs.

It is important for you to open and maintain the airway and to ventilate adequately any child with a respiratory condition. Otherwise, the child may go into respiratory arrest, followed by cardiac arrest because of the lack of oxygen to the heart. This is a different situation than adults, who usually experience cardiopulmonary arrest as a result of a heart attack.

Some of the specific causes of cardiopulmonary arrest in children include suffocation caused by the aspiration of a foreign body, infections of the airway such as croup and acute epiglottitis, sudden infant death syndrome (SIDS), accidental poisonings, and injuries around the head and neck. This chapter covers each condition in detail.

▶ Treating Respiratory Emergencies in Infants and Children

You need four types of skills to treat respiratory emergencies in children: opening the airway, basic life support, suctioning, and the use of airway adjuncts. Each of these skills is described below.

Table 17-4	**Normal Vital Signs in Children at Rest**	
Age	**Heart Rate (beats/min)**	**Respirations (breaths/min)**
Newborn (0 to 1 month)	90–180	30–60
Infant (1 month to 1 year)	100–160	25–50
Toddler (1 to 3 years)	90–150	20–30
Preschool age (3 to 6 years)	80–140	20–25
School age (6 to 12 years)	70–120	15–20
Adolescent (12 to 18 years)	60–100	12–20

Data from: American Heart Association. *2015 Guidelines for Cardiopulmonary Resuscitation and Emergency Cardiovascular Care*; Chameides L, Samson RA, Schexnayder SM, Hazinski MF, eds. *Pediatric Advanced Life Support Provider Manual*. Dallas, TX: American Heart Association; 2011.

Opening the Airway

When opening the airway of a child or an infant, use the same general techniques that you use for an adult patient. The head tilt–chin lift maneuver can be used for children who have not sustained an injury to the neck or head **Figure 17-5**. When using the head tilt–chin lift maneuver on a child, be sure that you do not hyperextend the neck when you tilt the head back. Hyperextending a child's neck can occlude the airway. Use a neutral or slight sniffing position. You can place a folded towel under the child's shoulders to help maintain this position. If the possibility of injury to the head or neck exists, try the jaw-thrust maneuver to open the airway. If the jaw-thrust maneuver does not open the airway, use the head tilt–chin lift maneuver because opening the airway is a top priority for an unresponsive patient.

Basic Life Support

Because children are smaller than adults, you must use specific techniques when you perform cardiopulmonary resuscitation (CPR) on children. There are special procedures for hand placement, compression pressure, and airway positioning.

CPR for children (1 year of age to the onset of puberty) is different from adult CPR in the following three ways:

1. If you are alone, without help, and no one has called EMS, perform five cycles or 2 minutes of CPR before activating the EMS system.
2. Use the heel of one hand or two hands to perform chest compressions, depending on the size of the child **Figure 17-6**.
3. Compress the sternum at least one-third the depth of the chest (about 2 inches [5 cm]).

CPR for infants (younger than 1 year) has the following five differences from adult CPR:

1. Check for responsiveness by tapping the infant's foot or gently shaking the shoulder.
2. Check the pulse by using the brachial pulse as shown in Figure 17-4.
3. Use your middle and ring fingers to compress the sternum just below the nipple line.
4. Compress the sternum to a depth of at least one-third the depth of the chest (about 1.5 inches [4 cm]).
5. Give gentle rescue breaths, using mouth-to-mouth-and-nose ventilations.

Suctioning

To clear secretions, vomitus, or blood from a patient's airway, turn the patient on his or her side and use your

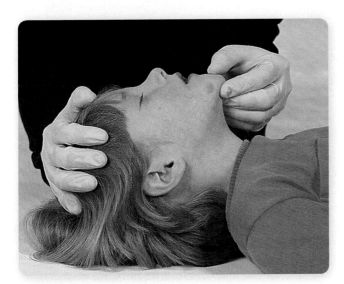

Figure 17-5 Open the child's airway using the head tilt–chin lift maneuver.
© Jones & Bartlett Learning. Courtesy of MIEMSS.

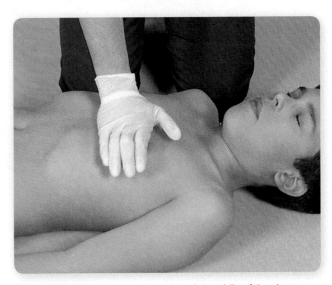

Figure 17-6 Place one or two hands in the middle of the chest, between the nipples.
© Jones & Bartlett Learning. Courtesy of MIEMSS.

gloved fingers to scoop out as much of the substance as possible. You can use **suctioning** (aspirating or sucking out fluid by mechanical means) to remove the foreign substances that cannot be removed with your gloved fingers. Suctioning to open a blocked airway can be a lifesaving procedure.

The procedure used for suctioning infants and children is generally the same as for adults, with the following exceptions:

1. Use a tonsil tip or rigid tip to suction the mouth. Do not insert the tip any farther than you can see.
2. Use a flexible catheter to suction the nose of a child; set the suction on low or medium power.
3. Use a bulb syringe to suction the nose of an infant. Remember that an infant can breathe only through the nose.
4. Never suction for more than 5 seconds at one time.
5. Try to ventilate and re-oxygenate the patient before repeating the suctioning.

For a complete description of how to use suctioning, review the material presented in Chapter 7, *Airway Management*, and Chapter 16, *Childbirth*.

Airway Adjuncts

An oral airway can maintain an open airway after you have opened the patient's airway by manual means. Use the steps in **Skill Drill 17-1** to insert an oral airway in a child or an infant.

1. Select the proper size oral airway by measuring from the patient's ear lobe to the corner of the mouth **Step 1**.
2. Position the patient's airway. If the emergency is medical, use the head tilt–chin lift maneuver, avoiding hyperextension. If the patient has a traumatic injury, use the jaw-thrust maneuver **Step 2**.
3. Depress the patient's tongue with two or three stacked tongue blades. Press the tongue forward and away from the roof of the mouth **Step 3**.
4. Follow the anatomic curve of the roof of the patient's mouth to slide the airway into place.
5. Be gentle. The mouths of children and infants are fragile.

Treatment

In pediatric patients, you must be careful not to overextend the neck. In infants and some small children, the overextension may actually obstruct the airway because of the flexibility of the child's neck. Smaller children may breathe easier if the neck is held in a neutral position rather than overextended. To maintain the neutral position, you can use a towel to support the patient's shoulders.

Skill Drill 17-1

Inserting an Oral Airway in a Child

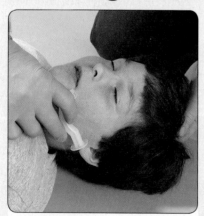

Step 1 Select the proper size oral airway by measuring from the patient's ear lobe to the corner of the mouth.

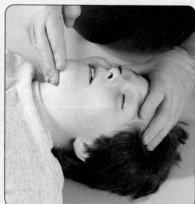

Step 2 Position the pediatric patient's airway with the appropriate method.

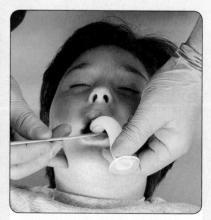

Step 3 Depress the patient's tongue and press the tongue forward and away from the roof of the mouth. Follow the anatomic curve of the roof of the patient's mouth to slide the airway into place.

EMRs usually do not use nasal airways for children. If you have questions about using nasal airways in pediatric patients, check with your medical director.

▶ Mild (Partial) Airway Obstruction

You can usually relieve a mild (partial) airway obstruction by placing the child on his or her back (supine), tilting the head, and lifting the chin in the head tilt–chin lift maneuver.

An airway blocked by an aspirated foreign object (eg, small toy, piece of candy, balloon) is a common occurrence in young children, particularly in children who are crawling. If the foreign object is only partially blocking the airway, the child will probably be able to pass some air around the object. You can remove the object if it is clearly visible in the mouth and you can remove it easily. However, if you cannot see the object or if you do not think you can remove it easily, do not attempt to remove it as long as the child can still breathe air around the object. Sometimes trying to remove an object that is partially blocking the airway can result in a severe airway blockage, which is an extremely serious situation.

Children with a partial (mild) airway obstruction should be transported to the emergency department. During treatment and transport, talk constantly to a child with a partially obstructed airway about what you are doing. Carrying on a conversation with the child oftentimes comforts the child and reduces the terror of having something stuck in the throat.

The presence of a parent during transport can provide emotional support to both the parent and the child. The parent's presence can often reassure and calm the child. Judge each situation carefully. Not all parents are able to remain calm during such a serious situation. However, most of the time, parents are able to realize the seriousness of the situation, redirect their emotions, and work with you to reassure and calm the child.

If you have oxygen available and are trained in its use, administer it by carefully placing the oxygen mask over the child's mouth and nose. Do not try to get an airtight seal on the mask; hold it 1 or 2 inches (3 to 5 cm) away from the child's face. If you tell the child what you are doing with the oxygen and how it will make breathing easier, you may be able to calm and relax the child. Carefully monitor this critical situation to ensure that the mild obstruction does not become a severe obstruction.

▶ Severe (Complete) Airway Obstruction in Children

A severe (complete) airway obstruction is a serious emergency. A severe airway obstruction exists when the child has poor air exchange, increased breathing difficulty, a silent cough, the inability to speak, or no air movement because of an obstruction. You have only a few minutes to act before permanent brain damage occurs. Use the Heimlich maneuver (abdominal thrusts) because it provides enough energy to expel most foreign objects that could completely block a child's airway **Figure 17-7**.

The steps for relieving an airway obstruction in a conscious child (1 year to the onset of puberty) are the same as for an adult patient. However, the anatomic differences between adults and children require that you make some adjustments in your technique. When opening the airway of a child or infant, tilt the head back just past the neutral position. Tilting the head too far back (hyperextending the neck) can actually obstruct the airway of a child or infant. If you are by yourself and a

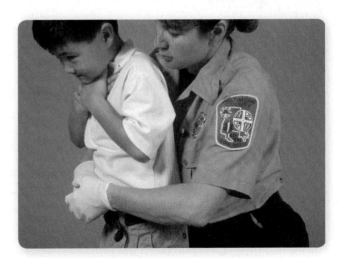

Figure 17-7 Performing abdominal thrusts on a child.
© Jones & Bartlett Learning. Courtesy of MIEMSS.

YOU ▶ are the Provider   CASE 2

At 2327, you are dispatched to a residence on the edge of your town for the report of a sick child. The house is located about 7 minutes from your location. While you are responding, the dispatcher tells you that the caller now reports that the child just had a seizure. When you arrive on the scene, a very excited man meets you at the curb and urges you to hurry into the house. In the living room, the mother is holding an 18-month-old toddler who is tightly wrapped in blankets. The mother tells you that the child has had a fever this evening and that they are waiting for a call back from their pediatrician.

1. What initial actions can you take to protect the child from harm?
2. What steps can you take to help cool the child?
3. What further care is needed to prevent this child from having another seizure?

child with an airway obstruction becomes unresponsive, perform CPR for five cycles (about 2 minutes) before activating the EMS system.

A skill performance sheet titled Child: Foreign Body Airway Obstruction is included for your review and practice Figure 17-8 .

▶ Complete or Severe Airway Obstruction in Infants

An infant (younger than 1 year) is very fragile. Infants' airway structures are very small and they are more easily injured than those of an adult. If you suspect an airway obstruction, first assess the infant to determine whether there is any air exchange. If the infant is crying, the airway is not completely obstructed. If no air is moving in or out of the infant's mouth and nose, suspect an obstructed airway. Find out what was happening when the episode of breathing difficulties began. Someone may have seen the infant put a foreign body into his or her mouth. To relieve an airway obstruction in a conscious infant, use a combination of back slaps and the **chest-thrust maneuver**. Be sure you are holding the infant securely as you alternate the back slaps and chest thrusts.

If there is no movement of air from the infant's mouth and nose, a sudden onset of severe breathing difficulty, a silent cough, or a silent cry, suspect a severe airway obstruction. To relieve a severe airway obstruction in an infant, use a combination of back slaps and chest thrusts. Review the following sequence until you can carry it out proficiently and automatically. To assist a conscious infant with a severe airway obstruction, perform the following steps:

1. Assess the infant's airway and breathing status. Determine that there is no air exchange.
2. Place the infant in a facedown position over your forearm and support your forearm with your thigh. Support the infant's head and neck with one hand and place the infant's head lower than the trunk. Use the heel of your hand and deliver five back slaps forcefully between the infant's shoulder blades Figure 17-9A .
3. Next, continuing to support the head, turn the infant faceup by sandwiching the infant between your hands and arms. Rest the infant on his or her back with the head lower than the trunk.
4. Deliver five chest thrusts in the middle of the sternum. Use two fingers and deliver the thrusts firmly Figure 17-9B .
5. Repeat the series of back slaps and chest thrusts until the infant expels the foreign object or becomes unresponsive.
6. If the infant becomes unresponsive, continue with the following steps.
7. Ensure that EMS has been activated.
8. Begin CPR:
   - Open the airway by using the head tilt–chin lift maneuver.
   - Look into the mouth for any foreign object. Use finger sweeps only if you can see a foreign object.

Child: Foreign Body Airway Obstruction

Steps	Adequately Performed
1. Ask "Are you choking?"	
2. Give abdominal thrusts.	
3. Repeat thrusts until foreign body is dislodged or until patient becomes unresponsive.	
If the patient becomes unresponsive:	
4. If a second rescuer is available, have him or her activate the EMS system.	
5. Begin CPR: • Open the airway by using the head tilt–chin lift maneuver. • Look into the mouth for any foreign object. Use finger sweeps only if you can see a foreign object. • Attempt to give one ventilation. If air does not go in, reposition the head and attempt another breath. • If air still does not go in, begin chest compressions. (See Chapter 8, *Professional Rescuer CPR*, for coverage of this part of the CPR sequence.)	
6. Continue CPR for five cycles (about 2 minutes) and then activate the EMS system if you are by yourself.	
7. Continue CPR until more advanced EMS personnel arrive.	

Figure 17-8 Skill Performance Sheet.

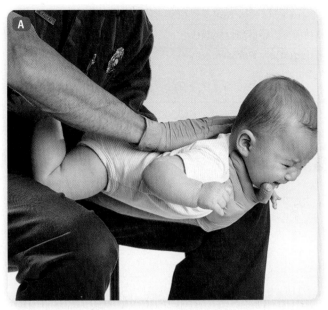
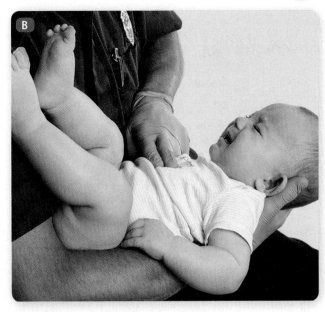

Figure 17-9 Administering back slaps and chest thrusts in an infant. **A.** Hold the infant facedown with the body resting on your forearm. Support the jaw and face with your hand without blocking the airway and keep the head lower than the rest of the body. Give the infant five back slaps between the shoulder blades, using the heel of your hand. **B.** Sandwich the infant between your hands, turn the infant over, and give the infant five quick chest thrusts, using two fingers placed on the lower half of the sternum (finger position should be the same as CPR for infants).
A&B: © Jones & Bartlett Learning.

- Attempt to give one ventilation. If air does not go in, reposition the head and attempt another breath.
- If air still does not go in, begin chest compressions. (See Chapter 8, *Professional Rescuer CPR*, for coverage of this part of the CPR sequence.)

9. Continue these CPR steps until more advanced EMS personnel arrive.

Note: If you are alone, administer CPR for five cycles (about 2 minutes) and then activate EMS.

Recent studies have shown that administering chest compressions to an unresponsive patient increases the pressure in the chest similar to administering chest thrusts and may relieve an airway obstruction. Therefore, performing CPR on an infant who has become unresponsive has the same effect as administering chest thrusts on a conscious patient.

A skill performance sheet titled Infant: Foreign Body Airway Obstruction is included in ⟨ **Figure 17-10** ⟩ for your review and practice.

▶ Swallowed Objects

Children often swallow small, round objects like marbles, beads, buttons, and coins. If these objects do not become airway obstructions, they usually pass uneventfully through the child and are eliminated in a bowel movement. However, sharp or straight objects such as open safety pins, bobby pins, and bones are dangerous if swallowed. Arrange for *prompt transport* to an appropriate medical facility because special instruments and techniques are required to locate and remove the object from the stomach and intestinal tract.

▶ Respiratory Distress

Respiratory distress indicates that a child has a serious condition that requires immediate medical attention. Often respiratory distress quickly leads to respiratory failure.

You must be able to recognize the following signs of respiratory distress:

1. A breathing rate of more than 60 breaths per minute in infants
2. A breathing rate of more than 30 to 40 breaths per minute in children
3. Nasal flaring on each breath
4. Retraction of the skin between the ribs and around the neck muscles
5. Stridor (a high-pitched sound on inspiration)
6. Cyanosis of the skin
7. Altered mental status
8. Combativeness or restlessness

If you see that any of the listed signs are present, try to determine the cause. Support the child's respirations by placing the child in a comfortable position, usually sitting. Keep the child as calm as possible by letting a parent hold the child if practical. Prepare to administer oxygen if it is available and you are trained in its use. Monitor the child's vital signs and arrange for *prompt transport* to an appropriate medical facility.

▶ Respiratory Failure/Arrest

Respiratory failure often results as respiratory distress proceeds. Many of the same factors that cause respiratory distress can cause respiratory failure.

Infant: Foreign Body Airway Obstruction	
Steps	**Adequately Performed**
1. Confirm severe airway obstruction. Check for sudden onset of serious breathing difficulty, ineffective cough, silent cough, or silent cry.	
2. Give up to five back slaps and up to five chest thrusts.	
3. Repeat Step 2 until the foreign body is dislodged or until the infant becomes unresponsive.	
If the infant becomes unresponsive:	
4. If a second rescuer is available, have him or her activate the EMS System.	
5. Begin CPR: • Open the airway by using the head tilt–chin lift maneuver. • Look into the mouth for any foreign object. Use finger sweeps only if you can see a foreign object. • Attempt to give one ventilation. If air does not go in, reposition the head and attempt another breath. • If air still does not go in, begin chest compressions. (See Chapter 8, *Professional Rescuer CPR,* for coverage of this part of the CPR sequence.)	
6. Continue CPR for five cycles (about 2 minutes) and then activate the EMS system if you are by yourself.	
7. Continue CPR until more advanced EMS personnel arrive.	

Figure 17-10 Skill Performance Sheet.
© Jones & Bartlett Learning.

Characteristics of respiratory failure include the following conditions:

1. A breathing rate of fewer than 20 breaths per minute in an infant
2. A breathing rate of fewer than 10 breaths per minute in a child
3. Limp muscle tone
4. Unresponsiveness
5. Decreased or absent heart rate
6. Weak or absent distal pulses

A child in respiratory failure is on the verge of experiencing respiratory and cardiac arrest. Immediately assess the child and take whatever steps are appropriate to support the patient. Support respirations by performing mouth-to-mask ventilations. Administer oxygen if it is available and you have been trained to use it. Begin chest compressions if the heart rate is absent or less than 60 beats per minute. Arrange for *prompt transport* to an appropriate medical facility. Continue to monitor the patient's vital signs and support the airway, breathing, and circulation functions as well as you can.

Circulatory Failure

The most common cause of circulatory failure in children is respiratory failure. Uncorrected respiratory failure in children can lead to circulatory failure, and uncorrected circulatory failure can lead to cardiac arrest. That is why it is so important for you to correct respiratory failure before it progresses to circulatory failure. However, this is not always possible, so you should learn the signs of circulatory failure and its treatment. An increased heart rate, pale or blue skin, and changes in mental status indicate circulatory failure. If the child or infant's heart rate is more than 60 beats per minute, your treatment should consist of completing the patient assessment sequence, supporting ventilations, administering oxygen if available, and observing vital signs for any changes. If the heart rate of a child or infant is less than 60 beats per minute and there are signs of poor circulation, such as cyanosis, you should begin chest compressions and rescue breathing.

Sudden Illness and Medical Emergencies

Not many illnesses occur suddenly in young children, but most of the medical calls for children will involve sudden illnesses. It is important that you be able to recognize and treat these key pediatric illnesses.

▶ Altered Mental Status

Altered mental status in children can be caused by a variety of conditions, including low blood glucose level, poisoning, postseizure state, infection, head trauma, and decreased oxygen levels. Sometimes you will be able to determine the cause of the altered mental status and take steps to correct the condition. For example, if the parent tells you that the child has diabetes and is experiencing insulin shock, you can administer glucose to increase the patient's blood glucose level. However, in many situations, you will not be able to determine the cause of the altered mental status and will have to treat the patient's symptoms.

Complete your patient assessment, paying particular attention to any clues at the scene. Question any bystanders or family about the situation and try to get as much of the medical history as possible. Pay particular attention to the patient's initial vital signs. Recheck vital signs regularly to monitor any changes. Calm the patient and the patient's family. Be prepared to support the patient's airway, breathing, and circulation if needed. Place an unconscious patient in the recovery position to help keep an open airway and to aid in drainage of any secretions.

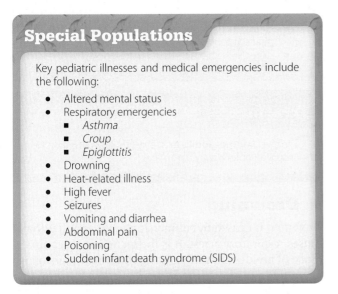

Special Populations

Key pediatric illnesses and medical emergencies include the following:

- Altered mental status
- Respiratory emergencies
  - *Asthma*
  - *Croup*
  - *Epiglottitis*
- Drowning
- Heat-related illness
- High fever
- Seizures
- Vomiting and diarrhea
- Abdominal pain
- Poisoning
- Sudden infant death syndrome (SIDS)

▶ Respiratory Illnesses

A respiratory condition in an infant or child can range from a minor cold to complete blockage of the airway. Because infants breathe primarily through their noses, even a minor cold can cause breathing difficulties. The excessive mucus in the nose resulting from a cold makes it more difficult for an infant to breathe than for an older child who can breathe through both the nose and mouth. Although colds cause most common respiratory conditions in children, you should also be able to recognize and treat the three more serious conditions: asthma, croup, and epiglottitis.

Asthma

A child who has **asthma** is usually already being treated for the condition by a physician and is taking a prescribed medication. In most situations, the child's parents call for assistance or transport only if the child is experiencing unusual breathing difficulties.

Asthma can occur in children older than 1 year; it rarely occurs during the first year of life. It is caused by a spasm or constriction (narrowing) and inflammation of the smaller airways in the lungs and usually produces a characteristic wheezing sound. Asthma attacks can range from mild to severe and can be triggered by many factors, including feathers, animal fur, tobacco smoke, pollen, respiratory infections, exercise, and even emotional situations.

A child who is experiencing an asthma attack is in obvious respiratory distress. During a severe attack, you can often hear the characteristic wheezing on exhalation—even without a stethoscope. The child can inhale air without difficulty but must labor to exhale the air. The effort to exhale is both frightening and tiring for the child.

Your primary treatment consists of calming and reassuring both the parents and the child. Tell them everything possible is being done and encourage them to relax.

Place the child in a sitting position to make breathing more comfortable. Ask the child to purse his or her lips, as if blowing up a balloon. Tell the child to blow out with force while doing this. Breathing through pursed lips helps in two ways: Both parents and the child feel that something is being done and this type of breathing relieves some of the internal lung pressures that cause the asthma attack Figure 17-11 .

If a child has asthma medication but it has not been administered, help the parent administer the medication. The parents should contact the child's physician for further advice. If the child's physician is not available, arrange for *prompt transport* to the emergency department.

Croup

Croup is an infection of the upper airway that occurs mainly in children who are between 6 months to 6 years. The lower throat swells and compresses (narrows) the airway, resulting in a characteristic hoarse, whooping noise during inhalation and a seal-like, barking cough.

Croup occurs often in colder climates (during fall and winter) and is frequently accompanied by a cold. The child usually has a moderate fever and a croupy noise that has developed over time. The worst episodes of croup usually occur in the middle of the night. A lack of fright or anxiety in the child and his or her willingness to lie down are important signs for you to note because they can help you distinguish croup from epiglottitis. Epiglottitis is a more serious condition that is discussed in the next section.

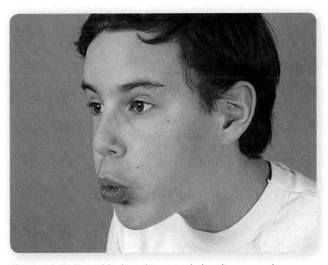

Figure 17-11 Pursed-lip breathing may help relieve an asthma attack.
© American Academy of Orthopaedic Surgeons.

> ### Signs and Symptoms
>
> Signs and symptoms of croup include the following:
> - Noisy, whooping inhalations
> - Seal-like, barking cough
> - History of a recent or current cold
> - Lack of fright or anxiety
> - Willingness to lie down

Although the signs and symptoms of croup are frightening for parents, it may not frighten the child. In many childhood emergencies, you must respond to the emotional needs and concerns of the parents as well as the medical needs of the child. Do not assume that croup is the cause of noisy breathing. Look to see if the child is choking on a toy, food, or foreign object lodged in the airway.

If the EMS unit is delayed, ask the parents to turn on the hot water in the shower and close the bathroom door. After the bathroom steams up, ask the parents to wait in there with the child until the EMS unit arrives. The moist, warm air relaxes the vocal cords and lessens the croupy noise. This effectively treats the child and reassures the parents. Have the parents contact the child's physician for further instructions or arrange for *transport* to an appropriate medical facility.

Epiglottitis

The third and most severe major respiratory condition is epiglottitis. **Epiglottitis** is a severe inflammation of the epiglottis, the small flap that covers the trachea during swallowing. In this condition, the flap is so inflamed and swollen that air movement into the trachea is completely blocked. Epiglottitis usually occurs in children between ages 3 to 6 years. Because of the widespread vaccination of infants against the bacteria (*Haemophilus influenzae* type b) that causes epiglottitis, the incidence of this disease is much less common now than in the past. This condition also occurs in adult patients who have not received the vaccination for *Haemophilus influenzae*.

> ### Safety
>
> Do not examine a child's throat if you suspect epiglottitis! An examination can cause more swelling of the epiglottis, resulting in a complete airway blockage.

While you conduct your initial examination, you may think the child has croup. However, because epiglottitis poses an immediate threat to life, you must be able to recognize the differences between croup and epiglottitis and know the signs and symptoms of epiglottitis; this is a very serious respiratory emergency. There is little that you can provide in the way of treatment except to make the child comfortable with as little handling as possible, keep everyone calm, administer oxygen (if you

have it available and have been trained to use it), and arrange for *prompt transport* to an appropriate medical facility. You may consider letting a parent hold the child during transport if the emotional attitudes of the child and parent are appropriate.

> ### Signs and Symptoms
>
> The signs and symptoms of epiglottitis include the following:
> - The child is usually sitting upright (he or she does not want to lie down).
> - The child cannot swallow.
> - The child is not coughing.
> - The child is drooling.
> - The child is anxious and frightened (he or she knows that something is seriously wrong).
> - The child's chin is thrust forward.

> ### Treatment
>
> The child with epiglottitis must have medical attention to ensure an open airway.

▶ Drowning

Drowning is caused by submersion in water and initially causes respiratory arrest. It is the second most common cause of accidental death among children 5 years of age or younger in the United States. Although swimming pools, lakes, streams, and oceans present significant risks of drowning, ordinary water sources around the home increase the risk of drowning for young children. Children left unattended in washbowls or bathtubs—for even a few minutes—can drown. Buckets of water and toilet bowls also pose threats to young children who put their heads down to look into the water, lose their balance, fall in, and are unable to get out.

The many sources of water around a home increase the chance that you may encounter a drowning situation when responding to a medical emergency involving a child. If you respond to a drowning situation, make sure that you do not put yourself in danger as you attempt a rescue. (See Chapter 20, *Vehicle Extrication and Special Rescue*, for more information on water rescues.)

After the child is removed from the water, begin assessment and treatment. Signs and symptoms of drowning include lack of breathing and no pulse. Begin by assessing the airway, breathing, and circulation. Make sure the airway is clear of water. Turn the child to one side and allow the water to drain out of the mouth. Use suction if it is available, start rescue breathing if necessary, and administer supplemental oxygen if it is available. If no pulse is present, start chest compressions. Because there is a chance that the patient has a cervical spine injury, stabilize the neck. To reduce the risk of hypothermia, dry the child with towels and cover the child with dry blankets or jackets.

Arrange for *prompt transport* of the patient to an appropriate medical facility. A physician needs to evaluate all patients who have experienced submersion, because serious respiratory conditions may develop several hours after submersion.

▶ Heat-Related Illnesses

Heat-related illnesses may range from relatively minor muscle cramps to vomiting, heat exhaustion, and heatstroke. The most dangerous heat-related illness in children is heatstroke. Any child who is in a closed, parked car on a hot day or in a poorly ventilated room and who has hot, dry skin may be experiencing heatstroke. This is a serious and potentially fatal condition that requires you to provide rapid treatment to cool the child and reduce his or her body temperature. Remove the child's clothing, sponge water over the child, and fan him or her to help lower the body temperature quickly. You may wrap the child in wet sheets (if they are available) to speed up the evaporation and cooling process, but do not let the child become chilled. Finally, be sure that you have arranged for *rapid transport* to an appropriate medical facility. (See Chapter 13, *Environmental Emergencies*, for a more detailed description of heatstroke.)

▶ High Fever

Fevers occur quite commonly in children and can be caused by many different infections, especially ear and gastrointestinal infections. Because the temperature-regulating mechanism in young children has not fully developed, a very high temperature (104°F to 106°F [40°C to 41°C]) can occur quickly even with a relatively minor infection. Most children can tolerate temperatures as high as 104°F (40°C), but a high fever may require that the child be hospitalized so that the underlying cause can be discovered and treated.

Your first step in treating a child with a high fever is to uncover the child so that body heat can escape. Layers of clothing or blankets retain body heat and can increase the patient's body temperature high enough to cause convulsions. About 10% of children between 1 and 6 years of age are susceptible to seizures brought on by high fevers. Remember that in attempting to reduce a high fever, you are treating only the symptom and not the source. A physician must see the child as soon as possible to determine the cause of the fever.

If you encounter a child with a temperature above 104°F (40°C), take these steps to treat the fever symptoms:

1. Make certain the child is not wrapped in too much clothing or too many blankets.
2. Attempt to reduce the high temperature by undressing the child.
3. Fan the child to cool him or her down.
4. Protect the child during any seizure (do not restrain the child's motion), and make certain that normal breathing resumes after each seizure.

▶ Seizures

Seizures (convulsions) can result from a high fever or from disorders such as **epilepsy** (see Chapter 10, *Medical Emergencies*). Seizures can vary in intensity from simple, momentary staring spells (without body movements) to generalized seizures in which the entire body stiffens and shakes severely.

Although seizures can be frightening to parents, bystanders, and rescuers, they are not usually dangerous. During a seizure, a child becomes unconscious, the eyes roll back, the teeth become clenched, and the body shakes with severe jerking movements. Often, the child's skin becomes pale or turns blue. Sometimes the child has a loss of bladder and bowel control and soils his or her clothing. Seizures caused by a high fever usually last about 20 seconds.

If a seizure occurs, place the child on a soft surface (sofa, bed, or rug) to protect the child from injury during the seizure. Reassure the child's parents who may be frightened by the seizure. If they become too emotional, ask them to leave the room. Carefully monitor the child's airway during and after the seizure.

As an EMR, you can provide the following treatment for seizures:

1. Place the patient on the floor or a bed to prevent injury.
2. Maintain an adequate airway after the seizure ends.
3. Provide supplemental oxygen after the seizure if it is available and you are trained to use it.
4. Arrange for *prompt transport* to an appropriate medical facility.
5. Continue to monitor the patient's vital signs and support the ABCs if necessary.
6. After the seizure is over, cool the patient if the patient has a high fever.

YOU ▶ are the Provider   CASE 3

You respond to a residential area for a child having trouble breathing. When you arrive, you find a young child sitting on the edge of the couch. The child has a respiratory rate of 46 breaths per minute, and you notice nasal flaring. You hear wheezing when listening to the child's lungs and notice neck muscle retractions. You are able to palpate a weak distal pulse and note the child appears to be getting tired.

1. What signs exhibited by the child indicate respiratory distress?
2. How should you treat this patient?
3. What is likely to happen to the child if you do not initiate treatment?

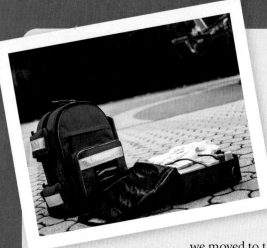

Voices *of* Experience

During my EMS training, my instructor always told me I needed to learn my skills until I could do them without thinking. When we moved to the pediatrics section of the curriculum, my instructors increased their prompting to engrain the basics in our minds. They kept teaching, I kept learning, but I never realized why I needed to focus so much on the repetition of skills. Then I became an instructor and I continued to tell my students much the same. We need to engrain the basics into you so that you can accomplish the needs of the scene without having to think about the basics. Why do we teach that?

> **❝ Suddenly, he made a loud noise, spit out his pacifier, and began full-body convulsions. ❞**

I recently was presented with a situation that would test my knowledge without me knowing. During a normal day, enjoying a nice lunch with family and friends, my son began to develop a fever. He was playing, having fun, and enjoying the company of close friends. However, by the time we finished lunch and made it home to place him down to take his afternoon nap, his fever had increased. My wife and I determined that he was probably developing another ear infection because he had been treated for three within the past 2 months. We decided to take him to the pediatrician's office during their daily sick call. We arrived at the office, signed him in, and then sat down awaiting his turn with the physician. Our son, who is normally a very active child, wanted simply to sit in our laps and watch the television. He was calm, but his temperature continued to increase.

Suddenly, he made a loud noise, spit out his pacifier, and began full-body convulsions. Without hesitation, I moved from the parental mode to that of an emergency medical provider. I carefully moved him from a sitting position to a carry and informed the receptionist at the window we needed to go to the examination area immediately. At that point we passed our physician, and I explained that my son was experiencing an active febrile seizure. The nursing staff and physicians quickly responded and together we were able to open and maintain his airway, assess his breathing rate and quality, and increase his oxygen levels through the administration of blow-by oxygen. The team ensured adequate circulation during the episode and continued a watch of the oxygen levels perfusing my son's body. We used multiple avenues of temperature control, active cooling procedures such as strategic placement of ice packs, passive cooling procedures (including removal of clothing), and medications, thereby preventing further seizure activity. During the coming minutes, he continued to experience a postseizure state, which required a constant watch over his airway, breathing, and circulatory status.

The amount of time that I have spent and continue to spend dedicated to the basics of emergency medical care resulted in my body's ability to take that information and translate it to immediate action without a conscious thought on my part. As emergency medical providers, we are not faced with pediatric patients requiring assistance as often as adult patients. Because we do not see them as often, and because pediatric patients decline quickly and drastically, emergency medical responders such as yourself should prepare for the worst and train to achieve the best outcome.

David S. Blevins
City of Knoxville Fire Department
Knoxville, Tennessee

► Vomiting and Diarrhea

Children are very susceptible to vomiting and diarrhea, which are usually caused by gastrointestinal infections. Prolonged vomiting and diarrhea may produce severe dehydration. The dehydrated child is lethargic and has very dry skin, which can be especially noticeable around the mouth and nose. Hospitalization may be required to replace fluids through the veins. If you suspect that a child may be dehydrated, arrange for *transport* to an appropriate medical facility.

► Abdominal Pain

One of the most serious causes of abdominal pain in children is appendicitis. Although it can occur at any age, appendicitis is often seen in people who are between 10 and 25 years. A cramping pain usually starts in the belly button area of the abdomen. Within a few hours, the pain moves to the right lower quadrant of the abdomen, becoming steady and more severe. Usually the child is nauseated, has no appetite, and occasionally will vomit.

Because there are several potential causes of abdominal pain, including appendicitis, do not try to make a diagnosis in the field. Even physicians may find it difficult to diagnose the cause of abdominal pain. A good rule for you to follow is to treat every child with a sore or tender abdomen as an emergency and arrange for *transport* to an appropriate medical facility for an appropriate diagnosis.

► Poisoning

Young children are curious and often like to sample the contents of brightly colored bottles or cans looking for something good to eat or drink. However, many common household items contain poisonous substances. The two most common types of poisonings in children are caused by ingestion and absorption.

Ingestion

An ingested poison is taken by mouth. A child who has ingested a poison may have chemical burns, odors, or stains around the mouth and be experiencing nausea, vomiting, abdominal pain, or diarrhea. Later symptoms may include abnormal or decreased respirations, unconsciousness, or seizures.

If you believe a child has ingested a poisonous substance, do the following:

1. Try to identify what the child has swallowed, attempt to estimate the amount ingested, and send the bottle or container along with the child to the emergency department.
2. Gather any spilled tablets if the child swallowed tablets from a medicine bottle and replace them in the bottle so they can be counted. The emergency physician may then be able to determine how many tablets the child has taken.

3. Contact your local poison control center if transportation to an appropriate medical facility is delayed. The poison control center will need to know the following information:
   - Age of the patient
   - Identification of the poison
   - Weight of the patient
   - Estimated quantity of the poison taken
4. Follow the directions provided by the poison control center. You may need to perform the following actions:
   - Dilute the poison by giving the child large amounts of water.
   - Administer activated charcoal if it is available and you have been trained in its use (the usual dose for pediatric patients is 12.5 to 25 grams).
5. Monitor the child's breathing and pulse closely. This is a critical step, and you must be prepared to provide emergency care, including rescue breathing and CPR.
6. Arrange for *prompt transport* to an appropriate medical facility for examination by a physician.

Treatment

Do not attempt to give liquids or induce vomiting in an unconscious or partially conscious child because of the danger of aspiration of the vomitus.

Absorption

Poisoning by absorption occurs when a poisonous substance enters the body through the skin. A child who has absorbed a poison may have localized symptoms, such as skin irritation or burning, or may have systemic signs and symptoms of the poisoning, such as nausea, vomiting, dizziness, and shock.

Safety

Be careful not to get any chemical on your skin.

If you believe a child has absorbed a poisonous substance, perform the following actions:

1. Ensure that the child is no longer in contact with the poisonous substance.
2. Protect yourself from exposure to the poison. Call for specially trained personnel if indicated.
3. Remove the child's clothing if you think it is contaminated.
4. Brush off any dry chemical. After you have removed all dry chemical, wash the child with water for at least 20 minutes.

5. Wash off any liquid poisons by flushing with water for at least 20 minutes.
6. Try to identify the poison and send any containers with the child to the emergency department.
7. Monitor the child for any changes in respiration and pulse. Be prepared to administer rescue breathing or CPR if needed.
8. If the child has vomited, save a sample in a clean container and send it with the patient to the hospital if you can perform this action without detracting from the care of the patient.
9. Arrange *transport* to an appropriate medical facility for examination by a physician.

See Chapter 11, *Poisoning and Substance Abuse*, for additional information on emergency treatment of poisoning.

> ## Treatment
>
> Chemical burns to the eyes cause extreme pain and injury. Gently flush the affected eye or eyes with water for at least 20 minutes. Hold the eye open to allow water to flow over its entire surface. Direct the water from the inner corner of the eye to the outward edge of the eye to avoid contaminating the other eye. After flushing the eyes for 20 minutes, loosely cover both eyes with gauze bandages and arrange for *prompt transport* to an appropriate medical facility.

▶ Sudden Infant Death Syndrome

A condition that is frequently mistaken for child abuse is sudden infant death syndrome (SIDS), also called crib death or sudden unexpected infant death (SUID). It is the sudden and unexpected death of an apparently healthy infant. SIDS usually occurs in infants between the ages of 3 weeks and 7 months. The infants are usually found dead in their cribs.

Currently, no adequate scientific explanation exists for SIDS. These deaths are not the result of smothering, choking, or strangulation. SIDS deaths often remain unexplained, even after a complete and thorough autopsy.

You can imagine the shock and grief felt by parents who find their apparently healthy infant dead in bed. Your actions and words can help relieve their feelings of remorse and guilt.

If the infant is still warm, begin CPR and continue until help arrives (infant CPR is described in Chapter 7, *Airway Management*, and Chapter 8, *Professional Rescuer CPR*). In many cases, the infant has been dead several hours and the body is cold and lifeless. Do not mistake the large, bruise-like blotches on the infant's body for signs of child abuse. The blotches are caused by the pooling of the infant's blood after death. Sometimes you may find a small amount of bloody foam on the infant's lips. If the child is obviously dead, follow the protocol in your community for the management of deceased patients.

Know your local guidelines for the management of SIDS. Remember that the parents could do nothing to prevent the death. Be compassionate and supportive during this tragic situation.

■ Pediatric Trauma

Trauma remains the number one killer of children. Each year, many young lives are lost because of accidental injury, particularly motor vehicle crashes.

Treat an injured child as you would treat an injured adult, but remember the following differences:

1. A child cannot communicate symptoms as well as an adult.
2. A child may be shy and overwhelmed by adult rescuers (especially those in uniform), so it is important to develop a good relationship quickly to reduce the child's fear and anxiety.
3. You may have to adapt materials and equipment to the child's size.
4. A child does not show signs of shock as early as an adult but can progress into severe shock quickly.

▶ Patterns of Injury

The type of trauma a child experiences, the type of activity causing the injury, and the child's anatomy affect the pattern of injuries sustained by the child. Motor vehicle crashes produce different patterns of injuries depending on whether the patient was using a seat belt, whether the patient was strapped into a car seat, and whether an air bag inflated in the crash. Unrestrained patients tend to have more head and neck injuries. Restrained passengers often sustain head injuries, spinal injuries, and abdominal injuries. Children struck while riding a bicycle often have head, spinal, abdominal, and extremity injuries. The use of bicycle helmets greatly reduces the number and severity of head injuries. Pedestrians who are struck by a vehicle often sustain chest and abdominal injuries with internal bleeding, injuries to the thighs, and head injuries. Falls from a height or diving accidents tend to cause head and spinal injuries and extremity injuries. Burns are a major cause of injuries to children. Sports activities cause a wide variety of injuries depending on the type of sports activity. By learning some of the basic patterns of injury, you can anticipate the injuries you may find when carefully examining pediatric patients.

If the child has been struck by a motor vehicle, look for the common types of injuries shown in Figure 17-12 . Major trauma in children usually results in multiple system injuries. No matter what the cause of injury, your first priority is always to check the patient's ABCs. Stop severe bleeding, treat the patient for shock, and proceed with the full-body assessment described in Chapter 9, *Patient Assessment*, to determine the extent of any other injuries Figure 17-13 . The full-body assessment is a hands-on procedure. A complete examination

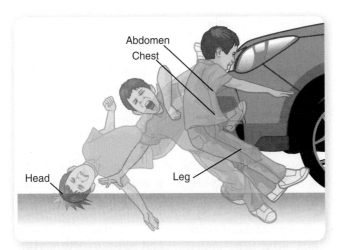

Figure 17-12 Look for these typical injuries when a child has been hit by a motor vehicle.
© Jones & Bartlett Learning.

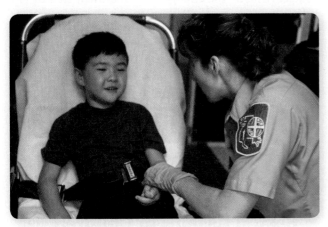

Figure 17-13 Examine every child thoroughly.
© Jones & Bartlett Learning. Courtesy of MIEMSS.

is especially important because a child cannot always communicate symptoms. Involve the child in the physical examination as much as possible. Ask the child simple questions. Complete the full-body assessment even if the patient is too young to understand what is happening. Then stabilize all injuries you find. Splint suspected fractures, bandage wounds, and immobilize suspected spinal injuries.

If your patient has head lacerations, remember that the generous blood supply to the scalp can result in severe bleeding. Treat these wounds with direct pressure

and appropriate bandaging techniques. See Chapter 14, *Bleeding, Shock, and Soft-Tissue Injuries*, for a review of effective bandaging techniques.

▶ Traumatic Shock in Children

Children show shock symptoms much more slowly than adults, but they progress through the stages of shock quickly. An injured child displaying obvious shock symptoms such as cool, clammy skin; a rapid, weak pulse; or rapid or shallow respirations is already experiencing severe shock. It is vital that you learn to recognize and treat shock quickly. Review the signs and symptoms of shock in Chapter 14, *Bleeding, Shock, and Soft-Tissue Injuries*.

Immediate treatment of an injured child experiencing shock includes controlling external bleeding, keeping the child warm, and administering oxygen if it is available. Children who show signs of shock should be transported as soon as possible to an emergency department. Seizures are relatively common in children who have sustained a serious head injury. Be prepared to manage this condition by maintaining the airway and protecting the child from further injury.

The greatest dangers to any patient who has sustained trauma are airway obstruction and hemorrhage. When caring for an injured child, the most important actions you should perform are as follows:

- Open and maintain the airway.
- Control bleeding.
- Arrange for *prompt transport* to an appropriate medical facility.

▶ Car Seats and Children

The impact of mandatory child restraint laws means that EMRs are finding more children still strapped into car seats after motor vehicle crashes. You should become familiar with child restraint seats and understand how to gain access to children restrained in them. If you find a child properly restrained in a car seat, leave the child in the car seat until the ambulance arrives **Figure 17-14**. In many situations, a child can be secured in the seat, the seat removed from the vehicle, and both the seat and the child transported together to the hospital **Figure 17-15**.

YOU ▶ are the Provider ⠀⠀⠀⠀⠀⠀⠀⠀⠀**CASE 4**

As you are leaving the local grocery store, you hear the loud screech of tires. A car leaving the parking lot struck a child on a bicycle. You notice a bystander calling 9-1-1 as you grab the first aid kit from your car. The child has a loud cry and you notice blood coming from her forehead. When you ask the child what hurts, she tells you her head, arms, and legs. The mother arrives on the scene and immediately wants to take the child to the local hospital in her personal vehicle.

1. Why is the sign of loud crying considered a useful finding in this patient?
2. What assessment and treatment steps can you perform while waiting for EMS to arrive?
3. Should the mother be allowed to transport the child in her personal vehicle?

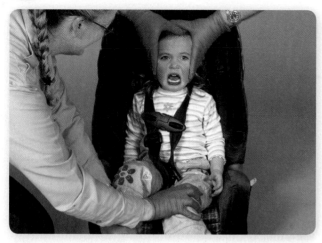

Figure 17-14 Leave the child in the car seat if possible.
© Jones & Bartlett Learning. Courtesy of MIEMSS.

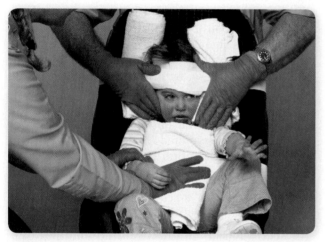

Figure 17-15 A child can be immobilized in the car seat.
© Jones & Bartlett Learning. Courtesy of MIEMSS.

Treatment

Children younger than 9 years who are not in a booster seat but are wearing a seat belt are at risk for sliding out of the lap belt during a crash. Rapid, jackknife bending of the child's body increases the chances of intra-abdominal, spinal cord, and brain injuries.

▶ Child Abuse

Child abuse is not limited to any ethnic, social, or economic group or to families with any particular level of education. Suspect child abuse if the child's injuries do not match the story you are told about how the injuries occurred. Child abuse is often masked as an accident. The abused or battered child may have many visible injuries—all at different stages of healing. The child may appear to be withdrawn, fearful, or even hostile. Be concerned if the child refuses to discuss how an injury occurred. Occasionally, the child's parents or caretaker will reveal a history of several "accidents" in the past.

Treat the child's injuries and, if you are suspicious that this may be a case of child abuse, ensure the safety of the child.

Make sure that the child receives *transport* to an appropriate medical facility. If the parents object to having the child examined by a physician, summon law enforcement personnel and explain your concerns to them. The safety of the child is your foremost concern in these situations.

Neglect is also a form of child abuse. Children who are neglected are often dirty or too thin or appear developmentally delayed because of a lack of stimulation. You may observe such children when you are making calls for unrelated problems. The parents of an abused child need help, and the child may need protection from the parents' future actions. Handle each situation in a nonjudgmental manner. Know whom you need to contact (usually the emergency department staff or law enforcement personnel), and report any instances of suspected child abuse.

Signs and Symptoms

Signs and symptoms of neglect include the following:
- Lack of adult supervision
- Malnourished-appearing child
- Unsafe living environment
- Untreated chronic illness

▶ Sexual Assault of Children

Sexual abuse occurs in children as well as adults. It may occur in both male and female infants, young children, and adolescents. In addition to sexual assault, the child may have been beaten and may have other serious injuries.

If you suspect sexual assault has occurred, obtain as much information as possible from the child and any witnesses. Realize that the child may be hysterical or unwilling to talk, especially if the abuser is a brother or sister, parent, or family friend. Providing a caring approach to these children is extremely important, and take appropriate action to shield them from onlookers.

All victims of sexual assault should receive *transport* to an appropriate medical facility. Sexual assault is a crime; cooperate with law enforcement officials during their investigation.

■ Emergency Medical Responder Debriefing

As an EMR, you will respond to many calls that involve children. These calls tend to produce strong emotional reactions. At times, you may experience a feeling of helplessness when an innocent child is seriously injured or gravely ill. An ill or injured child may remind you of your own children. You may feel especially angry or helpless when you suspect the neglect or abuse of a child.

After you have completed your treatment of the patient and transferred the responsibility for care to other EMS personnel, you may need to talk about your frustrations with a counselor or with another member of your department. After a major incident or an especially emotional incident involving children, it may be helpful for you to set up a critical incident stress debriefing session. Although you cannot change the types of traumatic events you will see, you can use your department's resources to work through your feelings about these events. By attending a debriefing session, you can express your feelings, learn some coping strategies, and maintain a healthy approach to future calls.

Signs and Symptoms

Signs and symptoms of child abuse include the following:

- Multiple fractures
- Bruises in various stages of healing (especially those clustered on the torso and buttocks) **Figure 17-16A**
- Human bites **Figure 17-16B**
- Burns (particularly cigarette burns and scalds from hot water) **Figure 17-16C**
- Reports of bizarre accidents that do not seem to have a logical explanation

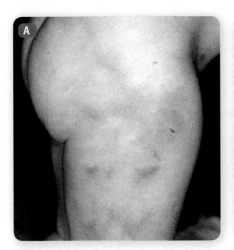
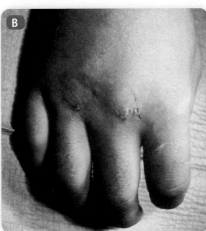
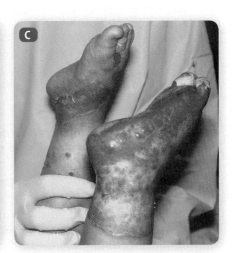

Figure 17-16 A. Bruises of different ages suggest physical maltreatment. New bruises are red or pink; over time, bruises turn blue, green, yellow-brown, and faded. **B.** A human bite wound has a characteristic appearance. **C.** Stocking/glove burns of the hands and feet in the infant or toddler are often inflicted injuries.

You are the Provider: CASE 1

1. **What factors do you need to consider as you evaluate the first side of the pediatric triangle?**

The first step, or side, of the pediatric assessment triangle is to carefully evaluate the appearance of the ill or injured child. When evaluating appearance look for the following characteristics: movement, interaction, reassurance, eye movement, speech, and cry. Is the child moving vigorously or is he or she listless or limp? Does the child reach for interesting things or is he or she uninterested? Can the child be reassured by his or her caregivers or does he or she remain agitated or crying? Does the child follow the movements of other people or toys or does he or she seem uninterested? Does the child use appropriate speech for his or her age or is his or her speech confused? If the child is crying, does he or she have a strong cry or is his or her cry weak or high pitched?

2. **What factors do you need to consider as you evaluate the second side of the pediatric triangle?**

The second step, or side, of the pediatric assessment triangle is to carefully evaluate the work of breathing of the ill or injured child. When evaluating the work of breathing, consider the following characteristics: abnormal breath sounds, abnormal positioning, retractions, and nasal flaring. Abnormal breath sounds include noisy breathing, snoring, grunting, or wheezing. Look for abnormal positioning, which includes leaning forward while using the arms for support. Are retractions present? Retractions can occur above the collarbones or between the ribs when the child inhales. Look for flaring of the nostrils as the child inhales and exhales. Putting all these factors together will give you a lot of information about the degree of difficulty the child is having breathing.

3. **What factors do you need to consider as you evaluate the third side of the pediatric triangle?**

The third step, or side, of the pediatric assessment triangle is to carefully evaluate the circulation to the skin of the ill or injured child. When evaluating the circulation to the skin, look for the following characteristics: the color or pallor of the skin, mottling of the skin, and cyanosis of the skin. White or pale skin may indicate decreased blood flow to the skin because of shock or dehydration. Look for mottling of the skin, which is caused by too little or too much blood flow to the skin. Look for cyanosis. Is there a blue discoloration of the skin or mucous membranes? Cyanosis is a sign of decreased blood flow to the skin. Putting all these factors together will give

you a lot of information about the status of the child's circulatory system.

You are the Provider: CASE 2

1. **What initial actions can you take to protect the child from harm?**

Seizures in a child are usually a very frightening event for parents and caregivers. Because there is a chance that the child will have another seizure and because you will need to unwrap the blankets and clothing from the child, it is usually a good idea to place the child on a soft surface such as a sofa or a carpeted floor. This prevents anyone from dropping the child in the event of another seizure and allows you to begin to examine and assess the child. In addition, if you need to open the airway or perform cardiopulmonary resuscitation, you are in a good position to do this.

2. **What steps can you take to help cool the child?**

Because the child has a high fever and this may be the cause of the seizure, it is important to take simple steps to cool the child. The first step in cooling a child with a high fever is to remove the blankets or covers from the child. Next, remove some clothing to help cool the child's skin. Another step that may assist the cooling process is to gently fan the child's skin. This will help to remove some of the excess heat from the child's body.

3. **What further care is needed to prevent this child from having another seizure?**

The preceding steps may begin to cool the child. However, additional steps are needed. Often the physician will prescribe medication to reduce the fever and to keep it from returning to a high level. This may include supportive measures to ensure that the child does not become dehydrated and sometimes it will require an antibiotic. Additionally, it is important to determine the cause of the fever. It is important that emergency medical responders arrange for a physician to see the child.

You are the Provider: CASE 3

1. **What signs exhibited by the child indicate respiratory distress?**

The child is exhibiting classic signs of respiratory distress. When you initially see the child, pay attention to his or her position. Children will naturally move to a position that allows for easier breathing. This position typically includes the child sitting up, possibly with his or her chest pushed out. The presence of nasal flaring and retraction of the neck muscles are clear indications that the child is not breathing adequately. Although these signs are sometimes subtle, it is important for you to visually inspect for these signs when treating a pediatric patient. The respiratory rate and breath sounds will also provide you with details about the child's respiratory status. Respiratory rates that are too fast or too slow may not provide sufficient oxygenation to a patient. Consider any abnormal breath sound a sign of possible respiratory distress.

2. How should you treat this patient?

The patient should receive immediate high-flow oxygen. This patient is likely to be experiencing an asthma attack. If the patient has a history of asthma, the parents may have administered a rescue inhaler to the patient. Arrange for immediate transport of this patient to the closest hospital equipped to care for pediatric respiratory emergencies. Advanced life support should be summoned as well. Be prepared for this child to decompensate and possibly need airway management and resuscitation.

3. What is likely to happen to the child if you do not initiate treatment?

The child is getting tired and has a weak pulse. If you do not initiate immediate treatment in this patient, the child will go into respiratory failure. Pediatric patients have a remarkable ability to physiologically compensate in times of distress. However, once those compensatory mechanisms fail, the child will decompensate quickly, resulting in respiratory failure and possibly cardiac arrest. Early recognition and intervention are essential components to the treatment of pediatric respiratory emergencies.

You are the Provider: CASE 4

1. Why is the sign of loud crying considered a useful finding in this patient?

Although the idea of a crying child does not sound appealing in most situations, it is a welcome sound when treating a pediatric patient. A loud cry is an important assessment tool and provides you with much vital information. A cry generally indicates that the patient has a patent airway and sufficient ability to breathe. The volume of the cry may be an indication of the mental status of the patient. A loud cry indicates the patient is irritated enough to provide a forceful cry and is associated with a higher level of consciousness; a weak cry may be an indication of a depressed mental status or a sign of shock.

2. What assessment and treatment steps can you perform while waiting for EMS to arrive?

It can be frustrating to be at the scene of an incident and have only minimal supplies to treat patients. However, even with basic supplies and equipment, you are still able to treat a number of conditions. For this particular patient, have a person maintain cervical spine stabilization as you assess the ABCs. Check for signs of external bleeding and provide direct pressure and/or dressings using gauze or a suitable substitute. Keep the child warm by placing blankets, jackets, or other materials over the child until emergency medical services (EMS) arrives. This will help in the treatment of shock. Even though these interventions may seem minimal to you, they can have a drastic effect on the overall outcome of this patient.

3. Should the mother be allowed to transport the child in her personal vehicle?

Although you cannot keep the mother from taking her child in her own vehicle, you should encourage her to wait for the arrival of EMS personnel. First, identify yourself as an emergency medical responder to the mother and explain to her the possible injuries involved. Tell her what to expect when the EMS team arrives and what treatment the EMS team may provide for her child. Explain to the mother the possible risks involved with moving a person with a possible spine injury. Once the mother understands the purpose of the EMS system and the risks involved, she is likely to cooperate and wait for EMS.

Prep Kit

► Ready for Review

- Sudden illnesses and medical emergencies are common in children and infants. Because the anatomy of children and infants differs from that of adults, emergency medical responders need special knowledge and skills to assess and treat pediatric patients.
- Managing a pediatric emergency can be a stressful situation for emergency medical responders. Because both the child and the parents may be frightened and anxious, you must behave in a calm, controlled, and professional manner.
- A child's airway is smaller in relation to the rest of the body; therefore, secretions and swelling from illnesses or trauma can more easily block the child's airway. Because the tongue is relatively larger than the tongue of an adult, a child's tongue can more easily block the airway. Hyperextension of a child's neck can occlude the airway.
- The pediatric assessment triangle is designed to give you a quick general impression of the child using only your senses of sight and hearing. The three components of the pediatric assessment triangle are overall appearance, work of breathing, and circulation to the skin.
- Carefully evaluate the child who is unresponsive, lackluster, and appears ill, because the lack of activity and interest signal serious illness or injury. After you conduct your primary assessment, carry out the routine patient examination, paying special attention to mental awareness, activity level, respirations, pulse rate, body temperature, and color of the skin.
- It is important for you to open and maintain the patient's airway and to ventilate adequately any child with a respiratory condition. Otherwise, the child may experience respiratory arrest, followed by cardiac arrest.
- Cardiopulmonary resuscitation for children and infants differs from adult cardiopulmonary resuscitation in several important ways. Be certain that you understand these differences and are able to perform the appropriate steps confidently in the field.
- Suctioning removes foreign substances that you cannot remove with your gloved fingers from the airway of a child. An oral airway can be used to maintain an open airway after you have opened the child's airway by manual means.
- Young children often obstruct their upper and lower airway with foreign objects, such as small toys or candy. If the object is only partially blocking the airway, the child should be able to pass some air around it. Attempt to remove the object only if it is clearly visible and you can remove it easily.
- In complete or severe airway obstruction in a conscious child, perform the Heimlich maneuver (abdominal thrusts). If the child becomes unresponsive, begin cardiopulmonary resuscitation.
- To relieve an airway obstruction in an infant, use a combination of back slaps and chest thrusts.
- Children in respiratory distress require immediate medical attention. Signs of respiratory distress include a rapid or slow breathing rate, nasal flaring, retraction of the skin between the ribs and around the neck muscles, stridor, cyanosis, altered mental status, and combativeness. Respiratory distress can lead to respiratory failure, which in turn can lead to circulatory failure.
- Three serious respiratory conditions in pediatric patients are asthma, croup, and epiglottitis. A child who has asthma is usually already being treated for the condition by a physician; your primary treatment consists of calming and reassuring the parents and the child. Croup is an upper airway infection that results in a barking cough. Although epiglottitis resembles croup, it is a serious respiratory emergency and you must arrange for prompt transport.
- Other pediatric medical emergencies include drowning, heat-related illnesses such as heatstroke, high fevers, seizures, vomiting and diarrhea, and abdominal pain.
- Children's natural curiosity may lead them to sample medications or household items that contain poisonous substances. The two most common types of poisonings in children are caused by ingestion (taken by mouth) and absorption (entering through the skin).
- Sudden infant death syndrome, also called crib death, is the unexpected death of an apparently healthy infant. Know your local guidelines for the management of sudden infant death syndrome. Remember that the parents could do nothing to prevent the death.
- When caring for pediatric trauma patients, remember that you may have to adapt materials and equipment to the child's size. Also remember that children do not show signs of shock as early as adults, although they can progress into severe shock quickly.
- Major trauma in children usually results in multiple system injuries. Your first priority is always to check the ABCs and then stop severe bleeding, treat for shock, and proceed with the physical examination.
- If you suspect child abuse or sexual assault, arrange for transport to an appropriate medical facility.

Prep Kit *Continued*

▶ Vital Vocabulary

asthma An acute spasm of the smaller air passages that results in narrowing and inflammation of these passages. It is marked by labored breathing and wheezing.

chest-thrust maneuver A series of manual thrusts to the chest to relieve upper airway obstruction; used in the treatment of infants, pregnant women, or extremely obese people.

croup Inflammation and narrowing of the air passages in young children, causing a barking cough, hoarseness, and a harsh, high-pitched breathing sound.

drowning Submersion in water or other fluids that results in suffocation or respiratory impairment.

epiglottitis Severe inflammation and swelling of the epiglottis; a life-threatening situation.

epilepsy A disease manifested by seizures, caused by an abnormal focus of electrical activity in the brain.

mottling Patchy skin discoloration caused by too little or too much circulation.

pediatric assessment triangle (PAT) An assessment tool that measures the severity of a child's illness or injury by evaluating the child's appearance, work of breathing, and circulation to the skin.

stridor A high-pitched sound heard during inspiration. It is a sign of a narrowing or partial obstruction.

suctioning Aspirating (sucking out) fluid in the mouth or airway by mechanical means.

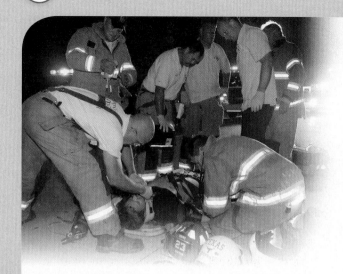

Assessment
in Action

You are called to a home where a 4-year-old girl is sitting in her mother's lap. The mother tells you that her daughter seemed hot and did not eat or drink much all day. She says that the child vomited once. You notice that the girl's forehead seems hot.

1. In what order should you examine this child?

   1. Level of consciousness
   2. Full-body assessment
   3. Airway, breathing, and circulation
   4. Determine the nature of illness
      - **A.** 3, 4, 2, 1
      - **B.** 3, 1, 4, 2
      - **C.** 4, 1, 3, 2
      - **D.** 4, 2, 3, 1

2. On the basis of the patient's history and your assessment of this child, which of the following conditions is least likely to be occurring?

   - **A.** Possibility of seizures
   - **B.** Possibility of gastrointestinal illness
   - **C.** Dehydration
   - **D.** Acute allergic reaction

3. Where is the best place to examine this child?

   - **A.** Lying on a table
   - **B.** Lying on the floor
   - **C.** In the mother's lap
   - **D.** Sitting on your partner's lap

4. If the child experiences a seizure, you should do all of the following EXCEPT:

   - **A.** place the child on a soft surface.
   - **B.** monitor the airway after the seizure ends.
   - **C.** cool the patient after the seizure is over.
   - **D.** restrain the child to prevent shaking.

5. What is the most appropriate management for this patient?

   - **A.** Apply cool compresses to the child's forehead.
   - **B.** Help arrange for transportation to an appropriate medical facility.
   - **C.** Tell the mother to call her physician in the morning.
   - **D.** Advise the mother that her child needs to drink some fluids.

6. Describe the information you get from each step of the pediatric assessment triangle.

7. How would you assess the pulse in this patient and what would be the expected rate?

8. In addition to the child having a gastrointestinal illness, what other condition can cause the child's signs and symptoms?

9. What is the normal respiratory rate for a 4-year-old child and what factors can influence the rate?

10. The child vomited once before you arrived and vomits again as you are talking with her mother. What further care does a child with these symptoms need?

Geriatric Emergencies

National EMS Education Standard Competencies

Trauma

Uses simple knowledge to recognize and manage life threats based on assessment findings for an acutely injured patient while awaiting additional emergency medical response.

Special Considerations in Trauma

Recognition and management of trauma in

> Pregnant patient (Chapter 16, *Childbirth*)
> Pediatric patient (Chapter 17, *Pediatric Emergencies*)
> Geriatric patient (pp 390–391)

Special Patient Populations

Recognizes and manages life threats based on simple assessment findings for a patient with special needs while awaiting additional emergency response.

Geriatrics

> Impact of age-related changes on assessment and care (pp 388–389)

Patients With Special Challenges

> Recognizing and reporting abuse and neglect (p 397)

Knowledge Objectives

1. Define geriatric patient. (p 388)
2. Discuss some of the physiologic changes that occur with aging. (pp 388–391)
3. Explain how to ensure more effective communication with geriatric patients who have hearing or vision impairment. (pp 389–390)
4. Explain why geriatric patients are at high risk for broken bones. (p 390)
5. Describe the types of cardiovascular and respiratory diseases that are prevalent among geriatric patients. (p 391)
6. List possible causes of altered mental status in geriatric patients. (pp 391–392)
7. Describe the general signs and symptoms of an infectious disease. (p 392)
8. Describe how to approach the assessment and treatment of patients who require long-term care. (p 392; p 394)
9. Explain the responsibility of emergency medical responders (EMRs) in caring for patients who show signs of depression, suicide, or dementia. (pp 395–396)
10. Describe the purpose of hospice care. (p 396)
11. Explain the purpose of advance directives and do not resuscitate orders. (p 396)
12. Describe the signs and symptoms of elder abuse. (p 397)

Skills Objectives

1. Demonstrate effective communication with geriatric patients who have hearing or vision impairment. (pp 389–390)

Introduction

A **geriatric patient** is commonly defined as a patient who is older than 65 years. The geriatric population of the United States is the fastest growing segment of society. According to the US Census Bureau, 13% of the US population (or 40.3 million people) were age 65 years or older in 2010. This chapter addresses concerns particular to geriatric patients, including sensory changes such as hearing loss and vision impairment, changes in mobility, and changes in medical conditions. Special considerations for the care of patients with chronic conditions are addressed. Mental health conditions that commonly affect older patients, such as depression and senility, are also covered. The chapter concludes with a discussion of end-of-life issues, hospice care, advance directives, and methods of recognizing signs of elder abuse.

The natural aging process results in a decline in the functioning of all body systems. This slowdown is gradual and begins shortly after the body reaches maturity. Heredity and lifestyle choices such as diet, alcohol and/or drug abuse, stress level, and amount of exercise influence the speed at which this decline occurs.

As an emergency medical responder (EMR), it is important not to prejudge the physical or mental health of older patients. Some people are vibrant and healthy at age 80 years, whereas others experience chronic debilitating diseases in their 50s. The same is true of mental capacity: Although you may encounter middle-aged patients who have become senile, many older people retain their full mental capacity.

Because older patients experience health complications more frequently than younger people do, most emergency medical services (EMS) systems respond to many calls involving geriatric patients. These calls will be much easier for you to handle if you understand some of the physical and mental changes involved in the aging process. As discussed in Chapter 5, *Communications and Documentation*, these calls will also be less stressful for the patient and for you if you understand how to effectively communicate with older patients. You will achieve a greater rapport with older patients if you interact with each person as an individual, rather than as a member of some stereotypical group defined by age Figure 18-1 .

Older people often wear more clothing than younger people do, even during warmer months. Do not use layers of clothing as an excuse to perform an incomplete examination. It is essential that you conduct a complete full-body examination on all patients.

Be especially careful as you examine geriatric patients. Their skin is thinner and more fragile than the skin of younger people. As a person ages, the layer of fat under the skin decreases. The skin becomes drier because the number of sweat glands decreases with age. These changes mean that older people have more fragile skin. They tend to bruise easily and tend to bleed more easily than younger patients. These changes also make older patients more prone to pressure sores (bedsores) if they are unable to change positions frequently or if they are left on a hard surface that is not padded.

The loss of bowel and bladder control occurs frequently in the geriatric population. This situation can be distressing and embarrassing to both you and the

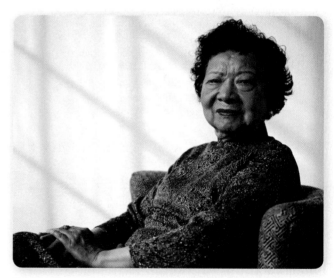

Figure 18-1 Treat every patient as an individual.
© Photodisc/Getty.

YOU are the Provider   CASE 1

At 1327 hours, you are dispatched to a local residence at 256 North Market Street for a report of an injured person. As you arrive at the modest house, you are met by an older woman who leads you inside to the kitchen. Her husband is sitting on a kitchen chair cradling his left arm, which is wrapped in a bath towel. It is partially soaked in blood. You introduce yourself and begin to assess the patient. Mr. Schuum is 76 years old and seems to be alert and fully oriented. You learn that the couple was preparing to leave for an appointment with his cardiologist when Mr. Schuum slipped in the kitchen and struck his left arm on a sharp corner of the kitchen counter. As you examine his arm, you note a 4-inch (10-cm) cut that continues to seep blood. Your medical history reveals that Mr. Schuum is taking medication for high blood pressure, heart conditions, and gout. He also uses eye drops. His wife tells you he had a heart bypass operation 3 years ago.

1. What is the first step you need to take in caring for this patient?
2. What factors should you consider as you treat this patient?

patient. Do not let this occurrence interfere with appropriate patient care.

When you respond to a call for an older patient, remember the patient's spouse is probably anxious as well. Try to keep the spouse informed of what is happening to ease some of his or her anxiety.

Sensory Changes

Two of the most socializing senses are hearing and sight. Many people experience some loss of hearing as they age, and the ability to see often diminishes as well. For some older people, decreased vision results in the need to wear eyeglasses for reading, and activities such as driving and walking can become more hazardous. Impaired vision and confusion often contribute to mistakes in taking medications. Other conditions, such as cataracts (a clouding of the lens of the eye) or macular degeneration (a disease that results in blurred or no vision), may develop.

Words of Wisdom

Suspect the possibility of medication errors in patients with decreased vision or mental confusion.

▶ Patients Who Are Hard of Hearing or Deaf

Hearing loss is an invisible disability. Hearing loss may be related to repeated exposures to loud noises or to heredity. Often hearing losses are more pronounced in the higher frequencies, meaning that a person may be able to hear a person with a low-pitched voice but not hear a person with a higher-pitched voice. Some older adults require the use of a hearing aid. As a person ages, there is also an increased chance for disorders of the inner ear. People with certain inner ear disorders are more prone to poor balance and falls than the general population.

Be certain an older patient can hear and understand what you say. Identify yourself by name and title and speak slowly and clearly. If you think the patient has difficulty hearing you, do not shout. Ask the patient if he or she can hear you. Speak directly into the patient's ear or talk while facing the patient and maintaining eye contact. If you determine that a patient has a hearing aid, ask the patient or caregiver to check to make certain it is in place and is functioning properly. Many older patients read lips to help compensate for hearing loss. If you are still having difficulties communicating, write down your questions and offer paper and a pencil to the patient to respond. Consider learning sign language so you can communicate with patients who know sign language Figure 18-2 . If you do not know sign language, use gestures to communicate.

▶ Patients Who Are Visually Impaired or Blind

During your scene size-up (initial assessment of the scene), look for signs indicating the patient may be visually impaired. These signs may include the presence of eyeglasses, a cane, or a service dog Figure 18-3 . As you approach, introduce yourself to the patient. If you think the patient is blind, ask, "Can you see?"

A patient who is visually impaired may feel vulnerable, especially during the chaos of an emergency incident. The patient may have learned to use other senses such as hearing, touch, and smell to compensate for the loss of sight. The sounds and smells of an emergency scene may be disorienting. The patient may rely on you to make sense of everything. Tell the patient what is happening, identify noises, and describe the situation and surroundings, particularly if you must move the patient. Find out what the patient's name is and use it throughout your examination and treatment, just as you would with a sighted patient. A reaffirming, supportive touch may provide emotional support.

If an older patient wears eyeglasses, keep them with the patient if at all possible. If the eyeglasses are lost during a medical emergency, make every effort to

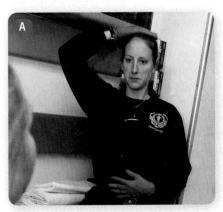
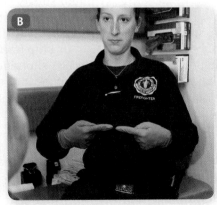
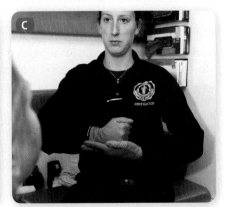

Figure 18-2 Simple phrases in sign language. **A.** Sick. **B.** Hurt. **C.** Help.
A, B, & C © Jones & Bartlett Learning. Courtesy of MIEMSS.

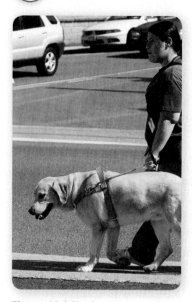

Figure 18-3 Blind patients may have a service dog.
Courtesy of the Guide Dog Foundation for the Blind. Photographed by Christopher Appoldt.

locate them because your patient may be severely handicapped and anxious without his or her eyeglasses. Knowing that the eyeglasses are not lost will be a great relief to the patient. Imagine how you would feel if you were in an emergency situation and could not see. If you bring that understanding and empathy to your interactions with patients who are visually impaired, it will help you provide compassionate care.

Words of Wisdom

Techniques for communicating with older patients include the following:

- Identify yourself by name and title.
- Look directly at the patient.
- Speak slowly and distinctly.
- Explain what you are going to do in clear, simple language.
- Listen to the patient.
- Show the patient respect.
- Do not talk about the patient in front of the patient.
- Be patient.

Musculoskeletal and Mobility Issues

As a person ages, several changes occur to the musculoskeletal system. Muscles decrease in strength. Part of this loss is the result of decreased physical activity, which can be offset by a good exercise program, and part is an inevitable outcome of the aging process. The disks between the vertebrae narrow; this change can cause a loss of height, curvature of the spine, and a loss of flexibility. The bones in the skeletal system decrease in strength because of a loss of calcium. This loss of bone strength is especially pronounced in postmenopausal women and can result in the development of **osteoporosis**. Osteoporosis is a decrease in the density of bone, and this condition affects both women and men. Many older people also experience some

loss of balance caused by a variety of issues. Together, the loss of muscular strength, weakened bones, and decreased balance result in an increased incidence of falls among older patients. Falls in older patients result in an increased risk for brain injuries because the blood vessels are more fragile and because the brain gets smaller as a person ages. As the brain gets smaller, the amount of space in the cranium increases, resulting in an increased chance of injury to the brain as the result of trauma.

▶ Slowed Movements

When you assist an older patient, remember that as a person ages, physical movements become slower. Lend a helping hand or supporting arm. Most older patients are afraid of falling and your support will help them overcome this fear. Allow enough time for patients to move safely; do not try to rush them.

▶ Fractures

Fractures occur frequently in the geriatric population because the loss of bone density often results in osteoporosis. Osteoporosis affects both women and men. Be aware that a simple fall at home can result in multiple severe fractures in an older patient who has weakened bones. Fractures of the wrist, spine, and hip are particularly common. Some of these fractures can occur with little trauma—even fractures of the vertebrae. Geriatric patients may also have a reduced awareness of pain. They may experience little pain, even with a major fracture, and they may not realize the seriousness of their injury. Splinting and spinal immobilization of a geriatric patient can be a challenge when a spinal curvature or osteoporosis is present. Handle these patients carefully.

Hip fractures are a common result of osteoporosis. They are usually caused by a fall and occur most frequently in older women. As you conduct your primary assessment, remember that other conditions may have contributed to the fall. Patients may have experienced a minor stroke, heart attack, or confusion before the fall or they may not have seen an obstacle that caused them to trip.

In a hip fracture, the injured leg is usually (but not always) shortened compared with the other leg. The toes of the injured leg are pointed outward (**externally rotated**), and pain may be so great that the patient cannot move the leg. An older patient who reports pain after a fall must be examined by a physician to identify any possible fractures. Splint the patient as described in Chapter 15, *Injuries to Muscles and Bones*, and arrange for *prompt transport* to an appropriate medical facility.

The types of conditions that may occur with age are listed in **Table 18-1**.

Table 18-1	Conditions That May Occur With Age

- Hearing loss or impairment
- Sight loss or impairment
- Loss of sensation
- Slowed physical movements
- Fractures
- Senility
- Loss of bowel or bladder control

© Jones & Bartlett Learning.

Treatment

Carefully examine geriatric patients for signs and symptoms of fractures.

■ Medical Considerations

With increasing age comes an increase in the incidence of many different medical conditions. Two types of medical conditions that cause the greatest number of deaths are cardiovascular diseases and respiratory diseases. As people get older, they are generally less able to fight off diseases. Their immune systems become less effective. They are unable to cough as effectively and may have increased difficulty handling secretions, thus increasing the need for suctioning.

▶ Cardiovascular Diseases

Cardiovascular diseases are conditions that affect the heart and blood vessels. As a person ages, the ability of the body to speed up the rate of contractions of the heart decreases. At the same time, the blood vessels become stiffer and narrowed by fatty deposits. These changes increase the occurrence of cardiac diseases such as heart attacks, angina, and congestive heart failure in geriatric patients. Strokes and abdominal aortic aneurysms are two common conditions related to blood vessels. The incidence of these diseases also rises with age.

Some patients may have experienced one of these conditions in the past. Their current medical emergency may be related to the ongoing results of a past stroke or heart attack. With other patients, the immediate cause of their medical emergency may be a heart attack or stroke that is occurring at that moment.

When caring for geriatric patients, it is important to understand that the signs and symptoms of medical conditions may be different from the classic signs and symptoms you would expect in a younger patient. Remember, older patients often have a decreased awareness or sensation to the pain of a medical or trauma condition. Older patients are more likely to have a so-called silent heart attack where they do not experience acute pain; hence,

they may not realize that they are experiencing a heart attack. Some patients who are experiencing a stroke will not be aware of the signs and symptoms that are present. Treat older patients with a high degree of suspicion. It is better to err on the side of overtreatment than it is to fail to treat and arrange for transport.

▶ Respiratory Diseases

Respiratory diseases are a major cause of sickness and death in older patients. As a person ages, the alveoli have a loss of elasticity. This condition makes it harder to inhale oxygen and to exhale carbon dioxide. Older patients usually have a reduced lung capacity, which means they do not exchange as much air with each breath as they did when they were younger. Also, the muscles associated with respiration become weaker with age. This condition makes it harder for older people to cough, which makes them more susceptible to a variety of respiratory infections. There are two major types of respiratory diseases: chronic respiratory diseases and acute respiratory diseases.

Patients with chronic obstructive pulmonary disease may live with this condition for many years. They call for EMS assistance when some type of change in their life causes them to experience shortness of breath. A cold or other respiratory infection can upset their normal equilibrium and result in a medical emergency.

Acute respiratory diseases can strike a patient quickly. Pneumonia is a common infectious disease in older patients. Because many older patients have a weakened immune system, they are especially susceptible to pneumonia. Pneumonia frequently kills older people. Minor symptoms can become a major illness in a short period of time. A physician should examine any older patient who has congestion and a possible fever.

Your role in caring for older patients with a possible respiratory condition is to carefully examine them, secure an accurate medical history (past and present), treat their presenting symptoms, and arrange for *transport* to an appropriate medical facility when indicated.

▶ Cancer

Cancer is a frequent cause of disability and death in older patients. Cancer can strike any part of the body. Patients do not call EMS because they have cancer. They call for help when complications from the cancer result in acute pain, shortness of breath, shock, or some other medical condition. These patients require prehospital support and then *transport* to a medical facility for stabilization. Patients with cancer and their families are experiencing a major crisis. Your support and understanding will help them to get through this difficult time.

▶ Altered Mental Status

Many of the medical conditions that commonly occur in older patients can result in **altered mental status** (decreased responsiveness). Recall from Chapter 10, *Medical Emergencies*, that patients may be confused or unresponsive for a wide variety of reasons, and knowledge of the common causes of altered mental status may help you in treating these patients. Three common causes of decreased responsiveness in older patients are (1) lack of adequate oxygen to the brain, (2) low blood glucose level, and (3) hypothermia. When you encounter a patient with an altered mental status, carefully assess the patient and provide treatment that is appropriate for his or her signs and symptoms. Ensure the patient is transported to an appropriate medical facility for further assessment and treatment.

> ### Words of Wisdom
>
> Complications with the transmission of nerve impulses can result in the loss of sensation in the arms or legs. This lack of sensation places the older patient at a higher risk for burns from hot water or from cooking accidents.

▶ Medications

Because older patients can have a variety of chronic conditions, many of them take multiple medications every day. They may see several physicians for different conditions. If the various physicians do not communicate effectively, there is a chance that some medications may interfere with the action of other medications. Many medications have negative side effects, such as dizziness, when taken in excess quantities. Many patients with heart conditions take blood thinners (anticoagulants) to prevent blood clots, which make them more likely to bleed from even minor cuts. Older patients may not take their medications as instructed, accidentally taking the wrong dosage of a particular medication or missing doses altogether **Figure 18-4** .

It is important for you to determine what types of medication a patient takes, including any over-the-counter drugs or supplements. While you cannot be expected to learn all the medications that a patient might take, you can learn a lot by asking the patient directly. Often the patient knows the conditions for which he or she is taking medications; for example, "The white pill is for my high blood pressure, and the green pill is a blood thinner." If the patient is being transported to a medical facility, gather up his or her prescription medications and bring them to the hospital with the patient.

> ### Words of Wisdom
>
> In addition to medications taken by mouth, some patients receive medication through skin patches (for example, nitroglycerin). It is important to ask the patient whether he or she is using any type of skin patch for medication administration.

▶ Infections and Sepsis

Infectious diseases are illnesses that are caused by bacteria, viruses, or fungi. They may affect different body systems or different organs of the body. Because older people have weakened immune systems, they are more susceptible to contracting infectious diseases, including pneumonia, abdominal infections, kidney infections, and urinary tract infections. Signs and symptoms of an infectious disease vary depending on the organism causing the infection and the body system primarily infected, but in general, common signs and symptoms include fever, fatigue, coughing, muscle aches, and diarrhea.

A severe, potentially life-threatening complication of infection is sepsis. Sepsis occurs when chemicals are released into the bloodstream as a result of infection and trigger an inflammatory response throughout the body. Sepsis is most common in older adults and people who have weakened immune systems. If untreated, sepsis can progress to septic shock, a condition in which the blood pressure drops dramatically. Septic shock often results in death. The most common types of infections that may cause sepsis include pneumonia, abdominal infections, bloodstream infections, kidney infections, and urinary tract infections.

The most effective way to prevent complications and death from infection is to recognize and treat an infection as soon as possible. As an EMR, you do not have the training and tools to diagnose or to treat patients who may have infections. Your job is to understand that older people are more likely to contract infections and develop sepsis than younger people and to recognize that older people often do not realize how sick they are. If an older patient shows signs or symptoms of an infection such as fever, diarrhea, fatigue, muscle aches, or coughing, he or she should be evaluated by a physician to rule out the possibility of an infection or sepsis.

■ Patients Who Require Long-Term Care

Modern medical science has made great advances in treating patients with chronic conditions. In the past, most patients with serious chronic medical conditions

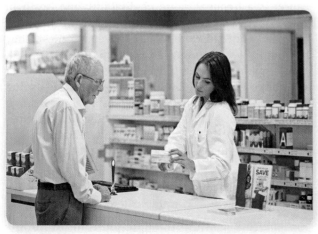

Figure 18-4 Older patients may take many different medications at the same time.
© Yuri_Arcurs/iStock/Getty.

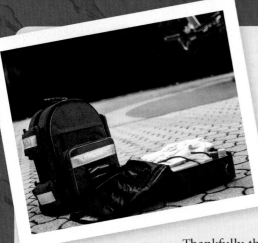

Voices *of* Experience

Many years ago, I responded to a motor vehicle collision in which an older couple's car collided with a gasoline tanker truck. Thankfully, the truck was not transporting fuel, but the incident was still devastating. We rapidly extricated both patients from the vehicle. The truck had struck the car on the passenger side. The man, who had been riding on the passenger side, was injured more severely than his wife who had been driving. He was struggling to breathe and had sustained numerous injuries, including chest injuries.

As a second ambulance arrived, my partner assisted me with caring for the man as the other crew took over care of his wife. I recall the older woman asking to be with her husband, and I informed her that we needed to transport them in separate ambulances to a trauma center. The man was struggling to breathe despite our aggressive care, and the curvature of his spine made it more difficult to immobilize him on the long backboard. I recall the wife begging me not to separate her from her husband.

> **He was struggling to breathe and had sustained numerous injuries, including chest injuries.**

My heart went out to this couple. To this day I am not sure why I did what I did, but I am thankful that I made the decision to transport these patients in the same ambulance. I instructed the crew of the other ambulance to load my patient's wife in my ambulance and have the paramedic of that ambulance come onboard to continue her care as I cared for her husband. The other crew questioned my request because of the severity of this collision but I insisted.

As we were transporting both patients to the trauma center, I continued care of the husband and I recall the wife reaching over with her right hand to hold the hand of her husband. I continued to assist ventilations of my patient as he responded to his wife's touch. Words of many years of love and companionship were spoken by the wife, and I realized that this couple had been together longer than I had been alive. They had shared many years together, and I feel sure that this older man had depended on his wife for most of his life. My patient knew his wife was by his side until the end.

When we arrived at the hospital trauma center, the husband stopped breathing. His heart stopped less than 5 minutes later. Because of the extent of his injuries, resuscitative measures were unsuccessful. Before we placed our patients in the ambulance, I had no idea that this would be the last time that this gentleman would feel the love of his wife's touch.

Several weeks later, I saw the wife of my patient in the local hospital where she was a volunteer. She came up to me and hugged me. She thanked me for allowing her to share the last 30 minutes of her husband's life. I knew then that I had made the right decision.

James B. Eubanks, NREMT-P, CCEMT-P
Piedmont Medical Center, Emergency Medical Services
Upstate Carolina Medical Center, Emergency Medical Services
Spartanburg Regional Medical Center, Transportation Services
South Carolina

were treated in hospitals or rehabilitation facilities; many died shortly after their conditions were diagnosed. Today, many patients are treated at home by nurses, home health aides, or family members. The life expectancy of people with chronic conditions has greatly increased. Patients with chronic conditions may be of any age. Because most patients with chronic conditions are older, this topic is being addressed in this chapter. However, remember that young children with complex chronic conditions are often treated at home as well.

A variety of complex medical devices are used with patients who require long-term care. Devices that help patients breathe include ventilators that push oxygen into the patients' lungs, oxygen-enrichment devices, surgically inserted breathing tubes, and monitors that sound an alarm if a patient stops breathing. Patients with certain heart conditions may have pacemakers and automatic defibrillators inserted under their skin. Tubes inserted into a patient's arm, neck, or stomach may provide fluids or food. Catheters drain urine from the patient's bladder. To make matters even more complex, patients who require long-term care must often take a variety of medications.

As an EMR, you may be called to assist with these patients for a variety of reasons, ranging from trauma or illness to mechanical failures or transport needs. A minor illness for a healthy person can be life threatening for a patient with a chronic condition. Some patients fall and sustain musculoskeletal trauma, whereas others simply need help getting back into bed. Medical equipment may stop working because the power or backup batteries failed. Patients may need transport to a hospital for assessment and treatment.

When you receive such a call, remember your role as an EMR is to assess the emergency and to use your training to take the appropriate steps in caring for the patient. Do not get overwhelmed or distracted by the complex equipment Figure 18-5 . You are not expected to understand how all these complex medical devices work. The people caring for the patient are familiar with the equipment they use each day. Do not be afraid to ask them about the equipment and the condition of the patient. Do not hesitate to question the patient and the patient's caregivers about the issue. They can probably tell you what the issue is and how you can help. Keep in mind the principles of your training. These patients need an open airway and adequate breathing and circulation. In most situations, you need to help stabilize the patient for only a few minutes until more highly trained EMS personnel arrive to provide care.

■ Mental Health Considerations

Three types of mental health conditions seen frequently in older people are depression, suicidal thoughts, and dementia or Alzheimer disease. It is helpful for you to have some understanding of why these conditions are

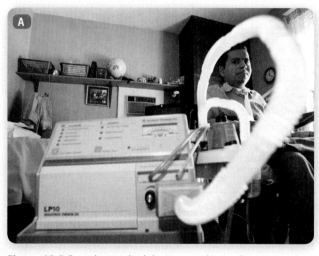
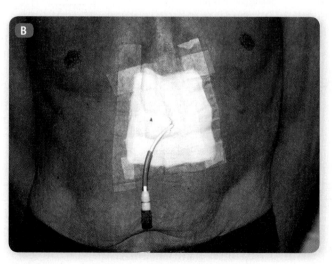

Figure 18-5 Complex medical devices may be used to treat patients who need chronic care. **A.** Ventilator. **B.** Feeding tube.
A: © Jim Slosiarek, Journal Times/AP Photo; B: © Dr. P. Marazzi/Photo Researchers, Inc.

YOU are the Provider   CASE 2

So far you have had a quiet shift on a cool October day. At 1847 hours, you are dispatched to the Fox Chase Retirement Community for a report of a 67-year-old woman who has fallen. Your response time is 6 minutes. As you arrive at the address given, you are flagged down by an older man who anxiously tells you that he and his wife were returning from dinner with friends at the local buffet. As his wife was getting out of the car, she fell and is unable to get up.

1. What are your first steps as you approach this patient and begin to care for her?
2. Given the age of his patient, what are your special concerns for her?

common in older people and what you can do when you encounter them.

▶ Depression

Depression is the most common psychiatric condition experienced by older adults. While the rates of depression are between 1% and 5%, for older people living on their own, the rates rise significantly with the loss of independence. Fourteen percent of people receiving home health care are estimated to suffer from depression and between 29% and 52% of older people living in nursing homes suffer from depression. This condition is more common in women than in men. The recent loss of a spouse or close friend can contribute to depression. People with declining health, chronic health conditions, or terminal illnesses are especially likely to experience depression. Be aware of the high incidence of depression in older patients and be alert for signs and symptoms of persistent feelings of sadness or despair. If you observe signs or symptoms of depression, bring this to the attention of other EMS providers or other medical professionals.

> **Special Populations**
>
> Do not overlook signs of mental health conditions in older patients.

▶ Suicide

Older men have the highest suicide rate of any age group in the United States, according to the American Foundation for Suicide Prevention. When older people attempt suicide, they choose more lethal means than younger people do. This factor results in more deaths from suicide than in some other age groups. Many factors contribute to the high suicide rate among older men. Physical illnesses, especially terminal ones, can lead to suicide. Loss of a loved one and alcohol abuse are also contributing factors. Listen carefully to the patient. Be alert for indications of hopelessness, depression, or attempts at suicide. If you think a patient may be considering suicide, arrange for *transport* to an appropriate medical facility **Figure 18-6**. Be alert for your safety because weapons may be present on the scene. Contact law enforcement for assistance if needed. Know the protocols in your department for handling this type of situation.

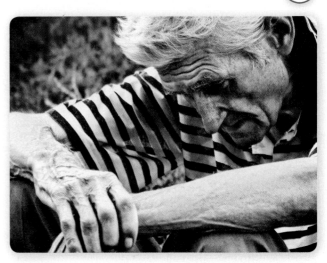

Figure 18-6 If you think a patient may be considering suicide, arrange for transport to an appropriate medical facility.
© dundanim/Shutterstock.

▶ Dementia

As people get older, some of them experience a decrease in mental function. A pattern of decline in mental function is called dementia. Dementia is a progressive and usually irreversible decline in mental functions. It is marked by impairment in memory and may result in decreases in reasoning, judgment, comprehension, and ability to communicate verbally. It is estimated that 20% to 40% of people older than age 85 have some degree of dementia. You may hear people use the term senile dementia when referring to patients with decreased mental function. Senile dementia is a general term used to describe an abnormal decline in mental functioning seen in older patients. Dementia can be caused by many different conditions including small strokes, hardening of the arteries, and/or heredity.

The most common type of dementia is Alzheimer disease. Alzheimer disease is a chronic degenerative disorder that attacks the brain and results in impaired memory, behavior, and thinking. According to the Alzheimer's Association, more than 5 million people in the United States are living with Alzheimer disease. During the course of this illness, the patient may experience mood swings and feelings that people are plotting against him or her. Patients with Alzheimer disease may wander at night and are at increased risk for falls. In the terminal stages of this disease, patients may be unable to walk, control their bowels and bladder, and swallow.

YOU ▶ are the Provider   CASE 3

You and your partner are called to a residence for an unknown emergency. When you arrive at the scene, a woman meets you at the door and tells you that her husband's intravenous pump is malfunctioning and the visiting nurse has already left for the day.

1. What can you do to help?
2. What other resources may be helpful?

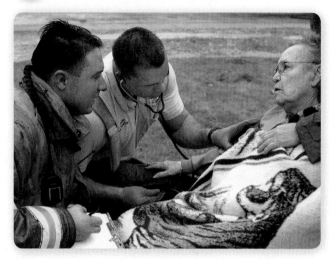

Figure 18-7 Use a kind and caring approach when caring for patients who have dementia.
© Glen E. Ellman.

When you care for patients with dementia, it is important to speak clearly to them and use their name. Let the patient know what you are doing at each step of your assessment and treatment. You will need to rely on family members or caregivers for a medical history. Because the patient's thought processes are impaired, communication may be difficult; therefore, inform the patient what you need to do. Be respectful and patient. Patients who are senile will pick up on your calm attitude and approach and respond accordingly. Use nonverbal communication to connect with patients who are unable to communicate verbally. Your kind and caring approach will make the patient more comfortable and will make your job easier Figure 18-7 .

End-of-Life Issues

It is important that you have an understanding of end-of-life issues when caring for geriatric patients. This section discusses the role of hospice care and advance directives.

▶ Hospice Care

A **hospice** is a health care program that brings together a variety of caregivers to provide physical, emotional, spiritual, social, and economic care for patients who have terminal illnesses and who are expected to die within the next 6 months. Hospice care is provided in the patient's home or in a special facility.

The hospice's interdisciplinary programs are designed to provide pain relief and other supportive care when there is no hope that the patient can recover from the illness. One of the goals of a hospice is to provide pain relief without the use of needles or intravenous (IV) lines. Pain relief is provided through oral medications, medication patches, and medicine placed in the mouth between the gum and the cheek. Most hospice patients have some type of cancer.

When the hospice care is working well, EMS providers are usually not called. However, if the patient experiences unexpected conditions such as shortness of breath, EMS may be requested by a family member or by a caregiver. In the event that you are called to care for someone who is under the care of hospice, it is helpful for you to know the purpose of the hospice and the types of care being provided. Patients who are under the care of hospice may have advance directives that request that they not be resuscitated (discussed next). If there is any question about whether you should begin treatment, begin treatment and let the physician at the hospital make any further decisions.

▶ Advance Directives

Patients who have a terminal condition may have drawn up a document to instruct physicians and other medical caregivers regarding the care they want to receive if they are unable to make their own medical decisions. These documents, called advance directives or living wills, were discussed in Chapter 4, *Medical, Legal, and Ethical Issues*. Recall that advance directives may include do not resuscitate (DNR) orders. A DNR order is a request to withhold cardiopulmonary resuscitation and other lifesaving measures if a person's heart stops or if he or she stops breathing. It is important for you to know the regulations and local protocols concerning these documents in your state. Some states have systems, such as bracelets, to identify patients with DNR orders. If you are unable to determine whether a DNR order is valid, begin appropriate medical care and leave the questions about living wills to physicians.

YOU ▸ are the Provider   CASE 4

You are called to a nursing home for an 86-year-old man with abdominal pain. When you arrive at the scene, the patient does not know why you are there. The staff tells you that the patient complained of abdominal pain and per their protocol they contacted EMS.

1. What is your assessment of this situation?
2. How are you going to take care of this patient?

■ Elder Abuse

Older adults who are physically weak or mentally compromised are at high risk for abuse by a spouse, other family members, friends, or caregivers. **Elder abuse** is hard to detect because those who are at the highest risk of abuse are also isolated from public view if they are confined to their homes or are living in an assisted care facility. As an EMR, you may be in a position to recognize physical or emotional abuse in geriatric patients. Elder abuse may be in the form of physical abuse, sexual abuse, emotional abuse, financial abuse, or neglect **Figure 18-8** . Patients with severe physical conditions or with senility may not be able to report abuse.

The signs and symptoms of abuse include bruises, especially on the buttocks, lower back, genitals, cheeks, neck, and earlobes. Look for pressure bruises caused by a human hand grabbing the patient. Look for multiple bruises in different states of healing. Burns are another means of abuse. These may be caused by cigarettes or hot fluids. Suspect sexual abuse if there is trauma in the genital area. Finally, look for signs of neglect. Does the patient appear to be malnourished? If you suspect abuse, you need to report it to the proper authorities. Learn the requirements for reporting elder abuse in your

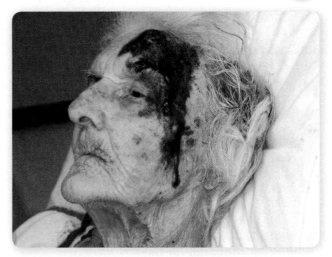

Figure 18-8 Physical abuse is one form of elder abuse.
Courtesy of Rhonda Hunt.

state and know how to follow the protocols for reporting within your department.

Many community-based programs assist in supporting geriatric patients who need physical assistance, nutritional support, or emotional help. It is only by reporting signs and symptoms of abuse to the proper authorities that the condition can be improved.

YOU are the Provider　　　　　SUMMARY

You are the Provider: CASE 1

1. What is the first step you need to take in caring for this patient?

It is important to complete a thorough patient assessment. Make sure the patient has not injured any other part of his body as a result of the fall. Complete your SAMPLE history. Bandage his injured arm with a thick dressing and a snug bandage. Take a complete set of vital signs because this patient is currently taking medications for high blood pressure, heart problems, and gout. If you are unsure what some of the medications are for, ask the patient or his wife for this information. Finally, provide reassurance to the patient and his wife; this event is traumatic for them.

2. What factors should you consider as you treat this patient?

This patient is 76 years old, has a history of high blood pressure and heart problems, and takes a variety of medications. His bones may be weaker than the bones of a younger patient. Make sure he does not have any signs or symptoms of a broken bone. Check his blood pressure and other vital signs. His primary injury, the cut on his arm, may be impacted by the medications he is taking. Ask the patient if he takes blood thinners

(anticoagulants), which increase the risk of bleeding from even minor cuts. Dress the wound with a thick dressing and a snug bandage. Finally, try to determine the cause of the fall. Ask the patient if he had blacked out when he tried to stand. This condition is not uncommon in older patients who are taking several different medicines. Even though this patient appears to have a single injury, you need to consider his full medical history. This patient needs further evaluation by a physician.

You are the Provider: CASE 2

1. What are your first steps as you approach this patient and begin to care for her?

Because this woman has fallen in a parking lot, make sure you have parked your vehicle in a manner that protects both emergency care providers and the patient from traffic hazards. Before you approach, survey the scene for other safety issues (scene size-up). Introduce yourself by name and title, and perform a primary assessment of the patient. If the patient is oriented and is able to talk with you, you know that her airway, breathing, and circulation are somewhat stable. Determine the patient's chief complaint. Perform a secondary assessment to verify her chief complaint and to identify and assess any injuries. Obtain a SAMPLE history. Obtain a set of vital signs and repeat them if EMS is delayed. If you are working with a partner, you may be able to perform a couple of these steps at the same time. Keep the patient as comfortable as possible. Remember, a patient who has fallen and is lying on pavement may become chilled. Cover her with warm blankets to keep her comfortable and to prevent hypothermia. If it is starting to get dark, make sure you have taken steps to light the incident scene.

2. **Given the age of this patient, what are your special concerns for her?**

Because of her age, this patient is more likely to have reduced bone density and brittle bones (osteoporosis). She is complaining of severe pain in the area of her right hip. Older people often experience fractures with relatively little trauma. Because a hip fracture can result in substantial internal blood loss, you need to keep this patient warm and monitor her vital signs for possible shock. Assess her for any other injuries. It is important to obtain a complete medical history in older patients because they often take multiple medications for a variety of conditions. You may need to specifically ask this patient whether she has heart-related diseases or diabetes; these conditions are more common in geriatric patients. Determine if the patient is taking blood thinners (anticoagulants) or aspirin, which would make her prone to increased blood loss. Provide reassurance to the patient as well as her family members; they are having a bad day. Finally, be certain that an EMS unit is responding to your location.

You are the Provider: CASE 3

1. **What can you do to help?**

A malfunctioning intravenous (IV) pump is not under the expertise of an emergency medical responder; however, it is not uncommon for people to call 9-1-1 for such issues. First determine whether the patient is experiencing any life-threatening conditions and address them as necessary. If the patient's airway, breathing, and circulation (ABCs) are intact and he reports no other issues, assess his vital signs and explain to the family that IV pump management is beyond your training. Do not attempt to manipulate or correct any issues with the device. Instead, offer to help the family by contacting

the visiting nurse's office or by obtaining additional resources that can assist with this situation.

2. **What other resources may be helpful?**

EMS has a variety of resources to help in these situations. Advanced life support units are trained in these areas and may be able to provide you with guidance. Many EMS systems have registered nurses and critical care ambulance crews that are also trained in IV pump management. It is important that you attempt to get help for this patient. The IV solution or medication being administered may potentially harm the patient if administered incorrectly.

You are the Provider: CASE 4

1. **What is your assessment of this situation?**

There may be a few reasons why the patient does not know why you are there. One simple reason could be that the staff did not inform the patient that EMS was called. A more serious reason could be that the patient has had a change in mental status or has an underlying dementia. To make a determination, assess the patient's mental status and compare it to information from the staff. It is important for you to investigate this situation further because a new change in mental status could be caused by a potentially life-threatening condition.

2. **How are you going to take care of this patient?**

Determine the patient's chief complaint. If the patient denies any complaints, ask him specifically about his abdominal pain. In any event, it is always safer to have the patient transported to a hospital for evaluation. If the patient refuses to go to the hospital, determine whether he is competent to make that decision and ask the staff if the patient has a family member or a person with a power of attorney who can be consulted for medical matters (see Chapter 4, *Medical, Legal, and Ethical Issues*). You may need to contact such a person to aid you in transporting the patient. It may be necessary to have additional help present, including law enforcement, to make sure the patient's rights are not violated. Consult your local protocols and department policies for these specific situations.

Prep Kit

▶ Ready for Review

- The natural aging process results in a decline in the functioning of all body systems, including sensory and musculoskeletal changes.
- Fractures occur often in older people because of the loss of bone density that can lead to osteoporosis. A simple fall at home can result in multiple severe fractures in a geriatric patient who has weakened bones. Fractures of the wrist, spine, and hip are particularly common.
- Common medical concerns for geriatric patients include cardiovascular and respiratory diseases.
- Many of the medical conditions that commonly occur in older patients can result in altered mental status. Three common causes of altered mental status are lack of adequate oxygen to the brain, low blood glucose level, and hypothermia.
- Older people and people with weakened immune systems are prone to contracting infectious diseases, including pneumonia, abdominal infections, kidney infections, and urinary tract infections. A severe, potentially life-threatening complication of infection is sepsis. If untreated, sepsis can progress to septic shock.
- You may be called to assist with patients who require long-term care for a variety of reasons, ranging from trauma or illness to mechanical failures or transport needs. A minor illness for a healthy person can be life threatening for a patient with a chronic condition.
- Do not overlook signs of mental health conditions in older patients. Three types of mental health conditions seen frequently in older people are depression, suicidal thoughts, and dementia.
- Older people who are physically weak or mentally compromised are at high risk for abuse by a spouse, other family members, friends, or caregivers. As an emergency medical responder, you may be in a position to recognize abuse in geriatric patients. Elder abuse may be in the form of physical abuse, sexual abuse, emotional abuse, financial abuse, or neglect.

▶ Vital Vocabulary

altered mental status A sudden or gradual decrease in the person's level of responsiveness. Measured using the AVPU scale.

Alzheimer disease A chronic, progressive dementia that accounts for 60% of all dementia.

dementia A progressive, irreversible decline in mental functioning; marked by memory impairment and decrease in reasoning, judgment, comprehension, and ability to communicate verbally.

depression A psychiatric disorder marked by persistent feelings of sadness, hopelessness, and decreased interest in daily activities. The person may have persistent thoughts of suicide.

elder abuse An action taken by a family member or caregiver that results in the physical, emotional, financial, or sexual harm to a person older than 65 years; also includes neglect.

externally rotated Rotated outward, as a fractured hip.

geriatric patient A patient who is older than 65 years.

hospice An interdisciplinary program designed to reduce or eliminate pain and address the physical, spiritual, social, and economic needs of terminally ill patients.

osteoporosis Abnormal brittleness of the bones caused by loss of calcium; affected bones fracture easily.

senile dementia General term for dementia that occurs in older people.

sepsis A severe, potentially life-threatening complication of infection that can progress to septic shock if left untreated; occurs when chemicals are released into the bloodstream and trigger an inflammatory response throughout the body.

septic shock A condition in which the blood pressure drops dramatically as a result of severe infection; often results in death.

suicide Intentionally causing one's own death. Suicide is especially common in older and chronically ill people.

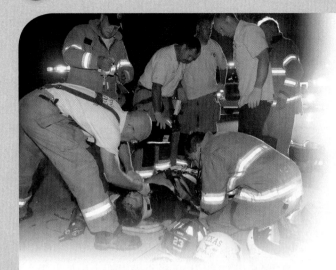

Assessment *in Action*

You are dispatched to a residence for the report of an older person with an unknown medical emergency. Your dispatcher indicates she does not have any further information because a neighbor made the 9-1-1 call. When you arrive at the house, you are met by the neighbor, who states that Mrs. Jones "does not seem to be herself" today.

1. As you begin to talk to your patient, her neighbor tells you that Mrs. Jones cannot hear very well. On the basis of this information, what should you do?

   A. Use sign language.
   B. Speak slowly and clearly while facing the patient.
   C. Shout so that the patient can hear you better.
   D. Have the neighbor talk to the patient.

2. During your examination of the patient, you notice that she is dressed in several layers of clothing even though it is 80°F (26°C) outside. What should you do?

   A. Take her vital signs only.
   B. Omit the physical examination and provide immediate transport.
   C. Remove as much of her clothing as you need to examine her properly.
   D. Perform an incomplete physical examination because she is wearing too much clothing.

3. Which of the following conditions increases the risk of an older patient sustaining a fracture?

   A. Diabetes
   B. Senility

   C. Arthritis
   D. Osteoporosis

4. If it becomes necessary to transport Mrs. Jones to a medical facility, the (EMS) crew should also take along which of the following items?

   A. Medical insurance policy
   B. Coat
   C. Address book
   D. Medications

5. How would you care for this patient if she were blind?

   A. Speak loudly so the patient knows where you are.
   B. Verbally explain everything you are doing during your assessment and treatment.
   C. Avoid touching the patient when not necessary because your unexpected touch may scare the patient.
   D. Secure the service dog in another area to prevent the dog from interfering with your assessment.

As you return to your station from the last call, you are dispatched to a nursing home for a patient who has fallen out of bed. When you arrive, a staff member takes you to the patient's room. Several complex medical devices surround the patient's bed and one of the machines is sounding an alarm.

6. What is your first step in your assessment of this patient?

7. What should you do about the sounding alarm?

8. How can you get a medical history of this patient?

9. The patient has an altered mental status. How will this affect your assessment and treatment?

10. What item(s) should be taken with the patient, if he or she needs to be transported to an appropriate medical facility?

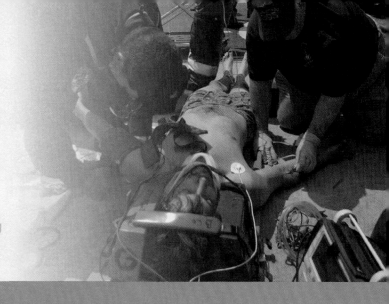

SECTION 7

EMS Operations

Transport Operations

National EMS Education Standard Competencies

EMS Operations

Knowledge of operational roles and responsibilities to ensure safe patient, public, and personnel safety.

Principles of Safely Operating a Ground Ambulance

> Risks and responsibilities of emergency response (pp 403–405)

Air Medical

> Safe air medical operations (pp 407–408)
> Criteria for utilizing air medical response (p 405)

Knowledge Objectives

1. Summarize the different phases of an emergency response. (pp 404–405))
2. Explain the importance of preparing for an emergency call. (p 403)
3. List the medical and nonmedical equipment needed to respond to a call. (p 403)
4. Explain the importance of reviewing dispatch information. (p 404)
5. Explain the safety precautions needed to ensure a safe emergency response. (p 404)
6. Describe the actions emergency medical responders (EMRs) should take on arrival at an emergency scene. (pp 404–405)
7. Describe the importance of transferring patient care to other emergency medical services (EMS) personnel. (p 405)
8. Explain the postrun activities that follow the completion of an emergency response. (p 405)
9. Describe the guidelines for safe helicopter operations. (pp 407–408)
10. Describe the steps of setting up a helicopter landing zone. (p 407)
11. Describe the steps of loading patients into a helicopter. (pp 407–408)

Skills Objectives

1. Demonstrate how to set up a helicopter landing zone. (p 407)
2. Demonstrate how to assist with loading a patient into a helicopter. (pp 407–408)

Introduction

To be an effective emergency medical responder (EMR), you need to prepare for an emergency medical services (EMS) call, review dispatch information, respond safely to the scene, perform a scene size-up, perform initial patient assessment and provide emergency care, update responding EMS units and transfer care to other EMS personnel, and complete postrun activities. This chapter describes the phases of an EMS call and the tasks required to complete each of these phases safely. The second part of this chapter describes your role in helicopter medivac operations. It describes helicopter safety guidelines, how to set up a landing zone, and how to assist with loading patients into a helicopter.

Preparing for a Call

In your primary role as a law enforcement officer, firefighter, lifeguard, or security guard, you are also on call as an EMR. In preparing yourself for a call, you must understand your role as a member of the emergency medical system. You may respond using a fire department vehicle, a law enforcement vehicle, your personal vehicle, or on foot. It is important to ensure these vehicles are ready to respond at all times. Follow a regular schedule to inspect and maintain all vehicles. Your department should provide a checklist to follow to ensure that everything is in working order, such as checking tire pressure, fluid levels, and fuel levels. Be prepared to respond promptly, using the most direct route available. Make sure you have the proper equipment to perform your job, including the medical equipment in your EMR life support kit, your personal safety equipment, and equipment to safeguard the incident scene. Suggested contents of an EMR life support kit are shown in **Figure 19-1** and listed in **Table 19-1**. This equipment must be stocked and maintained on a regular basis according to the schedule specified by your agency.

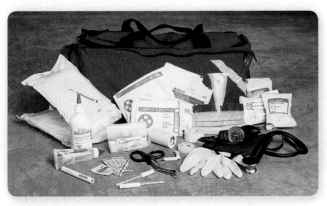

Figure 19-1 Suggested contents of an EMR life support kit.
© Jones & Bartlett Learning. Courtesy of MIEMSS.

Table 19-1	Suggested Contents of an EMR Life Support Kit
Patient examination equipment	1 flashlight
Personal safety equipment	5 pairs of gloves 5 face masks 1 bottle of hand sanitizer
Resuscitation equipment	1 mouth-to-mask resuscitation device 1 portable hand-powered suction device 1 set oral airways 1 set nasal airways
Bandaging and dressing equipment	10 gauze adhesive strips (1 inch [3 cm]) 10 gauze pads (4 inch × 4 inch [10 cm × 10 cm]) 5 gauze pads (5 inch × 9 inch [13 cm × 23 cm]) 2 universal trauma dressings (10 inch × 30 inch [25 cm × 76 cm]) 1 occlusive dressing for sealing chest wounds 4 conforming gauze rolls (3 inch × 15 feet [8 cm × 5 m]) 4 conforming gauze rolls (4.5 inch × 15 feet [11 cm × 5 m]) 6 triangular bandages 1 adhesive tape (2 inch [5 cm]) 1 burn sheet
Patient immobilization equipment	2 (each) cervical collars: small, medium, large, or 2 adjustable cervical collars 3 rigid conforming splints (SAM splints), or 1 set air splints for arm and leg, or 2 (each) cardboard splints (18 inch [46 cm] and 24 inch [61 cm])
Extrication equipment	1 spring-loaded center punch 1 pair of heavy leather gloves
Miscellaneous equipment	2 blankets (disposable) 2 cold packs 1 pair of bandage scissors 1 obstetric kit
Other equipment	1 set of personal protective clothing (helmet, eye protection, EMS jacket) 1 reflective vest 1 fire extinguisher (5 lb [2 kg] ABC dry chemical) 1 *Emergency Response Guidebook* 6 flares 1 pair of binoculars
Optional equipment (based on the protocols of your service)	Oral glucose Naloxone intranasal spray (for opioid overdoses)

© Jones & Bartlett Learning.

YOU are the Provider

CASE 1

At 2047 hours you are dispatched to 209 East Second Street for a report of a sick child with a high fever. You are informed the child is located in apartment 318. This address is about 7 minutes from your location.

1. Why is it important for you to understand the phases of an EMS call?
2. Why is it important to differentiate between East Second Street and West Second Street and confirm the apartment number?
3. What steps do you need to take if you do not understand the location of the address given to you by your dispatcher?

■ Phases of an EMR Call

When you respond to an EMS call, make sure each task is carefully completed to ensure a safe and positive outcome to the incident.

▶ Dispatch

The dispatch facility is a center that citizens can call to request emergency medical care. Most centers are part of a 9-1-1 system that is responsible for receiving emergency calls at a public safety answering point (PSAP) and then dispatching fire, police, and EMS. You should understand how the dispatch facility used by your department operates. Your job will be easier if the dispatcher obtains the proper information from the caller. Dispatchers should also be able to instruct callers on how to perform lifesaving techniques such as cardiopulmonary resuscitation until you arrive.

You may receive your dispatch information by telephone, radio, pager, computer terminal, or written printout. Regardless of the transmission method, the information should include the nature of the call, the name and location of the patient, the number of patients, and any special conditions at the scene. The dispatcher should also obtain a callback number in case you need more information from the caller. Without adequate dispatch information, you will not be able to respond properly.

▶ Response to the Scene

Your first priority in responding to the scene is to get there quickly and safely. Consider traffic patterns and the time of day before you select the best route to the scene. Before you begin to respond, be sure you know how to get to the location of the call. Be certain that all personnel are properly seated and secured with approved seat belts. Keep all equipment secured so it does not injure someone in the event of a sudden stop or crash. Use emergency lights and sirens according to your state laws and according to the regulations of your agency. Remember that emergency lights and sirens allow you to request the right of way; they do not guarantee it. Be especially careful at intersections and railroad crossings. Do not exceed a safe speed for the vehicle you are operating. Be aware that distractions such as radios, mobile devices, and global positioning systems (GPS) can contribute to vehicle crashes. Reduce your speed on unpaved roads, on wet or icy roads, and during periods of darkness or reduced visibility. Follow all safety procedures specified by your department. Above all else, drive defensively so you are not involved in a crash. Remember, your goal is to arrive on the scene safely.

> **Safety**
>
> Emergency lights and sirens allow you to request the right of way but do not guarantee it. Drive defensively and safely.

▶ Arrival at the Scene

When you arrive at the scene, remember to place your vehicle in a safe location to minimize the chance of injury. Consider how best to position your vehicle to effectively use your warning lights. Remember to perform a scene size-up as outlined in the patient assessment sequence (Chapter 9, *Patient Assessment*). Look for safety hazards such as downed power lines, leaking fuel, broken glass, and fire, as described in Chapter 20, *Vehicle Extrication and Special Rescue*, as well as potential biologic hazards. Control the flow of traffic to ensure the safety of responders, patients, and bystanders. Determine the number of patients and determine whether you need to call for additional resources. Be as efficient and as organized as you can. Provide patient care using the

YOU are the Provider

CASE 2

You arrive for work and find a new response vehicle in the garage. Your supervisor informs you that you will be using this vehicle during your shift. You have never seen this vehicle before and are not sure how everything works.

1. How can you verify this vehicle is ready for response?
2. When should you tell the dispatch center that you are ready for response?

knowledge and skills you have learned in this course. Call for additional resources if needed.

▶ Perform Patient Assessment and Provide Emergency Care

Many of the activities you perform at the scene of an emergency are related to the assessment and treatment of patients. The knowledge and skills needed to perform patient assessment and provide treatment are detailed throughout this book. These skills are mentioned here only to give you an idea of where they fit within the phases of responding to an emergency call.

▶ Transferring the Care of the Patient to Other EMS Personnel

As more highly trained EMS personnel arrive on the scene, you will have to transfer care of the patient to them. Update the responding EMS units by providing them a brief report of the situation as you initially observed it and tell them the results of your patient assessment and what care you have provided. Ask them if they have any questions for you. Finally, offer to assist other EMS personnel in caring for the patient.

▶ Postrun Activities

You may think you are done with a call after you have cared for the patient and provided assistance to other EMS personnel; however, your job is not done until you have completed the paper or electronic patient care report. Documentation is important, as emphasized in Chapter 1, *EMS Systems*, and Chapter 5, *Communications and Documentation*. In addition to completing the report, you must also clean your equipment and replace needed supplies. Only after you have completed these activities should you resume regular duties or notify your dispatcher or supervisor that you are ready for another call.

■ Helicopter Operations

Helicopters are used by EMS systems to reach patients, transport patients to medical facilities, and evacuate patients from otherwise inaccessible areas **Figure 19-2**. The use of helicopters to transport patients has several advantages. Helicopters can respond at speeds greater than 100 miles per hour (mph). They can travel above traffic congestion and into wilderness areas. They usually carry specialized equipment, and the personnel staffing them may include emergency medical technicians (EMTs), paramedics, registered nurses, and physicians. These personnel may be able to perform advanced life support (ALS) skills that are unavailable on ground ambulances. Helicopters are requested for patients with severe injuries or acute illnesses who may benefit from a higher level of care or more rapid transport to an appropriate medical facility. However, helicopters are limited by bad weather such as thunderstorms, blizzards, and other conditions that reduce visibility. In addition, the amount of weight helicopters can carry may be decreased in very hot temperatures and at high elevations. Adequate safe landing zones are necessary in order for helicopters to gain access to patients.

If your EMS system uses a helicopter, obtain a copy of the ground operations procedures or schedule an orientation session with helicopter personnel so you will be prepared during an emergency. As an EMR, you may be responsible for making the initial call for helicopter assistance or for setting up and preparing a landing site in the field. You need to know how to request a helicopter response as well as the criteria for calling a helicopter for trauma patients, medical patients, and wilderness response.

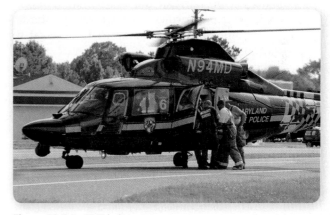

Figure 19-2 An EMS helicopter.
© Mark C. Ide.

YOU are the Provider CASE 3

You are dispatched to a motor vehicle crash at a busy intersection, which you recognize as the site of frequent crashes. When you arrive at the scene, you see two damaged vehicles in the middle of the intersection. Police officers have controlled traffic around the crash scene. All the occupants of the damaged vehicles appear to be standing near the crash scene.

1. How would you perform a scene size-up at this incident?
2. When should you request additional resources?

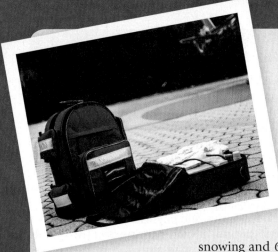

Voices *of* Experience

I had been an EMT for more than a year and worked for a local fire department in a mountain district outside of town. It was snowing and 6 inches (15 cm) of snow were already on the ground when we got a call for a 1-month-old infant with difficulty breathing. When I got to the house, the familiar red flashing lights marked the driveway and colored the falling snow.

Inside the home, the battalion chief looked relieved that I had arrived, but he was still very concerned. An infant girl, lying on her mother's lap, was having difficulty breathing. I administered high-flow oxygen and knew to sit the child upright. I auscultated her lungs and heard diffuse rhonchi. I gathered the SAMPLE history from the mother and recognized a possible return of recent pneumonia.

> **"Always do what is in the best interest of your patient."**

I continually reassessed the patient. The oxygen seemed to help initially, and the infant's color and respiratory effort improved. The ALS ambulance had come up from town, but was unable to make it up the steep 2-mile (3-km) hill to the house. We weighed the risks and benefits of bringing the paramedic up to us, but we still had to transport the patient down. We decided that the infant was doing better at this time and, because we were not supposed to transport patients, we would wait until the ambulance with four-wheel drive arrived. The ALS ambulance went back to town and the second four-wheel drive ambulance was en route.

Minutes kept passing and the patient was getting tired; the improving trend started to reverse and the infant was back to her original presentation. Anxiously awaiting the paramedics, I made a deal with myself that if the child had any change in respiratory rate or rhythm, I would begin positive-pressure ventilation. I opened the pediatric kit and assembled the appropriate bag valve mask.

When the paramedics arrived, I was just about to begin ventilating. I gave a quick report, and we dashed out to the ambulance. On the way to the hospital, we started to ventilate and administer bronchodilators with significant improvement.

The paramedic questioned why we did not take the patient down to the first ambulance. I explained that we made that decision because of the child's initial improvement, and the issue of not being a transporting agency. He told me it is good to prioritize patient and crew safety, but "Always do what is in the best interest of your patient." Then, he looked me squarely in the eyes and said, "In EMS, you must always move forward toward higher levels of care. You cannot count on your interventions to fix the problem." Lesson learned and never forgotten!

Michael Dann, NREMT-P, BSN
Remote Medical International
Boulder, Colorado

▶ Helicopter Safety Guidelines

Helicopters can provide lifesaving transport for patients with serious injuries to an appropriate medical facility. However, helicopters are also dangerous to untrained personnel. The main rotor of the helicopter spins at more than 300 revolutions per minute (rpm) and may be just 4 feet (1 m) above the ground. The tail rotor spins at more than 3,000 rpm and may be invisible to an unwary person. Additionally, the rotors can generate a "wash," or blast of air, equivalent to winds of 60 to 80 mph. If you approach without caution, you may be severely injured by walking upright or by raising an arm above the head. It is important to understand safe helicopter operations.

Setting Up Landing Zones

When choosing a landing site, remember that pilots usually land and take off into the wind. The size of a landing zone will vary and depends on the size of the helicopter. Most civilian helicopters need a landing zone of at least 100 feet × 100 feet (30 m × 30 m), or 10,000 square feet (929 square m) **Figure 19-3**. Military aircraft may need a larger area. The landing zone should be as flat as possible and free of debris that could become airborne in the 60-mph winds generated by the helicopter. Check carefully for any nearby electrical wires, which may be invisible to the pilot. If the site slopes or has any obstacles, notify the pilot.

Check with your helicopter service to see how you should secure and mark the perimeter of the site. Avoid using flags or other objects that can be blown away by the force of the helicopter rotor wash. Do not use **fusees** (red signal flares) because they create a fire hazard. Turn off unnecessary white lights and avoid flashing emergency lights because they interfere with the pilot's vision during

> ### Safety
> 1. Be alert for electrical wires when identifying a landing zone for a helicopter.
> 2. Always approach helicopters from the front so the pilot can see you. Approaching a helicopter from the rear is dangerous because the tail rotor is nearly invisible when spinning.
> 3. Do not approach the helicopter until the pilot signals that it is safe to do so.
> 4. Helicopters are very noisy and you may not be able to hear a shouted warning. Maintain eye contact with the pilot.
> 5. Keep low when you approach the helicopter to avoid the spinning rotor blades.
> 6. Follow the directions of the helicopter crew.

landing and takeoff. Keep vehicles clear of the landing zone. Close the windows and doors of any nearby vehicles and remove any loose objects on the vehicles that could become airborne. Some helicopter services request that a charged hose line be available for fire emergencies.

Loading Patients Into Helicopters

Certain safety precautions must be followed during the loading of a helicopter patient. Secure all loose clothing, sheets, and instruments such as stethoscopes. Use eye protection and a helmet, if available, to prevent debris from getting into your eyes. Approach a helicopter from the front and only after the pilot or a crew member signals that it is safe **Figure 19-4**.

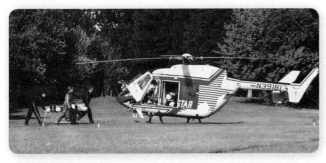

Figure 19-3 Landing zone with cones and warning devices in place.
© Thomas R. Fletcher/Alamy.

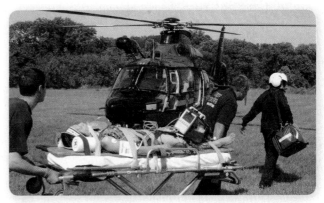

Figure 19-4 Approach helicopters from the front so the pilot can see you.
© Mark C. Ide.

YOU are the Provider   CASE 4

You are at the scene of a motorcycle crash. The EMS crew at the scene has decided to use a helicopter to transport the patient to the trauma center. You have been asked to help set up the landing zone.

1. What are some of the components of an ideal landing zone?
2. When would it be appropriate to use a helicopter for EMS transport?

Safety

Keep the following guidelines in mind during helicopter operations:

- DO NOT approach the helicopter landing zone unless necessary.
- DO NOT approach a helicopter from the upside if it is on a slope.
- DO NOT run near a helicopter.
- DO NOT raise your hand when approaching a helicopter.

The helicopter crew may need help carrying equipment to the patient. Follow their instructions. Give your patient care report to the crew, away from the helicopter's noise, and offer your assistance. It is more difficult to load a helicopter stretcher than an ambulance stretcher. Because loose sheets or blankets can blow off the stretcher, patients need to be packaged (prepared) properly and securely.

As an EMR, you can provide ground support and assistance during helicopter operations, provided that you take proper safety precautions.

YOU are the Provider   SUMMARY

You are the Provider: CASE 1

1. **Why is it important for you to understand the phases of an EMS call?**

Understanding the phases of an EMS call helps you to understand the order in which these steps occur. It gives you a framework to follow as an emergency call progresses. It also helps you to understand your role during each phase of the call. By understanding your role at each step of this sequence, you will become a valuable member of the EMS team.

2. **Why is it important to differentiate between East Second Street and West Second Street and to confirm the apartment number?**

During dispatch, listen carefully to the address of the emergency call. Do not begin responding until you are sure you understand where you need to go. Responding to West Second Street when the patient is at East Second Street or arriving at the wrong apartment number may significantly delay your response and could compromise your safety.

3. **What steps do you need to take if you do not understand the location of the address given to you by your dispatcher?**

If you do not understand the location given by your dispatcher, you need to call the dispatcher back to clarify the patient's address. Alternately, you can look it up in an address book or use a GPS. Do not begin responding until you know exactly where you are going.

You are the Provider: CASE 2

1. **How can you verify this vehicle is ready for response?**

Your service may have a list of minimum equipment or materials required for response. Check the vehicle and use the equipment checklist to verify that all the necessary equipment is present and operational. These actions help you verify the vehicle is ready for response and show you where all the equipment is located. In addition to checking the equipment, make sure the vehicle is adequately fueled and fully operational. If for any reason the vehicle is not functioning properly, do not use it for response until the issues have been corrected.

2. **When should you tell the dispatch center that you are ready for response?**

Whenever your service introduces new equipment or a different vehicle with new operational features, do not make yourself available for response until you have been properly trained in the use of the new items. Although you might be able to "figure it out," this casual approach would put you and your patients at an additional safety risk. After you have been properly trained on the new features and equipment, make sure the unit is cleaned and properly stocked. After all of those tasks have been accomplished, you are then ready for response.

You are the Provider: CASE 3

1. **How would you perform a scene size-up at this incident?**

Always begin with scene safety. Dispatch information can provide clues regarding the situation and may indicate the need for additional resources. After you arrive at the scene, assess for any safety hazards; this includes potential biologic hazards. In this case, law enforcement officers have already controlled the traffic flow; therefore, the next step is to determine the number of patients and the potential nature of illness or mechanism of injury. Be sure to get a report from the law enforcement officers and to check the inside of each vehicle for additional patients. After you have completed these steps and acquired that information, determine whether any additional resources are needed.

YOU ▶ are the Provider · SUMMARY *Continued*

2. When should you request additional resources?

After you have identified the need for additional resources, request them immediately. Do not wait to call for additional resources because you may find yourself in a situation that you are no longer able to handle by yourself. The delay could result in poor patient care. If it is determined that certain resources are no longer required, they can be easily recalled.

You are the Provider: CASE 4

1. What are some of the components of an ideal landing zone?

When you set up a landing zone, make sure the area is free of trees, electrical lines, and other obstructions. The area should be flat and free of debris. Most EMS helicopter services require a landing zone of at least 100 feet × 100 feet (30 m × 30 m). Check with your local EMS helicopter services for specific landing zone requirements. If you notice any unavoidable hazards, make sure you communicate that information to the pilot.

2. When would it be appropriate to use a helicopter for EMS transport?

Helicopters are typically used in situations where the patient has suffered severe trauma or a major illness and will benefit from more rapid transport to an appropriate medical facility. With trauma patients, it is ideal to get the patient to a trauma center within 1 hour from the initial incident. Many times this can be easily accomplished through ground transport; however, depending on the distance from the medical facility and traffic congestion, it may be beneficial to use a helicopter to transport the patient to definitive care.

Prep Kit

▶ Ready for Review

- In preparing yourself for a call, you must understand your role as a member of the emergency medical system and be prepared to respond promptly.
- As an emergency medical responder (EMR), you need the proper equipment on an emergency call, including the medical equipment in your life support kit, your personal safety equipment, and equipment to safeguard the incident scene.
- The phases of an emergency call include dispatch, response to the scene, arrival at the scene, performing an initial patient assessment and emergency care, updating responding emergency medical services (EMS) units and transferring care of the patient to other EMS personnel, and postrun activities.
- If you will be working with a medical helicopter, you need to know proper safety precautions and loading procedures for helicopter transport.
- By learning the simple but important skills involving EMS operations, you can become an effective member of the EMS system in your community.

▶ Vital Vocabulary

fusees Warning devices or flares that burn with a red color; usually used in scene protection at motor vehicle crash sites.

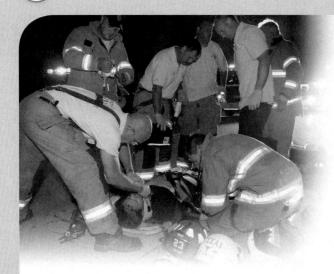

Assessment
in Action

You are dispatched to the Pleasant Elementary School at 125 School Street for a report of a 57-year-old man who is reporting chest pain and shortness of breath. Further information reveals that he is a janitor at the school. As you arrive on the scene, you are directed to the school boiler room. You find a man sitting in a chair. His skin is pale and he is sweating.

1. The dispatch center has all of the following responsibilities EXCEPT:

   A. determine the resources and personnel needed to handle the emergency.
   B. keep the caller on the line until the incident is over.
   C. notify responders of the type and location of the emergency call.
   D. receive calls from people needing emergency medical assistance.

2. What phase of an emergency call is most risky for you as an EMR?

   A. Arrival and scene size-up
   B. Response to the scene
   C. Transferring the care of the patient to other EMS personnel
   D. Each phase presents different hazards depending on the type of call. Any phase can be hazardous.

3. Hazardous conditions you might encounter at an emergency scene that would require you to request specially trained resources include all of the following EXCEPT:

   A. weapons.
   B. electrical hazards.
   C. chemical fumes.
   D. hemorrhaging.

4. All of the following information should be reported when transferring care of the patient to other EMS personnel EXCEPT:

   A. your partner's family problems.
   B. your observations of the initial situation.
   C. the care you provided.
   D. the patient's vital signs.

5. Place the phases of an EMS call in the order in which they occur.

   1. Arrival at the scene
   2. Updating responding EMS units and transferring care of the patient to other EMS personnel
   3. Response to the scene
   4. Perform initial patient assessment and provide emergency care
   5. Postrun activities
   6. Dispatch
      A. 6, 3, 1, 4, 2, 5
      B. 4, 6, 3, 1, 5, 2
      C. 1, 6, 4, 5, 3, 2
      D. 3, 1, 6, 2, 5, 4

6. The patient in this scenario is having chest pain. Would it be appropriate to use lights and sirens in your response?

7. On the basis of the dispatch information, what type of equipment might be necessary when you arrive at the scene?

8. What other resources might be necessary when treating this patient?

9. What are your responsibilities when higher-trained EMS providers arrive?

10. When should you make yourself available for another call?

Vehicle Extrication and Special Rescue

National EMS Education Standard Competencies

EMS Operations

Knowledge of operational roles and responsibilities to ensure safe patient, public, and personnel safety.

Vehicle Extrication

> Safe vehicle extrication (pp 412–421)
> Use of simple hand tools (pp 416–419)

Knowledge Objectives

1. Discuss the role of emergency medical responders (EMRs) during extrication. (p 412)
2. Identify the seven steps in the extrication process. (p 412)
3. List the various methods of gaining access to a patient. (p 416)
4. Describe the simple extrication procedures that an EMR can perform. (pp 416–419)
5. Identify the complex extrication procedures that require specially trained personnel. (p 420)
6. Discuss the role of EMRs in special rescue situations, including the following:
   - Water rescue (pp 421–423)
   - A patient with diving injuries (p 424)
   - Ice rescue (pp 424–425)
   - Confined space rescue (p 425)
   - Farm rescue (pp 427–428)
   - Bus rescue (p 428)

Skills Objectives

1. Demonstrate how to gain access to a patient through a vehicle window. (pp 418–419, Skill Drill 20-1)
2. Demonstrate how to provide airway management to a patient who is trapped in a vehicle. (pp 419–420, Skill Drill 20-2)
3. Demonstrate the role of EMRs in special rescue situations. (pp 412–413; pp 421–425; pp 427–428)
4. Demonstrate the steps EMRs can take in assisting with a water rescue. (pp 421–423)
5. Demonstrate the initial treatment of a patient in the water. (pp 422–424)
6. Demonstrate the initial treatment of a patient with diving injuries. (p 424)
7. Demonstrate the steps EMRs can take in assisting with an ice rescue. (pp 424–425)
8. Demonstrate the steps EMRs can take in assisting with a confined space rescue. (p 425)
9. Demonstrate the steps EMRs can take in assisting with farm rescue incidents. (pp 427–428)
10. Demonstrate the steps EMRs can take in assisting with bus crashes. (p 428)

Introduction

The first part of this chapter covers the steps you can take as an emergency medical responder (EMR) to perform simple extrication procedures and to assist other rescuers with patient extrication. The extrication process consists of seven steps, beginning with your arrival on the scene and ending with the removal of the patient from a position of **entrapment**. As an EMR, you are directly involved in the first four of the seven extrication steps, but you should be aware of the entire process. You cannot provide effective assistance unless you fully understand what must be done and how each step is accomplished. By learning these steps, you can provide valuable care for the patient until other rescuers arrive. After the arrival of additional rescuers, your role may change to assisting them in administering further care.

The second part of this chapter covers special rescue situations. These challenging situations can be life threatening to both the rescuer and the patient. Special rescue situations include water rescue, diving injuries, ice rescue, confined space rescue, farm emergencies, and bus crashes. This chapter provides you with the guidelines for handling these situations. In each situation, your first objective is to maintain your personal safety. Do not perform any rescue procedures that could endanger either yourself or the patient.

Extrication

This section describes simple techniques you can use to access, treat, and remove patients who are trapped inside crashed vehicles. As an EMR, it is essential for you to think quickly and to use the principles and guidelines that are presented here. You will also need several hours of practical exercises to become skilled in the process of **extrication**.

Your EMR course should include a demonstration of the entire extrication operation. Become familiar with extrication equipment, its use, and the hazards involved in the extrication process. You should know what equipment is available in your community and how to summon this equipment. Rescue personnel usually use extrication techniques for motor vehicle crashes, but many of these same principles are applicable in other situations. Resourcefulness, common sense, and a knowledge gained through training are key attributes of the EMR and underlie every act of patient care.

The safety of all rescuers and patients is an important consideration during the extrication process. Ideally, you should wear protective equipment similar to a firefighter's outfit: full bunker gear consisting of a coat, pants, boots, helmet with face shield, and gloves. Minimally, you should wear a helmet with a face shield or goggles and gloves.

A situation in which a patient is trapped in a motor vehicle can be complex enough to tax the skills and resources of even the most highly trained and well-equipped emergency medical services (EMS) system. To ensure the best patient care, many different agencies may need to cooperate: law enforcement, the fire department, EMS, and sometimes the utility company and a wrecker operator. It requires coordination and practice to achieve the cooperation and mutual understanding that is needed for a safe, smooth extrication effort.

As you read this section, keep in mind these basic guidelines:

- Know the limitations of your training, equipment, and skills.
- Identify any hazards (power lines, gasoline, or other **hazardous materials (HazMat)**).
- Control those hazards for which you are trained and equipped.
- Gain access to the patients.
- Provide patient care and stabilization.
- Move the patients only if absolutely necessary.

As an EMR, you have two primary extrication goals: (1) to obtain safe access to the patients and (2) to ensure patient stabilization. To achieve these goals, your role in the extrication process can be divided into the steps listed below. Think safety first so that you do not become injured. An injured rescuer becomes a second patient.

Safety

At an extrication scene, your objective is to help extricate and treat the patient efficiently, but do not rush. Moving too fast can be dangerous for you and for the patient. Experienced rescuers seldom run; they walk briskly.

As the first trained rescuer on the scene, the actions you take can make the difference between an organized and a disorganized rescue effort, perhaps even the difference between life and death! You set the stage and you have an essential role in the extrication process.

Words of Wisdom

The steps in the vehicle extrication process include the following:

1. Conduct a scene size-up or an overview of the incident and its surroundings.
2. Stabilize the scene, control any hazards, and stabilize the vehicle.
3. Gain access to the patients.
4. Provide initial emergency care.
5. Help disentangle the patients.
6. Help prepare the patients for removal.
7. Help remove the patients.

▶ Step One: Conduct a Scene Size-up

As soon as the dispatcher tells you of the incident, begin to plan for what you are likely to find on arrival. For instance, you may know that a certain type of crash frequently occurs at a particular intersection or along a specific stretch of highway. Do not, however, become complacent about responding to the "same old thing." Use your knowledge, but be flexible.

If the dispatch information is complete, you will know the types of vehicles involved (for example, two cars or a truck and motorcycle) and whether there are any injured or trapped people, burning vehicles, or HazMat present.

As you approach the scene and before you exit your vehicle, perform a scene size-up, which includes a visual overview of the entire incident and its surroundings Figure 20-1 . Remember, you must locate the patients before you can treat them! Rapidly determine the extent of the incident, estimate the number of patients, and try to locate any hazards that may be present. Then call for whatever additional resources you may need to manage the incident.

▶ Step Two: Stabilization of the Scene and Any Hazards

It is especially important to keep a sharp lookout for hazards that can result in injury, disability, or death to a patient, yourself, other emergency personnel, or bystanders. Some of the most common hazards found at motor vehicle crash scenes include infectious diseases, traffic, bystanders, spilled fuel or other HazMat, automotive batteries, downed electrical wires, unstable vehicles, and vehicle fires Figure 20-2 .

Infectious Diseases

Many patients involved in motor vehicle crashes will have soft-tissue injuries and active bleeding from open wounds or from their mouth or nose. Take standard precautions at all motor vehicle crash scenes. If sharp glass or metal is present, you should wear heavy-duty leather gloves over your latex or vinyl gloves; otherwise, vinyl or latex gloves should offer sufficient protection. If there is the danger of splattering blood, consider using face protection.

Traffic Hazards

First, park your vehicle and other emergency vehicles so that they protect the scene and warn oncoming traffic to avoid the crash site. In most situations, park your vehicle

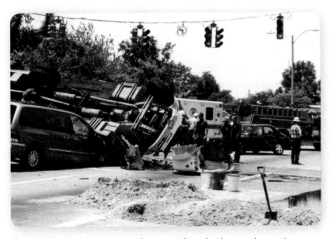

Figure 20-1 As you approach an incident, look over the entire scene.
Courtesy of District Chief Chris E. Mickal/New Orleans Fire Department, Photo Unit.

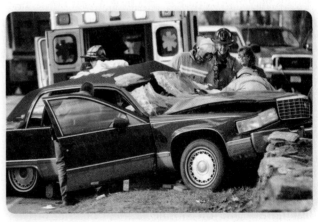

Figure 20-2 A single incident scene may contain many hazards.
© Mark C. Ide.

YOU are the Provider   CASE 1

At 2330 hours on a rainy night, you are dispatched for a report of a vehicle crash about 3 miles (5 km) from your location. As you are responding, your dispatcher tells you that this has been reported as a single vehicle crash. As you approach the scene, you note that the vehicle has struck a power pole and the pole has been sheared off close to the ground. Closer examination reveals that there are downed power lines. One power line is resting on the hood of the car. From a distance, you see one patient in the driver's seat. She appears to be dazed and slightly confused.

1. What initial actions do you need to take to stabilize the scene and ensure scene safety?
2. What other resources are needed for an incident like this?
3. What actions can you take once the scene is safe?

in a location that does not obstruct open traffic lanes, but do not hesitate to use your vehicle to block traffic to protect yourself, your patients, and other rescuers. If other emergency personnel are already on the scene, ask them where you should park your vehicle. Consider the design of your vehicle's warning lights and park so you can use them to their best advantage. Do not leave your trunk lid open after removing your emergency equipment as the lid may block your warning lights. Remember to wear an approved safety vest and other personal protective equipment.

Another way to protect the scene is to ignite **fusees** (or warning flares) as soon as possible. Place the fusees up and down the road to warn oncoming traffic and give other drivers time to slow down safely. After you have taken these protective measures, survey the scene for other hazards. Always keep fusees away from flammable liquids.

Bystanders

Keep bystanders away from the crash scene to minimize the danger to themselves and patients. It is not usually enough to ask everyone to stay away. Give specific directions such as, "Move back to the other side of the road," or "Move back onto the sidewalk." Sometimes you can pick one or two bystanders and ask them to assist you in keeping others away from the scene.

If available, either a rope or police or fire barrier tape is very effective for establishing an off-limits area. Bystanders respond appropriately to such barriers and usually will not cross them after they are set up.

Spilled Fuel

Gasoline or diesel fuel spills are common during motor vehicle crashes. Expect to find a fuel spill if a motor vehicle has been hit near the rear, is on its side, or is upside down. If a fuel spill is present (or if the vehicle is in a position that suggests a fuel spill could occur), call the fire department to minimize the fire hazard and to clean up any spilled fuel.

If the patient is trapped in a motor vehicle that is leaking fuel and the fire department has not arrived, consider covering the fuel with dirt. This reduces the amount of vapor coming from the spill, which, in turn, reduces the danger of fire. Fuel vapors tend to stay close to the ground and will travel with the wind. Be sure to call the fire department whenever you suspect a fuel spill. In addition to fuel, other potentially hazardous fluids may leak from a wrecked vehicle, including motor oil, transmission fluid, power steering fluid, and antifreeze.

Safety

Keep all sources of ignition, such as cigarettes and flares, well away from a fuel spill.

Motor Vehicle Batteries

Motor vehicle batteries are hazardous, and you must avoid contact with them. In a front-end crash, the battery may already be broken open and acid may be leaking. Reduce the possibility of an electrical short circuit by turning off the vehicle's ignition. Do not attempt to disconnect the battery unless you have received special training in the proper way to do this and have the necessary tools. You could be injured by a short circuit, explosion, or contact with battery acid. Remember that hybrid vehicles and electric vehicles have large quantities of batteries. These batteries operate at much higher voltage than regular automotive batteries and present a greater risk of electric shock. Approach hybrid and electric vehicles cautiously unless you have received special training.

Downed Electrical Wires

Downed electrical wires may be caused by high winds, ice buildup, a vehicle crashing into a utility pole, a fallen tree, or a building fire. Sometimes, downed electrical wires explode in arcs of spectacular flashes and sparks; other times, they simply lie across the vehicle, fully charged with electricity and capable of causing injury or death.

Locate the wires but avoid contact. If a vehicle has a downed wire across it and passengers are trapped inside, immediately instruct them to stay inside the vehicle. Then summon the utility company and fire department. Move bystanders back in all directions, to at least the distance between two power poles.

Do not forget that electrical hazards can come from other sources as well, including traffic light control boxes and underground power feeds. Be sure to check everywhere, including under the vehicles, for electrical hazards. However, do not attempt to manage electrical hazards at vehicle crash scenes.

Safety

Treat all downed wires as if they are charged (live) until you receive specific clearance from the electric company. Even if the lights are out along the street where the wires are down, never assume that the wires are de-energized. Be especially alert for downed wires after a storm that has blown down trees and tree limbs.

Words of Wisdom

Remember these guidelines when you encounter a motor vehicle that is in contact with electrical wires:

- If the wire is draped over the vehicle, instruct trapped persons to remain inside the vehicle. Any attempt to remove either the wire or the passengers may result in serious injury or death to yourself as well as the passengers.
- Keep all bystanders away from the vehicle.
- Call the utility company for assistance.
- Call the fire department for assistance.

Unstable Vehicles

Assume that every vehicle involved in a crash is unstable, unless you have manually stabilized it. A vehicle that is positioned on a hill, on its side, upside down, or teetering over the edge of an embankment or bridge is obviously unstable **Figure 20-3**. However, no matter how stable the vehicle appears to be, it may suddenly roll away or topple over. Be sure to check and ensure the stability of every vehicle before you attempt to enter it or treat the passengers inside.

Safety

Even vehicles that are positioned upright on all four wheels should be stabilized.

Vehicle on Its Wheels

If the vehicle is upright and on its wheels, you can ensure stability by **chocking** the front or back of each wheel with hubcaps or pieces of wood **Figure 20-4**. If you can gain access to the inside of the vehicle, place

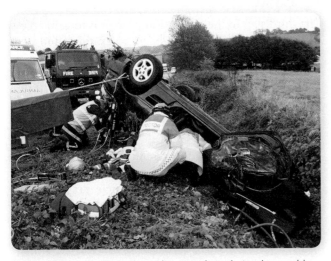

Figure 20-3 A vehicle positioned on its side is obviously unstable.
Courtesy of Mark Woolcock.

the transmission in park and set the parking brake to prevent the vehicle from moving. You can also deflate the tires by safely cutting or pulling the valve stems **Figure 20-5**.

Safety

If wooden blocks or hubcaps are not available for chocking the wheels, improvise by using materials found at the scene.

Vehicle on Its Side or Upside Down. A vehicle that is positioned on its side is extremely unstable. Fortunately, this position is unusual. Stabilizing a vehicle on its side is beyond the range of skills and equipment for many EMRs and should be handled by a specially trained rescue crew or the fire department. Many fire departments and rescue crews carry **wooden cribbing**, step chocks, or special jacks to manage this situation. If you must enter a vehicle that is on its side to respond to a life-threatening situation, do not climb on the vehicle. Carefully break the rear window glass and enter through the back of the vehicle. Bend over or crouch down to stay close to the ground. This will help prevent upsetting the vehicle's center of gravity. Your purpose is to keep the vehicle in the position found. Do not move it. Any movement could cause the vehicle to move. Gaining access to a patient is further discussed later in this chapter.

An upside-down vehicle is relatively stable. The primary hazard in this situation is spilled fuel, which must be handled by the fire department.

Vehicle Fires

Even though fires happen infrequently at motor vehicle crash sites, they are a cause of great concern among EMS personnel. There are two types of fires related to motor vehicle crashes: impact fires and postimpact fires.

Impact fires occur when the fuel tank ruptures during the crash. The vehicle is usually rapidly engulfed

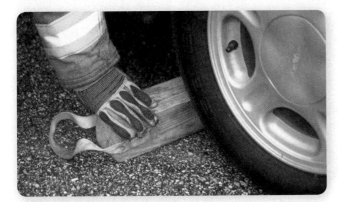

Figure 20-4 Chock the wheels.
© Jones & Bartlett Learning.

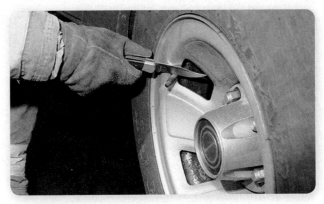

Figure 20-5 Deflate the tires to help to stabilize the vehicle.
© Jones & Bartlett Learning.

in flames, and it soon becomes impossible to approach it for a rescue attempt. Passengers rescued from this type of fire are usually saved by bystanders and witnesses to the crash who act immediately to remove them.

Postimpact fires are often caused by electrical short circuits and can be prevented by turning off the ignition, as discussed previously. These fires usually do not develop into major fires if prompt action is taken. Should a fire occur, first turn off the ignition. Then attempt to extinguish the fire with a portable fire extinguisher. Remove the passengers from the vehicle as soon as possible.

> ### Safety
>
> Be alert for vehicles that are powered by alternative fuels, which present special electrical and fire hazards. These include propane-powered vehicles, compressed natural gas-powered vehicles, battery-powered vehicles, and hybrid vehicles.

Emergency Actions for Motor Vehicle Fires. If you arrive at a crash scene and find a motor vehicle on fire with people trapped inside, remember the following procedures:

- Use your dry chemical fire extinguisher Figure 20-6 . Most dry chemical fire extinguishers can be used on ordinary combustibles, flammable liquids, or electrical fires. Be sure you know how to use the extinguisher in your vehicle.
- Immediately have someone else gather fire extinguishers from other vehicles at the scene. Do not wait until your extinguisher runs out.
- Use your extinguisher to keep flames out of the passenger compartment. Direct the extinguisher to the base of the fire—not at the passenger compartment.

- Do not be overly worried about discharging the extinguisher onto the passengers; the dry chemical powder is nontoxic. However, the dry chemical can be corrosive, so you should watch for respiratory conditions.
- Remove the patients as quickly as possible, but take care because they may have sustained injuries.
- Move everyone at least 50 feet (15 m) away from any vehicle that is on fire.
- Stay away from the front and rear ends of a burning vehicle. Modern bumpers contain air-filled cylinders that can explode forcefully when exposed to fire.

> ### Safety
>
> Do not mistake hot water vapor from a damaged radiator for smoke from an engine compartment fire. If the smoke disappears rapidly (10 feet to 15 feet [3 m to 5 m] away from the vehicle), it is probably steam and not smoke.

▶ Step Three: Gain Access to the Patients

The third step in the extrication process is to gain access to the patients. You cannot begin to examine and treat the patients until you have gained access to them. This section discusses the two methods you can use to achieve access. First, try to gain access through the doors. If this does not work, try to gain access through a window.

Access Through Doors

Before you can provide patient care, you must gain access to the patient. Between 85% and 90% of all patients involved in a motor vehicle crash can be reached simply by stabilizing the vehicle and then opening a door or window. Try all the doors first, even if they appear to be badly damaged. It is an

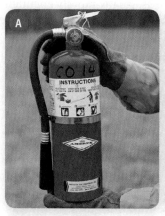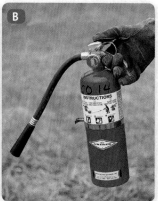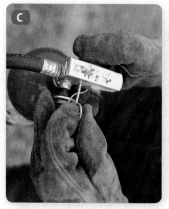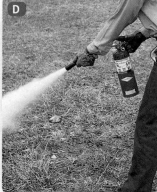

Figure 20-6 Use of a dry chemical fire extinguisher. **A.** Check the pressure gauge. **B.** Release the hose. **C.** Pull the locking pin. **D.** Discharge at the base of the fire.

embarrassing waste of time and energy to open a jammed door with heavy rescue equipment when another door can be opened easily and without any equipment. Attempt to unlock and open the least damaged door first. Make sure that the locking mechanism is released. Then try the outside and inside handles at the same time   Figure 20-7 .

Access Through Windows

If you believe that any passenger's condition is serious enough to require immediate care (for example, if the passengers are not sitting up and talking) and you cannot enter through a door, you should break a window.

Do not try to break and enter through the windshield because it is made of plastic-laminated glass   Figure 20-8 . The side and rear windows are made of **tempered glass** and will break easily into small pieces when hit with a sharp, pointed object such as a tire iron, spring-loaded center punch, or fire ax. Because these windows do not pose a safety threat, they should be your primary access route.

A spring-loaded center punch (available from many hardware stores) should be carried in your EMR life support kit   Figure 20-9 . It can be used rapidly, takes up little room in the kit, and is nearly always successful in breaking the side and rear windows on the first try.

If you must break a window to open a door or gain access, try to break one that is the farthest from the patient. However, if the patient's condition warrants your immediate entry, do not hesitate to break the closest side or rear window, even if the glass will fall onto a patient. If the patient can cover his or her own face when you are breaking glass, this may help to prevent injuries from glass shards.

> ### Words of Wisdom
>
> Remember: Try before you pry!

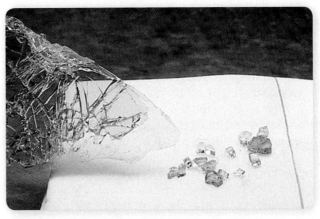

Figure 20-8 The two types of glass in vehicles are plastic-laminated glass (left) and tempered glass (right).
© Jones & Bartlett Learning. Courtesy of MIEMSS.

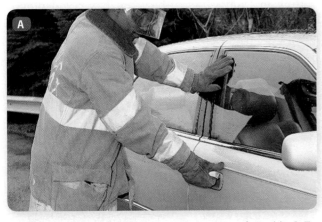 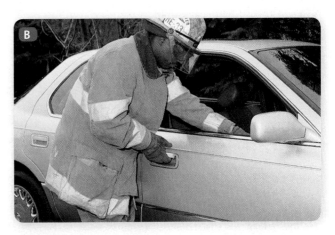

Figure 20-7 Access the vehicle through the doors, if possible. **A.** Try all doors first. **B.** Try the inside and outside handles at the same time.
A&B: © Jones & Bartlett Learning. Courtesy of MIEMSS.

YOU are the Provider   CASE 2

As you are returning to your station following a routine call, you notice tire skid marks on the road. You reduce your speed and discover a broken guardrail. You and your crew stop to investigate further. You find a sport utility vehicle (SUV) that has skidded from the roadway, catapulted through the guardrail, and traveled about 20 feet (6 m) down an embankment. The wrecked SUV is resting on the passenger side of the vehicle. A bystander says she thinks three passengers are inside.

1. What concerns you most about this scene?
2. What are the important aspects of the scene size-up for this particular scene?

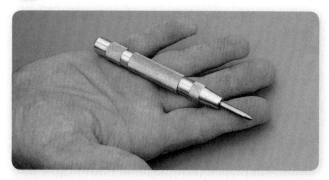

Figure 20-9 Spring-loaded center punch for breaking tempered glass.
© Jones & Bartlett Learning. Courtesy of MIEMSS.

Tempered pieces of glass do not usually pose a danger to people trapped in vehicles. Advise EMS personnel if a passenger is covered with broken glass so they can notify the hospital emergency department. If there is glass on a passenger, pick off the glass—do not brush it off.

After breaking the window, use your gloved hands to pull out the remaining glass from the window frame so it does not fall onto any passengers or injure any rescuers.

If you are using something other than a spring-loaded center punch to break the window, always aim for a lower corner. That way, the window frame will help prevent the tool (such as a tire iron, fire ax, or large screwdriver) from sailing into the vehicle and hitting the person inside.

> **Safety**
>
> Always warn trapped vehicle passengers that you are going to break the glass.

After you have broken the glass and removed the remaining pieces of glass from the frame, try to unlock the door again. Release the locking mechanism, and then use both the inside and outside door handles at the same time. This will often enable you to force a jammed locking mechanism, even in a door that appears to be badly damaged.

To access a vehicle through the window, follow the steps in **Skill Drill 20-1**:

1. Wear heavy-duty leather gloves and eye protection, if available.
2. Place the spring-loaded center punch at the lower corner of the window **Step 1** .
3. Press on the center punch to break the window **Step 2** .
4. With gloved hands, remove the broken glass to the outside of the vehicle **Step 3** .
5. Enter the vehicle through the window **Step 4** .

Using the simple techniques described and illustrated in this section, you should be able to gain access to nearly all patients involved in a motor vehicle crash, even those who are trapped in an upside-down vehicle.

When you gain access to a crashed vehicle, be alert for airbags that have not deployed. Airbags are mounted in the steering wheel on the driver's side and in the dashboard on the passenger's side. In some newer vehicles, supplemental airbags may also be mounted on the sides of the vehicle or around the rear seats. If the airbags did not deploy during the crash, they represent a hazard to rescuers because they may unexpectedly deploy and cause injuries. Avoid getting in front of an airbag that has not deployed until trained rescuers can assure you that it does not pose a hazard to you or to the patient.

Skill Drill 20-1

Accessing the Vehicle Through the Window

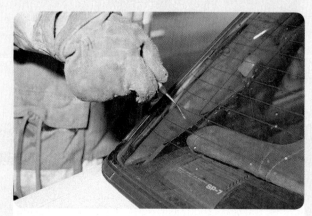

Step 1 Use a gloved hand to place the spring-loaded center punch at the lower corner of the window.

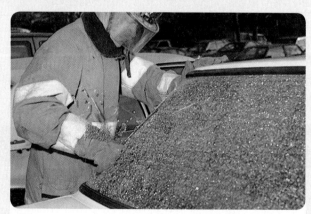

Step 2 Press on the center punch to break the window.

Skill Drill 20-1 *Continued*

Accessing the Vehicle Through the Window

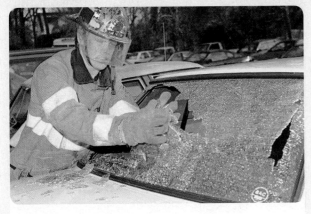

Step 3 Remove the glass to the outside of the vehicle.

© Jones & Bartlett Learning. Courtesy of MIEMSS.

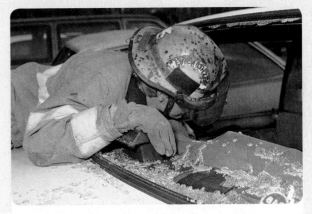

Step 4 Enter the vehicle through the window.

If you cannot gain access to the vehicle, you must do what you can to assist the patient. This means stabilizing the vehicle and protecting the scene until the proper equipment arrives.

Safety

Most cars and pickup trucks have both driver side and passenger side airbags. Some newer vehicles have supplemental airbags mounted in various places. Airbags that do not activate during a crash present a danger to rescuers until they are deactivated.

► Step Four: Initial Emergency Care

After you gain access to the passengers, immediately begin emergency medical care. Conduct a patient assessment on every patient. After you determine the status of each patient, you should monitor the ABCs (airway, breathing, and circulation), control bleeding, treat for shock, manually stabilize the cervical spine, and provide emotional support. Stay calm, and do not forget to maintain the patient's body temperature by covering the patient with a blanket. If you have time, you can conduct a secondary assessment (physical exam), as discussed in Chapter 9, *Patient Assessment*.

Leave the patients in the vehicle unless it is on fire or the patients are otherwise in immediate danger. Maintain manual stabilization until the patients are properly packaged (prepared) and can be removed from the vehicle by other trained rescuers.

Words of Wisdom

Do not forget to check the trunk of the vehicle. This step is especially important in border areas where significant numbers of illegal immigrants are transported in vehicle trunks to avoid detection **Figure 20-10**.

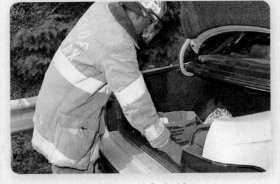

Figure 20-10 Check the trunk for hidden patients.
© Jones & Bartlett Learning. Courtesy of MIEMSS.

Skill Drill 20-2 shows how to perform initial airway management when the patient is in a vehicle:

1. Place one hand under the patient's chin and your other hand on the back of the patient's head **Step 1**.
2. Raise the patient's head to a neutral position to open the airway **Step 2**.

Skill Drill 20-2

Airway Management in a Vehicle

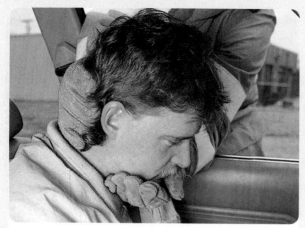

Step 1 Place one hand under the patient's chin and your other hand on the back of the patient's head.

Step 2 Raise the patient's head to a neutral position to open the airway.

© Jones & Bartlett Learning. Courtesy of MIEMSS.

▶ Step Five: Patient Disentanglement

Extrication operates on the principle of "removing the vehicle from around the patient." This process usually requires tools and specialized equipment, such as air chisels, manual or powered hydraulic rescue equipment, and airbags. In some serious extrication situations, disentanglement can take up to 30 minutes and requires advanced training   Figure 20-11 . In some situations, you can make the patient more comfortable and give yourself more room to work by carefully moving the front seat back or by raising the adjustable steering wheel.

Modern rescue crews use the concept of the Golden Hour when managing serious trauma situations. The concept of the Golden Hour (sometimes called the Golden Period) means that the less time spent at the scene with a seriously injured patient, the better. The patient's chance for survival increases if rescuers can get the patient to definitive medical care as soon as possible.

▶ Step Six: Preparation for Patient Removal

As disentanglement proceeds, help prepare the patient for removal from the vehicle by applying dressings, bandages, and splints as needed and maintaining manual stabilization of the head and cervical spine. If you are trained in the procedures and equipment for full spinal immobilization, you may be able to assist in this effort. For example, if you are properly trained and local protocols allow, you can help move and secure the patient

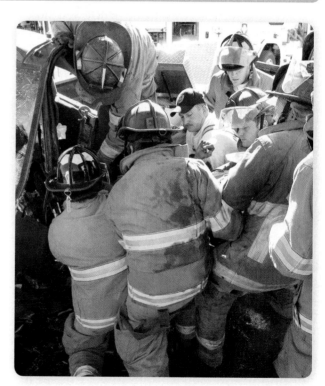

Figure 20-11 Serious entrapment situations require teamwork.
© Glen E. Ellman.

onto a long backboard for removal (see Chapter 3, *Lifting and Moving Patients*).

It is important to realize that the access route to the patient may not be adequate as an extrication route. The extrication route must be large enough to permit the safe removal of the packaged patient, whereas the access route may be relatively small.

Step Seven: Patient Removal

After the patient is packaged, he or she is removed from the vehicle and placed onto the stretcher of the transporting ambulance. Remember, although you are directly involved in only the first four of the seven extrication steps, your actions and assistance can have a vital impact on the entire operation.

▶ Review of the Extrication Process

Your familiarity with the phases of the extrication effort may enable you to assist the rescue and extrication crews. Take the time to find out about the rescue and extrication resources in your community. Ask the crews how you can assist them; they will probably be pleased to have your help and support.

Remember these steps when you arrive on the scene of a motor vehicle crash with trapped passengers:

- Call for additional resources and extrication help.
- Specify the number and types of vehicles involved.
- Do not stand idly by while waiting for help. You should:
  - Identify and contain safety hazards.
  - Park your vehicle so that its headlights and warning lights can be used to protect and light the scene.
  - Clear a working area around the site of the crash before you or rescue personnel attempt to stabilize the vehicle(s).
  - Use your head! Think and use what tools you already have.
  - Remember to try opening the doors first, rather than breaking windows.
  - After you gain access to the patient, assess and monitor his or her condition.
  - Above all, remain calm.

■ Water and Ice Rescue

You may encounter situations in which a person needs to be rescued from the water. The person may be fatigued, may have sustained an underwater diving injury, may have gotten caught in a strong current, or may have fallen through the ice in the winter. A book of this scope cannot teach you the skills of a certified lifesaver. However, the following information does describe some simple techniques you can use to perform a water or ice rescue without endangering your own safety.

▶ Water Rescue

When you see a person struggling in the water, your first impulse may be to jump in to assist. However, that action may not result in a successful rescue and can endanger your own life. If you are faced with a water rescue situation, remember to **reach, throw, row, go** Figure 20-12 . If you follow these steps, you may be able to perform a successful water rescue without entering the water. It may even be possible for someone who cannot swim to rescue a person who is drowning.

Safety

In many communities, a flash flood is a common occurrence. Flash floods occur as the result of sudden and continuing rainstorms that overwhelm the ability of streams and storm sewer systems to handle the runoff. Flash floods may cause water to quickly flow over roadways in low-lying areas. Most rescues during floods occur because motorists drive into low-lying areas that are flooded. Be cautious about driving through standing water, and be aware of the dangers posed by floodwaters that cover roadways. These floodwaters can contain strong currents and can be deadly. Do not venture into floodwaters without proper training and equipment.

Reach

Use any readily available object to reach the distressed person in the water. If the person is close to shore, a branch, pole, oar, or paddle may be long enough. If you are at a swimming pool, there may be a specially designed pole available for this purpose. Use it.

Throw

If you cannot reach the person, throw something that can float or that the victim can grab. At a swimming pool, dock, or supervised beach, a **flotation device** (such as a ring buoy) may be available. If a flotation device is

YOU are the Provider   CASE 3

You respond to the scene of a vehicle that has rolled over. The dispatcher informs you that the vehicle landed on its roof and two passengers are trapped inside. When you arrive at the scene, you find a minivan on its roof. As you approach the vehicle, you determine that the scene is safe and the vehicle is stable. You notice two patients in the vehicle; both appear unresponsive.

1. What could you do to assist in the extrication of these patients before rescue arrives?
2. What are the steps for using a spring-loaded center punch?

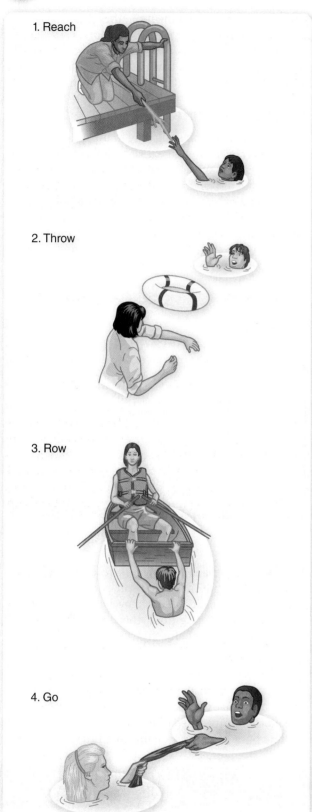

1. Reach

2. Throw

3. Row

4. Go

Figure 20-12 The rules for water rescue.
© Jones & Bartlett Learning.

available, throw it to the person in distress. Some public safety departments carry a specially constructed **rescue throw bag** that contains a rope that can be thrown to a distressed person in the water. If your department carries a throw rope, you need instruction and practice in its

use. If no buoy or throw bag is available, improvise. Throw a rope, plastic milk jug, or a sealed polystyrene plastic (Styrofoam) cooler. Even a spare tire can support several people in the water.

> ### Words of Wisdom
>
> If you use something like a plastic milk jug or picnic jug to throw to a person in the water, fill the container with about 1 inch (3 cm) of water to add weight before you seal it and throw it to the person.

Row

If you cannot reach the person by throwing something that floats, you may be able to row out to the drowning person if a small boat or canoe is available. Consider this option only if you know how to operate or propel the craft properly. Protect yourself by wearing an approved personal flotation device.

> ### Safety
>
> Currents in streams or strong currents (**riptides**) at ocean beaches can pull both the distressed person and the rescuer rapidly away from shore. In an area below a dam, rapids, or a waterfall, deadly currents may be present. Never attempt to enter the water under these conditions if you are untrained. If you do, it is likely that both you and the distressed person will need to be rescued.

Go

As a last resort, you may have to go into the water to save the person. Enter the water only if you are a capable swimmer trained in lifesaving techniques. Remove heavy clothing before entering the water. Take a flotation device with you if one is available.

▶ Initial Treatment of a Person in the Water

If you are involved in a water rescue situation, your primary concerns for the patient are to open an airway, establish breathing and circulation, and stabilize the head and neck in case of spinal cord injuries. Turn a patient faceup who is facedown in the water **Skill Drill 20-3** :

1. Support the back and head with one hand and place your other hand on the front of the patient to keep the head and neck stabilized **Step 1** .
2. Keep the head in the neutral position and carefully turn the patient as a unit **Step 2** .
3. Stabilize the patient's head and neck **Step 3** .

Skill Drill 20-3

Turning a Patient in the Water

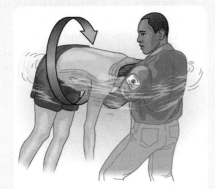
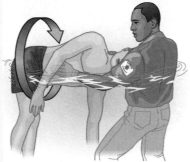
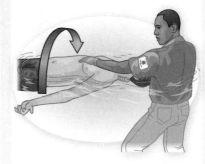

Step 1 Support the back and head with one hand. Place your other hand on the front of the patient.

Step 2 Carefully turn the patient as a unit.

Step 3 Stabilize the patient's head and neck.

© Jones & Bartlett Learning.

Use the jaw-thrust maneuver to open the airway. Do not hyperextend the neck because of the high risk of associated spinal cord injuries. Look, listen, and feel for signs of breathing. If the patient is not breathing, start rescue breathing while the patient is still in the water Figure 20-13. Ventilation will be much easier if you can stand on the bottom of the body of water.

If the patient has experienced cardiac arrest, quickly stabilize the head and neck, and remove the patient from the water. Place the patient on a hard surface before you begin cardiopulmonary resuscitation (CPR) (see Chapter 8, *Professional Rescuer CPR*).

Treat a patient who is unconscious in the water as if a spinal cord injury was present. Also assume the presence of a spinal cord injury if a conscious patient in the water reports numbness or tingling in the arms or legs, is unable to move the extremities, or reports neck pain.

Support the patient by floating a backboard in the water under the patient Figure 20-14. Strap the patient to the backboard, stabilize the head and neck, and remove the patient from the water. If a rigid device is unavailable and the patient must be removed from the water before EMS personnel arrive, six people can lift and support the patient using their hands Figure 20-15.

Words of Wisdom

If a backboard is unavailable, you can use a chaise lounge, door, or piece of plywood to provide rigid support under the patient. One rescuer should give the commands to lift, move, and set down the patient.

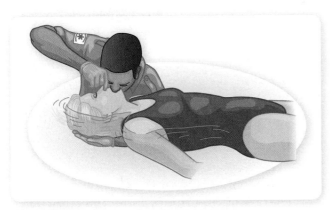

Figure 20-13 Begin rescue breathing in the water.
© Jones & Bartlett Learning.

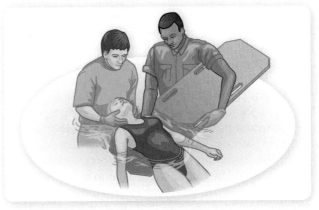

Figure 20-14 Apply the backboard while the patient is still in the water.
© Jones & Bartlett Learning.

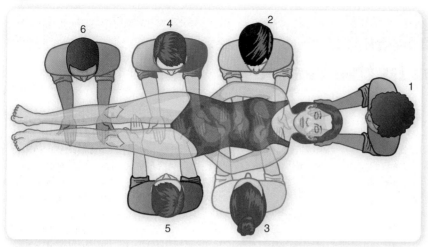

Figure 20-15 In emergency situations, a patient can be removed from the water using six people.
© Jones & Bartlett Learning.

► Diving Injuries

As an EMR, you may be called to care for people who are injured while diving. Most recreational divers use self-contained underwater breathing apparatus (scuba). Scuba gear consists of an air tank, a regulator, a mouthpiece, and a face mask. Commercial divers use either scuba gear or equipment that supplies air through a hose.

Most underwater diving emergencies occur in coastal regions or in areas with large lakes. Diving injuries can cause trauma, near drowning, or specialized injuries. In situations involving trauma or drowning, remove the patient from the water and treat the patient using information and skills you have already learned.

Two specialized injuries are associated with diving: **air embolism** and **decompression sickness (the bends)**. Usually, it will not be possible for you to differentiate between these two conditions. Both are caused by air bubbles being released in the body as a result of the changes in pressure while diving. If an air bubble affects the brain or spinal cord, the signs and symptoms may be similar to those of a stroke. These include dizziness, difficulty speaking, difficulty seeing, and a decreased level of consciousness. The patients may have difficulty in maintaining an open airway. If the air bubble causes a collapsed lung, the signs and symptoms will include chest pain, shortness of breath, and pink or bloody froth coming from the mouth or nose. If the air bubble obstructs blood flow to the abdomen, the patient will experience severe abdominal pain and may be bent over. If the air bubble involves a joint, there will be severe pain in that joint.

To treat a patient with a suspected air embolism or decompression sickness, maintain the patient's airway, breathing, circulation, and normal body temperature. Oxygen should be administered as soon as it is available. Only administer oxygen if you have received the proper training and have the approval of your medical director. Some physicians recommend placing the patient on his or her left side with the head of the patient slightly lowered. This may help to prevent further damage if there is an air bubble in the central nervous system. A patient with diving injuries may need to be transported to a hospital that is equipped with a hyperbaric (recompression) chamber. If you live in an area where diving injuries occur, you should receive specialized training and be familiar with the local protocols of your EMS system.

► Ice Rescue

Ice rescue is extremely hazardous because ice is changeable and should always be considered unsafe. Think safety first; do not exceed the limits of your training and do not put yourself at undue risk. You cannot save anyone if you fall through the ice yourself. As soon as you arrive at the scene of an ice rescue, visually mark the location where the person was last seen. This will enable other rescuers to concentrate their efforts on a limited area. Know who is responsible for ice rescue in your community and call this team as soon as possible.

The basic rules of ice rescue are the same as water rescue: reach, throw, row, go. Reach for the person using anything that will extend your natural stretch, such as a ladder, a pike pole, a tree branch, or a backboard. Next, throw a flotation device, throw rope, or anything that floats to pull in the person. Third, row or propel a small boat to the person if you can break through the ice, or use a toboggan to get across the ice. Using a toboggan will spread your weight over a wider area and reduce your chances of falling through the ice. Be sure that you have a rope and that the boat or toboggan is secured to the shore as well. Finally, if you must go, secure yourself to shore with a rope around your waist, lie on your stomach, and proceed across the ice. Spreading your weight over a wider area reduces your chances of falling through the ice **Figure 20-16** . Maintain good communication with other rescuers.

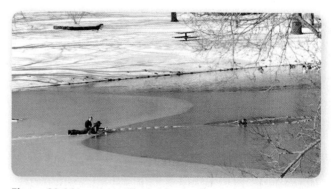

Figure 20-16 Ice rescue. The ladder distributes the rescuer's weight over a larger area, making it less likely that he or she will also fall into the water.
© Chris Rush, Bartlesville Examiner-Enterprise/AP Photo.

A motor vehicle on the ice presents a risky situation. Instruct the vehicle's occupants to avoid unnecessary movement. If the vehicle has not gone through the ice, instruct the occupants to open the vehicle's doors. This may help to slow the sinking of the vehicle if the ice breaks. If the doors cannot be opened, instruct the occupants to open the windows so they have a better escape route. If you must approach the vehicle, remember that the added weight of rescuers can cause movement of the vehicle. Do not place your head inside the vehicle because if it sinks, you may be unable to get out.

During ice rescues, both the people on the ice or in the water and the rescuers are at risk for hypothermia. Keep all rescuers as warm as possible. Rescue personnel who are not directly involved in the rescue operation should remain in a warm vehicle until they are needed. Remove wet clothing from rescued people, and dry off and warm them as soon as possible after they are removed from the water. Remember that people can survive for an extended period of time in cold water. If the patient has no pulse, start CPR and continue until the patient has been transported to a hospital. See Chapter 13, *Environmental Emergencies*, for more information on treating hypothermia.

Confined Space Rescue

Confined spaces are structures designed to keep something in or out. Confined spaces may be below ground, ground level, or elevated structures. Below-ground confined spaces include manholes, utility vaults or storage tanks, old mines, cisterns, and wells. Ground-level confined spaces include industrial tanks and farm storage silos. Elevated confined spaces include water towers and storage tanks.

Rescue situations involving confined spaces have two deadly hazards. The first hazard is respiratory. The confined space may have insufficient oxygen to support life, or it may be filled with a poisonous gas **Figure 20-17**. Never enter a confined space without the proper respiratory protection or else you risk becoming a patient yourself.

The second hazard in a confined space is the danger of collapse. In a mine, for example, rescuers may need to shore up (support) the confined space before they can safely enter. Confined space rescue requires a specially trained team. As soon as you determine there is a confined space situation, call for additional assistance and do not enter the space until help arrives.

If a worker in a confined space begins to feel sick because of a lack of oxygen or the presence of a poisonous gas, coworkers may assume the worker is having a heart attack. Therefore, the call you receive may be for a "sick person." When you arrive on the scene, take time to assess the scene carefully. If a patient is in a confined space, do not enter unless you are trained in confined space rescue and have adequate respiratory equipment to work in this deadly environment. Otherwise, wait for properly equipped and specially trained personnel to access, treat, and remove the patient.

> **Safety**
>
> More rescuers than patients die in confined space incidents. According to the Centers for Disease Control and Prevention, more than 60% of all deaths in confined space incidents involve rescuers. Do not enter a confined space without proper breathing apparatus and special training.

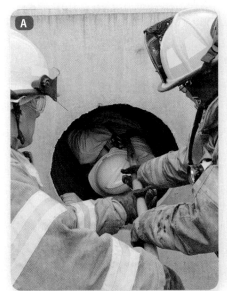
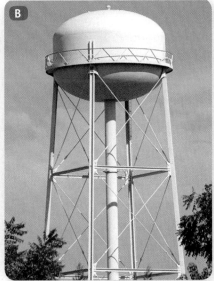
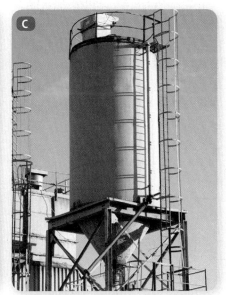

Figure 20-17 Confined spaces may have insufficient oxygen to support life without the use of a self-contained breathing apparatus.
A: © Jones & Bartlett Learning; B: © Harris Shiffman/Shutterstock; C: © Joe Gough/Shutterstock.

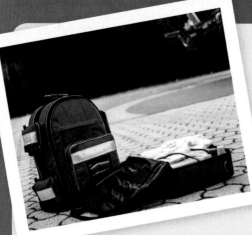

Voices *of* Experience

The call came in as a possible back injury. It seemed to be a routine call on an average day at a large manufacturing facility where I was working part time as a paramedic in the medical clinic. Routine, that is, until I found out that the patient was three stories high on a remote part of the roof with limited access. The report came from a coworker stating that an electrician had fallen approximately 15 feet (5 m) from a scaffold, striking a large pipe on the way to the roof.

> **" With everyone's help the patient was placed on oxygen, his fracture splinted, and a full spinal package completed. "**

En route to the scene, I met the plant safety officer. He told me that there was some confusion as to the exact location of the injured person and he was not sure which access would get us there. Because of the unknowns of the call and the access problems, we decided to call our local fire/rescue department; they are well trained in unusual patient evacuations. Meanwhile, I was on the radio with the coworker, trying to find out the status of the patient.

Fortunately, at this facility we have security personnel who are cross-trained as EMRs. The next report received was from a security/EMR staff member who had just arrived at the scene. He was able to tell us which access point to use and gave me a report stating that the patient was lying supine with a reduced level of consciousness. At this time, he was only responding to verbal stimulation. He had an open airway with no obvious bleeding. The secondary assessment showed a possible fracture to the left lower leg with stable vital signs.

I arrived at the scene along with two other security/EMR personnel. They had the long backboard, spinal packaging equipment, and a Stokes litter. My rapid trauma assessment found the patient just as the first EMR had reported. By now fire and rescue personnel had arrived and began to set up a vertical lower off the side of the structure. With everyone's help the patient was placed on oxygen, his fracture splinted, and a full spinal package completed. The patient was placed in the Stokes litter and successfully lowered as the EMS unit waited. He was transported to a local trauma center where he was treated and had a complete recovery from his injuries.

This was a great example, showing that having well-trained EMRs available with a good incident command system in place and local mutual aid response can lead to the best possible outcome for the patient.

Russ L. Miller, WEMT-Paramedic
Instructor/Coordinator
Past EMS Program Director, Cleveland State Community College
Director, Wilderness Safety Consultants
Delano, Tennessee

Farm Rescue

Farms are located in most parts of the country. They range from a few acres of land with limited machinery and a small number of animals to large complexes that contain many acres of land, heavy-duty machinery, and large animals. Farm emergencies pose a wide variety of challenges for rescuers. Because many farmers work by themselves, the reporting of emergencies may be delayed. Once notification of an incident is received, there may be a lengthy response in getting to a farm. After rescuers arrive at a farm, it may be hard to pinpoint the exact location of the emergency. Poorly maintained roads, nonexistent roads, and muddy soil may require you to leave your vehicle some distance from the patient. All of these factors can delay your response in getting to the patient.

Farms contain a wide variety of hazards. Animals can seriously injure farmers and pose a serious risk to rescuers. Be alert for the dangers posed by animals. Also, farms contain a wide range of chemicals that can be hazardous. These include pesticides, herbicides (weed-killing chemicals), and fertilizers such as anhydrous ammonia. Any of these chemicals, if improperly handled, can create a dangerous situation for farmers and rescuers. HazMat incidents are not always on highways. Additional information regarding pesticides can be found in Chapter 11, *Poisoning and Substance Abuse*. In addition, farms use a large number of electrically powered machines. Be alert for the shock hazard posed by the presence of electrical lines and electrical devices on any part of a farm.

Some injuries involve tall barns or silos and often require rescuers who are trained in high-angle rescue techniques Figure 20-18 . Some farm silos are sealed and are designed to operate in an oxygen-deficient atmosphere. Always treat silos as a hazardous confined space. Under certain conditions, gases given off by the contents of a silo can explode. Some farms also contain below-grade manure storage pits. These pits may be filled with poisonous gases or be deficient in oxygen. Do not enter any confined space or enclosed below-grade structure without proper self-contained breathing apparatus and proper training.

Farms also contain a wide variety of machinery. Machinery is used in every step of growing crops and raising animals. Accidents with farm machinery usually involve rollovers of farm tractors, entrapment in machinery, or severing of body tissue by sharp objects

Figure 20-19 . Tractor rollovers are more common with older tractors, which do not have roll bars or reinforced cabs. Rollovers most commonly occur on steep slopes and often result in the operator being pinned beneath

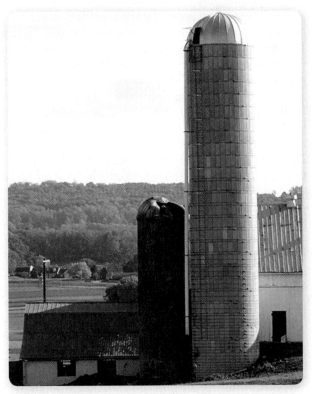

Figure 20-18 Farm silos represent high-angle hazards, confined space hazards, and explosive hazards.
© Nancy Hixson/Shutterstock.

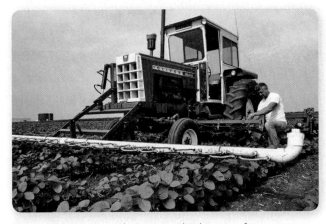

Figure 20-19 Farm machinery is involved in many farm rescue situations.
Courtesy of Lynn Betts/NRCS.

YOU are the Provider   CASE 4

You are dispatched to an emergency at a farm. On arrival at the scene, you are told a man was working outside when he heard an explosion inside the silo. He reports three people were inside the silo at the time of the explosion. You notice smoke coming from the silo.

1. What additional resources will you potentially need at this scene?
2. What are the potential hazards associated with farm rescue incidents?

the tractor. Entrapments can occur with a number of crop-harvesting equipment or mechanized animal feeding systems. Power take-off systems can catch clothing and can quickly entrap a person.

As an EMR, your role in farm rescues consists of stabilizing the scene and providing initial medical care for the patient. Follow the seven steps of extrication Table 20-1 . Perform a careful scene size-up to determine the scope of the incident. Shut off any electric power and turn off any machinery that is still running, if possible. Call for adequate assistance from fire, rescue, and EMS organizations. In some communities, rescue personnel use farm implement mechanics for assistance with complex farm rescues. Helicopter transport of the patient may be beneficial. Remember, it is better to call for help and not need it than it is to delay adequate help from arriving at the scene.

Stabilize any hazards that you can while keeping yourself and the patient safe. Realize that you do not have the training and equipment to stabilize all rescue scenes. If possible, gain access to the patient. Provide initial emergency care to the patient: establish responsiveness, support the patient's ABCs, control bleeding, and maintain the patient's body temperature. It is important to talk with the patient and provide emotional support. As other rescuers arrive on the scene, help them to disentangle the patient, prepare the patient for removal, and remove the patient.

Your actions at a farm rescue incident can make a lifesaving difference to the patient. Farm rescues can be challenging, but they require you to follow the same steps of patient care and extrication that you would use for other types of emergencies. Above all, remember your safety and the safety of the patient.

Bus Rescue

Buses operate in most communities. School buses transport students to school and to school-sponsored events. Cities operate fleets of municipal buses over established routes. Charter buses transport people of all ages to special events and on vacation trips. Specially equipped buses transport people with limited mobility. Interstate buses transport people all over the country.

Because of the large numbers of people being transported by buses, significant potential exists for bus crashes to occur in any community. Bus crashes range from minor incidents with no injuries to **mass-casualty incidents**; therefore, you need to understand some guidelines for providing care to patients involved in bus crashes. A mass-casualty incident refers to any accident or situation involving more patients than you can handle with the initial resources available.

If you are an EMR at a bus crash, perform a scene size-up or an overview of the scene and call for adequate police, fire, and EMS resources. Establish an incident command system if there are multiple casualties. Set up a one-way traffic pattern for responding vehicles to avoid congestion and gridlock at the emergency scene. For example, you might direct all responding emergency vehicles to approach the scene from the east and depart the scene traveling toward the west. If multiple patients must be removed from a bus, pass equipment into the bus through one door or window and remove the patients through a second door or window. This will improve the efficiency of the extrication process. If confronted with a large number of patients, triage the patients using the START triage system. This system is used for sorting and treating patients in mass-casualty situations. The START triage system is explained in Chapter 21, *Incident Management.*

You are not expected to handle the command functions at a bus crash involving multiple casualties. However, you may be the only trained person on the scene for the first several minutes of an incident. Knowing some of the basic elements of handling this type of incident will help to improve the efficiency and effectiveness of the care given to the patients Figure 20-20 .

Table 20-1	The Seven Steps of Extrication

1. Conduct a scene size-up or an overview of the incident and its surroundings and call for sufficient help.
2. Stabilize the scene, control any hazards, and stabilize the vehicle.
3. Gain access to the patients, if possible.
4. Provide initial emergency care.
5. Help disentangle the patients.
6. Help prepare the patients for removal.
7. Help remove the patients.

© Jones & Bartlett Learning.

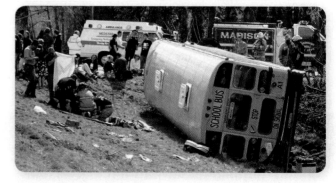

Figure 20-20 A bus crash requires an effective incident command system.
© Dena Libner, The Conway Daily Sun/AP Photo.

You are the Provider: CASE 1

1. What initial actions do you need to take to stabilize the scene and ensure scene safety?

Your first actions on the scene of an emergency incident should be to keep yourself and other rescuers safe and to ensure the safety of patients and bystanders at the scene. In this case, your active overview of the scene has determined that there are downed power lines, which create a deadly hazard for rescuers and for the patient. EMRs are not equipped or trained to determine if these lines are energized with electricity. Therefore, you must assume they are a life threat to the patient and to rescuers. One of your first actions after determining that there are power lines down is to notify dispatch that you need an emergency response from the power utility to disconnect the power to these wires. In addition, remember that downed lines present a hazard to motorists and bystanders entering the area. This is especially true under conditions of dark and inclement weather. Because your patient appears to be dazed and slightly confused, it is especially important talk with her from a safe location and instruct her to stay in her car until it has been confirmed that the downed wires are safe. Take steps to ensure that there is adequate traffic control to prevent drivers from entering the hazard area and that adequate resources have been requested to handle the situation.

2. What other resources are needed for an incident like this?

This incident represents a somewhat complex situation that requires additional resources. The additional resources needed include the following: the electric power utility company, emergency medical providers with transport capabilities, adequate law enforcement resources to handle traffic control, fire department to address fire hazards, and a rescue company if extrication services will be needed to remove the patient from the vehicle. Even though it is not possible to begin patient care and extrication until the electric wires have been rendered safe, it is important to get all needed resources en route to the scene as soon as possible. Remember that as a first responder you will often be the eyes and ears of your dispatcher. They will not always know what is needed until you give them an assessment of the conditions on the scene.

3. What actions can you take once the scene is safe?

Once the power has been rendered safe by the electric utility company and the traffic flow has been controlled, it is safe for you to begin the steps needed to further stabilize the scene and to begin to care for the patient and

to extricate her if necessary. In this situation, this might include the following steps:

1. Control any additional hazards.
2. Stabilize the vehicle to keep it from moving.
3. Gain access to the patient, if possible. Try the doors first; if access is not possible through a door, consider breaking and entering through a window to remove the patient.
4. Provide initial emergency care, spinal stabilization, external bleeding control, and maintaining body temperature.
5. Help disentangle the patient.
6. Help prepare the patient for removal.
7. Help remove the patient.
8. In the event that the patient is in continuing danger by remaining in the vehicle, it might be necessary to rapidly remove her from a position of danger.

For each rescue situation you will need to determine which steps you can undertake safely and how much you can do, but in general these same principles apply to help determine what actions you can take once the scene is safe.

You are the Provider: CASE 2

1. What concerns you most about this scene?

Unlike when you are officially dispatched to an emergency, you have discovered an unreported incident and do not have any information about it from your dispatcher. Your first step is to park your vehicle in a safe place where it protects the scene as much as possible from oncoming traffic. If other responders are with you, coordinate your activities with them. Based on your overview of this scene and information from the bystander, you have enough information to call dispatch and report that you are out of service at the scene of a vehicle crash. You will probably need law enforcement personnel for traffic control, EMS units to provide care and transportation for three patients, an extrication crew to remove the patients from the SUV, and additional personnel to help transport the patients up the embankment. Because there is an increased chance of flammable fluids escaping from the overturned SUV, you should also request fire suppression units although in most jurisdictions they are included in the response to all motor vehicle collisions with reports of injury. At some point, a tow truck (wrecker) operator will be needed to retrieve and remove the damaged vehicle. To provide the best possible care for these patients, request additional resources as soon as possible and get them en route to your location. After a more thorough overview of the scene, you may determine that some of those units will not be needed, at which time you can notify your dispatcher to

YOU are the Provider **SUMMARY** *Continued*

cancel their response. The additional units can return to service before they arrive on the scene.

2. What are the important aspects of the scene size-up for this particular scene?

Your first priority is to immediately identify any threat to your safety, other responders, and bystanders. In this case, realize that most overturned vehicles are unstable. As an EMR, you may not have the resources necessary to stabilize this vehicle before the arrival of additional resources. Sometimes you can help conscious patients to extricate themselves. At other times you may be able to use improvised resources to stabilize the vehicle. However, do not forget that the best course of action may be to wait for further assistance before attempting to enter an unstable, overturned vehicle, which would make the situation worse and endanger your own safety and potentially that of the patients. As mentioned previously, survey the scene and the patient(s) for the mechanism of injury and determine the need for additional resources. Determine the possible number of patients, and verify the appropriate EMS response. In addition, remember to treat every patient as potentially infectious and take standard precautions to prevent any exposure to blood or body fluids.

You are the Provider: CASE 3

1. What could you do to assist in the extrication of these patients before rescue arrives?

Because these two patients are unresponsive, consider them to be in critical condition. You have determined that the scene is safe and the vehicle is stable; therefore, attempt to gain access to the patients. Attempt to open the doors. Entrance through open windows is also an option. If the doors cannot be opened and the windows are closed, consider breaking a window with a spring-loaded center punch. Use caution when performing this task. The breaking of glass can cause injury to you and the patients. You should break the window that is farthest away from the patients.

2. What are the steps for using a spring-loaded center punch?

1. Wear heavy-duty leather gloves and eye protection, if available.
2. Place the spring-loaded center punch at the lower corner of the window.

3. Press on the center punch to break the window.
4. With gloved hands, remove the broken glass to the outside of the vehicle.
5. Enter the vehicle through the window.

You are the Provider: CASE 4

1. What additional resources will you potentially need at this scene?

Someone reported an explosion and smoke is coming from the silo; therefore fire suppression apparatus and personnel will be needed at the scene. Farms use a wide variety of chemicals in their operations, so be alert for the presence of pesticides, herbicides, and fertilizers, which may indicate the need for a HazMat team. This incident involves an enclosed silo, which means that you are dealing with a confined space rescue. Because no one should enter a confined space without proper training and self-contained breathing apparatus, a properly trained rescue crew is needed. You also need to be alert for electrical hazards, the need for ladders to access the silo, and the presence of dangerous equipment. Electric power needs to be disabled before rescue personnel begin operations. As with any emergency, request a sufficient number of EMS units for patient care and transportation. If the farm is located a long distance from an appropriate medical facility, you may need to request helicopter transport. While the rescue efforts progress, continue to monitor the operation for any additional resources that are needed.

2. What are the potential hazards associated with farm rescue incidents?

Farms are a major source of hazards for emergency workers. During your scene size-up, consider the presence of chemicals such as pesticides, herbicides, and fertilizers, which are commonly used on farms. Farmers also use heavy equipment with specialized functions. Unless you are trained to handle farm equipment or have received specialized rescue training, keep a safe distance from the equipment until trained help arrives and the power to this equipment has been disabled. In addition to their specialized functions, farm equipment is extremely heavy. Additional care needs to be taken when stabilizing these pieces of machinery before rescue attempts are made. Finally, whenever operating around a farm scene, be alert for animals that may be close to you.

Prep Kit

▶ Ready for Review

- As an emergency medical responder, you should be able to perform the first four steps in the extrication process and assist other rescuers with steps five through seven.
- Water rescue, ice rescue, underwater diving injuries, confined space rescue, farm rescue, and bus crashes are situations that require extensive skills and special training. It is important to help the patient, but not at the expense of your own safety.
- In water and ice rescue situations, there are four simple steps you can take to help the person without endangering yourself: reach out to the person with an object, throw a flotation device to the person, row to the person in a boat, or go to the person if you are adequately trained to do so (reach, throw, row, go).
- You may not be able to distinguish between the two major medical emergencies created by underwater diving incidents (air embolism and decompression sickness), but you can provide basic care and summon appropriate assistance.
- In confined space rescue, your primary goals are to call for additional assistance and prevent other people, including yourself, from becoming patients.
- Farm emergencies and bus crashes are complex rescue situations; however, if you follow simple steps, you can often stabilize these situations and provide initial aid to patients.

▶ Vital Vocabulary

air embolism A bubble of air obstructing a blood vessel.

chocking Placing a piece of wood or metal in front of or behind a wheel to prevent vehicle movement.

decompression sickness (the bends) A condition seen in divers in which gas, especially nitrogen, forms bubbles in blood vessels, obstructing them.

entrapment To be caught (trapped) within a vehicle, room, or container with no way out or to have a limb or other body part trapped.

extrication Removal from a difficult situation or position; removal of a patient from a wrecked vehicle or other place of entrapment.

flotation device A life ring, life buoy, or other floating device used in water rescue.

fusees Warning devices or flares that burn with a red color; usually used in scene protection at motor vehicle crash sites.

Golden Hour A concept of emergency patient care that attempts to place a trauma patient into definitive medical care in the shortest period of time to achieve the best possible outcome; also called the Golden Period.

hazardous materials (HazMat) Substances that are toxic, poisonous, radioactive, flammable, or explosive and can cause injury or death with exposure.

mass-casualty incidents Accidents or situations involving more patients than you can handle with the initial resources available.

reach, throw, row, go A sequence of four actions that should be taken in water rescue situations.

rescue throw bag A water rescue device consisting of a small cloth bag and a waterproof rope used for rescuing people from the water.

riptide Unusually strong surface currents flowing outward from a seashore that can present a hazard to swimmers.

tempered glass Safety glass that breaks into small pieces when hit with a sharp, pointed object.

wooden cribbing Wooden boards (either 2 inch × 4 inch [5 cm × 10 cm] or 4 inch × 4 inch [10 cm × 10 cm] used for vehicle stabilization or bracing.

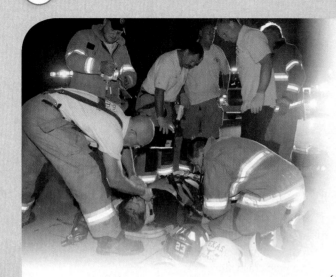

Assessment
in Action

You are dispatched to the intersection of Shelbourne Falls Road and State Route 324 for a motor vehicle crash. On arrival, you find a small pickup truck that has struck a utility pole. The power line is resting on the roof of the truck. Two occupants are in the vehicle. Both appear to be conscious and alert. It appears there is smoke coming from a nearby utility pole. (Questions 1 to 3 relate to this scenario.)

1. What is your first step in this situation?

   A. Perform a scene size-up.
   B. Call for additional assistance.
   C. Assess the patient's ABCs (airway, breathing, and circulation).
   D. Begin removing the patients from the vehicle.

2. What additional resources would probably not be needed at this scene?

   A. Electric company
   B. Hazardous materials (HazMat) team
   C. Fire department
   D. Additional ambulance

3. What is the greatest hazard at this scene?

   A. Battery acid
   B. Transmission fluid
   C. Fuel leakage
   D. Live power line

You and your family are at the local swimming pool enjoying a break from the summer heat when you notice two boys playing near the shallow end of the pool. A few minutes later, you hear a boy screaming, "Scott fell into the pool and hit his head on the bottom step! Help!" As you approach the side of the pool, you see a young boy floating with his face down in the pool. (Questions 4 through 10 relate to this scenario.)

4. What is your first priority in the treatment of this patient?

   A. Remove the patient from the water.
   B. Establish an airway.
   C. Turn the patient over.
   D. Begin chest compressions.

5. Performing rescue breathing on the patient while still in the water is easiest if:

   A. the patient is smaller than you.
   B. you can stand on the bottom.
   C. you are an expert swimmer.
   D. you are using a flotation device.

6. When opening your patient's airway, what maneuver should you use?

   A. Head tilt–chin lift
   B. Head tilt–jaw thrust
   C. Jaw thrust
   D. Head tilt–neck lift

7. What are the steps for turning the patient so that he is facing up?

8. After the patient is out of the water, how would you assess this patient?

9. If this patient is in cardiac arrest, what special precautions do you need to take when using an automated external defibrillator (AED)?

10. If a backboard is not available for use with this patient, what are possible substitutions?

Incident Management

National EMS Education Standard Competencies

EMS Operations

Knowledge of operational roles and responsibilities to ensure safe patient, public, and personnel safety.

Incident Management

> Establish and work within the incident management system. (pp 439–442)

Mass-Casualty Incidents

> Triage principles (pp 437–440)
> Resource management (pp 436–437; pp 439–442)

Hazardous Materials Awareness

> Risks and responsibilities of operating in a cold zone at a hazardous materials or other special incident. (pp 434–435)

Mass-Casualty Incidents due to Terrorism and Disaster

> Risks and responsibilities of operating on the scene of a natural or man-made disaster. (pp 439–443; pp 445–449)

Knowledge Objectives

1. State the responsibilities of emergency medical responders (EMRs) in incidents where hazardous materials are present. (pp 434–435)
2. Describe the actions EMRs should take in hazardous materials incidents before the arrival of specially trained personnel. (pp 434–435)

3. Discuss the different areas of a hazardous materials scene. (p 435)
4. Define a mass-casualty incident. (pp 435–436)
5. Describe the role of EMRs in a mass-casualty incident. (pp 435–440)
6. Explain the steps in the START triage system. (pp 438–440)
7. Describe the purpose of the National Incident Management System. (p 441)
8. Define terrorism and weapons of mass destruction. (p 442)
9. Describe potential terrorist targets and risks. (pp 442–443)
10. Explain the risks posed by explosives and incendiary devices. (p 443; p 445)
11. Explain the risks posed by the following chemical agents:
    - Pulmonary agents (p 445)
    - Metabolic agents (p 445)
    - Insecticides (pp 445–446)
    - Nerve agents (p 446)
    - Blister agents (p 446)
12. Explain the risks posed by biologic agents. (pp 446–447)
13. Explain the risks posed by radiologic agents. (p 448)
14. Describe the role of EMRs in a terrorist event. (p 449)

Skills Objectives

1. Demonstrate the actions EMRs should take in hazardous materials incidents before the arrival of specially trained personnel. (pp 434–435)
2. Demonstrate triage of a mass-casualty incident using the START triage system. (pp 437–439)

Introduction

This chapter covers hazardous materials incidents, mass-casualty incidents, the National Incident Management System (NIMS), and terrorism awareness. You should be able to identify the signs of a hazardous materials incident and prevent injury to yourself and to others in the first minutes of the incident. Because you may be called to assist with a mass-casualty incident, you should understand the purpose of an incident management system and the framework of the NIMS. Your knowledge of basic triage and your ability to use the START triage system are also important.

The last section of this chapter is designed to increase your awareness of terrorism. In addition to defining terrorism, you will learn the types of structures terrorists might target and how terrorists might use explosive, incendiary, chemical, biologic, and radiologic agents to cause mass destruction. You will also learn the importance of safety, preparedness, and the use of the incident command system (ICS).

Hazardous Materials Incidents

Hazardous materials (HazMat) are any substances that are toxic, poisonous, radioactive, flammable, or explosive and can cause injury or death with exposure. During a HazMat incident, your top priority is to protect yourself and bystanders from exposure and contamination.

A very important step when handling any HazMat incident is to identify the substances involved. Federal law requires all vehicles containing certain quantities of hazardous materials to display a HazMat placard, which is a large diamond-shaped indicator placed on all sides of transport vehicles that carry hazardous materials. When you see a HazMat placard, you know that a potential problem could exist. You will have to find the proper response to the problem before beginning patient treatment **Figure 21-1**. The placard should also have a four-digit identification number, which can be used to identify the substance and to obtain emergency information.

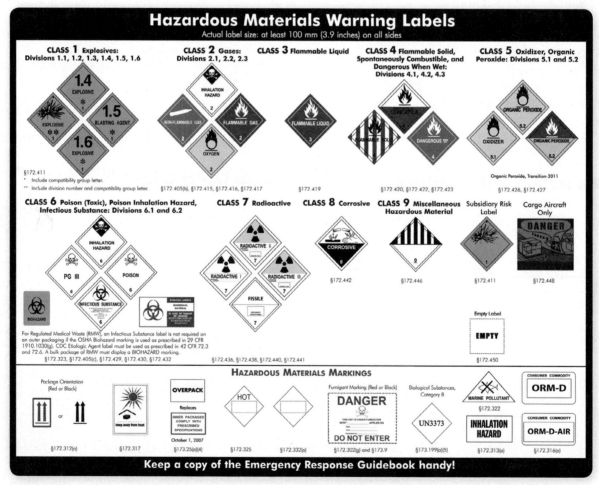

Figure 21-1 The Department of Transportation uses labels, placards, and markings (such as those found in the *Emergency Response Guidebook*) to give a general idea of the hazardous materials inside a particular container or cargo tank. Look for these placards when you arrive on an emergency scene. They are required when these hazardous materials are present. Be aware that shipments with only a small quantity of hazardous materials may not be required to be labeled with placards.
Courtesy of the U.S. Department of Transportation.

The *Emergency Response Guidebook*, published by the US Department of Transportation, lists the most common hazardous materials, their four-digit identification numbers, and the proper emergency actions to take to control the scene. It also describes the emergency medical care of patients who become ill or injured after exposure to these substances **Figure 21-2**. This guidebook is updated every 3 to 4 years. You should carry an up-to-date copy of this guidebook in your vehicle. You can download a free copy of the guidebook at the Pipeline and Hazardous Materials Safety Administration website.

Unless you have received specialized training in handling hazardous materials and can take the necessary precautions to protect yourself, you should keep away from the contaminated area or hot zone. As soon as you recognize that a hazardous materials incident exists, notify your dispatcher so other responders will be aware of the situation.

Once the trained HazMat rescuers have been properly protected, these rescuers need to identify the source of the hazardous materials and remove anyone who has been exposed to the hazard. Sometimes HazMat teams can stop the escape of the hazardous material by shutting off a leak or by absorbing spilled chemicals. Once people have been removed from the contaminated area, they need to be decontaminated by trained personnel, assessed for any injuries, given necessary emergency medical care, and transported to a hospital.

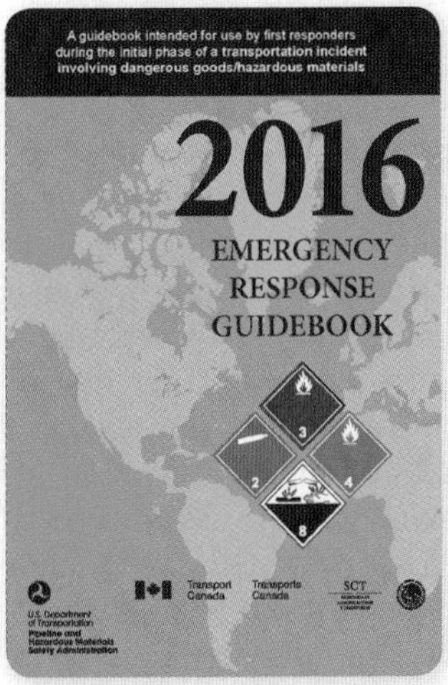

Very few specific antidotes or treatments exist for most HazMat injuries. Consequently, the emergency treatment you can provide to patients who have been exposed to hazardous materials is usually aimed at supportive care. Because most fatalities and serious injuries sustained in HazMat incidents result from breathing problems, you must constantly reevaluate the patient's vital

Figure 21-2 *Emergency Response Guidebook.*
Courtesy of the U.S. Department of Transportation.

signs, including breathing status, so that a patient whose condition worsens can be moved to a higher triage level.

Because of the unique aspects of responding to and working at a HazMat incident, as an emergency medical responder (EMR), you should receive specific additional training in hazardous waste operations and emergency response (often referred to as HAZWOPER) to the emergency medical response level.

Words of Wisdom

Anyone who is working at the scene of a hazardous materials emergency should understand the terminology used to differentiate separate parts of the HazMat scene:

- **Hot zone.** The contaminated area where people can be exposed to sharp metal edges, broken glass, toxic substances, lethal rays, or ignition or explosion of hazardous materials.
- **Warm zone.** The control area where personnel and equipment **decontamination** and hot zone support take place.
- **Cold zone.** The control safe area that contains the command post and other support functions needed in the incident.

Only specially trained and equipped personnel should be in the hot zone and the warm zone.

Safety

Your top priority in a possible HazMat incident is to protect yourself and any bystanders from exposure and contamination. Contaminated patients can contaminate unprotected rescuers!

■ Mass-Casualty Incidents

As an EMR, you may face situations in which there is more than one sick or injured person. These situations, known as **mass-casualty incidents** (or multiple-casualty incidents), may range from a serious motor vehicle crash with three or four injured people to a building explosion with dozens of injured people. A mass-casualty incident is

YOU are the Provider   CASE 1

In the middle of the night, you are dispatched for the report of a vehicle crash. A delivery truck lost control during a heavy rainstorm and hit a large oak tree. As you arrive at the scene, you find a package delivery truck that hit a tree on a residential road that runs through your community. There is still a light rain falling. Dispatch reports that because of the heavy volume of calls during the storm, the nearest emergency medical services (EMS) unit has an estimated arrival time of 8 to 9 minutes.

1. What is your principal role in this incident if hazardous materials are present?
2. What initial actions should you take if this incident turns out to be a mass-casualty incident?
3. What initial actions should you take if you identify this as a hazardous materials incident?

defined as any time there are more patients than resources (ambulances), either on scene or en route, ready to treat and transport patients. In these types of situations, how do you determine which patient to treat first?

You must first be able to recognize the situation as a mass-casualty incident. These incidents require a very different method of operation from routine emergency medical calls. During some mass-casualty incidents, you may be on the scene 15 to 20 minutes before additional assistance arrives, and it may be 45 to 60 minutes before enough rescue resources are available.

No easy formula exists for deciding when to shift from normal operations into the techniques of the mass-casualty incident. Simulations provide realistic situations, but there are many variables, including the severity of the crash, access routes, available resources, response times, levels of emergency training, and overall experience of the EMS system.

Your goal should be to provide the greatest medical benefit for the greatest number of people and to match patients' medical needs with appropriate treatment and transportation. To accomplish this goal, you must identify those patients most in need of treatment and those who can wait.

The Visual Survey: The Eye Sees It All

As you are on the way to the scene, you should mentally prepare yourself for what you may find **Figure 21-3**. Perhaps you have responded to other accidents at the same location. You should ask yourself the following

questions: Where will additional assistance come from? How long will it take for them to arrive?

When you arrive at the scene of a major incident, force yourself to stay as calm as possible. Make a visual assessment of the entire accident scene. This visual survey, as part of the scene size-up, gives you an initial impression of the overall situation, including the potential number of patients involved and, possibly, the severity of their injuries. The visual survey enables you to estimate how much and what kind of assistance you will need to handle the situation.

Your Initial Radio Report: Creating a Verbal Image

The initial radio report is often the most important radio message of a major emergency because it sets the emotional and operational stage for everything that follows. As you prepare for that first vital report, use clear language, be concise, be calm, and do not shout into the equipment. Give the communications center a concise verbal picture of the scene.

The key points to communicate are as follows:

1. Location of the incident
2. Type of incident
3. Any hazards
4. Approximate number of patients
5. Types of assistance required

Be as specific with your requests as possible. A good rule of thumb in mass-casualty situations is to request one ambulance for every five patients. For example, for 35 patients, request seven ambulances; for 23 patients, request five ambulances; and so forth. After taking several deep breaths (to give yourself time to absorb what you have seen and to try to calm your voice), you might give the following radio report about an intercity bus crash: "This is a major crash involving a truck and an intercity bus on Highway 233, about 2 miles west of Route 510. There are approximately 35 victims. There are multiple people trapped. Repeat: This is a major crash. I am requesting the fire department, rescue squad, and seven ambulances at this time. Dispatch additional police units to assist." Follow the protocols of your department when calling for additional resources.

1. Determine the perimeters for emergency vehicles only and exclude all other vehicles.
2. Establish a one-way route for emergency traffic to approach the scene and a separate one-way route for emergency traffic to exit the scene. This will prevent roads from becoming blocked for incoming units.
3. Allow adequate room for emergency vehicles that need to be close to the scene.
4. Keep vehicles and personnel at a designated staging area nearby, if they are not needed at the scene.

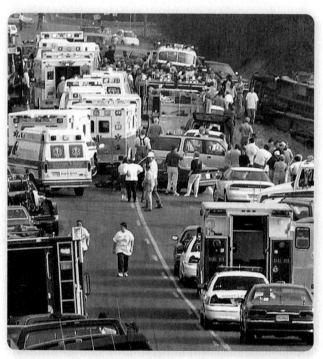

Figure 21-3 A mass-casualty incident requiring triage.
© David Crigger, Bristol Herald Courier/AP Photo.

▶ Casualty Sorting: Creating Order Out of Chaos

The sorting of patients into groups according to their need for medical treatment is called **triage**. Triage is a French word that has come to mean **casualty sorting** in the emergency medical care field. The purpose of casualty sorting is to determine the order in which patients should be treated based on the severity of their injuries so that the most good can be done for the most people.

Ideally, your casualty-sorting system should be simple and fast, based on the skills and knowledge you already have. Do not worry about making a specific diagnosis before categorizing patients; a casualty-sorting system is meant to provide the basis for a system of rapid, lifesaving actions. A casualty-sorting system focuses your activities in the middle of a chaotic and confusing environment. You must identify and separate patients rapidly, according to the severity of their injuries and their need for treatment.

Avoid spending undue time treating the first or second patient you see. Remember, your job is to get to each patient as quickly as possible, conduct a primary assessment, and assign patients to broad triage categories based on their need for treatment.

You should not stop during this assessment, except to correct airway and severe bleeding problems quickly.

Your job is to sort (triage) the patients. Other rescuers will provide follow-up treatment.

Different communities use many variations of triage systems, and you will need to learn the specific role that you have in your community's triage plan. Many EMS systems rely on the **START triage** system because it is simple and easy to remember and implement. The **S**imple **T**riage **A**nd **R**apid **T**reatment (START) system lets EMRs triage each patient in 60 seconds or less, based on three primary observations: breathing, circulation, and mental status.

The START triage system is designed to help rescuers find the most seriously injured patients. As more rescue personnel arrive, patients can be triaged again for further evaluation, treatment, stabilization, and transportation. This system also allows EMRs to open blocked airways and stop severe bleeding quickly.

Triage Tagging: Telling Others What You Have Found

Patients are tagged so that other rescuers arriving at the scene can easily recognize their triage level. Patients are tagged using colored surveyor's tape or colored paper tags, and this is based on the method determined by your local EMS system **Figure 21-4** .

The Four Colors of Triage. The START triage system consists of four categories of triage, each with its own color code:

- **Priority One (red tag).** Immediate care: injuries are life threatening. These patients cannot be stabilized at the scene and need to be transported to an appropriate medical facility as soon as possible. An example of a red tag patient might be a patient who has sustained severe chest trauma, is breathing at a rate of greater than 30 times a minute, and is pale and sweaty.
- **Priority Two (yellow tag).** Urgent care: care can be delayed up to 1 hour. These patients have sustained serious injuries, but they can survive a delay of up to 1 hour in getting to an appropriate medical facility. An example of a yellow tag patient might be a person who

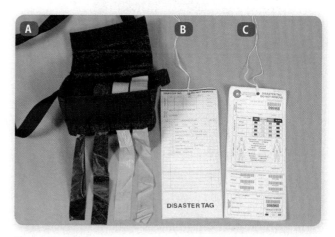

Figure 21-4 A. Triage tape. **B.** Triage tag (back). **C.** Triage tag (front).
© Jones & Bartlett Learning. Courtesy of MIEMSS.

is in pain from a deformity to the femur but is responsive to your verbal commands and is not showing signs and symptoms of shock.

- **Priority Three (green tag).** Delayed care, minor care, or hold (walking wounded): care can be delayed up to 3 hours. These patients are the ones who are able to walk to a designated area away from the immediate area of the incident. They may have isolated upper extremity injuries, cuts, and bruises, but they are responsive and are not showing signs and symptoms of shock.
- **Priority Four (gray or black tag).** Patient is dead; no care is required. These patients have suffered injuries that are obviously incompatible with life, or they have no pulse or respirations.

The First Step in START: Get Up and Walk

The first step in START is to ask everyone who can get up and walk to move away from the immediate rescue scene to a designated safe area. If patients can get up and walk, they rarely have life-threatening injuries. These patients are the walking wounded, designated as Priority Three (green tag/delayed care). A patient who reports pain when he or she attempts to walk or move should not be forced to move. Now you can concentrate on the patients who are left in the rescue scene.

The Second Step in START Triage: Begin Where You Stand

Begin the second step of the START triage system by moving from where you stand. Move in an orderly and systematic manner through the remaining patients, stopping at each patient to provide a quick assessment and tagging. The stop at each patient should never take more than 1 minute.

Your job is to find and tag the Priority One patients—those who require immediate attention. Examine these patients, treat life-threatening airway and breathing conditions, tag the patients with a red tag, and move on.

How to Evaluate Patients Using Breathing, Circulation, and Mental Status

The START triage system is based on the three observations: breathing, circulation, and mental status. Each patient must be evaluated quickly, in a systematic manner, starting with breathing **Figure 21-5**.

Breathing: It All Starts Here. If the patient is breathing, you need to determine the breathing rate. Patients with breathing rates of greater than 30 breaths per minute are tagged Priority One or Immediate (red tags). These patients are showing one of the primary signs of shock and need immediate medical care as soon as it is available.

If the patient is breathing at a rate of less than 30 breaths per minute, move on to the circulation and mental status observations to complete your 60-second survey.

If the patient is not breathing, quickly clear the mouth of any foreign matter. Use the head tilt–chin lift maneuver to open the airway. In a mass-casualty situation, you may have to ignore the usual cervical spine guidelines when you are opening airways during the triage process. This is the only time in emergency medical care when you may not have time to stabilize every injured patient's spine properly. Open the airway, position the patient to maintain the airway, and—if the patient breathes—tag

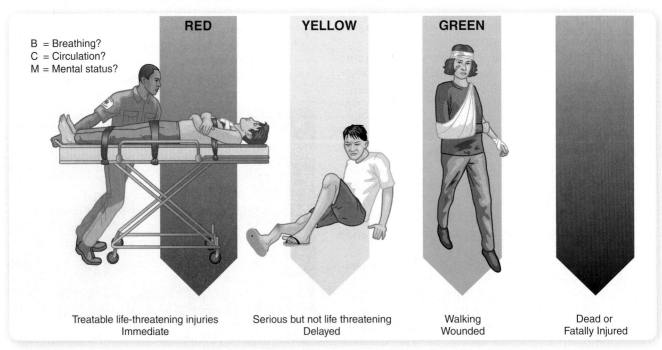

B = Breathing?
C = Circulation?
M = Mental status?

RED — Treatable life-threatening injuries / Immediate

YELLOW — Serious but not life threatening / Delayed

GREEN — Walking Wounded

Dead or Fatally Injured

Figure 21-5 Use the START triage system to sort patients into appropriate groups for treatment.
© Jones & Bartlett Learning.

the patient Priority One, Immediate (red tag). Patients who need help maintaining an open airway are Priority One (red tags). If you are in doubt as to the patient's ability to breathe, tag the patient as Priority One (red tag). If the patient is not breathing and does not start to breathe with simple airway maneuvers, tag the patient Priority Four, Deceased (gray/black tag).

Circulation: Is Oxygen Getting Around? The second part of the triage test is the patient's circulation. The best field method for checking circulation (to see if the heart is able to circulate blood adequately) is to check the patient's carotid pulse. The carotid pulse is close to the heart. It is large and easily felt in the neck. To check the carotid pulse, place your index and middle fingers on the larynx and slide your fingers into the groove between the larynx and the muscles at the side of the neck. You must keep your fingers there for 5 to 10 seconds to find and measure the pulse rate (see Chapter 8, *Professional Rescuer CPR*). If the carotid pulse is weak or irregular, tag the patient Priority One, Immediate (red tag). If the carotid pulse is strong, or a radial pulse is present, move on to the mental status observation, the third step of the triage system.

Treat patients with a weak carotid pulse for shock by laying the patient supine. Then try to stop any severe bleeding. Do not spend time controlling the bleeding yourself. Get the patient to assist with controlling the bleeding or ask one of the walking wounded, Priority Three (green tag) patients, to help. These patients are often eager to assist with emergency treatment. If the pulse is absent, tag the patient with a Priority Four, Deceased (gray/black tag).

Mental Status: Open Your Eyes. The final part of the triage test is the mental status of the patient. This observation is performed on patients who have adequate breathing and adequate circulation. First, determine whether the patient responds to verbal stimuli. Ask the patient to follow a simple command: "Open your eyes;" "Close your eyes;" "Squeeze my hand." Patients who can follow these simple commands and have adequate breathing and adequate circulation are tagged Priority Two, Delayed (yellow tag). According to the AVPU scale, which is described in Chapter 9, *Patient Assessment*, such patients are considered to be alert and responsive to verbal stimuli. A patient who cannot follow this type of simple command is unresponsive to verbal stimuli, according to the AVPU scale. Tag these patients as Priority One, Immediate (red tag).

START Is Just the Beginning

In every situation involving the sorting of casualties, your goal is to find, stabilize, and move Priority One patients first. The START triage system is designed to help you find the most seriously injured patients. As more rescue personnel arrive at the scene, the patients will be triaged again for further evaluation, treatment, stabilization, and transportation. As more EMS personnel arrive, you

should turn over the responsibilities of triage to a person with more training. Each mass-casualty scene should have a person designated as the triage officer.

Remember, injured patients do not always remain in the same condition. The process of shock may continue and some conditions will become more serious as time goes by. As time and resources permit, go back and reassess the condition of Priority Two and Priority Three patients to detect changes in their conditions that may require upgrading the patients to Priority One (red tag) attention Figure 21-6 .

Special Populations

Patients with life-threatening internal injuries may be quiet patients. Do not think that all quiet patients are stable or uninjured.

▶ Working at a Mass-Casualty Incident

You may or may not be the first person to arrive at the scene of a mass-casualty incident. If other rescuers are already at the scene when you arrive, be sure to report to the incident commander before going to work. Because many activities are going on at the same time, the incident commander will assign you to an area where your help and skills can best be used. The incident commander, based on training and local protocols, is in charge of the rescue operation. An effective **incident command system (ICS)** depends on integrated, agreed-upon protocols and procedures involving fire department, law enforcement, and EMS personnel. An explanation of the NIMS is presented in the next section of this chapter.

If you are the first on the scene, you will have to make the initial overview, clearly and accurately report the situation to your dispatcher, and conduct the initial START triage. In addition, you most likely will be called on to participate in many other ways during mass-casualty incidents.

As more highly trained rescue and EMS personnel arrive at the scene, accurately report your findings to the person in charge by using a format similar to that used in the initial arrival report. Note the following information:

- Approximate number of patients
- Number of patients you have triaged into each of the four levels
- Additional assistance required
- Other important information

After you have reported this information, you may be assigned to provide emergency medical care to patients, to help move patients, or to assist with ambulance or helicopter transportation. You may also be asked to assist with traffic control or to help provide fire protection, depending on your training.

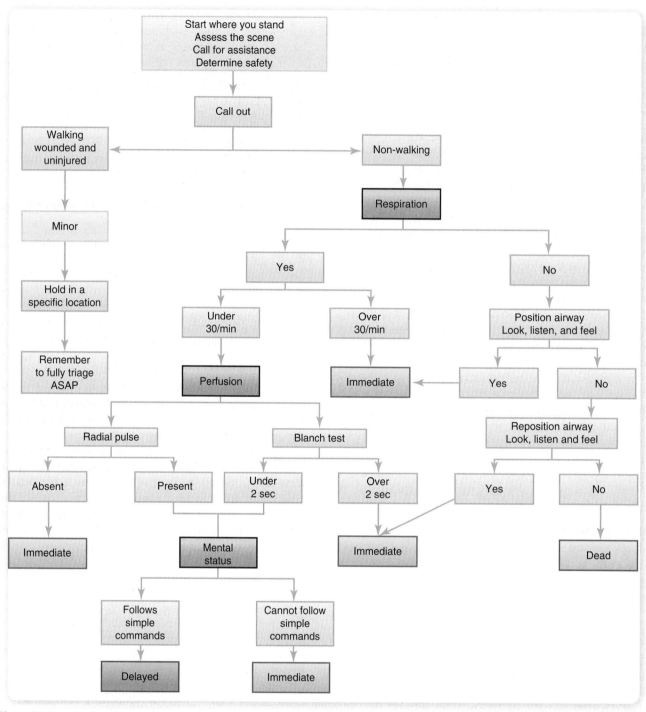

Figure 21-6 START algorithm.
Courtesy of Los Angeles Fire Department - Disaster Preparedness Section.

YOU are the Provider CASE 2

You respond to a motor vehicle crash involving three vehicles. You arrive at the scene after EMS, and you are assigned to assist with triage. All the patients who are able to walk were triaged as green prior to your arrival. As you approach your first patient, you kneel beside her and assess her breathing. You note she has a respiratory rate of 24 breaths per minute and the respirations are nonlabored. She has a weak carotid pulse, and no peripheral pulses are felt in her wrists.

1. In what triage category does this patient belong?
2. What is the appropriate treatment for this patient?

Treatment

At a mass-casualty incident, remember you are trying to do the most good for the most patients. Do not get sidetracked by spending too much time treating the first patient you encounter.

▶ National Incident Management System

The **National Incident Management System (NIMS)** has been developed by the US Department of Homeland Security to provide a comprehensive, consistent, and unified approach to handling emergency incidents. NIMS is designed to effectively and efficiently handle the immediate response, mitigation, and long-term recovery of small and massive natural and man-made incidents. Effective implementation of NIMS helps local government agencies work with regional, state, and federal agencies during all phases of a major emergency incident.

NIMS expands on the ICS in your department, which may cover only one type of agency. NIMS is designed to address a unified command structure that includes all types of agencies responding to any type of man-made or natural disaster. To accomplish this, NIMS is flexible and yet contains standardized components.

The five components of NIMS and ICS are:

1. Preparedness
2. Communications and information management
3. Resource management
4. Command and management
5. Ongoing management and maintenance

These components are illustrated in **Figure 21-7**. The incident command system is part of the command and management component of NIMS. The incident command system consists of six major features. These are:

1. Standardization
2. Command
3. Planning/organizational structure
4. Facilities and resources
5. Communications information management
6. Professionalism

An overview of the ICS features is shown in **Figure 21-8**.

As an EMR, your role falls within the command and management component of NIMS. You should understand the function of the ICS and understand your role within the ICS. In large incidents, you may be working with people from other agencies, so you need to understand how the Multiagency Coordination Systems ensure unified operating procedures. You should also understand the function of public information systems in releasing information about an emergency incident. The other components shown in Figure 21-7 are vital parts of NIMS, but your role as an EMR is not as directly related to these functions.

The federal government requires many agencies to use NIMS, and you may be required to become trained in this system. Different levels of training are offered through traditional and online courses. It is recommended that EMRs be certified in the following courses: ICS-100: Introduction to ICS, or FEMA IS-700: NIMS, An Introduction. Additional information on NIMS is

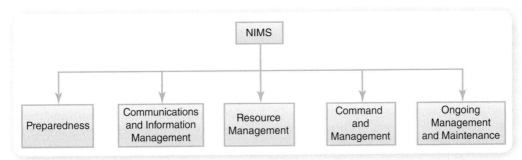

Figure 21-7 Components of the NIMS.
© Jones & Bartlett Learning.

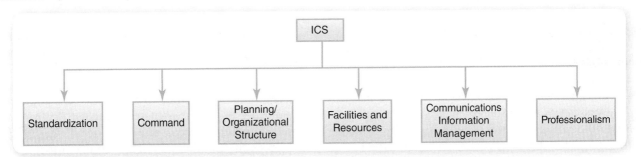

Figure 21-8 An overview of the six ICS features.
© Jones & Bartlett Learning.

available at the Federal Emergency Management Agency (FEMA) website. Take advantage of training in incident management. It helps you understand and work within the incident management system.

Terrorism Awareness

Terrorism is the systematic use of violence by a group to intimidate a population or government to achieve a political goal. Terrorism receives considerable public attention and is a high-profile crime. Domestic terrorism is caused by a country's own citizens. International terrorism is cause by people from another country. The bombing of an abortion clinic by an American citizen is considered a domestic terrorist event. The attacks on the World Trade Center and the Pentagon on September 11, 2001, were international terrorist events. A terrorist event may involve limited property damage with no injuries or it may involve the deaths of many people. The success of terrorist events is measured by the intimidation produced, not just by the value of the property lost or the number of lives lost. Terrorists might use a wide variety of methods to incite terror, including the use of guns, explosives, fire, chemicals, viruses, bacteria, and radiation.

As you study the agents and methods used by terrorists, realize that the type of events created intentionally by terrorists can also occur accidentally. For example, on April 15, 2013, the Boston Marathon bombings were the result of terrorists intentionally detonating two pressure cooker bombs. This event killed three people and injured an estimated 264 others. Compare that event with the one that occurred 2 days later on April 17, 2013, in West, Texas, at the West Fertilizer Company, where an accidental fire detonated about 30 tons of fertilizer grade ammonium nitrate, resulting in the death of 15 people and injuring more than 260 others.

The causes of these two events were very different, but the result of both incidents was multiple fatalities and injuries to a large number of people. Both incidents required a cautious approach and evaluation of the scene, a large response of emergency personnel, the triage of a large number of victims, and a carefully executed plan for treatment and transportation of many injured people.

Most agents used by terrorists are many of the same agents that produce hazards for EMRs in everyday accidents and emergencies. A building collapse caused by a natural gas explosion and a building collapse caused by a terrorist attack are both collapsed buildings. They share many of the same hazards and require many of the same safety precautions for rescuers. The accidental release of a chemical causes a HazMat emergency; an intentional release of the same chemical by terrorists becomes a terrorist event. Still, the safety precautions required for rescuers at both events are the same. A radiation leak from a nuclear power plant releases the same type of radiation

that would be released by a terrorist. It is important to understand the agents and methods that are used by terrorists and to compare them with the agents that normally exist in communities. Many of the safety precautions used in accidental emergencies are the same precautions needed when dealing with terrorist events.

▶ Weapons of Mass Destruction

A **weapon of mass destruction (WMD)** is any agent designed to bring about mass death, casualties, and/or massive damage to property and infrastructure (such as bridges, tunnels, airports, electrical power plants, and seaports). These instruments of death and destruction include explosive, chemical, biologic, and nuclear weapons. To date, the preferred WMD for terrorists has been explosive devices. Terrorist groups have favored tactics that use truck or car bombs or pedestrian suicide bombers. Many previous terrorist attempts to use either chemical or biologic weapons to their full capacity have been unsuccessful. Nonetheless, as an EMR, you should understand the destructive potential of these weapons.

▶ Potential Targets and Risks

To understand the threat that terrorists pose to people and places, you need to consider the places that terrorists might identify as targets for terrorist activities. Remember, terrorists strive to incite fear to achieve a political or ideological goal, and their motives do not limit their choice of targets. Bridges, tunnels, pipelines, and harbors constitute infrastructure targets. The Washington Monument and the Statute of Liberty are examples of symbolic targets. Housing developments and automobile dealerships have been targeted by ecoterrorists. Computer networks and data systems might be targets for cyberterrorists. Farms and agricultural installations might be targets for terrorists trying to destroy or taint the nation's food sources. Civilian targets such as schools, government buildings, churches, and shopping centers represent high-visibility targets for terrorists. Taken collectively, a wide variety of places, representing most components of society, might be considered as targets **Figure 21-9**. In an open society in which people are largely free to move around as they wish, a person committed to performing a terrorist act can access most of the components of the infrastructure and turn any one of them into a target.

Despite measures to heightened security, a terrorist event can occur at any time. You should always be alert for hazards—those associated with a terrorist event as well as those connected to any other emergency. In any discussion of the risks of terrorist attacks, it is important to consider the number of terror-related deaths compared with other major causes of death. **Table 21-1** compares the number of deaths from terrorist events with deaths from other common causes. This comparison is not intended to minimize the tragedies of

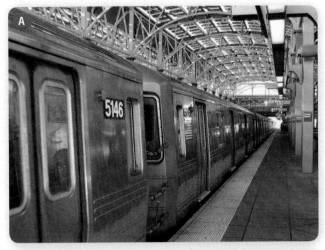
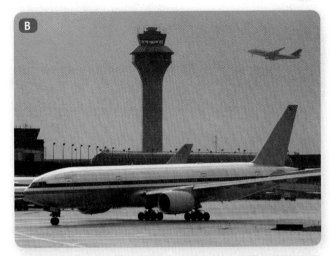
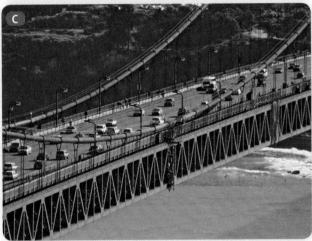
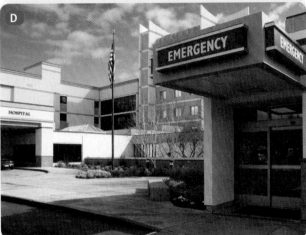

Figure 21-9 Terrorists could target a variety of places.
A: © Susan Tansil/Shutterstock; B: © Steve Allen/Brand X Pictures/Alamy; C: © phdpsx/Shutterstock; D: © Galina Barskaya/Shutterstock.

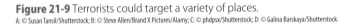

Table 21-1	Deaths in 2013
Cause of Death	**Number of Deaths in US**
Heart disease	611,105 per year
Cancer	584,881 per year
Accidents	130,557 per year
Suicide	41,149 per year
Murders	16,121 per year
All terrorism events in the US between 2001 and 2013	3,030

Data Source: Centers for Disease Control and Prevention.
© Jones & Bartlett Learning.

September 11, 2001; rather, it is intended to help you gain some perspective and realize that terrorist events do not occur every day. Although you should be prepared for terrorist events, the majority of the emergency medical calls you answer will be for the other types of events listed in Table 21-1.

▶ Agents and Devices

A wide variety of agents and devices can be used to incite terror, including explosive devices, incendiary devices, chemical agents, biologic agents, and radiologic agents. You need to understand how these devices are used and what safety precautions you need to take to ensure scene safety for yourself, other rescuers, and bystanders.

Explosives and Incendiary Devices

Explosives are used to produce a concussion that destroys property and inflicts injury and death. Some explosive devices, also known as **incendiary devices**, are designed to start fires. Incendiary devices can be

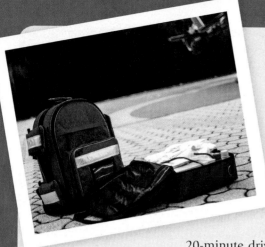

Voices *of* Experience

I had just finished my regular 8-hour paramedic shift in Lorain, Ohio. It was 2400 hours, and I was about halfway through my 20-minute drive home, when I heard a distant thud to the south, toward Elyria. When I looked in the direction of the sound, I thought I saw a glow reflecting off the clouds in the distance. The EMS agency I worked for covered both Lorain and Elyria, so I took the next right turn and headed toward the glow.

> **" When the time comes, you must do what you have been trained to do. "**

There had been an explosion at the Aztec chemical plant, which was inconveniently located in the middle of a city of about 50,000 residents. This occurred in the days before everyone had cell phones, and I didn't want to interfere with priority traffic by talking on the radio. One of the most important rules to remember as an emergency medical responder, and one of the most easily forgotten in the excitement of the moment is: Don't make things worse!

As I drove toward the scene, I looked for flags or smoke to check the wind direction. I was in luck; I was upwind. When I got into town, I could hear from the radio traffic that both fire and medical incident command were up and running. When there was a lull in radio traffic, I called dispatch and was directed to report to dispatch at the central station.

When I arrived at dispatch, I was told to wait for an assignment with several other off-duty personnel who were already there. After about an hour, we were sent to various schools where evacuation shelters were being set up by the Red Cross. Although the fire department had not been able to identify the chemicals released, there were reports of respiratory distress.

My partner and I took a squad and reported to one of the designated schools. What we saw on our arrival was amazing. Volunteers from the Red Cross were calmly and efficiently setting up things. They had already designated areas for decontamination, canteen, families, and intake. They had set up coolers, water, chairs, and cots, and they were bringing in food—and the explosion had occurred less than 2 hours before. Most of the volunteers were older adults, and they operated in a calm, friendly, and professional manner.

We were asked to set up a medical station to evaluate people who weren't feeling well. The chemical released was eventually reported to be a mild respiratory irritant. The explosion was caused by a worker, who was the only one to die in the blast. By morning, everyone was allowed to go back home.

It doesn't matter what caused a mass-casualty incident—accident, terrorism, or criminal violence—the principles remain the same. Emergency medical responders must respond quickly, but more importantly, they must respond wisely, calmly, and efficiently. The greatest service you can perform at a disorganized scene is to create order out of chaos, calm out of calamity. To do so, you must consciously work to control your emotions as well as your physiologic response to stress. Slow down, breathe slowly and deeply, and lower your voice. Tunnel vision is your worst enemy. Force yourself to look around, in all directions and dimensions, and use all of your senses. These skills do not come naturally—to be good in a crisis you must train and retrain, and when the time comes, you must do what you have been trained to do.

Guy H. Haskell, PhD, NREMT-P
Firefighter, Benton Township Volunteer Fire Department, Unionville, Indiana
Paramedic, Brown Township Fire and Rescue, Mooresville, Indiana
Director, Emergency Medical and Safety Services Consultants, Bloomington, Indiana

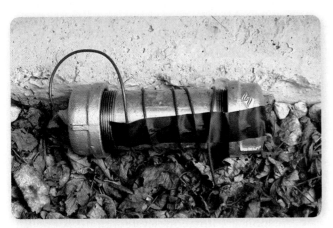

Figure 21-10 A pipe bomb is a simple explosive device.
Courtesy of Captain David Jackson, Saginaw Township Fire Department.

as simple as a homemade firebomb or as complex as a highly technical device that may have been stolen from the military **Figure 21-10**. An explosive device can be hand carried or transported in a heavy truck. Often the first indication that an explosive or incendiary device is present is the explosion or fire that results from the deployment of the device. In some parts of the world, suicide terrorists carry explosive devices on their person and set them off to kill themselves and others.

WMD Safety Considerations

In times of increased concern about terrorist activity, travelers and the general public are urged to be alert for bags or luggage left unattended. Be aware of suspicious vehicles and report them to the proper law enforcement officials. If you are called to respond to an explosion, be alert for safety hazards that may have been created by the explosion or by a terrorist. Do not enter any area that may be unsafe until properly trained personnel are able to assess the risks. Be alert for the possibility of a second explosive device that is timed to explode when rescuers are on the scene. Use the same safety skills you developed for other types of emergency situations to keep yourself safe.

When dealing with a WMD scene, it is safe to assume you will not be able to enter where the event has occurred—nor do you want to. The best location for staging is upwind and uphill from the incident. Wait for assistance from those who are trained in assessing and managing WMD scenes.

Chemical Agents

Many different types of chemicals can be used as terrorist weapons. Industrial-process chemicals can be used to intentionally inflict harm on people. For example, chlorine is a gas that is used in many industrial processes and in water purification, but it was also used as a poisonous gas in World War I. Many of the **chemical agents** that could be used by terrorists are the same chemicals that create HazMat incidents when accidentally released.

Chemical agents are liquids or gases that are used to kill or injure and can be divided into the following categories:

- Pulmonary (choking) agents
- Metabolic agents
- Insecticides
- Nerve agents
- Blister agents

Pulmonary Agents. Pulmonary agents are gases that cause immediate harm and injury. Their primary route of entry into the body is through the airway into the lungs. Once these chemicals are inhaled, they damage lung tissue, which causes fluid to escape into the lungs and leads to pulmonary edema. Pulmonary agents cause intense coughing, gasping, shortness of breath, and difficulty breathing. Two common pulmonary agents are chlorine and phosgene. Phosgene gas is produced by burning Freon, which is found in most domestic air conditioners. The odor of this gas is similar to freshly mowed grass. The symptoms of phosgene gas exposure may be delayed for several hours after inhalation of the gas.

Although pulmonary agents could be weapons of choice for terrorists, these chemicals are also present in a variety of domestic and industrial settings and might also be encountered following an accidental release. The safety precautions for an accidental release are the same as the precautions for an intentional release by terrorists: keep a safe distance away until properly trained HazMat personnel can handle the situation.

Metabolic Agents. Metabolic agents affect the body's ability to use oxygen at the cellular level. The most common metabolic agents are cyanides. Cyanides are produced in large quantities and used in gold and silver mining, photography, and plastics processing. Cyanide is also produced by the combustion of plastics and textiles, so there is the potential for cyanide poisoning in any house fire. Contact with cyanides produces shortness of breath, flushed skin, rapid heartbeat, seizures, coma, and cardiac arrest. The safety precautions for an accidental release of cyanide are the same as the precautions for an intentional release by terrorists: keep a safe distance away until properly trained HazMat personnel can handle the situation.

Insecticides. Insecticides are a class of poisonous chemicals that are inhaled or absorbed through the skin. Many insecticides belong to a class of chemicals called organophosphates. Absorption of these chemicals produces the following symptoms: salivation, sweating, lacrimation (excessive tearing), urination, diarrhea, gastric upset, and emesis (vomiting). The acronym for these symptoms is the word SLUDGE **Table 21-2**. Because insecticides are readily

Table 21-2	Symptoms of Exposure to an Organophosphate Insecticide or Nerve Agent
S	Salivation, sweating
L	Lacrimation (excessive tearing)
U	Urination
D	Defecation, diarrhea
G	Gastrointestinal upset and cramps
E	Emesis (vomiting)

© Jones & Bartlett Learning.

available, they could be used as agents by terrorists. It is important to realize that far more emergency providers have experienced accidental contact with insecticides in routine calls than during terrorist-related events. If you encounter an incident involving an insecticide, keep bystanders far enough away to prevent additional contact with the chemical. If you encounter an emergency involving multiple people with SLUDGE-like symptoms, assume you are dealing with poisoning from this type of chemical and call for assistance from a trained HazMat team. Do not make contact with contaminated patients until they have been through decontamination by trained personnel to prevent the spread of contamination.

Nerve Agents. Nerve agents are among the most deadly chemicals developed. These chemicals can kill large numbers of people with small quantities and cause cardiac arrest within seconds to minutes of exposure. Discovered by scientists in search of a superior pesticide, nerve agents are much stronger organophosphates than those found in insecticides. Nerve agents, like insecticides, block an essential enzyme in the nervous system and cause the SLUDGE-like symptoms listed in Table 21-2. Four of the most commonly mentioned nerve agents are sarin, soman, tabun, and V agent (VX).

In an emergency situation, your primary responsibility is to keep yourself, other rescuers, and bystanders from becoming contaminated. A well-trained HazMat team in special protective equipment is needed to remove and decontaminate people exposed to these agents. The DuoDote kit is a nerve agent antidote kit (NAAK) that contains two drugs in a single auto-injector, which counteract the effects of nerve agents.

Blister Agents. When blister agents come in contact with the skin, they produce burn-like blisters. If the vapors of these agents are inhaled, they cause burns of the respiratory system. Blister agents produce pain, skin irritation, eye irritation, severe shortness of breath, and severe coughing. Blister agents include sulfur mustard and Lewisite. As with other chemical agents, blister agents pose a threat to rescuers. Only well-trained and properly dressed rescuers with self-contained breathing apparatus should approach a scene that might contain these agents. Table 21-3 lists characteristics of some chemical agents.

This brief summary about chemical agents will not make you an expert; rather, it is intended to provide you with enough information to help you realize the chemicals that might be used by terrorists, while deadly, are in the same classes as many of the chemicals encountered by HazMat teams. Any time there are multiple people experiencing unexplained symptoms, you should suspect a common agent as the cause. Your primary role is to recognize that a problem exists and to avoid contaminating yourself, other rescuers, and bystanders. Stay upwind from any potential source and call for assistance from a properly trained HazMat team.

Biologic Agents. Biologic agents are naturally occurring substances that produce diseases. They may be bacteria, such as anthrax or the plague, or viruses, such as smallpox or hemorrhagic fever. Many biologic agents caused epidemics of disease in the past. Some of these agents, such as smallpox, have been wiped out; the last natural case of smallpox was seen in 1977. However, the smallpox organism has been maintained in laboratories and could be used intentionally to infect people. Although biologic agents are hard to disperse to large

YOU are the Provider   CASE 3

You are called to assist an EMS team at the scene of a fire at a plastics factory. When you arrive you are informed that a smoky fire inside the building has almost been extinguished by the fire department. As you approach the scene, you are directed by the incident commander to assist with the treatment of three patients in a treatment area. The patients all report shortness of breath, flushed skin, and a rapid heart rate. The patients tell you they were working in the plastics factory when some of the materials caught fire, and they breathed in some smoke while escaping from the fire.

1. On the basis of the patients' signs and symptoms and the history surrounding the incident, what type of agent do you think is involved?
2. How would you ensure you are in a safe location?

Table 21-3	Characteristics of Chemical Agents				
Name	**Military Designations**	**Odor**	**Lethality**	**Onset of Symptoms**	**Primary Route of Exposure**
Pulmonary agents	Chlorine (Cl) Phosgene (CG)	Bleach (Cl) Cut grass (CG)	Causes irritation, choking (Cl) Severe pulmonary edema (CG)	Immediate (Cl) Delayed (CG)	Vapor hazard
Metabolic agents	Hydrogen cyanide (AC) Cyanogen chloride (CK)	Almonds (AC) Irritating (CK)	Highly lethal chemical gases; can kill within minutes; effects are reversible with antidotes	Immediate	Vapor hazard
Nerve agents	Tabun (GA) Sarin (GB) Soman (GD) V agent (VX)	Fruity or none	Most lethal chemical agents; can kill within minutes; effects are reversible with antidotes	Immediate	Both vapor and contact (GA and GD) Vapor hazard (GB) Contact hazard (VX)
Blister agents	Mustard (H) Lewisite (L) Phosgene oxime (CX)	Garlic (H) Geranium (L)	Causes large blisters to form on victims; may severely damage upper airway if vapors are inhaled; severe, intense pain and grayish skin discoloration	Delayed (H) Immediate (L, CX)	Primarily contact with some vapor hazard

© Jones & Bartlett Learning.

Safety

Remember, hazardous chemical releases and terrorist events often result in large numbers of patients who are experiencing the same symptoms at the same time. For example, the report of multiple patients reporting difficulty breathing in the subway at rush hour, when no hint of smoke is evident, is cause for suspicion. You must resist the urge to rush into scenes when there are multiple victims from an unknown cause.

numbers of people, there is some concern that they could be used as a deadly weapon by terrorists.

If terrorists intentionally dispersed a biologic agent, the organism would have to come in contact with people in sufficient quantities to produce an illness. These diseases have an incubation period, which is the time between exposure to a disease organism to the time the person begins to show symptoms of the disease. This means that if people were exposed to an infectious organism today, it might be several days before they would show signs of the disease. The first awareness of

a biologic terrorist incident would probably come from hospital emergency departments and public health departments. Your role in biologic incidents is to report unusual patterns of illness and keep up to date on current information from your medical director and public health department.

Safety considerations for EMRs include being alert for unusual patterns of diseases with flulike symptoms. You should make every effort to review current information about disease trends from your medical director and public health department. Practice appropriate standard precautions for the signs and symptoms exhibited by every patient. If you have any indications that a call might involve a biologic agent, call for specially trained assistance and wait in a safe location.

You need to be aware of when you should suspect the use of biologic agents. If the agent is in the form of a powder, such as in the October 2001 attacks involving anthrax mailed in letters, the incident must be handled by HazMat specialists. Patients who have come into direct contact with the agent need to be decontaminated before any EMS contact or treatment is initiated.

Safety

Remember to use standard precautions—including wearing gloves, gowns, and HEPA masks—any time there is a chance that an infectious disease organism might be present. Many biologic materials are transmitted by air or indirect contact.

Table 21-4	Common Signs of Acute Radiation Sickness
Low exposure	Nausea, vomiting, diarrhea
Moderate exposure	Superficial burns, hair loss, depletion of the immune system (death of white blood cells), cancer
Severe exposure	Partial- and full-thickness burns, cancer, death

© Jones & Bartlett Learning.

Radiologic Agents

Ionizing radiation is a kind of energy that is formed by the decay of a naturally occurring or man-made radioactive source. **Radiation** is used in hospitals, research facilities, and nuclear power plants, and it is also used for military weapons. Exposure to excess amounts of radiation can cause delayed illnesses, such as an increase in the rate of certain cancers. Exposure to large amounts of radiation can cause people to become violently ill within a few hours of exposure and may cause death within hours or days. **Table 21-4** lists some signs and symptoms of radiation sickness.

Radiation is a hidden hazard that is similar to electricity. You cannot see, feel, or detect radiation with any of your normal body senses. Special instruments are needed to detect and measure the amount of radiation that is present **Figure 21-11**.

Some concern exists that terrorists could detonate an explosive device containing a small amount of radioactive material (known as a **dirty bomb**). Such an explosion would spread radioactive material over the area of the explosion, and thereby contaminate anyone in the vicinity. In a situation like this, rescuers would have no means of determining whether radioactivity was present unless special monitors were used to check for radiation. Unless there was a warning issued about such an event, rescuers might not know about the presence of radiation.

As an EMR, you need to be alert to warnings about incidents involving radiation. If the presence of radiation is suspected, you should stay away from a blast or suspicious site until specially trained teams check for the presence of radiation with special monitoring devices. Know what agencies in your community are equipped to handle such an event.

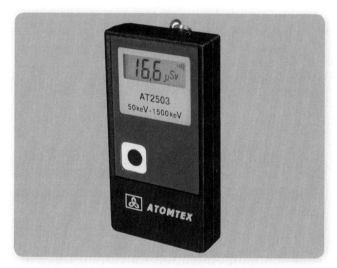

Figure 21-11 A personal dosimeter measures the amount of radioactive exposure received by an individual.
Courtesy of Atomex Scientific and Production Enterprise (www.atomex.com).

Words of Wisdom

One way to remember the classes of substances that could be used by terrorists is with the acronym B-NICE:

B Biologic
N Nuclear
I Incendiary devices
C Chemicals
E Explosives

YOU are the Provider
CASE 4

You are responding to an explosion in the downtown area. As you approach the scene, you see a cloud of smoke coming from a building. While you wait for the HazMat team at a safe distance, you see people walking out of the building toward your vehicle. The people are coughing, have blisters on their skin, and look like they are having difficulty breathing.

1. What agent is most likely causing these signs and symptoms?
2. What other resources will potentially be needed at this scene?

▶ Your Response to Terrorist Events

The threat of terrorist activity is frightening to most people. It is important that all emergency responders have some awareness and knowledge of the various tactics and agents terrorists might use. Emergency response personnel need to develop an all-hazards approach for managing these emergencies. Keep in mind that agents used by terrorists could be the same agents that you are already trained to deal with: explosions, fires, toxic chemicals, hazardous materials, infectious diseases, and radiation. Although you may feel apprehensive about dealing with a terrorist event, remember the same safety rules apply in all emergencies: good scene safety and diligent use of standard precautions.

To prepare for a terrorist event, master the skills that enable you to be a good EMR. Be prepared and know the limits of your training. Many types of terrorist events require you to stay a certain distance away to avoid contaminating additional people. Teams with special training are required to manage incidents involving special hazards. Be alert for secondary devices placed by a terrorist and set to detonate after emergency responders arrive at the scene.

> ### Safety Tips
>
> Be alert for a secondary explosive device at a terrorist incident. If you are called to a terrorist incident, be aware of places where a secondary device could be hidden, including abandoned vehicles, trash dumpsters, debris piles, newspaper boxes, mailboxes, and storm sewers.

Terrorist events can affect large numbers of people. Establish an ICS as soon as possible **Figure 21-12**. Know your role in working within the ICS. Treat these incidents as mass-casualty situations. Establish good working relationships with appropriate local, state, and federal agencies.

EMRs have a vital role in working at terrorist events. You can do the most good by following your training and not exceeding the level of skills you have. Always be alert for your safety, the safety of other rescuers, and the safety of patients. Remember, you cannot be an effective rescuer if you become a victim yourself.

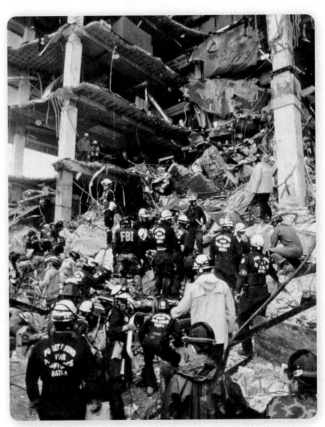

Figure 21-12 An incident command system needs to be set up for large-scale terrorist and mass-casualty events.
Courtesy of FEMA.

> ### Words of Wisdom
>
> Terrorism is no longer something that happens "somewhere else," as the bombing in Oklahoma City and the attacks on the World Trade Center and the Pentagon proved. As an EMR, be aware of the possibility of a terrorist event. Realize that a major incident may be dispatched as a routine call. Your skill in assessing scene safety could be vital in saving lives. Be especially alert for clues that point toward special hazards and take advantage of training offered in your local community.

YOU are the Provider

You are the Provider: CASE 1

1. What is your principal role in this incident if hazardous materials are present?

Your role in an incident that may involve hazardous materials is to look for and identify, from a safe distance, any hazardous materials involved while protecting yourself and keeping yourself and others away from the hazardous materials. The actual mitigation of a hazardous materials incident needs to be accomplished by a specially trained hazardous materials team.

2. What initial actions should you take if this incident turns out to be a mass-casualty incident?

Your role as an EMR in a mass-casualty incident is to:

- Determine the approximate number of patients.
- Determine the number of patients that you have triaged.
- Report any additional assistance required.
- Report any other important information.

3. What initial actions should you take if you identify this as a hazardous materials incident?

If you suspect this scene involves hazardous materials, you should take immediate steps to remove yourself from the danger zone to a safer place. In determining a safe location, keep in mind that liquids do not run uphill and fumes do not travel upwind. Keep other people from entering any area that might be hazardous. Quickly call for assistance from law enforcement for traffic control and possible evacuation. Request your hazardous materials team to assume overall control of the scene. They will identify the hazard, locate any patients, remove them from the hazardous zone, decontaminate them, and treat any injuries.

You are the Provider: CASE 2

1. In what triage category does this patient belong?

The patient's respirations are 24, which is within acceptable limits, and by itself is not a reason for concern. This patient did not walk to the green triage area, so you can suspect she has some type of injury that kept her from joining this group. As you assess her circulatory status you note a weak carotid pulse and no palpable radial pulse in the wrist. These findings place this patient in the immediate category. This patient should receive a red tag and be immediately taken to the treatment area

and prepared for transport. At this point an assessment of the patient's mental status would not serve to change her triage assessment from the red category. Take spinal precautions into consideration when attempting to move this patient.

2. What is the appropriate treatment for this patient?

There appears to be a decrease in the patient's circulation; therefore, you should begin immediate treatment for shock. After taking spinal precautions into consideration, lay the patient supine. Attempt to identify and correct any sources of external bleeding. Cover the patient with a blanket to maintain body temperature. Transport as soon as possible.

You are the Provider: CASE 3

1. On the basis of the patients' signs and symptoms and the history surrounding the incident, what type of agent do you think is involved?

The burning or combustion of materials involving plastics has the potential to release numerous toxins. The most likely type of agent affecting these patients is a pulmonary agent that they have inhaled. A wide variety of chemicals are present in plastics and can be released during the fire. It is impossible to identify specific toxins without sophisticated testing. You need to treat the symptoms the patients are experiencing. Also, you need to confirm with the HazMat team that you are in a location that is removed from toxic fumes and that you will not be contaminated by the patients.

2. How would you ensure you are in a safe location?

You need to check with the HazMat team. One of the responsibilities of the HazMat team is to designate areas or zones at an incident involving hazardous materials. Hot zones are designated for the area immediately involved with the hazardous material. Warm zones are outside the immediate hazardous area but still pose a risk to people who are not properly protected. This is typically an area where patients exposed to the agent are decontaminated. Once decontamination has taken place, patients are sent to the cold zone. Cold zones are safe areas for non-HazMat personnel to operate without fear of exposure to the agent. Although safety considerations still need to be exercised, this is a safe area for the triage and treatment of patients.

YOU are the Provider **SUMMARY** *Continued*

You are the Provider: CASE 4

1. **What agent is most likely causing these signs and symptoms?**

Many agents can cause respiratory distress; however, agents that cause blistering of the skin and trouble breathing are not that common. These patients are likely experiencing an exposure to a blistering agent, such as mustard gas or Lewisite. These agents produce burn-like blisters and can cause burns of the respiratory system, resulting in respiratory distress.

2. **What other resources will potentially be needed at this scene?**

HazMat is going to be your primary resource at this scene. However, there are other resources that may be necessary. The fire department may be needed to work in conjunction with HazMat and EMS. Police may be needed to help control the scene and to assist in area evacuation. In addition, your local health department and the Red Cross may be needed as well.

Prep Kit

▶ Ready for Review

- Because you may be the first trained person on the scene of an incident involving hazardous materials, you must be able to identify the signs of a potential hazardous materials incident and respond appropriately.
- During a HazMat incident, your top priority is to recognize that a hazard is present and protect yourself and bystanders from exposure and contamination from the hazardous material.
- You should understand the role of an EMR during the first few minutes of a mass-casualty incident.
- The START triage system is a simple triage system that you can use at mass-casualty incidents. It serves to sort patients into groups so that the most serious patients are treated and transported first.
- The National Incident Management System is designed to provide a unified approach to emergency incidents of any size that involve multiple agencies anywhere in the United States. All emergency responders need to have some understanding of this system.
- Terrorist attacks, although rare, are a concern for emergency providers. The goal of terrorists is to intimidate a population or government to achieve a goal. Terrorists may use a wide variety of methods to incite terror, including the use of explosives, fire, chemicals, viruses, bacteria, and radiation.
- Chemical agents are man-made substances that can have devastating effects on living organisms. These agents consist of pulmonary, metabolic, insecticides, nerve, and blister agents.
- Biologic agents are organisms that cause disease. They are generally found in nature and can be weaponized to maximize the number of people exposed to the germ.
- Radiologic weapons can create a massive amount of destruction. This type of weapon includes radiologic dispersal devices, also known as dirty bombs.
- EMRs need to consider their safety, the safety of other rescuers, and the safety of bystanders whenever dealing with a terrorist-related event. Your responsibility as an EMR in many of these situations is to identify potential threats, ensure safety, and call for specially trained personnel to deal with these threats.

▶ Vital Vocabulary

biologic agents Naturally occurring substances that cause disease. Terrorists may use bacteria, viruses, or toxins to intentionally cause epidemics of disease.

blister agents Chemicals that cause the skin to blister.

casualty sorting The sorting of patients to determine the order in which patients should be treated and transported.

Prep Kit *Continued*

chemical agents Compounds that can be used by terrorists to inflict harm.

cold zone The control area that contains the command post and other support functions needed in the incident.

decontamination The process of reducing or preventing the spread of contaminants at a hazardous materials event.

dirty bomb An explosive device using conventional explosives that is designed to spread radioactive material over a wide area.

explosives Substances that release energy in a sudden and uncontrolled manner when detonated.

hazardous materials (HazMat) Substances that are toxic, poisonous, radioactive, flammable, or explosive and can cause injury or death with exposure.

hot zone A contaminated area.

incendiary devices Substances or weapons designed to start a fire.

incident command system (ICS) A system of people, procedures, and equipment designed to improve emergency response operations at situations of all types and complexities.

incubation period The time between exposure to a disease organism to the time the person begins to show symptoms of the disease.

insecticides Chemicals that are formulated to kill insects but that can intentionally or accidentally cause injury or death to humans when inhaled or absorbed through the skin.

mass-casualty incidents Accidents or situations involving more patients than you can handle with the initial resources available; also known as multiple-casualty incidents.

metabolic agents Substances that are intended to produce injury or death by disrupting the body's ability to use oxygen and chemical reactions at the cellular level.

National Incident Management System (NIMS) A system developed by the US Department of Homeland Security for managing an emergency incident, which may require the response of many different agencies; designed to provide a comprehensive, efficient, and effective management approach from initial response through recovery.

nerve agents Deadly toxic substances that attack the central nervous system.

pulmonary agents Substances that produce respiratory distress or illness.

radiation The electromagnetic energy that is released from a radioactive material or a dirty bomb.

START triage A system of casualty sorting using Simple Triage And Rapid Treatment.

terrorism A systematic use of violence to intimidate or to achieve a political goal.

triage The sorting of patients into groups according to the severity of their injuries; used to determine priorities for medical treatment and transport.

warm zone The control area where personnel and equipment decontamination and hot zone support take place.

weapon of mass destruction (WMD) Any agent designed to bring about mass death, casualties, and/or massive damage to property and infrastructure (bridges, tunnels, airports, electrical power plants, and seaports).

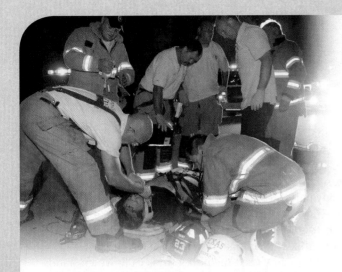

Assessment
in Action

You are dispatched for the report of several students who are short of breath and coughing at a local high school. As you arrive at the school, you find several students in the parking lot who are experiencing difficulty breathing.

1. Which of the following should NOT be one of your first actions?

   A. Park upwind of the school.
   B. Call for additional assistance.
   C. Enter the school building to investigate.
   D. Transmit an initial report to the dispatcher.

2. What type of assistance is probably not needed right away?

   A. Fire department support
   B. HazMat team
   C. Law enforcement personnel
   D. Highway department

3. What type of substance should you suspect might be involved in this incident?

   A. Blister agent
   B. Pulmonary agent
   C. Insecticide
   D. Chemical agent

4. What is the first step in the START triage system?

   A. Begin tagging patients.
   B. Walk among the injured patients.
   C. Instruct patients who can walk to move to a specified area.
   D. Ask each patient if he or she can walk to a different area.

5. Match each of the following colors with the appropriate level of triage in the START system.

   A. Green
   B. Black
   C. Red
   D. Yellow

   _____ Immediate care/life threatening
   _____ Urgent care/can be delayed up to 1 hour
   _____ Patient is dead; no care required
   _____ Care can be delayed up to 3 hours

6. What are the key points to communicate to the dispatcher when you are at the scene of a mass-casualty incident?

7. What are your primary goals when assessing patients in a mass-casualty incident?

8. What types of treatment do you want to avoid in a mass-casualty incident?

9. Do you need consent to begin treatment on these patients?

10. What are the possibilities for additional people to become symptomatic at the scene?

Appendix A: Medical Terminology

As an emergency medical responder (EMR), it is important that you have some knowledge of medical terminology. The medical terms you will most often use as an EMR are identified throughout the text. This appendix provides some rules for breaking down medical terms, some simple rules to help you identify additional terms that you may encounter, and some additional information for certain terms.

Understanding key terms, acronyms, symbols, and abbreviations is important for effective communication and documentation. Understanding how terms are formed and the definitions for the various parts of a medical term will help you determine the meaning of an unknown term by breaking the word apart. Once you understand medical jargon, you will be able to communicate more effectively with other members of the emergency medical services (EMS), health care, and public safety teams.

Anatomy of a Medical Term

Medical terms are made of distinct parts that perform specific functions. Changing or deleting any of those parts can significantly change the function (or meaning) of a word. Components that comprise medical terms include the:

- **Word root:** the foundation of the word
- **Prefix:** what occurs before the root word
- **Suffix:** what occurs after the root word
- **Combining vowels:** vowels that join one or more word roots to other components of a term

How the parts of a term are combined determines its meaning. Accurate spelling, especially when some words are pronounced almost the same way, is essential in medical terminology. For example, the suffix -*phasia* means speaking, whereas -*phagia* means eating or swallowing. The prefix *dys*- means difficult or painful. Combining those two parts, *dysphasia* means difficulty speaking, while *dysphagia* means difficulty eating or swallowing. These are very different terms and the two words, although spelled differently, sound almost identical. Likewise, the terms *ilium* and *ileum* are pronounced exactly the same but refer to different anatomic parts. The ilium is the largest bone of the pelvis, and the ileum is the last part of the small intestine. Knowing anatomy and the context of how these words are used will help you correctly determine (and spell) the term in a given situation.

▶ Word Roots

The main part or stem of a word is called a word root. Some books use the term *word root*; others use *root word*. The terms are synonymous. A word root conveys the essential meaning of the word and frequently indicates a body part. Most terms have at least one word root, and some have more than one word root. Adding a prefix or suffix to the word root creates a term. Changing the prefix or suffix will change the meaning of the term.

A frequently used medical term is CPR, which stands for cardiopulmonary resuscitation. *Cardiopulmonary* breaks down as follows: *cardio* is a word root meaning "heart," and *pulmon* is a word root meaning "lungs." By performing CPR, you introduce air into the lungs and circulate blood by compressing the heart to resuscitate the patient. Some word roots may also be used as prefixes or suffixes for other terms.

Examples of some word roots are shown in **Table A-1**.

▶ Prefixes

A prefix is the part of a term that appears at the beginning of a word. It generally describes location and intensity. Prefixes are frequently found in general language (ie, *auto*pilot, *sub*marine, *tri*cycle), as well as in medical and scientific terminology. Not all medical terms have prefixes.

Table A-1	Common Word Roots in EMS		
Root	**Meaning**	**Example**	**Definition of Example**
cardi	heart	tachycardia	fast heart rate
hepat	liver	hepatomegaly	enlargement of the liver
nephr	kidney	nephropathy	disease of the kidney
neur	nerves	neurologist	physician who specializes in diseases of the nervous system
psych	mind	psychology	study of the mind
thorac	chest	thoracic	pertaining to the chest or thorax

A prefix gives the word root a specific meaning. When a medical word contains a prefix, the meaning of the word is altered. For example, *pnea* is the word root for breathing. Adding the prefix *a-* (without), *brady-* (slow), or *tachy-* (rapid) to a word creates three very different terms:

- a/pnea – without breathing
- brady/pnea – slow breathing
- tachy/pnea – rapid breathing

Some common prefixes are shown in **Table A-2**.

▶ Suffixes

Suffixes are placed at the end of words and usually indicate a procedure, condition, disease, or part of speech.

A commonly used suffix is *-itis*, which means "inflammation." When this suffix is paired with the word root *arthro-*, meaning "joint," the resulting word is *arthritis*, an inflammation of the joints.

Some common suffixes are listed in **Table A-3**.

Table A-2 Common Prefixes in EMS

Prefix	Meaning	Example	Definition of Example
hyper-	over, excessive, high	hyperventilation	fast ventilations
hypo-	under, below normal	hypoperfusion	below normal blood flow to vital organs
tachy-	rapid, fast	tachycardia	fast heart rate
brady-	slow	bradypnea	slow breathing
pre-	before	prenatal	occurring before birth
post-	after, behind	postsurgical	occurring after surgery

© Jones & Bartlett Learning.

Table A-3 Common Suffixes in EMS

Suffix	Meaning	Example	Definition of Example
-al	pertaining to	syncopal	pertaining to syncope
-algia	pertaining to pain	arthralgia	joint pain
-ectomy	surgical removal of	appendectomy	surgical removal of the appendix
-ic	pertaining to	diaphoretic	pertaining to diaphoresis
-itis	inflammation	epiglottitis	inflammation of the epiglottis
-logy	study of	cardiology	the study of the heart
-logist	specialist	pulmonologist	specialist in diseases of the lung
-megaly	enlargement	cardiomegaly	enlargement of the heart
-meter	measuring instrument	sphygmomanometer	instrument to measure blood pressure
-oma	tumor (usually referring to cancer)	lymphoma	cancer of the lymphatic system
-pathy	disease	nephropathy	diseases of the kidneys

© Jones & Bartlett Learning.

▶ Combining Vowels

A combining vowel is the part of a term that connects a word root to a suffix or other word root. In most cases, the combining vowel is an *o*; however, it may also be an *i* or an *e*. A combining vowel is usually used when joining a suffix that begins with a consonant or when joining another word root. For example, take the term *gastroenterology*, the study of diseases of the stomach and small intestines:

- gastr/o + enter/o + logy
- stomach + small intestines + the study of

In this term, *gastr* and *enter* are both word roots, *-logy* is the suffix, and *o* is the combining vowel (used twice). The combining vowel helps ease the pronunciation of the term. Without the vowel, the term would be rather difficult to pronounce—*gastrenterlogy*.

A combining vowel shown with the word root is called a combining form. Here are a few of the most common combining forms you will see:

- cardi/o (heart)
- gastr/o (stomach)
- hepat/o (liver)
- arthr/o (joint)
- oste/o (bone)
- pulmon/o (lungs)

■ Word Building Rules

When building or taking apart a medical term, it is helpful to understand some basic rules. The following summarizes the rules covered thus far:

1. The prefix is always at the beginning of a term; however, not all terms will have a prefix.
2. The suffix is always at the end of the term.
3. When a suffix begins with a consonant, a combining vowel is used between the word root and suffix to make pronunciation easier.
4. When a term has more than one word root, a combining vowel must be placed between the two word roots, even if the second root begins with a vowel.

■ Plural Endings

To change a term from a singular to plural form, certain rules apply. In some cases, you simply add an *s* to the word (*lung* becomes *lungs*). However, for some medical terms, making the plural form is more complicated.

Rules you may encounter when converting terms from singular to plural are:

1. Singular words that end in *a* change to *ae* when plural.
   - Example: *vertebra* becomes *vertebrae*.
2. Singular words that end in *is* change to *es* when plural.
   - Example: *diagnosis* becomes *diagnoses*.
3. Singular words that end in *ex* or *ix* change to *ices*.
   - Example: *apex* becomes *apices*.
4. Singular words that end in *on* or *um* change to *a*.
   - Examples: *ganglion* becomes *ganglia*; *ovum* becomes *ova*.
5. Singular words that end in *us* change to *i*.
   - Example: *bronchus* becomes *bronchi*.

■ Special Word Parts

As already described, prefixes appear at the beginning of a word, before the word root. Prefixes used to indicate numbers, colors, and directions are described as follows. Look at the prefixes, meanings, and examples. Can you think of other terms using the same prefix with another root? Do you see how it changes the meaning?

▶ Numbers

Several prefixes are used to indicate if a term involves a number such as half, one, or two or more parts or sides. Common prefixes for numbers are listed in **Table A-4**.

▶ Colors

Several word roots are used to describe color. The most common include those listed in **Table A-5**.

▶ Positions and Directions

Prefixes can also be used to describe a position, direction, or location. The most common include those listed in **Table A-6**.

■ Movement Terms

The following terms relate to movement **Figure A-1**:

- **Flexion:** the bending of a joint
- **Extension:** the straightening of a joint
- **Adduction:** motion toward the midline
- **Abduction:** motion away from the midline

| Table A-4 | Common Number Prefixes | | |

Prefix	Meaning	Example	Definition of Example
uni-	one	unilateral	one side
dipl-	two; double	diplopia	double vision
null-	none	nullipara	never given birth
primi-	first	primigravida	pregnant for the first time
multi-	many	multiparous	giving birth to more than one offspring at a time
bi-	two	bilateral	pertaining to both sides
tri-	three	trigeminy	irregular heartbeat of two normal beats followed by one premature beat
quad-	four	quadriplegic	paralysis of all four extremities
tetra-	four	tetralogy of Fallot	a congenital defect involving four anatomic abnormalities of the heart
semi-	half; partial	semiconscious	partially conscious
hemi-	half; one sided	hemiplegia	paralysis on one side of the body
ambi-	both	ambidextrous	able to use either hand equally well
pan-	all, entire	pandemic	an epidemic over a wide area

© Jones & Bartlett Learning.

| Table A-5 | Word Roots That Describe Color | | |

Root	Meaning	Example	Definition of Example
cyan/o	blue	cyanosis	blue discoloration of the skin
leuk/o	white	leukocyte	white blood cells that fight infection
erythr/o	red	erythrocyte	red blood cells that contain hemoglobin to carry oxygen
cirrh/o	yellow-orange	cirrhosis	inflammation of the liver causing yellow-orange pigmentation of the liver
melan/o	black	melena	black, tarry stool typically caused by upper gastrointestinal bleeding

© Jones & Bartlett Learning.

Table A-6	Prefixes That Describe Position		
Prefix	**Meaning**	**Example**	**Definition of Example**
To/From			
ab-	away from	abduction	away from the point of reference
ad-	to, toward	adduction	toward the center
Above/Below/Around			
de-	down from, away	decay	to waste away
circum-	around, about	circumferential burn	a burn around an entire area (arm, chest, abdomen, etc.)
peri-	around	pericardium	the sac around the heart
trans-	across, through, beyond	transvaginal	across or through the vagina
epi-	above, upon, on	epigastric	above or over the stomach
supra-	above, over	suprasternal notch	top of the sternum
retro-	behind	retroperitoneal	the area behind the peritoneum
sub-	under, beneath	subcutaneous	beneath the skin
infra-	below, under	infraclavicular	below the clavicle
para-	near, beside, beyond, apart from	parasternal	beside the sternum
contra-	against, opposite	contraindicated	something that is not indicated
Outside/Inside			
ecto-	out, outside	ectopic pregnancy	pregnancy where the embryo attaches outside of the uterus
endo-	within	endoscopy	examining inside someone's body (with an endoscope)
extra-	outside, in addition	extraneous	outside the organism and not belonging to it
intra-	inside, within	intrauterine	within the uterus
ipsi-	same	ipsilateral	on or affecting the same side

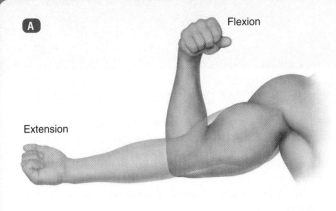

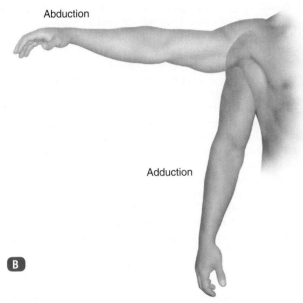

Figure A-1 A. Flexion and extension at the elbow. **B.** Adduction and abduction at the shoulder.

A, B: © Jones & Bartlett Learning.

■ Breaking Terms Apart

Just as you use parts of terms to build new words, you can use knowledge of the meaning of parts to decipher the meaning of a term. When trying to define a term, begin with the suffix and work backward. If the term also contains a prefix, define the suffix, followed by the prefix, and then the word root. Here are some examples:

- nephropathy
  nephr/o/pathy
  -pathy (suffix meaning "disease")
  o (combining form)
  nephr (word root meaning "kidney")
  nephropathy = disease of the kidney
- dysuria
  dys/ur/ia
  -ia (suffix meaning "condition of")
  dys- (prefix meaning "difficult, painful, or abnormal")
  ur (word root meaning "urine")
  dysuria = painful urination (pain when urinating) or difficulty urinating
- hyperemesis
  hyper/emesis
  hyper- (prefix meaning "excessive")
  emesis (word root meaning "vomiting")
  hyperemesis = excessive vomiting
- analgesic
  an/alges/ic
  -ic (suffix meaning "pertaining to")
  an- (prefix meaning "without" or "absence of")
  alges (word root meaning "pain")
  analgesic = pertaining to no pain

Glossary

abandonment Failure of the emergency medical responder to continue emergency medical treatment until relieved by someone with the same or a higher level of training.

abdomen The body cavity between the thorax and the pelvis that contains the major organs of digestion and excretion.

abdominal aortic aneurysm (AAA) A condition in which the layers of the aorta in the abdomen weaken. This causes blood to leak between the layers of the artery, causing it to bulge and sometimes rupture.

abdominal breathing Breathing using only the diaphragm.

abrasion Loss or damage of skin as a result of a body part being rubbed or scraped across a rough or hard surface.

absence seizures Seizures that are characterized by a brief lapse of attention. The patient may stare and not respond; formerly known as petit mal seizures.

acceptance The stage of the grieving process when the person experiencing grief recognizes the finality of the grief-causing event.

acid A chemical substance with a pH level of less than 7.0 that can cause severe burns.

acute abdomen The sudden onset of abdominal pain caused by disease or trauma that irritates the lining of the abdominal cavity and requires immediate medical or surgical treatment.

advance directive A legal document that indicates what a person wants done if he or she cannot make his or her own medical decisions. Advance directives include living wills, durable powers of attorney for health care, and do not resuscitate orders.

advanced emergency medical technician (AEMT) A person who is able to perform basic life support skills and limited advanced life support skills.

advanced life support (ALS) The use of specialized equipment (such as cardiac monitors and defibrillators) and specialized techniques (such as intravenous fluid administration, drug infusion, and endotracheal intubation) to stabilize a patient's condition.

air embolism A bubble of air obstructing a blood vessel.

airway The passages from the openings of the mouth and nose to the air sacs in the lungs through which air enters and leaves the lungs.

airway obstruction Partial (mild) or complete (severe) obstruction of the respiratory passages resulting from blockage by food, small objects, or vomitus.

altered mental status A sudden or gradual decrease in the person's level of responsiveness. Measured using the AVPU scale.

alveolar ventilation The exchange of oxygen and carbon dioxide that occurs in the alveoli.

alveoli The air sacs of the lungs where the exchange of oxygen and carbon dioxide takes place.

Alzheimer disease A chronic, progressive dementia that accounts for 60% of all dementia.

amphetamines Stimulants that produce a general mood elevation, improve task performance, suppress appetite, or prevent sleepiness.

anaphylactic shock Severe shock caused by an allergic reaction to food, medicine, or insect stings.

anger The stage of the grieving process when the person experiencing grief becomes upset or angry at the grief-causing event or other situation.

angina pectoris Chest pain with squeezing or tightness in the chest caused by an inadequate flow of blood to the heart muscle.

anterior The front surface of the body.

antivenin A serum that counteracts the effect of venom from an animal or insect.

anus The distal or terminal ending of the gastrointestinal tract.

appropriate medical facility A hospital or medical clinic with adequate medical resources to provide continuing care to sick or injured patients who are transported after field treatment by emergency medical responders.

arm The part of the upper extremity that extends from the shoulder to the elbow.

arm-to-arm drag An emergency move that consists of the rescuer grasping the patient's arms from behind; used to remove a patient from a hazardous environment.

arterial bleeding Serious bleeding from an artery in which blood frequently pulses or spurts from an open wound.

aspiration Breathing in foreign matter such as food, drink, or vomitus into the airway or lungs.

aspirator A suction device.

assessment-based care A system of patient evaluation in which the chief complaint of the patient and other signs and symptoms are gathered. The care given is based on this information rather than on a formal diagnosis.

asthma A disease in which the airway becomes narrowed and inflamed, resulting in episodes of shortness of breath because of air being trapped in the small air sacs of the lungs.

atherosclerosis A disease characterized by thickening and destruction of the arterial walls and caused by fatty deposits within them; the arteries lose the ability to dilate and carry blood.

atria The two upper chambers of the heart.

auscultation Listening to sounds with a stethoscope.

automated external defibrillator (AED) A portable, battery-powered device that recognizes ventricular fibrillation and advises when a countershock is indicated. The device delivers an electric shock to patients with ventricular fibrillation.

AVPU scale A scale to measure a patient's level of consciousness. The letters stand for Alert, Verbal, Pain, and Unresponsive.

avulsion An injury in which a piece of skin is torn completely loose or is left hanging as a flap.

backboard A straight board used for splinting, extricating, and transporting patients with suspected spinal injuries.

bag of waters The amniotic sac and fluid that surround the fetus before birth.

bag-valve mask (BVM) A patient ventilation device that consists of a bag, one-way valves, and a face mask.

bargaining The stage of the grief reaction when the person experiencing grief barters to change the grief-causing event.

base A chemical with a pH level of greater than 7.0. Bases are also called caustics or alkalis.

base station A powerful two-way radio that is permanently mounted in a communications center.

basic life support (BLS) Emergency lifesaving procedures performed without advanced emergency procedures to stabilize the condition of patients who have experienced sudden illness or injury.

bath salts The common name for certain types of synthetic stimulant-type drugs.

behavioral emergency A situation in which the patient exhibits abnormal behavior that is unacceptable or cannot be tolerated by the patient him- or herself or by family, friends, or the community.

biologic agents Naturally occurring substances that cause disease. Terrorists may use bacteria, viruses, or toxins to intentionally cause epidemics of disease.

birth canal The vagina and the lower part of the uterus.

blanket drag An emergency move in which a rescuer encloses a patient in a blanket and drags the patient to safety.

blister agents Chemicals that cause the skin to blister.

blood pressure The pressure of the circulating blood against the walls of the arteries.

bloody show The plug of mucus that is discharged from the vagina when labor begins.

bounding pulse A strong pulse (similar to the pulse that follows physical exertion such as running or lifting heavy objects).

brachial artery pressure point Pressure point located in the arm between the elbow and the shoulder; also used in taking blood pressure and for checking the pulse in infants.

brachial pulse The pulse on the inside of the upper arm located between the elbow and shoulder; used for checking the pulse in infants.

breech presentation A delivery in which the newborn's buttocks appear in the birth canal first, rather than the head.

bronchi The two main branches of the trachea that lead into the right and left lungs. Within the lungs, they branch into smaller airways.

bronchitis Inflammation of the airways in the lungs.

bruise Injury caused by a blunt object striking the body and crushing the tissue beneath the skin. Also called a contusion.

capillaries The smallest blood vessels that connect small arteries and small veins. Capillary walls serve as the membrane to exchange oxygen and carbon dioxide.

capillary bleeding Bleeding from the capillaries in which blood oozes from the open wound.

capillary refill The ability of the circulatory system to restore blood to the capillary blood vessels after it has been squeezed out by the examiner.

carbon dioxide The gas formed as a waste product of metabolism and excreted through the respiratory system during exhalation.

carbon monoxide A colorless, odorless, tasteless, poisonous gas formed by incomplete combustion, such as in a fire.

cardiac arrest Sudden cessation of breathing and heart function.

cardiogenic shock Shock resulting from inadequate functioning of the heart.

cardiopulmonary resuscitation (CPR) The artificial circulation of the blood and movement of air into and out of the lungs in a pulse-less, nonbreathing patient.

carotid artery The principal arteries of the neck; they supply blood to the face, head, and brain.

carotid pulse A pulse that can be felt on either side of the neck where the carotid artery is close to the skin.

cartilage A tough, elastic form of connective tissue that covers the ends of most bones to form joints; also found in some specific areas such as the nose and the ears.

casualty sorting The sorting of patients to determine the order in which patients should be treated and transported; also called triage.

central nervous system (CNS) The brain and spinal cord.

cerebrospinal fluid (CSF) A clear, watery, straw-colored fluid that fills the space between the brain and spinal cord and their protective coverings.

certification The process by which a person, institution, or program is evaluated and recognized as meeting certain predetermined standards to ensure safe and ethical patient care.

cervical collar A neck brace that partially immobilizes the neck following injury.

cervical spine That section of the spinal column consisting of the seven vertebrae located in the neck.

channel An assigned frequency or frequencies that are used to carry voice and/or data communications.

chemical agents Compounds that can be used by terrorists to inflict harm.

chemical burns Burns that occur when any toxic substance comes in contact with the skin. Most chemical burns are caused by strong acids or alkalis.

chest compression A means of applying artificial circulation by applying rhythmic pressure and relaxation on the lower half of the sternum; also called external cardiac compressions.

chest-thrust maneuver A series of manual thrusts to the chest to relieve upper airway obstruction; used in the treatment of infants, pregnant women, or extremely obese people.

chief complaint The patient's response to questions such as "What happened?" or "What's wrong?"

child A person between the age of 1 year and the onset of puberty (age 12 to 14 years).

chocking Placing a piece of wood or metal in front of or behind a wheel to prevent vehicle movement.

chronic obstructive pulmonary disease (COPD) A slow process of destruction of the airways, alveoli, and pulmonary blood vessels caused by chronic bronchial obstruction (emphysema).

circulatory system The heart and blood vessels, which together are responsible for the continuous flow of blood throughout the body.

clavicle The collarbone.

closed fracture A fracture in which the overlying skin has not been damaged.

closed head injury Injury where there is bleeding and/or swelling within the skull.

closed wound Injury in which soft-tissue damage occurs beneath the skin but there is no break in the surface of the skin.

clothes drag An emergency move used to remove a patient from a hazardous environment; performed by grasping the patient's clothes and moving the patient head first from the unsafe area.

cocaine A powerful stimulant that induces an extreme state of euphoria. Legitimately, it is a potent local anesthetic. On the street, it is commonly known as coke. Crack cocaine, crack, or rock is a solid, smokable form of cocaine.

coccyx The tailbone; the small bone at the base of the spinal column.

cold zone The control area that contains the command post and other support functions needed in the incident.

coma A state of unconsciousness from which the patient cannot be aroused.

communication The transmission of information to another person.

competent Able to make rational decisions about personal well-being.

concussion A closed head injury that alters the way the brain functions; symptoms of a concussion include headache, loss of memory, and confusion.

congestive heart failure (CHF) Heart disease characterized by breathlessness, fluid retention in the lungs, and generalized swelling of the body.

consent In the context of emergency medical services, permission to provide care.

contractions Muscular movements of the uterus that push the newborn out of the birth canal.

cradle-in-arms carry A one-rescuer patient movement technique used primarily for children; the patient is cradled in the hollow formed by the rescuer's arms and chest.

cravat A triangular swathe of cloth used to hold a body part splinted against the body.

critical incident stress debriefing (CISD) A system of psychological support designed to reduce stress on emergency personnel after a major stress-producing incident.

critical incident stress management (CISM) A process that confronts the responses to critical incidents and defuses them, directing the emergency services personnel toward physical and emotional equilibrium.

croup Inflammation and narrowing of the air passages in young children, causing a barking cough, hoarseness, and a harsh, high-pitched breathing sound.

crowning Appearance of the newborn's head during a contraction as he or she is pushed outward through the birth canal.

cyanosis Blue discoloration of the skin resulting from poor oxygenation of the circulating blood.

decompression sickness (the bends) A condition seen in divers in which gas, especially nitrogen, forms bubbles in blood vessels, obstructing them.

decontamination The process of reducing or preventing the spread of contaminants at a hazardous materials event.

defibrillation Process of delivering an electric shock through a person's chest wall and heart for the purpose of ending lethal heart rhythms such as ventricular fibrillation and to help establish normal heart contraction rhythms.

delirium tremens (DTs) A severe, often fatal, complication of alcohol withdrawal that most commonly occurs 3 to 4 days after withdrawal (though it can occur as late as 10 days after withdrawal). It is characterized by restlessness, fever, sweating, confusion, disorientation, agitation, hallucinations, and convulsions.

dementia A progressive, irreversible decline in mental functioning; marked by memory impairment and decrease in reasoning, judgment, comprehension, and ability to communicate verbally.

denial A stage of a grief reaction when the person experiencing grief rejects the grief-causing event.

dependent lividity Blood settling to the lowest point of the body after death, causing discoloration of the skin.

depression A stage of the grief reaction when the person expresses despair—an absence of cheerfulness and hope—as a result of a grief-causing event. Also a psychiatric disorder marked by persistent feelings of sadness, hopelessness, and decreased interest in daily activities; the person may have persistent thoughts of suicide.

diabetes A disease in which the body is unable to use glucose normally because of a deficiency or total lack of insulin.

diabetic coma A state of unconsciousness that occurs when the body has too much glucose and not enough insulin.

diaphragm A muscular dome that separates the chest from the abdominal cavity. Contraction of the diaphragm and the chest wall muscles brings air into the lungs; relaxation expels air from the lungs.

diastolic pressure The measurement of pressure exerted against the walls of the arteries while the left ventricle of the heart is at rest.

digestive system The gastrointestinal tract (stomach and intestines), mouth, salivary glands, pharynx, esophagus, liver, gallbladder, pancreas, rectum, and anus, which together are responsible for the absorption of food and the elimination of solid waste from the body.

digital messaging Technology that includes email, text messages, and social media, which are increasingly used by emergency medical responders to send and receive various types of information.

dirty bomb An explosive device using conventional explosives that is designed to spread radioactive material over a wide area.

dislocation Disruption of a joint so that the bone ends are no longer in alignment.

distal Describing structures that are farther from the trunk (or torso) or nearer to the free end of an extremity. Opposite of proximal.

do not resuscitate (DNR) order A written request giving permission to medical personnel not to attempt resuscitation in the event of cardiac arrest.

documentation The recorded portion of the emergency medical responder's patient interaction, either written or electronic.

dressing Any of various materials placed directly on a wound to control bleeding and prevent further contamination.

drowning Suffocation or respiratory impairment because of submersion in water or other fluids.

durable power of attorney for health care A legal document that allows a patient to designate another person to make medical decisions for him or her if the patient is unable to make his or her own treatment decisions.

duty to act An emergency medical responder's legal responsibility to respond quickly to an emergency scene and provide medical care (within the limits of training and available equipment).

dyspnea Shortness of breath or difficulty breathing.

ectopic pregnancy A pregnancy that occurs outside the uterus, usually in a fallopian tube; usually terminates with the rupture of the fallopian tube.

elder abuse An action taken by a family member or caregiver that results in the physical, emotional, financial, or sexual harm to a person older than 65 years; also includes neglect.

electrical burns Burns caused by contact with high- or low-voltage electricity. Electrical burns have an entrance and an exit wound.

emergency medical responder (EMR) The first medically trained person to arrive on the scene.

emergency medical technician (EMT) A person who is trained and certified to provide basic life support and certain other noninvasive prehospital medical procedures.

emergency response communications center A fire, police, or emergency medical services agency; a 9-1-1 center; or a seven-digit telephone number used by one or all of the emergency agencies to receive and dispatch requests for emergency care; also called a public safety answering point.

emotional shock A state of shock caused by a sudden illness, an accident, or the death of a loved one.

empathy The ability to share another person's feelings or ideas.

entrance wound Point where an object such as a bullet enters the body.

entrapment To be caught (trapped) within a vehicle, room, or container with no way out or to have a limb or other body part trapped.

epiglottis The valve located at the upper end of the voice box that prevents food from entering the larynx.

epiglottitis Severe inflammation and swelling of the epiglottis; a life-threatening situation.

epilepsy A disease manifested by seizures, caused by an abnormal focus of electrical activity in the brain.

esophagus The tube through which food passes. It starts at the throat and ends at the stomach.

exhalation Breathing out.

exit wound Point where an object such as a bullet passes out of the body.

explosives Substances that release energy in a sudden and uncontrolled manner when detonated.

expressed consent Consent actually given by a person, either verbally or nonverbally, authorizing the emergency medical responder to provide care or transportation.

external cardiac compressions A means of applying artificial circulation by applying rhythmic pressure and relaxation on the lower half of the sternum; also called chest compressions.

externally rotated Rotated outward, as a fractured hip.

extremities The arms and legs.

extrication Removal from a difficult situation or position; removal of a patient from a wrecked vehicle or other place of entrapment.

face mask A clear plastic mask used for oxygen administration that covers the mouth and nose.

fax machine A device used to send or receive printed text documents or images over a telephone or radio communications system.

femoral artery pressure point Pressure point located in the groin, in the middle of the bottom crease of the groin, between the groin and the upper thigh.

femoral pulse The pulse taken at the groin.

fetus A developing newborn in the uterus or womb.

firefighter drag A method of moving a patient without lifting or carrying him or her; used when the patient is heavier than the rescuer.

flail chest A condition that occurs when three or more ribs are each broken in two places and the chest wall lying between the fractures becomes a free-floating segment.

floating ribs The eleventh and twelfth ribs, which do not connect to the sternum.

flotation device A life ring, life buoy, or other floating device used in water rescue.

flowmeter A device on oxygen cylinders used to control and measure the flow of oxygen.

forearm The lower portion of the upper extremity; from the elbow to the wrist.

fractures Breaks in a bone.

frostbite Partial or complete freezing of the skin and deeper tissues caused by exposure to the cold.

full-thickness burns Burns that extend through the skin and into the underlying tissues; the most serious class of burns.

fusees Warning devices or flares that burn with a red color; usually used in scene protection at motor vehicle crash sites.

gag reflex A strong involuntary effort to vomit caused by something being placed or caught in the throat.

gastric distention Inflation of the stomach caused when excessive pressures are used during artificial ventilation and air is directed into the stomach rather than the lungs.

generalized seizures Seizures characterized by contractions of all the body's muscle groups that may last for 1 to 2 minutes; formerly known as grand mal seizures.

genitourinary system The organs of reproduction, together with the organs involved in the production and excretion of urine.

geriatric patient A patient who is older than 65 years.

Golden Hour A concept of emergency patient care that attempts to place a trauma patient into definitive medical care in the shortest period of time to achieve the best possible outcome; also called the Golden Period.

Good Samaritan laws Laws that encourage citizens to voluntarily help an injured or suddenly ill person by minimizing the liability for any errors or omissions in providing good faith emergency care.

gunshot wound A puncture wound caused by a bullet or shotgun pellets.

hallucinogens Chemicals that cause a person to see visions or hear sounds that are not real.

hazardous materials (HazMat) Substances that are toxic, poisonous, radioactive, flammable, or explosive and can cause injury or death with exposure.

head tilt–chin lift maneuver A method of opening the airway by tilting the patient's head backward and lifting the chin forward, bringing the entire lower jaw with it.

heat cramps Painful muscle spasms that usually occur after vigorous exercise in hot weather and are generally relieved by rest and drinking water.

heat exhaustion A form of shock that occurs from significant fluid loss and too many electrolytes through very heavy sweating after exposure to heat.

heatstroke A condition of rapidly rising internal body temperature that occurs when the body's mechanisms for the release of heat are overwhelmed. Untreated heatstroke can result in death.

Heimlich maneuver A series of manual thrusts to the abdomen to relieve an upper airway obstruction.

hemorrhage Excessive bleeding.

hemostatic agent A chemical compound that slows or stops bleeding by assisting with clot formation.

hives An allergic skin disorder marked by patches of swelling, redness, and intense itching.

hospice An interdisciplinary program designed to reduce or eliminate pain and address the physical, spiritual, social, and economic needs of terminally ill patients.

hot zone A contaminated area.

humerus The upper arm bone.

hypertension High blood pressure.

hypoglycemia A condition of low blood sugar that occurs in a person with diabetes who has taken too much insulin or has not eaten enough food.

hypotension Low blood pressure.

hypothermia A condition in which the internal (or core) body temperature falls below 95°F (35°C) after prolonged exposure to cool or freezing temperatures.

immobilize To reduce or prevent movement of a limb, usually by splinting.

impaled object An object such as a knife, splinter of wood, or glass that penetrates the skin and remains in the body.

implied consent Consent to receive emergency medical care that is assumed because the individual is unconscious, underage, or so badly injured or ill that he or she cannot respond.

incendiary devices Substances or weapons designed to start a fire.

incident command system (ICS) A system of people, procedures, and equipment designed to improve emergency response operations at situations of all types and complexities.

incubation period The time between exposure to a disease organism to the time the person begins to show symptoms of the disease.

infant A person younger than 1 year.

inferior Nearer to the feet than the head.

inhalation Breathing in.

insecticides Chemicals that are formulated to kill insects but that can intentionally or accidentally cause injury or death to humans when inhaled or absorbed through the skin.

insulin A hormone produced by the pancreas that enables glucose in the blood to be used by the cells of the body; supplementary insulin is used in the treatment and control of diabetes mellitus.

intravenous (IV) fluids Fluids other than blood or blood products infused into the vascular system to maintain an adequate circulatory blood volume.

jaw-thrust maneuver A method of opening the airway by bringing the patient's jaw forward without extending the neck.

joint The point where two bones come into contact with each other.

labor The process of delivering a newborn.

laceration An irregular cut or tear through the skin.

laryngospasm A spasm of the muscles of the larynx or vocal cords resulting in an inability to breathe.

larynx A structure composed of cartilage in the neck that guards the entrance to the windpipe and functions as the organ of voice; also called the voice box.

lateral Away from the midline of the body.

leg The lower extremity; specifically, the lower portion, from the knee to the ankle.

ligaments Fibrous bands that connect bones to bones and support and strengthen joints.

living will A legal document that states the types of medical care a person wants or wants withheld if he or she is unable to make his or her own treatment decisions. Living wills may include do not resuscitate orders.

log rolling A technique used to move a patient onto a long backboard.

lower extremity Consists of the thigh, leg, ankle, and foot.

lumbar spine The lower part of the back formed by the lowest five nonfused vertebrae.

lungs The organs that supply the body with oxygen and eliminate carbon dioxide from the blood.

mandible The lower jaw.

manual suction devices Hand-powered devices used for clearing the upper airway of mucus, blood, or vomitus.

mass-casualty incidents Accidents or situations involving more patients than you can handle with the initial resources available; also known as multiple-casualty incidents.

mechanical suction device A battery-powered pump or an oxygen-powered aspirator used for clearing the upper airway of mucus, blood, or vomitus.

mechanism of injury (MOI) The means by which a traumatic injury occurs.

medial Closer to the midline of the body.

metabolic agents Substances that are intended to produce injury or death by disrupting the body's ability to use oxygen and chemical reactions at the cellular level.

metered dose inhaler (MDI) A miniature spray container used to direct medications through the mouth and into the lungs.

midline An imaginary vertical line drawn from the head to toe that divides the body into equal left and right sides.

minute ventilation The amount of air pulled into the lungs and removed from the lungs in 1 minute.

miscarriage Delivery of an incomplete or underdeveloped fetus before it is mature enough to survive outside the womb (about 20 weeks of pregnancy); also called spontaneous abortion.

mobile data terminal (MDT) A computer terminal mounted in a vehicle that sends and receives data through a radio communications system.

mobile radio A two-way radio that is permanently mounted in an emergency vehicle that draws electricity from the electrical system of the vehicle.

mottling Patchy skin discoloration caused by too little or too much circulation.

mouth-to-mask ventilation device A piece of equipment that consists of a mask, a one-way valve, and a mouthpiece. Rescue breathing is performed by breathing into the mouthpiece after placing the mask over the patient's mouth and nose.

mouth-to-stoma breathing Rescue breathing for patients who, because of surgical removal of the larynx, have a stoma.

multi-system trauma An injury that affects more than one body system.

nasal airway An airway adjunct that is inserted into the nostril of a patient who is unable to maintain a natural airway; also called a nasopharyngeal airway.

nasal cannula A clear plastic tube, used to deliver oxygen, that fits onto the patient's nose.

nasopharynx The posterior part of the nose.

National Incident Management System (NIMS) A system developed by the US Department of Homeland Security for managing an emergency incident, which may require the response of many different agencies; designed to provide a comprehensive, efficient, and effective management approach from initial response through recovery.

negligence Deviation from the accepted standard of care resulting in further injury to the patient.

nerve agents Deadly toxic substances that attack the central nervous system.

nerves Fiber tracts or pathways that carry messages from the spinal cord and brain to all body parts and back; sensory, motor, or a combination of both.

nervous system The brain, spinal cord, and nerves.

nitroglycerin A medication used to treat angina pectoris; increases blood flow and oxygen supply to the heart muscle and reduces or eliminates the pain of angina pectoris.

occlusive dressing An airtight dressing or bandage for a wound.

one-person walking assist A method used if the patient is able to bear his or her own weight.

one-rescuer CPR Cardiopulmonary resuscitation performed by one rescuer.

on-scene peer support Stress counselors at the scene of stressful incidents who help emergency personnel deal with stress.

open fracture Any fracture in which the overlying skin has been damaged.

open wound Injury that breaks open the skin or mucous membrane.

opioids Medications that relieve pain, including prescription drugs such as morphine, oxycodone, and hydrocodone and illicit drugs such as heroin, which is produced from the morphine in poppy plants.

oral airway An airway adjunct that is inserted into the mouth to keep the tongue from blocking the upper airway; also called an oropharyngeal airway.

oropharynx The posterior part of the mouth.

osteoporosis Abnormal brittleness of the bones caused by loss of calcium; affected bones fracture easily.

oxygen A colorless, odorless gas that is essential for life.

pack-strap carry A one-person carry that allows the rescuer to carry a patient while keeping one hand free.

paging systems Communications systems used to send voice or text messages over a radio system to specially designed radio receivers.

palpation To examine by touch.

paralysis Inability of a conscious person to move voluntarily.

paramedic A person trained and certified to provide advanced life support.

partial-thickness burns Burns in which the outer layers of skin are burned; these burns are characterized by blister formation.

pathogens Microorganisms that are capable of causing disease.

pediatric assessment triangle (PAT) An assessment tool that measures the severity of a child's illness or injury by evaluating the child's appearance, work of breathing, and circulation to the skin.

pelvis The closed bony ring, consisting of the sacrum and the pelvic bones, that connects the trunk to the lower extremities.

pharynx The throat.

placenta Life support system of the fetus; also called the afterbirth.

plasma The fluid part of the blood that carries blood cells, transports nutrients, and removes cellular waste materials.

platelets Microscopic disc-shaped elements in the blood that are essential to the process of blood clot formation; the mechanism that stops bleeding.

pneumatic antishock garments (PASGs) Trouser-like devices placed around a shock victim's legs and abdomen and inflated with air.

pocket mask A mechanical breathing device used to administer mouth-to-mask rescue breathing.

poison Any substance that may cause injury or death if relatively small amounts are ingested, inhaled, absorbed, applied to, or injected into the body.

portable radio A handheld, battery-operated, two-way radio.

portable stretcher A lightweight, nonwheeled device for transporting a patient; used in small spaces where the wheeled ambulance stretcher cannot be used.

posterior The back surface of the body.

posterior tibial pulse Ankle pulse.

posttraumatic stress disorder (PTSD) A mental health or behavioral condition triggered by experiencing or witnessing a terrifying event.

preincident stress education Training about stress and stress reactions conducted for public safety personnel before they are exposed to stressful situations.

premature newborn A newborn delivered before 36 weeks of gestation or who weighs less than 5 pounds (2 kg) at birth.

pressure points Points where a blood vessel lies near a bone; pressure can be applied to these points to help control bleeding.

primary assessment The first actions taken to form an impression of the patient's condition; to determine the patient's responsiveness and introduce yourself to the patient; to check the patient's airway, breathing, and circulation; and to acknowledge the patient's chief complaint. The primary assessment is sometimes called the initial patient assessment.

prolapsed umbilical cord A condition in which the umbilical cord appears before the newborn does; the newborn's head may compress the cord and cut off all circulation.

proximal Closer to the trunk (or torso). Opposite of distal.

psychogenic shock Commonly known as fainting; caused by a temporary reduction in blood supply to the brain.

psychotic behavior Mental disturbance characterized by abnormal thought processes and/or the loss of contact with reality.

public safety answering point (PSAP) A fire, police, or emergency medical services agency; a 9-1-1 center; or a seven-digit telephone number used by one or all of the emergency agencies to receive and dispatch requests for emergency care; also called an emergency response communications center.

pulmonary agents Substances that produce respiratory distress or illness.

pulse The wave of pressure that is created by the heart when it contracts as a result of forcing the blood out and into the major arteries.

pulse oximeter A machine that consists of a monitor and a sensor probe that measures the oxygen saturation in the capillary beds.

pulse oximetry An assessment tool that measures oxygen saturation in the capillary beds.

puncture A wound resulting from a bullet, knife, ice pick, splinter, or any other pointed object.

pupils The circular openings in the middle of the eye.

rabies An acute viral infection of the central nervous system transmitted by the bite of an infected animal.

radial pulse Pulse located on the inside of the wrist on the thumb side.

radiation The electromagnetic energy that is released from a radioactive material or a dirty bomb.

radius The bone on the thumb side of the forearm.

reach, throw, row, go A sequence of four actions that should be taken in water rescue situations.

recovery position A sidelying position that helps an unconscious patient maintain an open airway.

redirection A means of focusing the patient's attention on the immediate situation or crisis.

repeater A radio system that automatically retransmits a radio signal on a different frequency.

rescue breathing Artificial means of breathing for a patient.

rescue throw bag A water rescue device consisting of a small cloth bag and a waterproof rope used for rescuing people from the water.

respiratory arrest Sudden stoppage of breathing.

respiratory burn Burn to the respiratory system resulting from inhaling superheated air.

respiratory rate The speed at which a person is breathing (measured in breaths per minute).

respiratory system All body structures that contribute to normal breathing.

restatement Rephrasing a patient's own statement to show that he or she is being heard and understood by the rescuer.

ribs The paired arches of bone, 12 on either side, that extend from the thoracic vertebrae toward the anterior midline of the trunk.

rigid splint Splint made from firm materials such as wood, aluminum, or plastic.

riptide Unusually strong surface currents flowing outward from a seashore that can present a hazard to swimmers.

road rash An abrasion caused by sliding on pavement. Usually seen after motorcycle or bicycle accidents.

rule of nines Used to calculate the amount of body surface burned; the body is divided into sections, each of which constitutes approximately 9% or 18% of the total body surface area.

sacrum One of three bones (sacrum and two pelvic bones) that makes up the pelvic ring; forms the base of the spine.

saline Salt water.

SAMPLE history A patient's medical history. The letters stand for Signs and Symptoms, Allergies, Medications, Pertinent past medical history, Last oral intake, Events associated with or leading up to the illness or injury.

scene size-up A step within the patient assessment process that includes a visual survey, or an overview of the incident and its surroundings, and a quick assessment of the scene and the surroundings to provide information about scene safety and the mechanism of injury or nature of illness before you enter and begin patient care.

scoop stretcher A firm device used to carry a patient; can be split into halves and applied to the patient from both sides.

secondary assessment The step in the patient assessment sequence in which you carefully examine the patient from head to toe and measure vital signs.

seizure Sudden episode of uncontrolled electrical activity in the brain.

self-contained breathing apparatus (SCBA) A complete unit for delivery of air to a rescuer who enters a contaminated area; contains a mask, regulator, and air supply.

senile dementia General term for dementia that occurs in older people.

sepsis A severe, potentially life-threatening complication of infection that can progress to septic shock if left untreated; occurs when chemicals are released into the bloodstream and trigger an inflammatory response throughout the body.

septic shock A condition in which the blood pressure drops dramatically as a result of severe infection; often results in death.

shock A state of collapse of the cardiovascular system; the state of inadequate delivery of blood to the organs of the body.

shoulder girdles The three bones of the upper extremity; each shoulder supports the clavicle, the scapula, and the humerus.

sign A condition that you observe in a patient, such as bleeding or the temperature of a patient's skin.

situational crisis A state of emotional upset or turmoil caused by a sudden and disruptive event.

skull The bones of the head, collectively; the protective structure for the brain.

sling A bandage or material that helps to support the weight of an injured upper extremity.

soft splint A splint made from supple material that provides gentle support.

splint A means of immobilizing an injured part by using a rigid or soft support.

spontaneous nosebleed A nosebleed with no apparent cause.

sprain A joint injury in which the joint is partially or temporarily dislocated and some of the supporting ligaments are either stretched or torn.

stair chair A small portable device used for transporting a patient in a sitting position.

standard of care The manner in which an individual must act or behave when giving care.

standard precautions An infection control concept that treats all body fluids as potentially infectious.

standing orders Written documents, signed by the emergency medical service system's medical director, that outline specific directions, permissions, and sometimes prohibitions regarding patient care; also called protocols.

START triage A system of casualty sorting using Simple Triage And Rapid Treatment.

sternum The breastbone.

stoma A surgical opening in the neck that connects the windpipe (trachea) to the skin.

straddle lift A method used to place a patient on a backboard if there is not enough space to perform a log roll.

straddle slide A method of placing a patient on a long backboard by straddling both the board and patient and sliding the patient onto the board.

stridor A high-pitched sound heard during inspiration. It is a sign of a narrowing or partial obstruction.

stroke A brain attack caused by a blood clot or a broken blood vessel in the brain. Strokes can result in trouble speaking, inability to move parts of the body, confusion, or unconsciousness.

submersion injury An injury resulting from being beneath the surface of water or another liquid.

suction To aspirate (suck out) fluid by mechanical means.

suctioning Aspirating (sucking out) fluid in the mouth or airway by mechanical means.

suicide Intentionally causing one's own death; self-inflicted death. Suicide is especially common in older and chronically ill people.

superficial burns Burns in which only the superficial part of the skin has been injured; an example is a sunburn.

superior Closer to the head or above a body part.

symptom A condition the patient tells you, such as "I feel dizzy."

systolic pressure The measurement of blood pressure exerted against the walls of the arteries during contraction of the heart.

telemetry A process in which electronic signals are transmitted and received by radio or telephone; commonly used for sending electrocardiogram tracings.

tempered glass Safety glass that breaks into small pieces when hit with a sharp, pointed object.

tendons Tough, rope-like cords of fibrous tissue that attach muscle to bone.

terrorism A systematic use of violence to intimidate or to achieve a political goal.

thermal burn Burn caused by heat; the most common type of burn.

thighbone The upper portion of the lower extremity; from the hip joint to the knee.

thoracic spine The 12 vertebrae that attach to the 12 ribs; the upper part of the back.

thready pulse A weak pulse.

topographic anatomy The superficial landmarks on the body that serve as location guides to the structures that lie beneath them.

toxic Poisonous.

trachea The windpipe.

traction splint A splint that holds a lower extremity fracture in alignment by applying a constant, steady pull on the extremity.

trauma A wound or injury, either physical or psychological.

triage The sorting of patients into groups according to the severity of their injuries; used to determine priorities for medical treatment and transport; also called casualty sorting.

trunked communications system A computer-controlled radio system that allows the sharing of a few radio frequencies among a large group of users.

two-person chair carry A method of carrying a patient in which two rescuers use a chair to support the weight of the patient.

two-person extremity carry A method of carrying a patient out of tight quarters using two rescuers and no equipment.

two-person seat carry A method of carrying a patient in which two rescuers link arms behind the patient's back and under the patient's knees; requires no equipment.

two-person walking assist A method used when a patient cannot bear his or her own weight; two rescuers completely support the patient.

two-rescuer CPR Cardiopulmonary resuscitation performed by two rescuers.

ulna The bone on the little-finger side of the forearm.

umbilical cord Ropelike attachment between the pregnant woman and fetus; nourishment and waste products pass to and from the fetus and the woman through this cord.

upper extremity Consists of the arm, forearm, wrist, and hand.

uterus (womb) Muscular organ that holds and nourishes the developing fetus.

vacuum splint A soft splint that becomes rigid when air is removed from the splint.

vagina The opening through which the newborn emerges.

venous bleeding External bleeding from a vein, characterized by steady flow; the bleeding may be profuse and life threatening.

ventilation The movement of air in and out of the lungs.

ventricles The two lower chambers of the heart.

ventricular fibrillation An uncoordinated muscular quivering of the heart; the most common abnormal rhythm causing cardiac arrest; also called V-fib.

vertebrae The 33 bones of the spinal column: 7-cervical, 12 thoracic, 5 lumbar, 5 sacral, and 4 coccygeal vertebrae.

vital signs Measurements or critical parameters used to assess the patient's immediate health condition including pulse, capillary refill, skin condition, temperature, respirations, and blood pressure.

warm zone The control area where personnel and equipment decontamination and hot zone support take place.

weapon of mass destruction (WMD) Any agent designed to bring about mass death, casualties, and/or massive damage to property and infrastructure (bridges, tunnels, airports, electrical power plants, and seaports).

wooden cribbing Wooden boards (either 2 inch × 4 inch [5 cm × 10 cm] or 4 inch × 4 inch [10 cm × 10 cm]) used for vehicle stabilization or bracing.

xiphoid process The flexible cartilage at the lower tip of the sternum.

Index